Rehabilitation Robotics

Edited by
Sashi S Kommu

Rehabilitation Robotics
Edited by Sashi S Kommu

This is a reprint of the book published in 2007

Published by InTech
Janeza Trdine 9, 51000 Rijeka, Croatia

Technical Editor Teodora Smiljanic

Cover Design InTech Design team

Additional hard copies can be obtained from orders@intechopen.com

Rehabilitation Robotics, Edited by Sashi S Kommu
p. cm.
ISBN 978-3-902613-04-2

For EU product safety concerns:
IN TECH d.o.o., Prolaz Marije Krucifikse Kozulić 3, 51000 Rijeka, Croatia,
info@intechopen.com or visit our website at intechopen.com.

Preface

The coupling of several areas of the medical field with recent advances in robotic systems has seen a paradigm shift in our approach to selected sectors of medical care, especially over the last decade. Rehabilitation medicine is one such area. The development of advanced robotic systems has ushered with it an exponential number of trials and experiments aimed at optimising restoration of quality of life to those who are physically debilitated. Despite these developments, there remains a paucity in the presentation of these advances in the form of a comprehensive tool. This book was written to present the most recent advances in rehabilitation robotics known to date from the perspective of some of the leading experts in the field and presents an interesting array of developments put into 33 comprehensive chapters. The chapters are presented in a way that the reader will get a seamless impression of the current concepts of optimal modes of both experimental and applicable roles of robotic devices.

Robotic instrument designs are combined with the results of experiments and trials in an applicable and practical way. The ethos of the book is unique in that there is a considerable emphasis on practical applicability in making real time changes to patient care. The book begins by exploring the inherent and unique challenges of paediatric rehabilitation and presents the robotic platforms upon which promising preliminary results were noted. It then explores the key elements of robotic safety critical systems and risk management issues, an area of great concern in the medical field at present. There is also an in depth look at the role of robotics from a mechanotronics and virtual reality standpoint. The concept of high safety rehabilitation systems using functional fluid is explored and the platform for further studies is introduced. The concept of powered wearable assistance and the role of exoskeleton devices pave the brink of an exciting era in rehabilitation robotics. Additional concepts explored involve the interaction-control between robot, patient and therapist.

'Rehabilitation Robotics' promises to be a valuable supplementary tool to all those involved in rehabilitation from the standpoint of the patient and affected families, the therapist and the robot. It also acts as a platform upon which researchers can gain a solid and evidence based approach towards the initiation of future projects.

Editor
Sashi S Kommu

The Derriford Hospital and The Bristol Urological Institute
Devon, United Kingdom
E-mail: sashurol@gmail.com

Contents

1

Robotic Solutions in Pediatric Rehabilitation

Michael Bailey-Van Kuren
Miami University
USA

1. Introduction

The rehabilitation of pediatric patients involves unique constraints in comparison to adult rehabilitation. Therefore, the utilization of robotic technology in the rehabilitation of pediatric patients provides unique challenges. Research focusing on the application of robotic technology to pediatric cerebral palsy patients with spasticity is searching for flexible solutions that can address a wide range of patient capabilities. A variety of solutions are being investigated that place robotics in different roles in relation to the patient.

Cerebral palsy describes a group of neuro-muscular disorders that are caused by injury to the brain during the brain's developmental period. Cerebral palsy hinders motor skills and control of movement. According to the United Cerebral Palsy Research and Educational Facility, there are at least 550,000 persons in the United States with the disorder. Furthermore, there are approximately 9,750 new cases per year. Substance abuse and other factors also help increase the chances of the affliction (Matthews and Wilson, 1999; Styer-Acevedo, 1999).

Cerebral palsy affects the Basal Ganglia which is responsible for coordinating motion in the muscles. This affects all muscles of the body. The most noticeable muscles affected in children with cerebral palsy are the arm and leg muscles resulting in reduced motor skills, and the tongue which affecting speech and swallowing (Matthews and Wilson, 1999; Styer-Acevedo, 1999).

Cerebral palsy is usually diagnosed within the first two years after birth. Therefore, rehabilitative therapy for cerebral palsy patients may initiate shortly after birth. Although there are three main types of cerebral palsy: spastic, athetoid, and ataxic, the most common form of cerebral palsy is spastic cerebral palsy where high muscle tone constrains motion. Rehabilitation for pediatric cerebral palsy patients includes physical therapy, occupational therapy, and interventional medicine such as the injection of Botulinum-A Toxin paired with serial casting. Physical therapy early in the child's development prevents contractures and help to keep the muscles from becoming weakened or from deteriorating due to lack of use. Pediatric physical therapy differs from adult therapy in that patients often can not (or may not be willing to) follow direct instructions of a therapy routine thus therapy is incorporated in play. Furthermore, therapists must consider the natural progression of fine and gross motor skills in conjunction with developmental delays caused by cerebral palsy as a patient grows from infancy to adolescence.

2. Previous Work Related to Robotic Pediatric Rehabilitation

Robotics provide a reprogrammable flexible platform for manipulation and interaction with the robot's environment. The role of robotics in adult rehabilitation is well established. Robotic applications in adult rehabilitation have centered on the neuro-muscular difficulties experienced by stroke patients. Robotic devices to assist patients with their gait have been used to re-establish neuro-muscular pathways (Sawicki et al., 2006). Furthermore, robots have been developed that increase the bilateral range of motion of patients performing reach tasks (Burgar et al., 2000). In other related work, there is a variety of research investigating the use of gaming (Merians et al., 2002) or virtual reality to motivate adult patients in performing rehabilitative tasks. This research points to three capabilities that robotics can provide to pediatric patients with cerebral palsy: aiding the establishment of neuro-muscular pathways, extending range of motion, and providing patient motivation.

Previous pediatric devices have focused on the motivational capability of robots with children. Robots have been designed to target children with speech, learning, and physical disabilities (Plaisant et al., 2003). These robots mimic the actions of pediatric patients based on signals from armbands or leg bands. In addition, the robots used games and activities to encourage the children to continue their exercises.

The use of autonomous robots has been studied with autistic children (Michaud et al., 2003). It was hypothesized that "mobile robots can serve as an appropriate pedagogical tool to help children with PDD[autism] develop social skills because they are more predictable and less intimidating" than an adult or therapist. The project consisted of six different robots, each with a unique look and set of abilities. Three of the prototype robots are shown in Fig. 1. It was found that positive reinforcement was an affective tool for the children to improve their skills. They explain; "having the robots behave in particular ways (like dancing, playing music, etc.) when the child responds correctly to requests made by the robot becomes an incentive for the child to continue playing with the robots". The research found that the best and most effective robots appealed to the children's visual sense, auditory sense, sense of touch, spatial perception and use of language. The use of lights, music, and short vocal messages excited the children and encouraged continued play. Unique problems were found in dealing with the pediatric population including possible damage to the robots and the danger of small parts as choking hazards with younger children.

In further research, a robot named "Roball", shown in Fig. 2, was designed to develop the language, affective, motor, intellectual and social skills for children ages 12 to 24 months (Michaud et al., 2004). The robot has the ability to perform autonomous movement, sense, illuminate, and generate sound. A study of eight children investigated the development of each child's motor skills, stimulation of intellectual skills, social interaction and language skills. This study focuses on the development of healthy children; however, the similar research could be compared and applied to children with disorders such as autism and various physical disabilities.

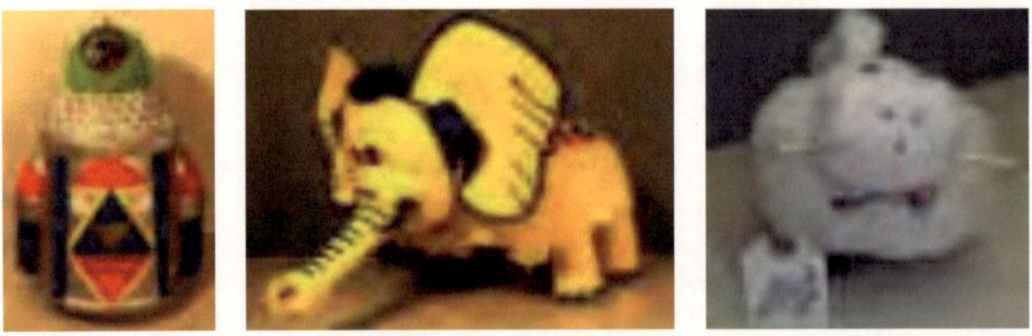

Fig. 1. Three Robots Used in Therapy for Autistic Children (Michaud et al., 2003).

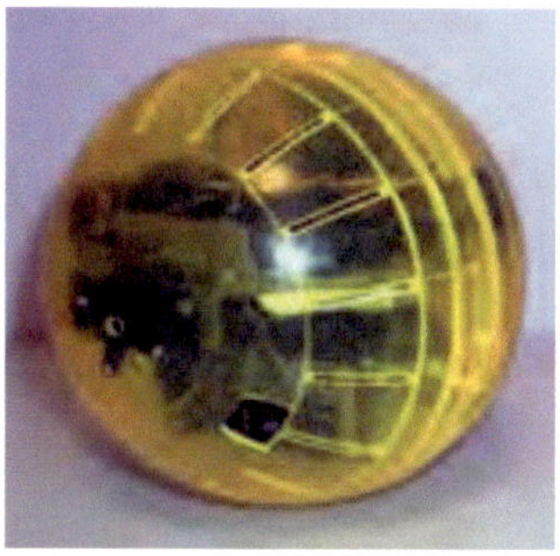 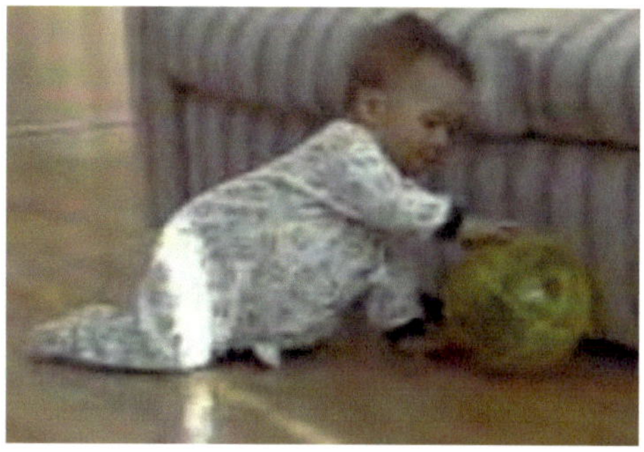

Fig. 2. Prototype Roball and infant interacting with Roball (Michaud et al., 2004).

Pediatric related robotic systems that extend beyond motivational capability include the blocks assembly robot that provides the ability for blocks play children without the physical capability to manipulate blocks with their hands (Plaisant et. al., 2003). This system utilizes customized interfaces to provide children with a command structure that can be used to control a prismatic actuator. Some children with cerebral palsy may be a candidate for this type of robotic interaction. However, this is not directly a therapy related activity.

Although robotics has been successfully applied to rehabilitation and interaction with children, these systems have not been designed to meet the specific needs of children with cerebral palsy. Therefore, three different pediatric robotic therapy approaches are being investigated to take of advantage of reprogrammable platforms including an active rehabilitative boot, motivation robots, and an assistive robotic trainer.

3. An Active Rehabilitative Boot

An active rehabilitative boot is the application of a programmable platform to the stretching of the lower leg to maximize range of movement for children with spastic cerebral palsy. The most commonly occurring form of CP is spastic CP. Spastic refers to high muscle tone (tightness) which constrains motion. When both legs are affected by this condition it is classified as spastic diplegia. Children with spastic diplegia often will walk on their toes. This is caused by the contraction of the gastronemus muscle in the leg.

The most common rehabilitative method for spastic diplegia is interaction with a physical therapist to stretch the muscle in order to increase the range of motion for the patient's gait. Physical therapy early in the child's development prevents contractures and helps to keep the muscles from becoming weakened or from deteriorating due to lack of use.

A second rehabilitation method is an ankle foot orthosis. An ankle foot orthosis forces the ankle into a preferred position while the patient wears the device. This is often achieved through the use of fastening straps. It has been found that ankle-foot orthosis are beneficial to children with spastic diplegia during sit to stand transitions (Park et. al., 2004).

Another method of therapy is the use of Botulinum-A Toxin, also called Botox, paired with serial casting. The Botox safely and effectively reduce spasticity in specific muscle groups. Botox is administered by direct injection into a shortened muscle (for example a spastic calf muscle causing a tight heel cord) to temporarily weaken that muscle and allow it to stretch. The effects of Botox are not permanent; weakness typically lasts for a few months. In some cases, patients may require repeated injections to treat a shortened muscle. The Botox helps relax the muscles so the therapist can stretch the muscle group by securing the foot into position with a standard plaster or fiberglass cast. After approximately one week, the cast is removed, the ankle is stretched to the new limits, and a new cast is applied. This process is repeated throughout a period of four to six weeks. The serial casting procedure can be uncomfortable and modify the patient's behavior. A set of casts restricts the child's gait, which may lead young patients to revert to crawling. A set of serial casts for a 3 year old child was weighed and the average weight of a cast was 377g per foot. Cast materials can also lead to skin irritations causing the cast to be removed and the effective therapy window for the Botox injection may be wasted.

A new active orthotic boot is being constructed to assist in the rehabilitation of children with cerebral palsy that have spastic diplegia typically manifested by toe-walking. A new dynamic or active orthotic boot can assist in walking and gradual rehabilitation of the associated muscle group. The programmability of a microcontroller based device provides the boot with the flexibility to address the needs of different patients as well as different therapeutic applications.

In previous work, an active ankle foot orthoses to treat drop-foot has been devised (Blaya and Herr, 2004). The actuator modulates the stiffness of the low muscle tone ankle joint. Although this work proved the feasibility of an active orthotic boot, the actuator mounting on the back side of the calf would be problematic for pediatric patients. Furthermore, this previous boot required fast actuator response times in order to facilitate active ambulation of the patient. Our proposed boot for pediatric rehabilitation requires a much slower system response which enables the investigation of different actuation solutions. By incorporating new materials and technology, the boot can be more compact and lightweight resulting in increased patient comfort. Some important functional requirements of this new boot are the ability to adapt to changing rehabilitation requirements, the ability to store a history patient/boot interaction data for the therapist, and safety for daily use.

Thus, the rehabilitation of patients with spastic diplegia can benefit from the development of a new active orthotic boot that can provide a more flexible alternative to serial casts and also provide in home stretching therapy.

3.1 Rehabilitative Boot Design Concept

The active boot design targeted a thin wall boot similar to current orthoses with integrated actuators and feedback sensors to provide the proper stretch or set to a fixed "cast" position. Feedback on the patient is collected in terms of the foot angle and the pressure that the foot exerts against the boot and is monitored by a microcontroller. The microcontroller analyzes input signals and provides output voltage to the system actuators. The magnitude and duration of the system output can be tuned and customized for each patient. Based on the input of a pediatric physical therapists, an approximation of three times the patient's body weight provides an upper bound for the magnitude of force needed to be exerted on the patient's foot. The relationship of system components is depicted in Figure 3.

The boot design is based on existing DAFO configurations. Current manufacturing methods can be utilized to custom fit durable, lightweight plastic to the geometry of the foot and ankle. Figure 4 shows the final design and the original prototype. A thin film pressure sensor is located at the ball of the foot to detect the pressure resulting from the patient's tendency to walk on their toes. The sensor pads depicted in Figure 4 provide a stiffened package to improve the repeatability of the signal from thin film sensors. The objective of the pressure sensor is to determine whether the foot is bearing weight so that the brace flexibility can be increased to facilitate ambulation. An angle sensor is located at the hinge point of the boot. This can be used for dynamic feedback or verification that the boot is in a set "cast" position. Pediatric physical therapists have stated that +/- 10 degree range is typical for the target population.

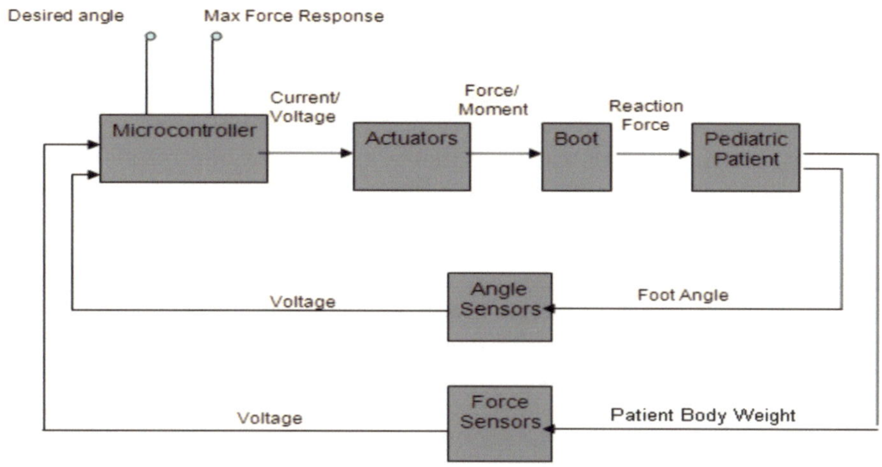

Fig. 3. System Block Diagram for a Pediatric Rehabilitative Boot.

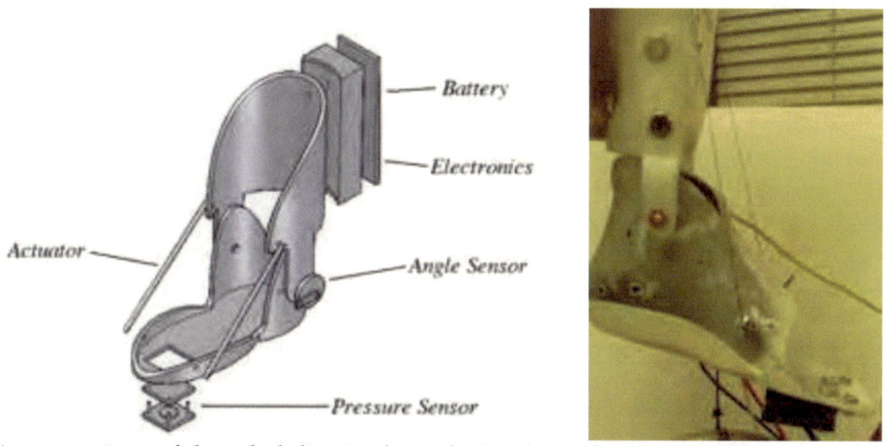

Fig. 4. A comparison of the rehabilitative boot design (a) and prototype (b).

Further development of a lightweight compact design integrates the actuators into the boot materials. Actuation can be achieved through contraction or bending. The microcontroller, interface circuitry, and battery are located on the back side of the boot to create an autonomous wearable device.

3.2 Prototype Rehabilitative Boot Design

System actuators must be able to move and stretch the leg muscles as part of a daily physical therapy routine. The concept of smart materials for use in orthotic and prosthetic devices has been investigated (Herr and Kornbluh, 2004) but not implemented. The use of electroactive polymer artificial muscles for assisting ambulation is discussed. Whereas the

ambulatory system requires a high speed system response, the rehabilitation system benefits from a slow actuator response.
A smart material that meets the design requirements well is Shape Memory Alloys. Their unique pseudo-elastic and shape memory effects would provide the structure and motion needed in the therapy, along with the flexibility desired for safety. The heat being supplied to the wire is essentially the power that drives the molecular arrangement. This particular effect would be useful in the orthotic device as a way to change and set the desired distortion (length and angle). However, the pseudo-elastic properties are only exhibited when the alloy is composed of austenite phase and a load is applied. As the load is increased, the alloy transforms from austenite to martensite. The load strain is absorbed by the softer martensite, then as the load is reduced, the martensite transform back into austenite and returns to its original shape. In conjunction with the shape memory effect, the pseudo-elastic effect would be useful in the orthotic device as a general comfort and safety level assurance since the material would ideally give flexibility in its movement while still maintaining the needed shape. Some advantages the shape memory alloys have over other actuators include high power density (>1000 W/kg), large stress (>200 MPa), and large strain (~5%).
System sensors monitor the interaction between the patient and the boot. Force sensors are required to monitor that actuation forces are stretching the leg muscles while ensuring that the muscle is not torn. This is performed indirectly by measuring the force applied by the brace on the patient's foot. The sensor will be placed at the ball of the foot because the spasticity is often exhibited by the extension of the child's foot, as when the child is walking on his/her toes.
Since the boot is controllable it is possible to facilitate walking when the patient is ambulating by reducing the boot stiffness. In order to perform this function, the sensor must be able to differentiate when the patient is standing versus when the patient is sitting.
By placing sensors at the ball of the foot, the type of sensors that can be used are limited by the comfort of the user. Therefore a thin flexible sensor is required. Second, it should give consistent readings over a range of temperatures. As an approximation, the lowest temperature the sensor will experience would be during the winter months (0°C) and the highest temperature the sensor will experience would be during the summer months (45 °C). Finally, the sensor must give accurate measurements over the required range of forces, 0-108kg. Negative force measurements are not required since we are only concerned when pressure is being applied. The highest force will occur either when the patient is standing or when the brace is applying forces to the patient to stretch the leg muscles. The highest force will vary from patient to patient however an estimate of the force needed to stretch the leg muscles is no more than three times the body weight of the child. This gives a maximum force of 108 kg.
A thin film force sensitive resistor can meet the design requirements. This sensor was chosen because it has a thickness of 0.2 mm, high durability, and low cost. The ability of the sensor to detect small forces, indicating the patient is sitting, versus large forces, indicating the child is standing, will require the sensor to give a measurement within approximately 0 to 5 kg of the actual force. This can be achieved because the sensor has a repeatability of 2.5%, a hysteresis of 4.5%, a linearity of 5%, and a temperature error of 0.36% / °C.
The angle of the foot relative to the leg is an important measurement in the therapy. The objective is to stretch the leg so that the range in foot angle of the patient will match the range

of a person who does not have spastic diplegia. Currently the angle of the foot is measured during visits to the therapist using a goniometer. The active boot will track the angle for active control of the boot. Furthermore, the availability of this data over time greatly enhances the physical therapist's insight into the ankle behavior. This information will give a more accurate picture of the patient's progress and can be used in future diagnosis.

An angle measurement sensor needs to be constrained to planar motions. Since the ankle joint can move with three degrees of freedom, the boot needs to measure a planar movement containing the calf and foot. In addition to this, the brace itself should be designed to limit rotation of the foot to only one axis. For this application, the range of angles is between -10° to $+10^{o}$.

Finally, in order to meet the design objective for comfort, the sensor should be as small as possible and easily attached to the boot. Potentiometers provide a simple solution that meets the design objectives. This results in resistive elements for both the pressure sensor and the angle measurement sensor. The use of resistive elements provides for easy interface with a system microcontroller.

In order to provide a boot that can adapt to different patient requirements and support a wearable device, an embedded programmable controller is required. The system microcontroller has two modes: serial casting and therapeutic stretching. In the serial casting mode, a desired angle is maintained until the force sensor detects that the foot is supporting a load, such as walking. The boot then allows flexure of the angle by the patient to facilitate walking. Once, the boot comes to rest, the desired angle for stretching the calf muscles is restored. In home therapy mode, a therapy sequence can be initiated when the patient is at rest. The boot is slowly cycled through a stretching exercise that has been set by the physical therapist. The safety functions of the boot system require a fast monitoring rate, so there will be no muscle damage. However, a high speed microcontroller is not required. The Parallax BS2-IC microcontroller was selected for development of a prototype rehabilitation boot based on familiarity with the device, no need for numerous I/O pins, cost and ease of programming.

3.3 Rehabilitative Boot Conclusions

Bench testing of the boot proved that the proposed actuator is sufficient for the stretching task. However, the prototype achieved a range of motion of 8-10 degrees short of the device goal of +/- 10 degrees. This discrepancy can be accounted for by changes to the actuator and boot geometry. Furthermore, heat generated by the actuator presents safety concerns which are being addressed.

Overall, it can be concluded that the concept of a wearable active rehabilitative boot is feasible. Continuation of the project will model and test candidate materials with and without embedded sensors.

4. Physical Therapy Robot Study

As stated earlier, there have been instances of motivational robots in physical therapy. However, it does not appear that the design of robot activities has been designed as a tool for the pediatric physical therapist. Therfore, motivational robot sessions were investigated by reprogramming commercially available robots to perform some standard therapy routines and instructing children to mimic the robots actions. These robots were designed for children who suffer from Cerebral Palsy. It should be noted that these children tend to have more physical difficulties. Everyday activities such as walking, crawling, or stretching are a struggle for these children. A child's physical impairments can lead to a low perception of self-efficacy and self-competence due to having difficulties engaging in play activities (Miller and Reid, 2003). To address these issues, proposed therapy routines for CP patients will focus on walking, stretching, and positive reinforcement for motivation.

After preliminary interviews with pediatric physical therapists, it was revealed that therapists often have difficulty keeping a child's attention during physical therapy sessions. Furthermore, they often have difficulty persuading the child to perform his or her required exercises. The goal of this project is to fully create, program, and implement therapy routines using the Sony AIBO robotic dog (model ERS-220) focused on the needs of Cerebral Palsy and Autism patients in the age range of 3 to 12. More specifically, the robotic dog will be used to improve children's motor skills and social interactions during physical therapy sessions.

The group has thoroughly investigated several pediatric disorders and found that both Autism and Cerebral Palsy (CP) will benefit most from AIBO's capabilities. Therapists and professionals were consulted to aid in developing several proposal routines that can be programmed into AIBO and implemented during therapy sessions. These proposals consist of motivational games, stretches, exercises, and social activities designed to enhance the current sessions. The Sony AIBO, a robotic dog, was chosen as prototype due to its vast capabilities, intricate programmability, and its highly sophisticated components. The autonomous robot is fully programmable and responds to its surroundings. Its performance is enhanced with colorful LEDs and the ability to play music and sound clips.

A user friendly interface will ensure ease of use for the therapist and parents. Overall, the project hopes to aid children suffering from these diseases by improving their physical, cognitive, and social skills, all while enhancing their overall well-being.

4.1 Physical Therapy Robot Activity Design Concept

The physical therapist centered design methodology was implemented using seven design criteria. These criteria required the final designs to: 1) be within AIBO's physical capabilities, 2)correspond with the desired age group, 3) address a pertinent or common physical, cognitive, or emotional problem, 4) have a high predicted effectiveness, 5) be relatively simple to program, 6) pose no risk of harm to the child, and 7) be easy to evaluate the effectiveness. These criteria wereapplied to activities targeting two distinct populations of children: children with autism and children with cerebral palsy. The proposed therapy routines for autistic children focus on speech, interaction, and play. The proposed therapy routines for cerebral palsy patients will focus on walking, stretching, and positive reinforcement for motivation.

Under the guidance of professional therapists, several Autism routines have been developed and each evaluated based on the seven feasibility criteria described above. One proposed activity is a voice activation game in which the child can command the dog to perform a certain action such as "sit," "stand," "move forward," "walk right," etc. Children with Autism typically have trouble asking questions or with speech in general. This will encourage the child to not only speak, but also ask a question or make a command. The child will be further motivated to play with AIBO when he or she sees AIBO successfully perform the desired action.

Another proposed activity is a game that involves throwing and kicking AIBO's pink ball (a special ball that comes with the robot). The child will gently throw or kick the ball to AIBO and the robot will locate the ball and kick it back to the child. This activity could involve more than one child to further encourage social interaction for the Autistic child.

The last activity is a sensory exercise that utilizes AIBO's pressure sensors. Autistic children often cannot distinguish between touching something hard and touching it lightly. This activity begins with the therapist (or adult) telling the child to touch one of AIBO's buttons "hard." If the child touches lightly and lifts his or her finger, AIBO will shake his head "no" and the child can try again. If the child succeeds, AIBO performs a celebration dance.

Several routines for cerebral palsy patients were developed. The first routine is a game that will be used to motivate children to walk. Most cerebral palsy patients have trouble walking and many patients do not have any motivation or desire to try to walk. To address this, AIBO can be programmed to walk in front of the child a set distance (approximately 1 meter). AIBO will then turn around and face the child. The robot will use its distance sensor to determine whether the child has walked closer (within ¾ of a meter from AIBO). Next, AIBO will complete a celebration dance if the child succeeds or sit and wait until the child does. This process can be repeated the desired number of times as specified by the therapist or parent.

To aid the cerebral palsy patient in his or her stretches, a "Follow the Leader" set of activities is proposed. This set of activities will involve AIBO performing a stretch and the child mimicking the robot for the desired number of repetitions as specified by the therapist. One example stretch is referred to as the "Airplane," which requires the child to lie on his or her stomach. The child will then lift all four limbs into the air. This stretches and works the abdominal muscles and is often recommended for cerebral palsy patients (see Figures 5 and 6). Other proposed mimicking activities include arm extensions, balancing, hamstring curls, leg extensions, sitting up tall, pushups, rolling over, and stair climbing.

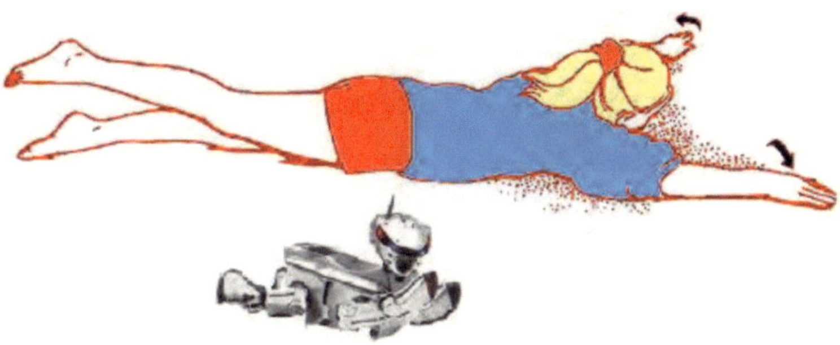

Fig. 5. A physical therapy document showing the airplane stretch along with the robot implementation.

An important aspect of the robotic therapy tool is ease of use for the therapist. A colorful user interface with detailed directions and an instructional computer program ensure that the therapist can perform the desired routine without delaying a therapy session (see Figure 7). Each routine can be accessed by pressing a combination of colored buttons on AIBO's back side. For instance, to instruct AIBO to perform the leg extension activity, the user must simply push the blue button and then the red button.

Evaluations of the project will be based on each child's level of motivation to participate in the activity, overall emotional effect that the activity has on the child, and the child's performance and overall improvement when completing a routine.

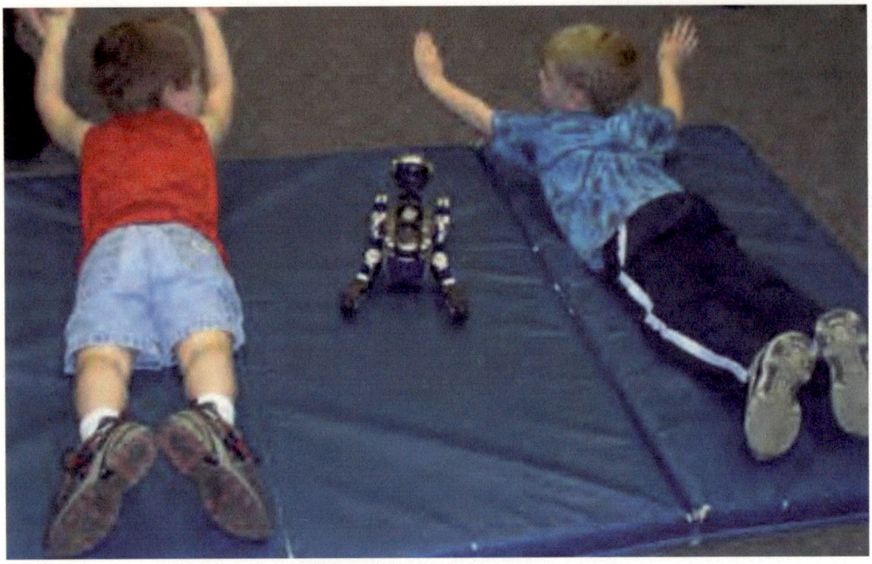

Fig. 6. Children Performing Airplane Stretch with AIBO.

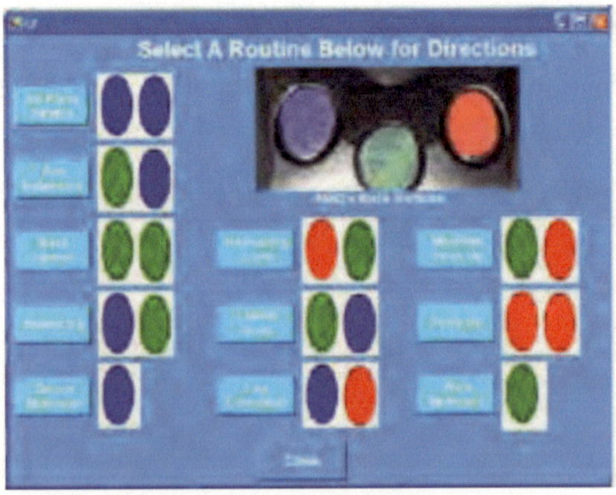

Fig. 7. Color code routine selection designed for therapist use.

4.2 Physical Therapy Robot Testing

After selecting various routines to be implemented, several programming designs were created for each routine. Smooth, human-like movements were desirable for each routine. When determining the best program design, robot positioning and stability were considered. This initial testing ensured that AIBO would remain stable throughout the routines and would look life-like to the users.

Pilot testing was conducted for the cerebral palsy routines during therapy sessions at a preschool, which is designed for children ages three to five with various developmental delays. Half of the test population at the preschool were typically developed. Testing was conducted by a physical therapist familiar with the project who also evaluating the robotic tool. Five groups were tested for 10-15 minute sessions. The sessions were video taped. A second set of sessions was performed a month after the first.

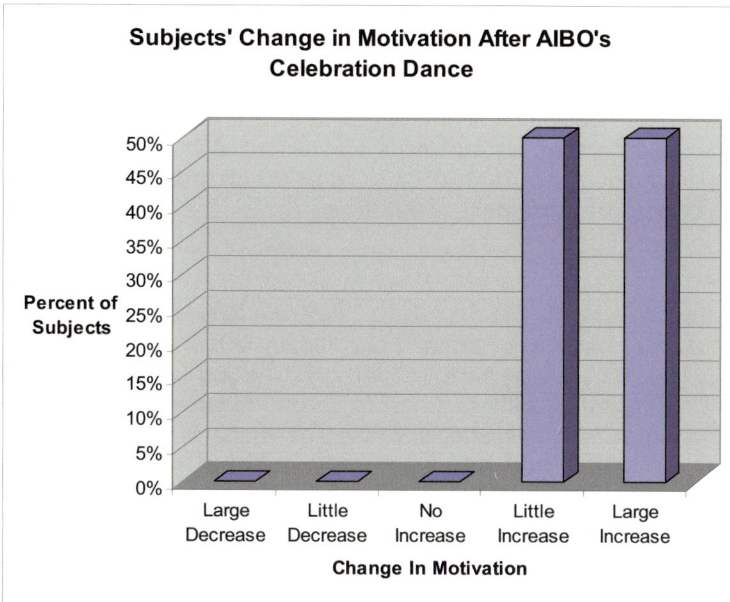

Fig. 8. Pilot study results regarding motivation.

Therapist evaluation of the tool was collected with a survey. Furthermore, video tape of the sessions were reviewed for visual cues. Results presented in Figure 8 and Figure 9 include a increased willingness to imitate body positions and a high level of enthusiasm for all participants. Most participants correctly mimicked the robot movements. In exercises that separately moved limbs on the right and left, some participants moved the wrong limb. Participants that were exposed to the robot therapy a second time did not lose motivation or enthusiasm with the second exposure.

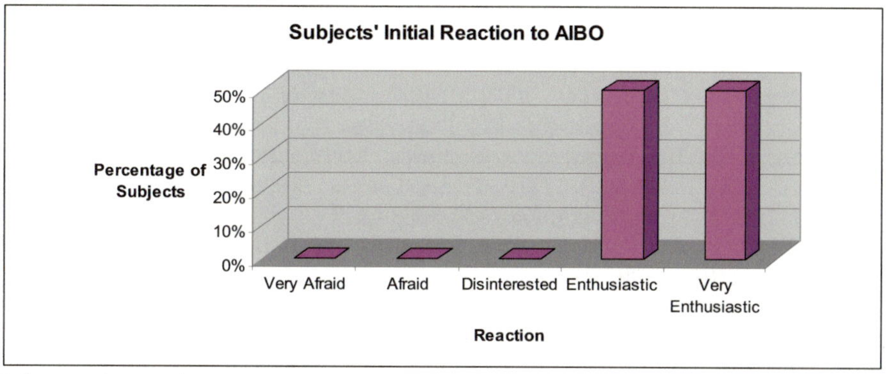

Fig. 9. Pilot study results regarding enthusiasm.

3.3 Physical Therapy Robot Conclusions

Programming a robot to aid pediatric physical therapists provides an effective tool for the therapist. The programmable platform can be used to provide an alternate method of performing existing therapy tasks. A robotic solution provides a tool that can be applied to a wide range of patients with little set up time. Further studies need to be conducted in order to test the long term effects in therapy.

4. Final Conclusions

The results of the two studies provide evidence that there are wide ranging opportunities in the area of pediatric rehabilitation for the application of robotic platforms. Two very different platforms were presented addressing two distint therapy outcomes. In both cases, the inclusion of rehabilitation professionals was essential in the deign of the device or activity. System design considerations need to be based on direct therapy goals and robotic systems need to be evaluated on medical outcomes.

5. References

Matthews, D.J. and Wilson, P., Cerebral Palsy. *Pediatric Rehabilitation,* 3rd ed., G. E. Molnar and M. A. Alexander, Ed. Philadelphia: Hanley & Belfus, 1999, pp. 193-217.

Styer-Acevedo, J., Physical Therapy for the Child with Cerebral Palsy. *Pediatric Physical Therapy,* 3rd ed., J. S. Tecklin, Ed. Philadelphia: Lippincott Williams & Wilkins, 1999, pp. 107-162.

Sawicki, G. S., Domingo, A., and Ferris, D. (2006) The effects of powered ankle-foot orthoses on joint kinematics and muscle activation during walking in individuals with incomplete spinal cord injury. *Journal of Neuroengineering and Rehabilitation*, Vol. 3, 1743-0003 (Electronic)

Burgar, C.G., Lum, P. S., Shor, P.C., and Van der Loos, H.F.M. (2000) Development of robots for rehabilitation therapy: The Palo Alto VA/Stanford experience. *Journal of Rehabilitation Research and Development,* Vol . 37 No . 6 (November/December 2000), 663-673, 03425282.

Merians, A.S., Jack, D., Boian, R., Tremaine, M., Burdea, G.C., Adamovich, S.V., Recce, M., and Poizner, H. (2002) Virtual Reality-Augmented Rehabilitation for Patients Following Stroke. *Physical Therapy*, Vol. 82 No. 9 (September 2002), 898-915, 00319023

Plaisant , C., Druin, A., Lathan, C., Dakhane, K., Edwards, K., Maxwell Vice, J., and Montemayor, J. (2000) A Storytelling Robot for Pediatric Rehabilitation. Proceedings *of ASSETS'00: The Fourth International ACM SIGCAPH Conference on Assistive Technologies,* pp. 50-55, 1-58113-314-8, Arlington, Virginia, November, 2000, ACM, New York.

Michaud, F., Duquett, A. and Nadeau, I. (2003) Characteristics of Mobile Toys for Children with Pervasive Developmental Disorders. *Proceedings of IEEE International Conference on Systems, Man and Cybernetics, Vol.3,* pp. 2938-2943, 0-7803-7952-7, Washington, D.C., Ocotober, 2003, IEEE, Piscataway, NY

Michaud, F., Laplante, J-F., Larouche, H., Duquette, A., Caron, S., Letourneau, C. and Masson, P. (2004) Autonomous Spherical Mobile Robot for Child Development Studies. 34(4) (2004) 1-10. , *IEEE Transactions on Systems, Man and Cybernetics, Part A*, Vol. 35, No. 4 (July 2005), 471- 480, 1083-4427

Park, E. S., Park, C. I., Chang, H. J., Choi, J. E. and Lee, D.S. (2004) The effect of hinged ankle-foot orthoses on sit-to-stand transfer in children with spastic cerebral palsy. *Archives of physical medicine and rehabilitation*, Vol. 85, No. 12 (December 2004), 2053-2057, 0003-9993

Blaya, J. A. and Herr, H., (2004) Adaptive Control of a Variable-Impedance Ankle-Foot Orthosis to Assist Drop-Foot Gait. *IEEE Trans. Neural Systems and Rehabilitation Engineering*, Vol. 12, No. 1 (March 2004), 24-31, 1534-4320

Herr, H. M. and Kornbluh, R. D. (2004) New horizons for orthotic and prosthetic technology: artificial muscle for ambulation. *Proceedings of SPIE -- Volume 5385 Smart Structures and Materials 2004: Electroactive Polymer Actuators and Devices*, pp. 1-9, 2004, pp. 1-9 , 07393717, San Diego, CA, March 2004,

Miller, S. and Reid, D. (2003) Doing Play: Competency, Control, and Expression. *Cyber Physiology and Behavior, Vol.* 6, No. 6 (December 2003): 623-630, 10649506

2

Biomechanical Constraints in the Design of Robotic Systems for Tremor Suppression

Juan-Manuel Belda-Lois, Álvaro Page, José-María Baydal-Bertomeu, Rakel Poveda, Ricard Barberà
Instituto de Biomecánica de Valencia (Spain)

1. Introduction

The *Movement Disorder Society* defines tremor as an involuntary rythmical oscillation of a body part (Deuschl et al. 1998). This definition excludes other movement disorders with a less cyclic character such as chorea or ataxia. Tremor is the most frequent movement disorder in clinical practice with an estimated prevalence between 3-4% of the population over 50 (Manto et al. 2004).

Everybody has some tremor component, usually invisible for the naked eye, called *physiological tremor*. However, there are other forms of pathological tremor that can be very disabling, and often a cause of social exclusion (Rocon et al. 2004). There are many pathologies that can cause pathological tremor, among others Essential Tremor, Parkinson Disease, brain trauma or multiple sclerosis.

Common treatments of tremor are pharmacological and surgical. Pharmacological treatments depend on the specific pathology that causes tremor. For instance *Parkinson disease tremor* is treated with L-dopa, and common treatments for *Essential Tremor* are β-blockers (Deuschl et al. 1998). Surgical classical treatment for tremor is thalamic thermocoagulation (Deuschl et al. 2000). However from mid 90's Deep Brain Stimulation (DBS) is preferred to thermocoagulation (Deuschl et al. 2000).

Despite these therapies, there are still an important number of people with pathological tremor resistant to the common treatments (Deuschl et al. 1998). Thus, other alternatives are of interest to help people suffering from different kinds of pathological tremor. Many of these alternatives focus on removing the consequences of tremor rather than its origins. Among others the following approaches can be mentioned:

(a) Removing the tremor from a tremorous signal (Riviere & Thakor, 1996; Gonzalez et al. 2000) (b) Design of assistive devices based in dampers (such as the NeaterEater® or the MouseTrap® (c) Design of robotics systems to suppress tremor.

This chapter focuses the attention on the design of robotics systems to suppress tremor. First of all, we will introduce different strategies to suppress tremor using robotic approaches, then we will show the biomechanical and ergonomics issues to take into consideration in the design of these robotic systems, finally we will introduce a set of guidelines to take into account in the design of robotics systems for tremor suppression.

2. Robotic systems to suppress tremor

Robotic systems allow mechanical tremor suppression while preserving the component of voluntary movement. This approach has been attempted previously by several authors considering different strategies, and using different robotic configurations.

2.1 Methodological introduction

In this chapter we will consider the mechanical system of a body segment with a robotic system attached to it from the perspective of dynamic systems theory. Given a simple mechanical system such as the one in figure 1, we can express the relationship between force and displacement in the form of a differential equation that includes the components of inertia (M), stiffness (K) and viscosity (c) (1)

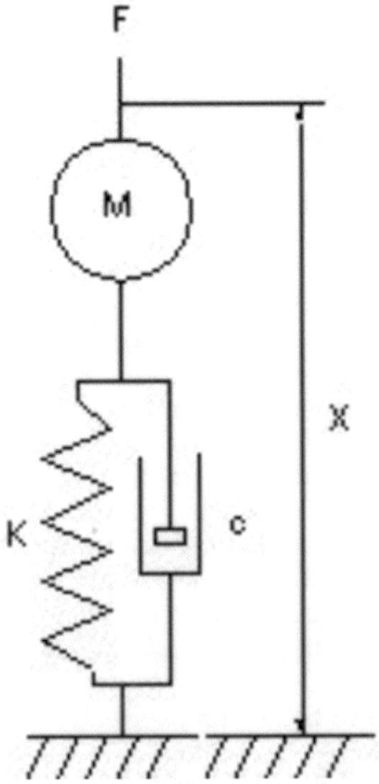

Fig. 1. Simple mechanical system to exemplify the relationship between force (F) and displacement (ΔX) depending on the mechanical characteristics of the system.

$$F(t) = M \cdot \frac{\partial^2(\Delta x)}{\partial t^2} + c \cdot \frac{\partial(\Delta x)}{\partial t} + K \cdot \Delta x \tag{1}$$

Using the Laplace transform (2) we can change a differential equation such as (1) into an expression dependent on the operator s (3), and this kind of transformation allows to obtain expressions in which we can separate the physical charateristics of the system from the inputs and outputs (4). We can refer to these physical characteristics as *dynamic stiffness* (5) in the sense that is an expression of the complex relationship between the force applied and the position of the system.

$$L[f(t)] = F(s) = \int f(t)e^{-st}\,dt \quad (2)$$

$$F = M \cdot s^2 x + c \cdot sx + Kx \quad (3)$$

$$F = \left(M \cdot s^2 + c \cdot s + k\right)x \quad (4)$$

$$F = B(s) \cdot x \quad (5)$$

Besides, the use of the Laplace transformation has two extra benefits: a) it allows a relationship between an input signal (i.e. force) and an output signal (i.e. displacement) in a mathematical expression known as *transfer function*. b) it allows the identification of the mechanical system from its frequency response.

2.2 Strategies for tremor suppression

One obvious way to supress tremor consists in damping the tremor component: adding viscosity to a joint makes the joint speed dependent. Thus, since a tremor movement is faster than common voluntary movements, the addition of damping should attenuate tremor. This approach has been tested through the use of dampers (Kotovsky & Rosen, 1998) or through the use of actuators based on magneto-rheological fluids (MRFs) (Loureiro et al. 2006).

From a wider perspective, adding viscosity to a joint changes the dynamic stiffness of the joint. But we can change dynamic stiffness by not only adding viscosity but also adding stiffness and inertia.

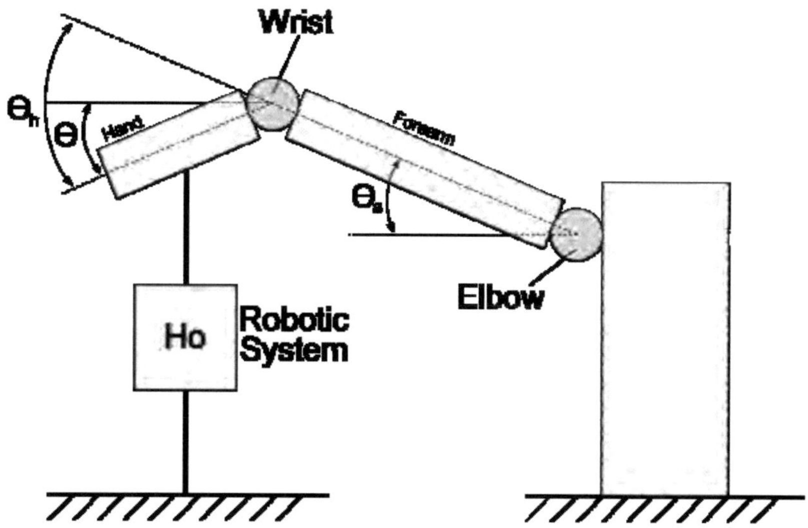

Fig. 2. Simplified diagram of grounded robotic system for tremor suppression.

Pledgie et al. (2000), suggested the use of changes in the dynamic stiffness in order to attenuate tremor. Adding dynamic stiffness the overall bandwith of the system can be changed, if the band of tremor is let out of the band of the overall system (human joint and robotic system) then the tremor should attenuate. This is the approach shown in (6), where B_a is the dynamic stiffness of the body system and B_o is the dynamic stiffness of the robotic system.

$$\theta(s) = \frac{1}{B_a + B_o} \cdot T(s) \tag{6}$$

Another feasible strategy consists in the implementation of a filter in a mechanical system. This has been one of the approaches of Rocon et al. (2005). The main idea of these authors was to track the frequency of tremor using the Weighted Linear Fourier Transform suggested by Riviere & Thakor (1996) and designing a zero-lag notch filter tuned to remove the tremor frequency component.

2.3 Grounded robotic systems

Grounded systems are those which create a mechanical linkage from a body segment to the ground or a fixed external system such as a desktop or a wheelchair. Figure 2 shows a simplified diagram of a grounded robot attached to the hand. For the sake of simplicity we have assumed a 2D model of the arm with only two joints the wrist and the elbow.
A system of these characteristics can efficiently suppress the tremor at the level of the hand. We can simplify the behaviour of the overall system to the diagram blocks of figure 3. We are considering that an input torque at the wrist joint of T_w , H_o is the dynamic response of the robotic system (i.e. the transfer function), and B_e and B_w are respectively the dynamic stiffness of elbow and wrist joints.

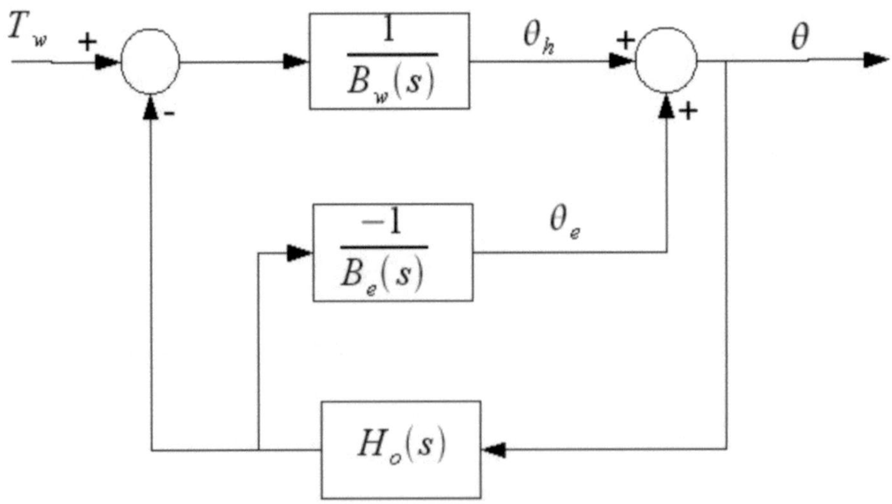

Fig. 3. Linearised model of the grounded robotic system shown in figure 2.

(7) is the be the expression of the overall movement of the hand according to figure 3. As it can be observed in (7) the response of the robotic system can modify the response of the hand.

$$\theta(s) = \frac{B_e}{B_w \cdot B_e + B_w \cdot H_o + B_e \cdot H_o} \cdot T_w(s) \tag{7}$$

However, due to the mechanical coupling introduced by the robotic system, a component of tremor will appear at elbow level such as shown in (8).

$$\theta_e(s) = \frac{-H_o}{B_w \cdot B_e + B_w \cdot H_o + B_e \cdot H_o} \cdot T_w(s) \tag{8}$$

In other words, keeping the tip of the hand steady with a grounded system will introduce a tremor component in the proximal joints. This component of tremor can be potentially dangerous when users perform movements oriented to his/her body such as eating or dressing.
If we considered an strategy based on the addition of dynamic stiffness instead of a generic suppressing strategy represented by a transfer function, we can compare (7) with the approximation of tremor suppression through impedance control suggested by Pledgie et al. (2000) which is shown in (6). At first sight both expressions are very different, but we can rearrange the terms of (7) as shown in (9), and substitute the response of the system, a generic transfer function ,represented by H_o , for a dynamic stiffness represented by B_o .

$$\theta(s) = \frac{1}{B_w + \left(1 + \frac{B_w}{B_e}\right) B_o} \cdot T_w(s) \tag{9}$$

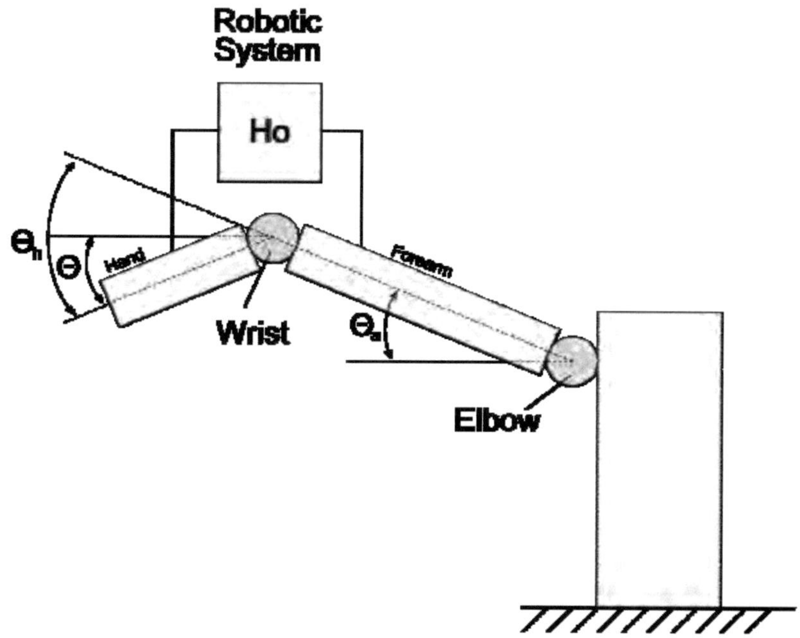

Fig. 4. Simplified diagram of a wearable robotic system for tremor suppression attached to the wrist joint.

But, according to Acosta et al. (2000) the dynamic stiffness of the arm should be considered as a whole due to the coupling of body structures and in particular to the existence of biarticular muscles. This hypothesis provides consistency to the approach of Pledgie et al. (2000) who identify the overall response of the arm as a generic linear second order system. Therefore, if frequency response of the arm is unitary, the dynamic stiffness of different joints can only differ, approximately, in the gain. Consequently, we can simplify further (9) to (10), where K is a positive real number representing the relationship of stiffness of wrist and elbow joints.

$$\theta(s) = \frac{1}{B_w + K \cdot B_o} \cdot T_w(s) \tag{10}$$

As it can be seen, (10) is very similar to (6), and therefore the approximation of Pledgie et al. (2000) can be considered as a special case of the approach shown.

2.4 Exoskeletons and wearable systems

The principles of exoskeletons are very different from grounded robotic systems. figure 4, shows a simplified diagram of exoskeleton to suppress tremor at the wrist joint. As it can be inferred from the figure, in this case there are not mechanical couplings (other than inertial coupling characteristics) able to transmit tremor from distal to proximal joints.
However, this approximation has two main drawbacks: firstly the system doesn't have control over the global position of the hand, just in the movement performed by the joint under control, (in the case of figure 4 the wrist angle), and secondly the system is unable to compensate tremor coming from other joints.
The block diagram for this approximation is much simpler (figure 5).

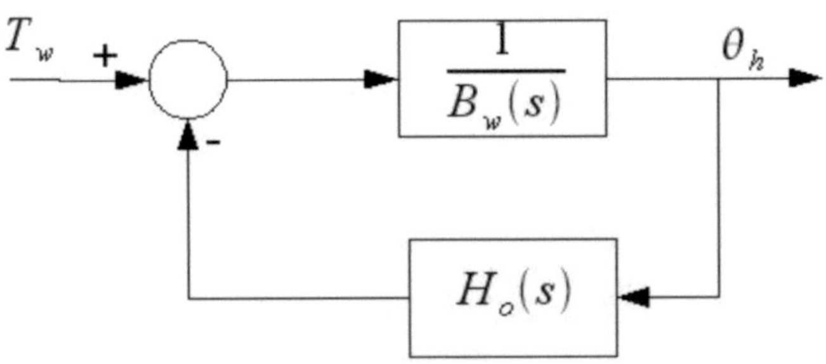

Fig. 5. Linearised model of the exoskeleton system.

Consequently the expression of the position of the hand with respect to the forearm is also simpler (11).

$$\theta_h = \frac{1}{B_w + H_o} \cdot T_w \tag{11}$$

Comparing (11) with (6) we can see that both expressions are identical, therefore the same type of tremor supressing strategy is possible in this configuration.

3. Biomechanical requirements

In the last point we have considered how different strategies and approximations can be effective for tremor suppression. However, in all the development, we have considered ideal conditions in relation to the compatibility between the robotic system and the body segments. Human body segments impose their own constraints to the system and these constraints must be kept into account in order to construct useful devices able to suppress tremor.
One of the key factors when designing these systems is the management of the contact between the body and the system. The systems attached to the body require the

transmission of the loads to the skeletal system, but this transmission is only possible through the layers of soft tissues between the device and the skeleton.
Common orthotic practice has developed procedures for load transmission based mainly on safety and comfort issues. However, many common orthotic procedures are not applicable in the design of systems to suppress tremor because they are successful only in static or quasiestatic conditions, but tremor is a pure dynamic effect and therefore requires other approaches.

3.1 Contact pressures

The transmission of loads from the systems to the skeleton produces contract pressure that can compromise safety and comfort.
Regarding safety, the usual guideline is avoiding pressures above the ischaemia level (the level at which the capillary vessels are not able to conduct blood compromising the tissue). This level has been estimated in 30 mmHg (Landis, 1930).
The relation between pressures and comfort is much more complicated. Touch receptors are sensitive to the deformation of the layers of tissue where they are located (Dandekar et al. 2003), therefore the perception of pressure is indirect: pressure deforms tissues and this deformation is sensed by skin receptors. Besides, the type, density and distribution of skin receptors varies significantly depending on the part of the body implied. Finally, the skin receptors have a dynamic response to the excitation (receptor adaptation). This dynamic response makes the pressure perception dependent on the dynamics of the process of applying pressure.
In orthotic practice the main guideline is reducing the contact pressure as much as possible increasing the contact surface between the system and the body, and reducing the risk of injury for maintained high pressures.
However, this guideline couldn't be appropriate from the point of view of comfort. According to Goonetilleke (1998) there exists an optimal surface to distribute a load and this value is a balance between pressure and number of touch receptors excited, also known as spatial summation theory (Goonetilleke, 1998). Furthermore, in the case of system for tremor suppression, as we will see later, the use of big supports to distribute the load worsen the performance of the system, consequently some kind of increase of contact pressure is needed in comparison with conventional orthoses.
To assess the tolerance of pressure of different parts of the body some authors made indentations to the point where the user feels pain or discomfort (Byström et al. 1995). However, the results of these experiments should be considered as a general indication of discomfort threshold since they depend on dynamics, shape and area of application.

3.1 Shear forces

Shear forces are together with pressure, the most important cause of skin injuries. Besides, compliance of skin in the shear plane is higher than in normal plane and this can cause loss of alignment in actuators which have an action line parallel to the body segment.

3.2 Kinematic compatibility

Body joints never act as pure hinge or ball joints, the geometry of body joints is usually very complex and can differ substantially depending on the person. On the other hand, robotics are commonly composed of inferior pair joints. Therefore, when we place a robotic system acting parallel to a body segment there are loss of alignments between the robotic system joint and body joint Instant Helical Axis (IHA). This loss of alignment is partially

compensated for the flexibility of body soft tissues and partially is transmitted as loads to the structures of the joint, and this can ultimately lead to an injury.
These injuries are relevant in powerful joints which manage an important amount of load such as the knee. In these cases the design of a mechanism able to follow-up as close as possible the body joint IHA is very important.

3.3 Protection of body structures

When applying loads to a body segment it is important to be careful with some structures in order to avoid discomfort, pain or the risk of injuries: Superficial vessels and nerves and bone prominences. Besides, we should keep free the area close to the joints.

3.4 Dynamic stiffness in the contact

In point 2, we have considered ideal contact conditions between the robotic system and the body segment. However, these conditions determine the overall performance of the system.

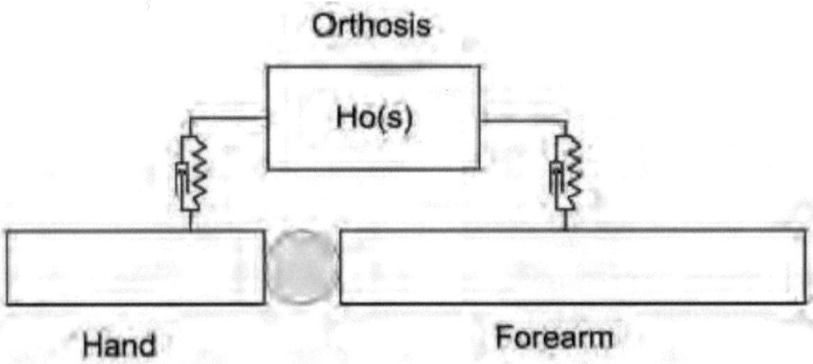

Fig. 6. Simplified view of a robotic system considering the dynamic stiffness in the contact.

If we consider the dynamic stiffness between the system and the body when we model the response of the system (figure 6), and we assume that the effect of the system is to apply a certain amount of dynamic stiffness (B_o), then the overall equivalent stiffness of the system is (12). The dynamical stiffness of the contact points between the robotic system and the body segments, as well as the dynamical stiffness of the actuator are all in serial mode and consequently the overall dynamical stiffness has been reduced.

$$B_t = \frac{B_{s1} \cdot B_{s2} \cdot B_o}{B_{s1} \cdot B_{s2} + B_{s1} \cdot B_o + B_{s2} \cdot B_o} \qquad (12)$$

If we consider that dynamic stiffness in both body segments is the same and we neglect the viscous component, then we can simplify (12) into (13) where K is the stiffness of the soft tissues under the contact of the system.

$$B_t = \frac{\frac{K}{2} \cdot B_o}{\frac{K}{2} + B_o} \qquad (13)$$

To understand how the contact conditions can affect the performance of a robotic system for tremor suppression the response of an effective system and a sitffness in the contact of

$0.47 N/m$ can be considered. As it can be seen in figure 7, the dynamic response of the system has changed considerably. If we consider the contact conditions, even for a well designed system we can lose all the attenuation in the frequency of pathological tremor (4 Hz) due to the stiffness of soft tissue. Thus the system is no longer capable of suppressing tremor due to the conditions of the contact.

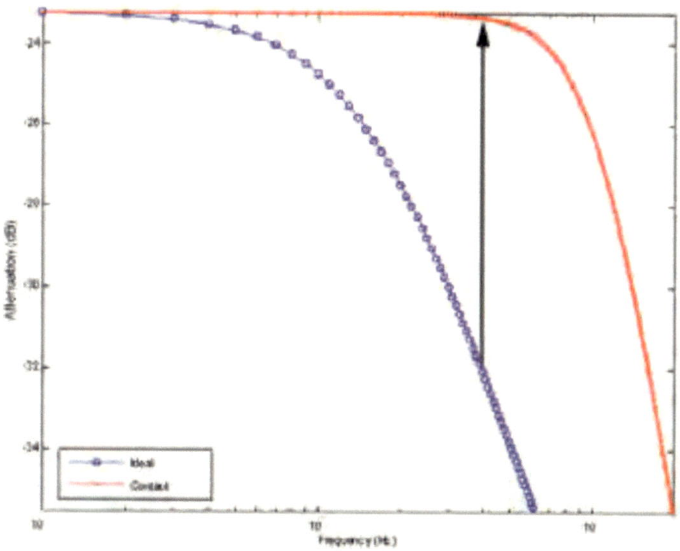

Fig. 7. Effect of the contact. The curve with circles is the response of the system considering an ideal contact between the system and the body segment. The curve with crosses is the response of the system considering the stiffness of the soft tissues. The arrow shows the loss of attenuation at 4 Hz (typical frequency of many pathological tremors) when stiffness of the contact is considered.

If we are able to increase the stiffness of the contact by a factor of 10 (overall stiffness $4.7 N/m$), the response of the system (figure 8) will come closer to the ideal behaviour. The system is able to suppress tremor.

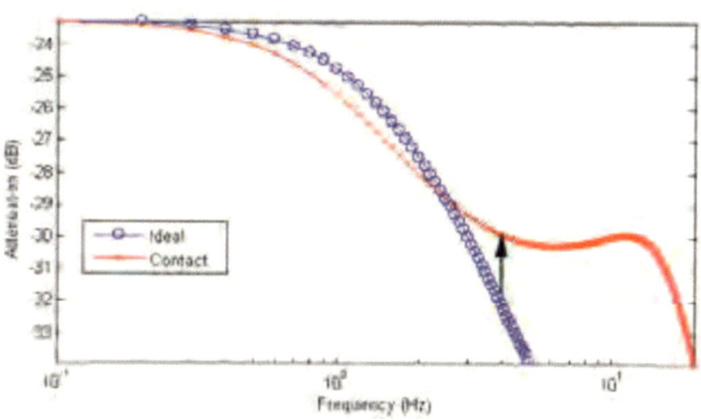

Fig. 8. The effect of increasing the stiffness in the contact. The arrow represents the loss of attenuation at 4 Hz when we consider the stiffness of the contact.

Moreover, the stiffness in the shear plane is considerably lower than in the normal plane. Thus, the response of the system will be worse in the shear plane.
In addition, the loss of alignment between the body segment and the orthosis can also produce a reduction of effectiveness. The stiffness of the soft tissues can produce this loss of alignment (figure 9). In the figure 9(a), the gap between the support system and the body segment is a representation of the contact of stiffness. When the segment corresponding to the hand moves, the orthosis does not act due to the loss of alignment between the fixation and the hand –Fig. 9(b)–

4. Design principles

All the above considerations imply restrictions in the design of robotic systems for tremor suppression. We have summarised these constraints in three design principles:

a) Length restriction
b) Increase of contact pressure
c) Alignments with body segments

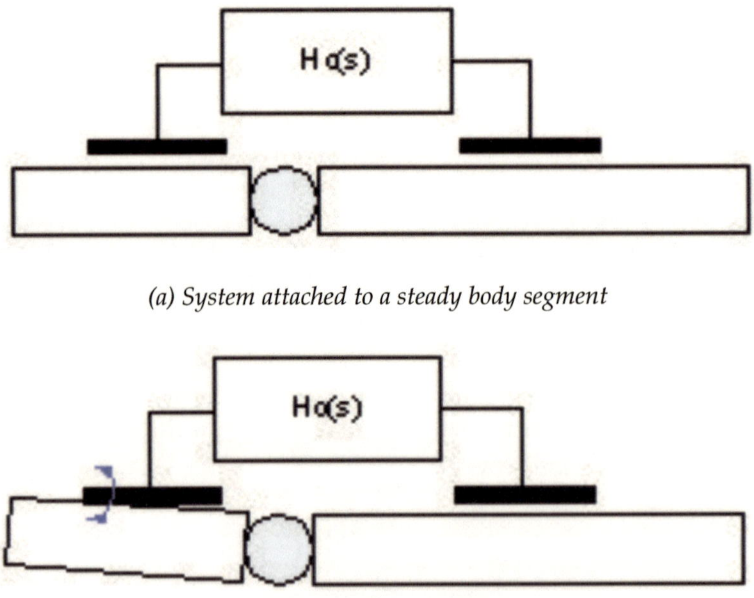

(a) System attached to a steady body segment

(b) Loss of alignment when the body segment moves

Fig. 9. The effect of loss of alignment due to a low impedance.

4.1 Length restriction

This principle is intended to deal with the low stiffness associated with the shear component of stiffness. A constraint in length between the fixation devices (figure 10) increases the overall stiffness of the contact in a factor of 4.
Without this restriction the supports corresponding to each segment can move separately. Therefore, their dynamical stiffness is in serial mode. However, if we restrict the distance between the supports (figure 10), now both supports can only move coordinately.

Consequently, both contacts are now in parallel and the overall dynamical stiffness is higher (14). Therefore, the length restriction affects the overall dynamic stiffness of the system.

$$B_t = \frac{B_o \cdot (B_{s1} + B_{s2})}{B_o + B_{s1} + B_{s2}} \tag{14}$$

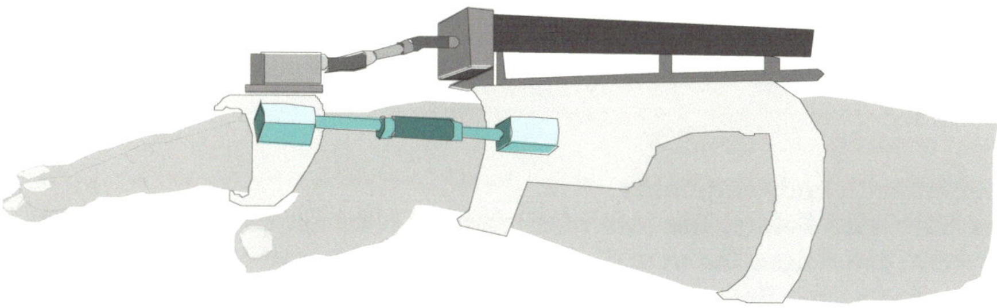

Fig. 10. Length restriction in a device to suppress tremor in the wrist flexion-extension based in a linear actuator.

Using the same simplifications as in (13) (equal impedance in both fixations and neglecting the viscous component), (14) converts to (15).

$$B_t = \frac{2\mathrm{K} \cdot B_o}{2\mathrm{K} + B_o} \tag{15}$$

Comparing (15) with (13) we can seen that now the equivalent stiffness of the contact is four times higher.

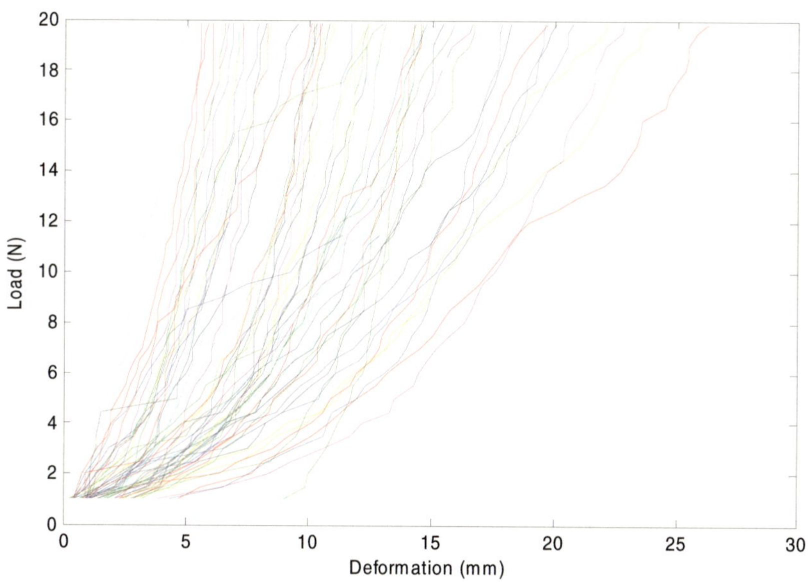

Fig 11. Force deformation characteristics of soft tissues in the forearm.

4.2 Increase of contact pressure

The tenso-deformational characteristics of the soft tissues under the arm are highly non-linear. The stiffness of the tissues increases as contact pressure increases. Figure 11 shows the force-displacement curve measured in the forearm of 10 different young people (5 males and 5 females) measured in 6 points of the forearm (3 in the palmar side and 3 in the volar side).

As we can infer from figure 11, one way to increase contact impedance is increasing contact pressure and moving upwards in the tenso-deformational curve. This strategy has two constraints of safety and comfort that have been dealt with in point 3.1.

4.3 Alignment with body segments

As it has been said before, the loss of alignment between the body segment and the robotic system can reduce the overall performance of the system. One way to ensure the alignment is increasing the number of contact points of each support. Each support part of the system should have at least three contact points to ensure the alignment (figure 12).

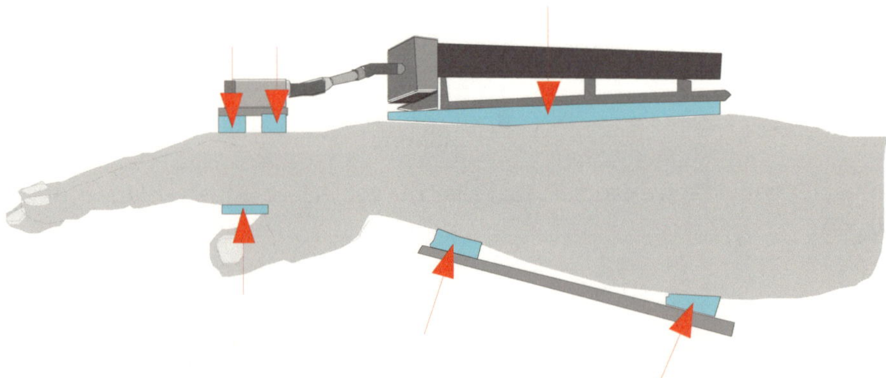

Fig 12. Alignment of the support devices with the body segments once the number of contact points have been increased.

5. Conclusions

Tremor suppression with robotic devices can be an alternative for people with pathological tremor resistant to conventional treatments.

Common orthotic principles don't fit well for tremor suppression due to the inherent dynamic characteristics of tremor.

In the design of robotic systems for tremor suppression the correct design of load transmission to the bones through the soft tissues is one of the key aspects for successful performance.

We have summarised the design specifications into three guidelines:

a) Length restriction to avoid the low stiffness associated in the shear plane.
b) Increase of contact pressure to increase contact stiffness.
c) Increase of the number of contact points to keep the alignments between the orthosis and the body segment.

6. References

Acosta, A M; Kirsch, R F & Perreault, E F (2000) A robotic manipulator for the characterization of two-dimensional dynamic stiffness using stochastic displacement perturbations. *Journal of Neuroscience Methods*, Vol. 102, (177–186), ISSN 0165-0270

Byström, S; Hall, C; Welander, T & Kilbom, A (1995) Clinical disorders and pressure-pain threshold of the forearm and hand among automobile assembly line workers. *Journal of Hand Surgery*, Vol. 20, No. 6, (782–790). ISSN 1753-1934.

Dandekar, K; Raju B I & Srinivasan M A (2003). 3-D Finite-Element Models of Human and Monkey Fingertips to Investigate the Mechanics of Tactile Sense. *Journal of Biomechanical Engineering*, Vol. 125, (682-691), ISSN 0148-0731

Deuschl, G; Bain, P & Brin, M (1998) Consensus Statement of the Movement Disorder Society on Tremor. *Movement Disorders*, Vol. 13, Supplement 3, (2–23), ISSN 0885-3185

Deuschl, G; Wenzelburger, R & Raethjen, J (2000) Tremor. *Current Opinion in Neurology*, Vol. 13, (437–443), ISSN 13507540

Gonzalez, J C; Heredia, E A; Rahman, T; Barner, K E & Arce, G R (2000) Optimal Digital Filtering for Tremor Suppression. *IEEE Transactions on Biomedical Engineering*, Vol. 47, No. 5, (664–673), ISSN 0018-9294

Goonetilleke, R S (1998). The Comfort "Slip". *Proceedings of the First World Congress on Ergonomics for Global Quality and Productivity*, July 8-11, 1998, R Bishu; W Karkowski y R Goonetilleke (Eds.), Hong Kong University of Science and Technology, Hong Kong, pp. 290–293

Kotovsky, J & Rosen, M (1998) A wearable tremor suppression orthosis. *Journal of Rehabilitation Research and Development*, Vol. 35, No. 4, (373–384), ISSN 0748-7711

Landis, E (1930) Micro-injection studies of capillary blood pressure in human skin. *Heart*, Vol. 15, (209–228).

Loureiro, R C V; Belda-Lois, J M; Rocon, E; Pons, JL; Normie, L & Harwin, WS (2006) Upper Limb Tremor Suppression Through Viscous Loading - Design, Implementation and Clinical Validation. *International Journal of Assistive Robotics and Mechatronics*, Vol. 7 No. 2, (11-19), ISSN 1975-0153

Manto, M; Rocon, E; Pons, J; Davies, A; Williams, J; Belda-Lois, J M & Normie, L (2004). An Active Orthosis To Control Upper Limb Tremor: The Drifts Project (Dynamicly Responsive Intervention For Tremor Suppression). *EURO-ATAXIA Newsletter*, No. 26, (2–6)

Pledgie, S; Barner, K E; Agrawal, S K & Rahman, T (2000) Tremor suppression through impedance control. IEEE Transactions on Rehabilitation Engineering, Vol. 8, No 1, (53–59), ISSN 1063-6528

Riviere, C N & Thakor, N (1996) Modelling and cancelling tremor in human-computer interfaces. *IEEE Engineering in Medicine and Biology Magazine*, Vol. 15, No 3, (29–36), ISSN 0739-5175

Rocon, E; Belda-Lois, J M; Sanchez-Lacuesta, J J & Pons, J L (2004) Pathological tremor management: Modelling, compensatory technology and evaluation. *Technology and Disability*, Vol. 16, No. 1, (3–18), ISSN 1055-4181

Rocon, E; Ruiz, A F; Pons, J L; Belda-Lois, J M & Sanchez-Lacuesta, J J (2005) Rehabilitation Robotics: a Wearable Exo-Skeleton for Tremor Assessment and Suppression. *ICRA 2005. Proceedings of the 2005 IEEE International Conference on Robotics and Automation*, pp. 2271 - 2276, ISBN 0-7803-8915-8, Barcelona (Spain), April 2005.

3

Robotics and Virtual Reality Applications in Mobility Rehabilitation

Rares F. Boian[1], Grigore C. Burdea[2] & Judith E. Deutsch[3]
[1] *Department of Mathematics and Computer Science, Babeş-Bolyai University, Romania*
[2] *CAIP Center, Rutgers University, New Jersey, USA*
[3] *Rivers Lab SHRP, University of Medicine and Dentistry, New Jersey, USA*

1. Introduction

Gait training is a method to reduce mobility dysfunction. Diverse patient populations exhibit mobility impairments that can be ameliorated with gait training. Two such populations are people post-stroke and post-spinal cord injury.
The ability to walk is one of several functions affected by stroke. Immediately after the stroke only 37% of the survivors are able to walk (Jorgensen et al., 1995). Of the patients with initial paralysis only 21% regain walking function (Wandel et al., 2000).
Another patient population that can benefit from gait training (Dietz et al., 1998; Nicol et al., 1995) is the spinal cord injury victims. According to the Travis Roy Foundation there are currently between 250,000 and 400,000 Americans living with spinal cord injury.
Gait training or locomotion therapy uses several devices to assist the patient move and maintain balance. Canes, crutches, walkers, and platforms are simple ambulatory assistive devices that modify a patient's independence and functional mobility. Treadmills often equipped with un-weighing devices are used for training walking at various speeds on a straight flat surface or small incline. These features, along with treadmills' simple design and affordable costs are sufficient reasons for their popularity. Treadmills, however, cannot render more complex walking surfaces which patients encounter daily, such as: stairs, curves, uneven surfaces (e.g. cobblestone paths), or surfaces with various stiffness or friction coefficients.
Training patients to negotiate complex walking surfaces can be done either through in-vivo training assisted by a physical therapist, or through using devices able to simulate such surfaces. The former approach often takes the patient out of the controlled clinic environment, which is not always feasible and may raise safety concerns. The latter approach may offer an alternative to real environment training. It would allow patients to exercise in controlled and safe conditions in the clinic, which could potentially be more time and personnel efficient than real environment training, In this context, numerous research projects have approached gait simulators trying to create robotic devices that could render complex walking surfaces.
The integration of such robotic systems with virtual environments may, in theory, expand the range of applications to entertainment and real-life task training of patients with walking dysfunction. The appealing reasons for using such systems are the flexibility and

transparent data collection offered by virtual environments over real environments (Iwata, 1999; Sveistrup, 2004). In addition, the ability to train for a task in a controlled environment, away from the potential hazards of a real environment makes such simulators viable choices in medical or military applications.

2. Locomotion Simulators

Locomotion simulators, which attempt to simulate the sensations of walking, have been the focus of many researchers due to their applicability in simulating real-life tasks. Beside the medical reasons presented above, gait simulators are an attractive subject due to their applicability for military training or gaming. However, the design of a locomotion simulator for therapeutic purposes must consider and possibly solve several aspects raised by the people using it and by the environment where it will be used.

- *Safety* - The first and most important aspect is safety. Gait simulators are usually complex robotic devices on which the patient stands and moves. To avoid accidents, the simulator must be constrained to move only within the physiological limits of the human body. It also must provide the patient with means to quickly reach safety should anything wrong happen with the simulator.
- *Environment* - A gait simulator must also be suitable for usage in a clinic or home environment. Given the size, these devices are most often used in clinics, but there are research projects (the simulator presented in the last part of this chapter included) that aim to reduce the simulator's size. The environment also imposes restrictions on the actuators. Hydraulic actuators are appropriate for balancing the weight of a person, but they are unsuitable for medical usage, because they are impossible to keep clean, and also pose the risk of dangerous leakages.
- *Interference with patient* - Although not always possible, a simulator should allow the patient to move freely, without constraining him or her. This implies supporting normal step lengths, various locomotion speeds, and changes of direction. Solutions for this requirement usually impose compromises on the size of the simulator.
- *Mechanical bandwidth* - The human haptic sensory capabilities require a force display to rendering bandwidth of about 1 KHz (Burdea, 1996), while the human motor actions require around 10 Hz bandwidth. Thus, a walking simulator needs to render forces at 10 Hz to be able to follow the patient's motion. In order to simulate more complex walking surfaces, forces should ideally be applied at 1 KHz bandwidth. However, these forces are usually felt through shoes, so there is no need of such high fidelity.
- *Surface simulation* - The interaction between a gait simulator and the patient is defined by the surface to be rendered. In order to render complex surfaces realistically, the contact between the simulator and the patient's foot should include multiple active points that define the shape of the surface. Ideally, the simulator should also support changes of walking direction and surface inclination. The solutions to all these issues depend primarily on the design and mechanical limits of the simulator.

- *Assistive mode* - The design of walking simulators for physical therapy also needs to consider assistive mode functioning. As the patients are likely to have difficulty walking, it can be useful to actively guide their feet while walking.
- *Data collection* - One benefit of involving robotics in the rehabilitation procedures is the possibility of collecting data about the patient actions and motions. Data measured during exercises can then be processed and serve as objective base for progress evaluation.

The design of a gait simulator poses numerous issues to be solved, besides those listed above. However, all designs must address one essential requirement: to create the sensation of walking on an infinite surface. The treadmill design solves this problem with a straight forward approach, but is limited to simulating an infinite straight smooth path. To rendered surfaces richer in features, researchers devised several designs, which Hollerbach (Hollerbach, 1999) classifies into three categories: walk-in-place devices, treadmills, and foot platforms.

2.1 Walk-in-Place Devices

These devices require the user to walk in place without advancing while his or her motions are tracked by sensors. The recorded data are then interpreted by a driving workstation that computes the direction and speed of the virtual avatar and changes the view in the virtual environment. These systems do not output any haptic feedback to the user. The only forces the user feels is the contact with the floor.

Templeman et al (Templeman et al, 1999) and Parsons et al. (Parsons et al., 1998) developed such systems using magnetic trackers to measure the user's motion and infer the direction and speed of walking.

Iwata tried the same approach using slippery shoes and asked the user to walk normally (Iwata & Yoshida, 1999). An improved walk-in–place device is presented in Bouguilla et al. (Bouguilla & Sato, 2002). The user walked on a turntable that counteracted the user's change of direction by rotating in the opposed direction.

Compared to a regular treadmill, the walk-in-place systems bring the possibility of changing the walking direction but do not allow the patients to actually walk with normal gait. Iwata's approach with slippery shoes may be risky when dealing with people with disabilities.

2.2 Treadmills

The treadmill category includes devices that allow the user to walk normally on top of a mobile surface that slides in the direction opposed to that of walking.

Such a treadmill is the Sarcos Treadport (Christensen et al., 2000) which can simulate steep up-hill walking and inertial forces.

The Torus treadmill (Iwata, 1999) allowed the user to walk in any direction at a maximum speed of 0.5m/sec.

Another omni-directional treadmill is presented in (Wang et al., 2003). The device developed by Wang et al. used a low friction cloth on top of a rigid board. The cloth was moved in the direction opposite to that of walking by high-friction casters pressed against the board.

The ATR-GSS device presented in (Miyasato, 2000) is a regular treadmill instrumented with mobile plates under the belt. Various walking surface shapes can be simulated by moving the plates up and down.

The advantages brought by these systems when compared with regular treadmills are readily apparent. The change in direction and up-hill walking are frequent daily life scenarios, for which the patients could be trained for. The disadvantage of these devices is that they were not designed for physical rehabilitation, thus their deployment in a clinic is problematic due to size and actuator choices.
The Lokomat System and the Robomedica BWS System are walking simulators developed specifically for clinical usage. Both of them rely on a regular treadmill and provide an actuated systems for dynamically supporting the patient's weight. The Lokomat system, designed for paraplegic rehabilitation, also features an exoskeleton that can guide the patient's legs through the normal gait cycle.

2.3 Foot Platforms

This category includes devices that use one actuated platform for each foot. Depending on the degrees of freedom of the platforms, these systems may be able to simulate complex surfaces, by controlling the position and orientation of the surface at each foot.
Examples of foot platforms are the Sarcos Biport (Hollerbach, 1999) that uses 2DOF platforms and the GaitMaster (Iwata et al., 2001) that uses 3DOF platforms. Just like the treadmills above, the foot platform system presented in this section feature flexibility for rendering more complex surfaces, but their design was not meant for clinical usage.

2.4 Other Walking Simulators

A very realistic simulation of uneven terrain is the Terrain Surface Simulator ALF presented in (Noma et al. 2000). The simulator is a rectangular surface made of small tilt-able plates that can be controlled in real-time. By changing the orientation of the plates, the walking surface can be set in a large variety of shapes. This device is not a treadmill so the user can only walk in any direction within the actuated area.
E-motek Inc. (Amsterdam, Netherlands) has developed the CAREN system, a hydraulically actuated Stewart platform robot supporting a 2-meter diameter board for simulating surfaces with any tilt angle.
VirtuSphere Inc. (Redmond, WA) develops a virtual sphere large enough for a person to fit in. The sphere is made of low-friction material and is supported by a system of casters that allow it to rotate as the user walks.

3. Virtual Environments

The integration of gait simulators with virtual environments makes possible task specific training in the clinic. A patient immersed in a virtual world while exercising may find the therapy less tedious and may also be more motivated (Riva, 2000).
A gait simulator integrated with a VR simulation has to accomplish two main tasks:
map the user's motion into virtual environment navigation and calculate the haptic feedback to be applied to the user's feet or legs as a result of the interactions in the virtual world. The extent to which these tasks are implemented depends mainly on the limitations imposed by the simulator system.
In most situations, the applicability and success of a virtual reality simulation is conditioned by the degree of video and audio feedback. For physical-based simulations, the realism is

also defined by how close the haptic feedback feels compared to the real life experience. In the case of gait simulators, the haptic feedback is calculated from the interaction between a virtual avatar and a virtual surface and applied primarily to the feet.

4. Dual Stewart Platform Mobility Simulator

The main hardware components of the Mobility Simulator are two 6DOF prototype Rutgers Mega-Ankle (RMA) pneumatic robots (see Figure 1). Each robot has a Stewart platform configuration with six dual-acting pneumatic pistons. Each piston is mounted in parallel with a linear potentiometer, which provides information of the smaller mobile platform position vs. the larger fixed one. The mobile platform has a foot attachment plate and a 6DOF force sensor. Force data are used when the Rutgers Mega-Ankle robot is in force control mode. The Mobility Simulator also incorporates an electro-pneumatic control interface, an un-weighting frame (Biodex Co.), a graphical workstation and a large screen custom display. The design of the simulator fits in the "foot platforms" category defined by Hollerbach (Hollerbach, 1999). The user stands with each foot secured with straps to the top of a platform, while the VR simulation (Boian et al., 2004b) is displayed on the large screen facing the user. To improve performance and safety, the user's body is strapped in the un-weighting frame placed above the two platforms. For lightweight users unloading is not necessary, safety being provided by the handlebars mounted on the frame's posts. In this setup, the user can walk on top of the RMA platforms with small steps limited by the platform's workspace (Boian et al., 2003).

During walking, each foot either supports the weight of the body or swings freely while taking a new step. Accordingly, each RMA platform can function in load compensation mode or in free motion mode. In free motion mode the RMA platform follows the swinging foot and compensates for its own mobile platform weight. During this mode, the platform applies very low to zero forces to the foot. In load compensation mode, the platform holds the supporting foot weight and slides backward simulating the behavior of a treadmill. In both modes, the robots can apply additional 6DOF forces or vibrations to the user's foot as commanded by the simulation running on the workstation. The two functioning modes mentioned above are a subset of the actual implementation, sufficient for the purpose of this paper. A more detailed description of the RMA platform's functioning modes can be found in (Boian, 2005).

The simulator software is distributed on two computers: the graphics workstation and the electro-pneumatic control interface (an embedded PC) as illustrated in Figure 2. The graphics workstation handles the graphic and haptic rendering. Based on the information received from the control interface, it calculates the interaction between the virtual feet and the virtual environment and sends back to the control interface commands regarding the forces to be applied or the functioning mode to be used.

The control interface handles the low-level servo control of the two robots, and provides the simulator with the position of each foot calculated through forward kinematics. For performance purposes, the control interface also takes care of switching between certain functioning modes based on the forces applied by the foot as measured by the Rutgers Mega-Ankle 6DOF force sensor. The current functioning mode of each RMA platform is also sent to the graphics workstation. A more detailed presentation of the tasks executed by the control interface can be found in (Boian et al. 2003).

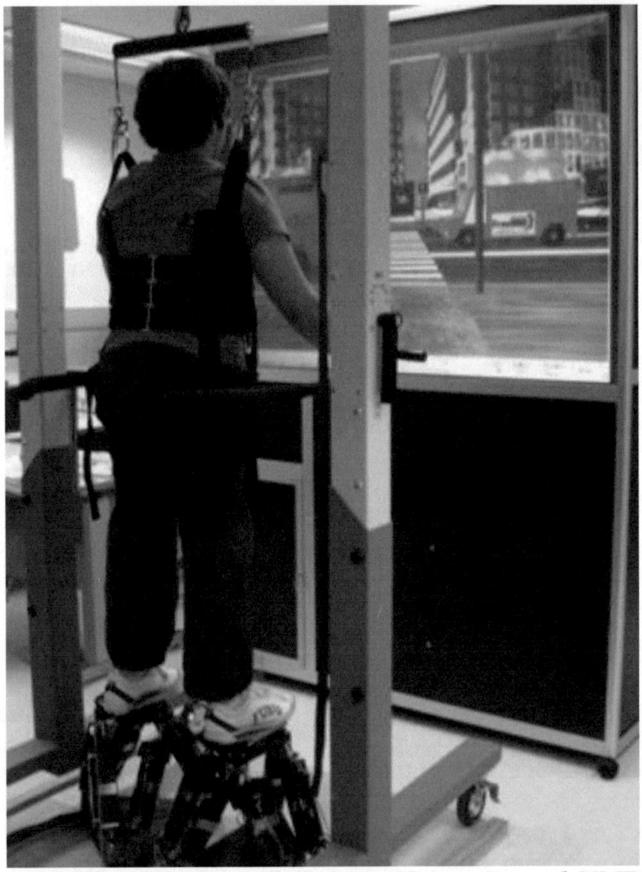

Fig. 1. The Rutgers Mobility Simulator. © Rutgers University and UMDNJ. Reprinted by permission.

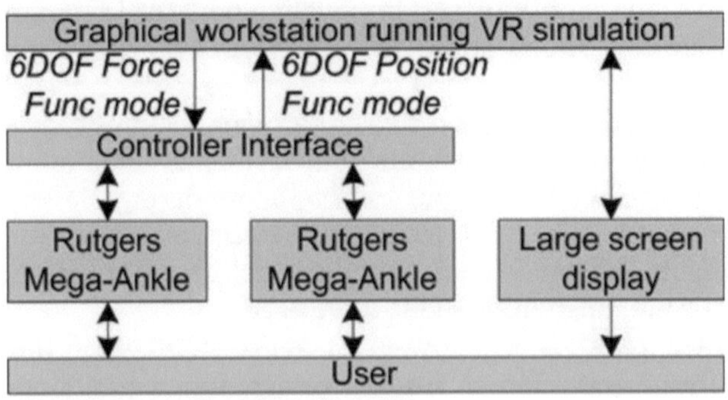

Fig. 2. The Mobility Simulator connection diagram.

4.1 The Rutgers Mega-Ankle servo control

The servo controller design is split over three loops represented as shaded areas in Figure 3. From top to bottom, the loops are: task control loop, dynamics loop, and pressure loop.

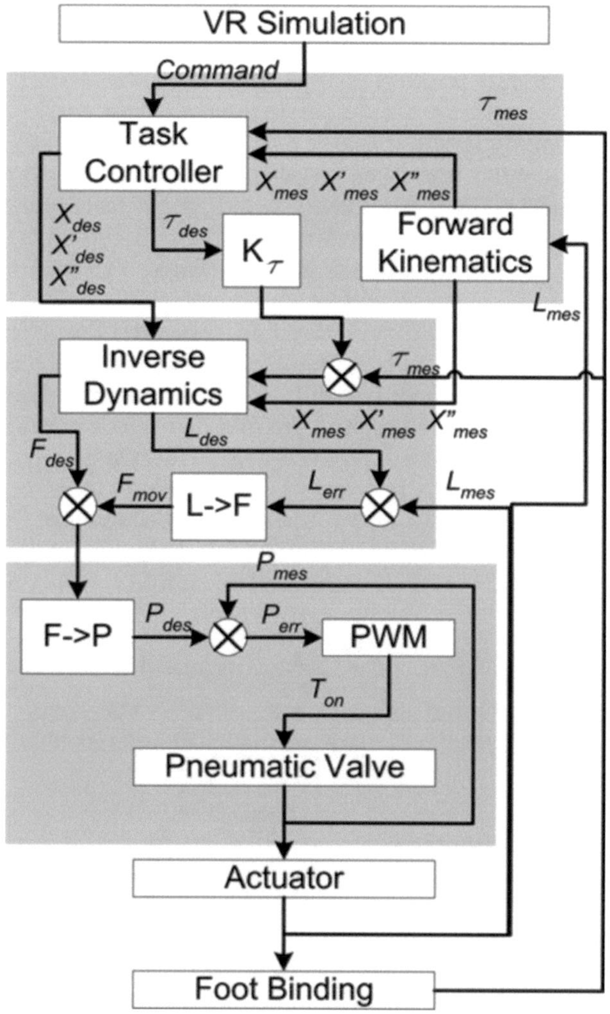

Fig. 3. Controller architecture. © Rutgers University and UMDNJ. Reprinted by permission.

The task control loop is responsible for processing the commands coming from the VR simulation and converting them into Stewart platform desired position, velocity, acceleration and forces. The commands coming from the simulation specify the functioning mode to be used (i.e. weight support mode or free motion mode), and haptic effects and forces to be applied to the users feet. This loop is executed alternatively for each platform. The task controller converts the simulation command using as additional input the measured positions and forces, read by the linear potentiometers and the force sensor of each robot. The dynamics loop transforms the desired Cartesian positions and forces into actuator level forces. The inverse dynamics implementation takes into account the current state of the robot, including position, velocity, acceleration and external forces. The measure external forces T_{mes} are added with the desired forces T_{des} calculated by the task control loop, hence the final force being applied will be the force necessary to counteract the user's action added with the desired force to be applied to the user's foot.

The actuators used by the RMA robots are dual-acting pneumatic pistons, hence the force applied by the cylinder can by controlled by adjusting the air pressure in the upper and lower chambers. The actuator position control transforms the desired change in position into a desired force. The calculated cylinder lengths L_{des} are added with the measured length L_{mes}, and the resulting length difference L_{err} is transformed into a force through the L→F control block. This control uses a proportional derivative (PD) strategy.
Finally, the pressure loop takes the desired actuator force, transforms it into upper and lower chamber pressures. The desired pressures are controlled in Pulse Width Modulation (PWM). The PWM strategy transforms the desired change in pressure P_{err} into the time interval T_{on} during which the valve should be kept open.
F→P is a direct transformation of actuator force into upper and lower pressures designed to minimize the change in pressures in both chambers, hence achieving a better response time. In cases when the desired force cannot be achieved through minimization, the pressures are determined so that they are balanced around the middle of the controllable pressure range.
The PWM is implemented using an adaptive strategy. The change in pressure in a cylinder chamber is not linear in time, and the shape of the curve depends on the volume of the actuated cylinder chamber. Another factor taken into consideration is the intake airflow, which is affected by the number of actuator chambers accepting or exhausting air simultaneously. The PWM duty cycle is calculated taken into consideration all these factors using the equation below.

$$T_{on} = kP_{err}(1 + k_V V_{air})(1 + k_N N_{chamber})(1 + k_F F_{flow})$$

V_{air} is the volume of uncompressed air necessary to achieve the change in pressure. $N_{chamber}$ is the number of chambers accepting or exhausting air simultaneously. F_{flow} is the curve of the airflow over time.

4.1.1 Simulator Mechanical Bandwidth

The mechanical bandwidth of the mobility simulator was measured for translations in the horizontal plane and rotations around the front/back axis. The motions are the most commonly used by our system to render haptic effects as discussed in the last section of the paper. The measurements were done with both RMA robots active simultaneously. While the bandwidth of each individual robot is higher when measured separately, when both robots are active the intake airflow is reduced, thus the bandwidth is lowered. The results are presented in Table 1.

X translation 0.1m amplitude	**Y translation** 0.18m amplitude	**Y rotation** 5 deg amplitude
1.56 Hz	1.79 Hz	1.5 Hz

Table 1. RMA robot mechanical bandwidth.

4.1.2 Robot Stability in Foot Support Mode

One of the first problems encountered during the development of the system was the stability of the RMA platforms under load. The robots were stable when subjected to external forces if there was no load attached to them. However, the working regime for which they were developed, involves resisting forces while supporting the weight of the user. Figure 4 shows the response of the robot to sinusoidal input. Under a 50 lbs load, the motion was distorted and the amplitude of the robot increased slowly eventually becoming unstable.

The cause of this problem was the addition of the desired cylinder force F_{des} with the cylinder motion force F_{mov}. Under load, the resulting forces were too high and caused the robot to become unstable. Increasing the derivative gain slowed down the instability but it didn't solve it. The solution was to reduce the proportional gains by a minimum of 42%. With lower gains, the platform was stable under load, but had very little power to move the user's foot backward during the foot support phase, hence making the system unusable. Also, when the system was unloaded, the steady state error was significantly larger. The use of an integrator term was avoided because the usage of the system caused it to windup consistently.

Two adaptive gains were used to bring the robot to respond properly under load. The gains added a fraction of the measured cylinder load to the proportional and derivative gains respectively. The proportional adaptive component helped increase the moving force of the platform when under load, while the derivative adaptive component was increased to compensate for the high proportional gains and insure the stability of the system.

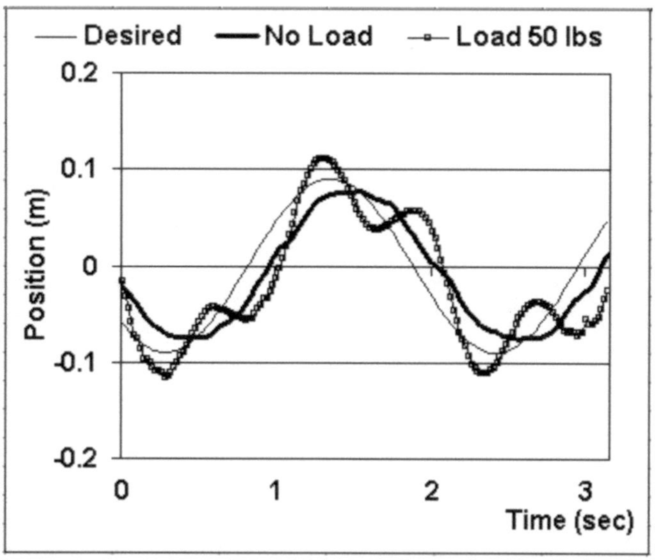

Fig. 4. RMA platform response to a sinusoid input along the Y axis (back-front) with 0.5Hz frequency and 0.18m amplitude. © Rutgers University and UMDNJ. Reprinted by permission.

Figure 5 presents the response of the platform to the same sinusoidal input signal, under a 50 lbs load, with and without the adaptive component added to the lowered proportional and derivative gains. While both the constant and the adaptive response were stable, the adaptive strategy provided the necessary power to move the load closer to the desired position, and reducing the error by approximately half. The adaptive gains did bring a side effect slightly visible in Figure 5; at higher velocity, the adaptive derivative gains increases the damping of the system slowing it down and the releasing it as the load n the robot shifts and the force is reduced. This can be seen as a change in the slope of the adaptive curve in Figure 5.

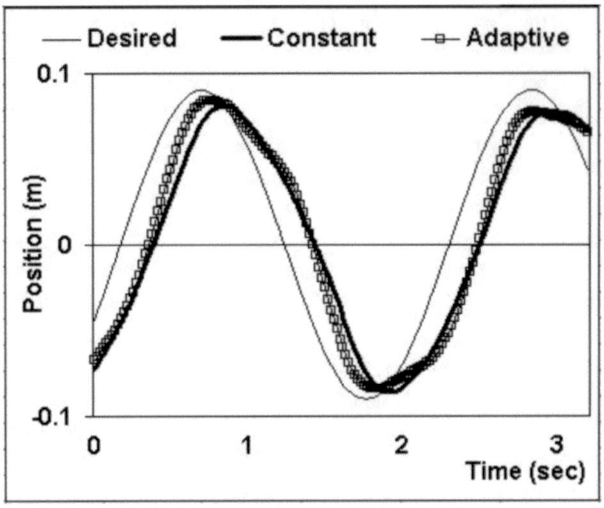

Fig. 5. Response comparison lower constant gains with and without the adaptive component. © Rutgers University and UMDNJ. Reprinted by permission.

4.1.3 Force Minimization in Free Motion Mode.

The second major functioning mode of the RMA robot is following the foot during the swing phase of the gait. In this mode, the platform has to compensate for its own weight and for the forces applied by the user to the end-effector, hence not making itself felt to the foot. To achieve this, the servo controller disables the cylinder position control by canceling out the moving force F_{mov}, and by switching the measured forces signs by changing the value of K_t from 1 to -1. While these changes cause the RMA robot to follow the user's foot, the motion is very slow and large forces are felt at the foot. Figure 6 shows the forces measured at the foot during one swing phase.

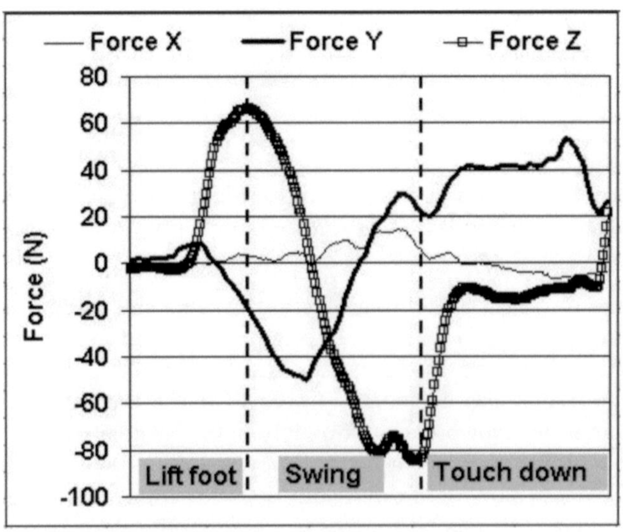

Fig. 6. Free mode forces during swing for K_t = -1.

The source of these large forces has been determined to be the damping created by the pneumatic actuators. While a K_t of 1 is sufficient to resist forces in foot support mode, in free mode, besides responding with a force to the user's force, the robot also has to move, which involves a much large air intake/exhaust activity. The damping is mostly coming from the airflow limitations imposed by the small intake and exhaust sections of the cylinder chambers. To overcome this problem, K_t was increased in absolute value. The increase was done for each of the robot's 6 DOF. The Z-axis (up-down) translation gain was approximately four times larger than the rest of the gains, because the motion on that direction required all the cylinders to either intake or exhaust, hence putting more airflow in a single direction. The measured forces for the increased K_t gains are shown in Figure 7. The forces are now reduced approximately 8 times to a maximum of 11N, which is comparable to the weight of a snow boot.

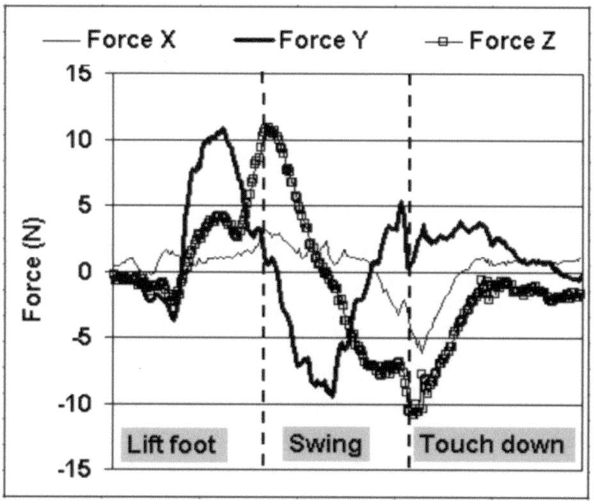

Fig. 7. Free mode forces during swing for larger K_t. © Rutgers University and UMDNJ. Reprinted by permission.

4.2 Haptic rendering for walking over virtual terrain

The Mobility Simulator transforms the input position, force and functioning mode of each RMA platform into haptic feedback to the feet and visual update of the virtual scene using the virtual surface specifications. The virtual ground model is stored on the graphics workstation, as a polygonal mesh with areas characterized by a haptic material. The haptic output data consists of two sets of values specifying the functioning mode to be used by each platform, the 6DOF forces and the vibrations to be applied to the user's foot.

4.2.1 Haptic Material

The ground surface is specified as a polygonal mesh that matches the shape of the visual 3D geometries in the virtual environment. The physical properties of the surface are specified using haptic materials, which are applied in layers that can be either distinct or mixed. The polygonal surface is unbreakable and the haptic materials can be placed on top of it in layers. This approach insures that the foot stepping down will always be supported if it penetrates through all the materials stacked on the surface.

A haptic material is defined as a collection of numerical parameters describing the physical properties of the surface. Given the requirements of an interactive virtual reality simulation, the haptic modeling computations need to be efficient. Thus, the model is not intended to be physically accurate but rather a good approximation of reality. Hence, the set of variables used is limited to stiffness, damping, friction, haptic texture, and breaking coefficient.

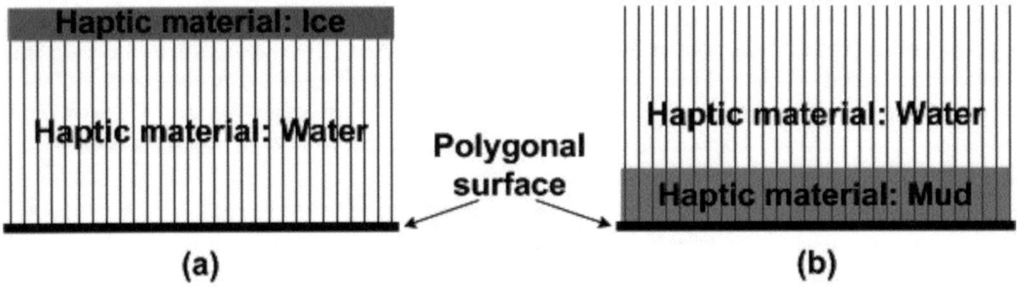

Fig. 8. Layered haptic materials: (a) distinct layers; (b) mixed layers.

The stiffness and damping coefficients are used for defining the material based on Hooke's law. Stepping on elastic materials is very common in every day life, however, the stiffness coefficient can be used to simulate Archimedes's law if considering the foot section constant when stepping into a liquid. The damping coefficient can be used to simulate the slow sinking sensation of walking on a thick carpet. A low friction coefficient can be used for simulating ice. If the foot applies horizontal forces to the material larger than the friction coefficient, the contact will break.

The haptic texture is defined as a vibration with a given amplitude and frequency. The breaking coefficient multiplied with the thickness of the material specifies the maximum force that the material can support. A haptic material is not rendered if the applied force is larger than its breaking force. The breaking coefficient makes it easy to simulate stepping on a thin layer of ice on top of a puddle of water.

4.2.2 Motion Rendering Stages

The processing necessary to calculate the graphics and haptic feedback can be divided into several stages that are executed at every simulation cycle (Figure 9). Only the swinging foot (free motion) is considered for the entire rendering process. The fixed foot (load compensation mode) is addressed only in the last stage of the process.

The process starts by reading the feet positions and functioning modes from the control interface. The functioning mode value is used to decide whether a foot should be moved or not. A foot in load compensation mode is kept fixed although the platform slides it backward.

The next stage requires the calculation of the change in real foot position to be added to the virtual feet. Because the simulator's workspace cannot cover the entire range of motion of the legs, it was necessary to scale the change in each foot's position to increase the virtual walking velocity so that the simulation felt real. The scale is also applied to the vertical displacement making it possible to negotiate realistic virtual obstacles that are visually larger than the platform work envelope.

The next phase updates the positions of the virtual feet with the calculated change. The changes are applied in a frame of reference aligned with the virtual avatar's walking direction calculated in the previous cycle.

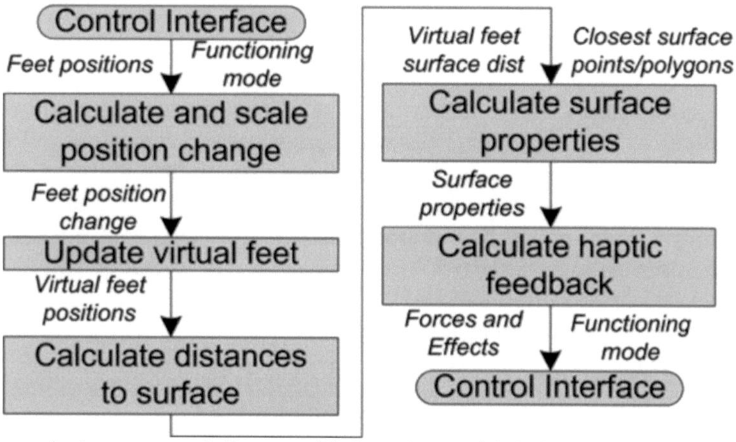

Fig. 8. Haptic rendering stages © Rutgers University and UMDNJ. Reprinted by permission.

After the feet have been mapped into the virtual world, the viewpoint has to be moved accordingly. Positioning the virtual camera above the center of the segment defined by the two feet yields good results although it is not what really happens with the center of gravity of a walking person.

The next stage is calculating the distance between the foot and the surface. This stage will also find the closest surface points to the foot and their corresponding polygons. Similar to the real case, certain surface properties are manifested above the surface (e.g. mud or snow) hence the distance to the surface is relevant to the haptic feedback even if there is no collision with the underlying ground. Based on the results of the previous stage the simulator can find the surface properties around the closest points on the surface.

The last stage of the process is the calculation of forces and haptic effects to be applied to the user's foot, based on the surface properties and the depth of the collision.

4.2.3 Virtual Foot Modeling

The interaction between the virtual foot and the virtual ground surface is based on the haptic mesh concept developed by Popescu (Popescu et al., 1999) as an extension to Ho's simpler haptic point concept (Ho et al., 1997). The virtual foot implemented for the Mobility Simulator is modeled as a mesh of points positioned on the shoe sole. From a haptic point of view, the RMA platforms can only render forces in one point. The use of a mesh of points to calculate the interaction of the foot with the surface is necessary for realistic surface contact calculation.

The number of points in the mesh should be minimized because it is directly proportional to the amount of collision detection calculations, and it increases factorially the number of contact stability calculations. The minimum number of mesh points has been determined to be five. One point is positioned in the center of the mesh, while the rest are positioned on a rectangle around it. The dimensions of the rectangle match the shape of the end-effector foot attachment plate to which the user's foot is secured.

4.2.4 Ground Contact Evaluation

When a foot touches the haptic surface the swinging phase of the foot is over and the support phase is about to begin. The switch between these two phases is tightly connected

to the functioning of the servo-controller, which has to be notified to start sliding the support foot backward.
The foot/surface interaction is evaluated by calculating the forces applied by the surface (through the layers of haptic materials) to each of the points in the virtual foot mesh. The vertical components of these forces are then compared with the vertical components of the forces applied by the user's foot to the simulator. The latter forces are calculated by transforming the output of the force sensor mounted on top of the RMA platforms to each point in the mesh. A point of the foot haptic mesh is "supported" if the resultant of these vertical components is pointing upward.
The three contact possibilities that can be differentiated based on the "supported" status of the haptic mesh points are presented in Table 2 and Figure 10.

Contact Status	Description
No contact	None of the mesh points are supported
Stable	Minimum three non-collinear points are supported
Unstable	Remaining cases

Table 2. Contact status based on the haptic mesh point support.

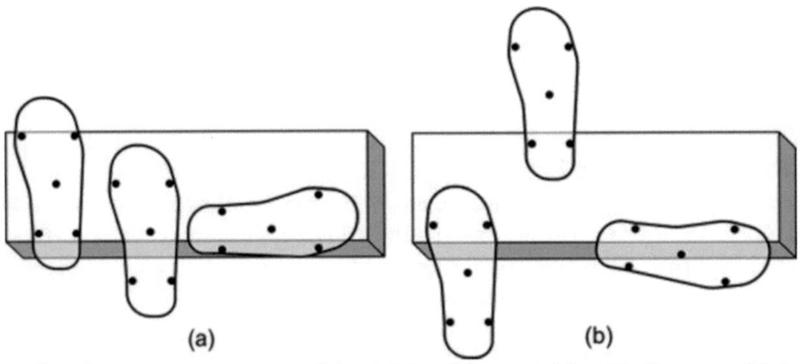

Fig. 10. Foot/surface contact types: (a) stable, (b) unstable. © Rutgers University and UMDNJ. Reprinted by permission.

The resultant of the haptic point forces is transmitted to the control interface to be applied to the swinging foot. If the swinging foot made a stable contact with the surface, the controller is notified to switch the functioning mode. The friction and surface textures are sent to the controller for both feet, regardless of their state.

4.2.5 Low-level Haptic Effects

The mobility simulator system is designed to execute most of the haptic calculations on the workstation, and render the results on the Stewart platforms using a reduced set of basic level effects:

- Apply a 6DOF force
- Change in position (positional jolt)
- Vibrations

These low level haptic effects are extensions of the haptic effects developed for a similar system using smaller Stewart platform robots, and designed for stroke rehabilitation in sitting (Boian et al., 2004a).

The simulation can request the controller to apply a certain force during both free or foot support functioning modes. If the request is made while in free motion mode, the given forces are scaled using positive values of the free mode gains and then applied. The scaling is necessary to counteract the same damping behavior mentioned above. If a force request is made during the foot support mode, the given forces become essentially τ_{des} in Figure 3.
The changes in position are used as an alternative force requests during foot support mode. For instance, to simulate slipping on the ice, a lateral displacement is used instead of applying a lateral force. This is preferred because a known displacement is more controllable and can be adjusted to a comfortable level easier than applying a force which will have a different effect from a user to another, mainly due to differences in weight.
The vibrations are used to simulate surface textures. The frequency and amplitude of the vibrations are calculated on the graphical workstation and sent to the controller. The vibrations are rendered only as changes in orientation around the Y-axis (back-front direction) because it interferes the least with the rest of the foot measurements necessary to calculate the direction of motion, or intersection with the virtual surface.

5. Acknowledgment

The research reported here was supported by grants from the National Science Foundation (BES 0201687 and BES 9708020) and from the New Jersey Commission for Science and Technology.

6. References

Boian, R.F.; Deutsch, J.E.; Lee, C.S.; G.C., Burdea & Lewis J.A. (2003). Haptic Effects for Virtual Reality-based Post-Stroke Rehabilitation. *Proceedings of the Eleventh Symposium on Haptic Interfaces For Virtual Environment And Teleoperator Systems*, pp. 247-253, Los Angeles, CA, March 2003.

Boian, R.F.; Bouzit, M.; Burdea, G.C. & Deutsch, J.E. (2004a). Dual Stewart Platform Mobility Simulator. *Proceedings of IEEE EMBS 2004*, September 2004.

Boian, R.F.; Burdea, G.C.; Deutsch, J.E. & Winter, S. H. (2004b). Street Crossing Using a Virtual Environment Mobility Simulator. *Proceedings of IWVR 2004*, pp. 27-33, Lausanne, Switzerland, 2004.

Boian, R.F. (2005). *Robotic Mobility Rehabilitation System Using Virtual Reality*. Electrical and Computer Engineering, Rutgers University, January 2005.

Bouguilla, L. & Sato, M. (2002). Virtual locomotion system for large-scale virtual environment. *Proceedings of the IEEE Virtual Reality Conference*, pp. 291–292, March 2002.

Burdea, G. (1996). Force and Touch Feedback for Virtual Reality. John Wiley & Sons, New York, NY, USA, 1996.

Christensen, R.R. ; Hollerbach, J.M.; Xu, Y. & Meek, S.G. (2000). Inertial-force feedback for the treadport locomotion interface. *Presence*, vol. 9, no. 1, pp.1–14, February 2000.

Dietz, V.; Wirz, M.; Curt, A. & Colombo, G. (1998). Locomotor pattern in paraplegic patients: training effects and recovery of spinal cord function. *Spinal Cord* 1998; 36: pp. 380-390.

Ho, C.; Basdogan, C. & Srinivasan, M. (1997). Haptic Rendering: Point- and Ray-Based Interactions. *Proceedings of the Second PHANToM Users Group Workshop*, October 2007, Dedham, MA.

Hollerbach, J.M. (1999). Locomotion interfaces. In: *Handbook of Virtual Environments Technology*, Stanney, K.M., (Ed.), pp. 239-254, Lawrence Erlbaum Associates, Inc., 2002.

Iwata, H. (1999). Walking about virtual environments on infinite floor. *Proceedings of IEEE Virtual Reality'99*, pp. 286-293, 1999, Houston, TX.

Iwata, H. & Yoshida, Y. (1999). Path reproduction tests using a torus treadmill. *Presence: Teleoperators and Virtual Environments*, vol. 8, pp. 587–597, 1999.

Iwata, H.; Yano, H. & Nakaizumi F. (2001). Gaitmaster: A versatile locomotion interface for uneven virtual terrain. *Proceedings of the IEEE VR2001 Conference*, pp. 131-137, 2001.

Jorgensen, H.S. ; Nakayama, H.; Raaschou, & Olsen, T.S. (1995). Recovery in walkingcfunction in stroke patients: The copenhagen stroke study. *Archives of Physical Medicine and rehabilitation*, vol. 76, no. 1, pp. 27–32, 1995.

Miyasato T. (2000). Tele-nursing system with realistic sensations using virtual locomotion interface. *Proceedings of the 6th ERCIM Workshop User Interfaces for All*, October 2000, Florence, Italy.

Nicol, D.J.; Granat, M.H.; Baxendale, R.H. & Tuson, S.J. (1995). Evidence for a human spinal stepping generator. *Brain Res* 1995; 684: pp. 230-232.

Noma, H.; Sugihara, T. & Miyasato T. (2000). Development of Ground Surface Simulator for Trl-E-Merge System. Proceedings of IEEE Virtual Reality 2000, pp. 217-224, March 2000.

Parsons, J.; Lampton, D.R.; Parsons, K.A.; Knerr, B.W.; Russell, D.; Martin, G.; Daly, J.; Kline, B. & Weaver. M. (1998) Fully immersive team training: A networked testbed for ground based training missions. *Proceedings of Interservice/Industry Training, Simulation and Education Conference*, Orlando, FL, 1998.

Popescu, V.; Burdea, G. & Bouzit, M. (1999). Virtual Reality Simulation Modeling for a Haptic Glove. *Computer Animation'99*, pp. 195-200, May 1999, Geneva, Switzerland.

Riva, G. (2000). Virtual Reality In Rehabilitation Of Spinal Cord Injuries: A Case Report. *Rehabilitation Psychology*, 45 (1), pp. 1-8, 2000

Sveistrup, H. (2004). Motor rehabilitation using virtual reality, *Journal of NeuroEngineering and Rehabilitation 2004.*

Templeman, J.N.; Denbrook, P.S. & Sibert. L.E. (1999). Maintaining spatial orientation during travel in an immersive virtual environment. *Presence: Teleoperators and Virtual Environments*, Vol 8, pp. 598–617, 1999.

Wandel, A.; Jorgensen, H.S.; Nakayama, H.; Raaschou, H.o. & Olsen, T.S. (2000). Prediction of walking function in stroke patients with initial lower extremity paralysis: the copenhagen stroke. Archives of Physical Medicine and rehabilitation, Vol. 81, No. 6, pp. 736–738, 2000.

Wang, Z.; Bauernfeind, K. & Sugar. T. (2003). Omni-direactional treadmill system. *Proceedings of the Symposium on Haptic Interfaces for Virtual Environment and Teleoperator Systems*, pp. 367–373, Los Angeles, CA, March 2003.

4

Designing Safety-Critical Rehabilitation Robots

Stephen Roderick[1] & Craig Carignan[2,1]
[1]*University of Maryland* & [2]*Georgetown University*
U.S.A.

1. Introduction

In recent years, robots have made substantial in-roads in the medical field and are gradually finding their way into clinical practice. Intuitive Surgical's *da Vinci® surgical robot* broke ground in 1998 by performing the first tele-robotic surgery to repair a heart valve (Salisbury, 1998; Guthart & Salisbury, 2000). Accuray's *CyberKnife* radiotherapy robot began treating head, neck and upper spine tumors in 1999 by combining image guidance with a robotically-directed radiation beam (Adler et al., 1997). In 2002, Interactive Motion Technology began therapy of stroke patients with the *InMotion*[2] robot, also known as the MIT-Manus (Krebs et al., 2002). These devices and many others under development have provided researchers and doctors alike with capabilities not previously available.

These additional capabilities, however, have also brought with them the issue of safety – these are *safety critical systems* in which a single malfunction can endanger the life of the patient. In contrast with traditional robotic systems, medical robots must enforce the safety of the patient as an object within its workspace, while also being able to treat the patient. This dichotomy creates the need for a *safety system* that can allow the robot to interact with the patient, while also enforcing all necessary safety precautions.

Human fatalities resulting from medical treatment with machines is unfortunately all-to-real. The *Therac 25,* a radiation therapy machine developed by the Atomic Energy Commission of Canada, was involved in six known accidents between 1984 and 1987. Five patients died as a result of massive overdoses of radiation when a high power electron beam was activated without the target tumor having been rotated into place (Leveson & Turner, 1993). Had the machine's software detected the fault, the accident would have been averted. Radiation therapy machines are now required to have hardware interlocks to prevent activation of the high-energy electron-beam unless the target is in place.

A similar tragedy occurred at the National Oncology Institute in Panama during 2000 and 2001. Twenty-eight patients were overexposed during radiation therapy for cancer treatment, after use of a computerized treatment planning system. Dosage calculations from the planning system had errors of up to 105%. By August 2005, 23 out of 28 overposed patients had died, of which at least 18 were attributed to radiation effects (Borras, 2006).

Dangers in medical robotics are not confined to surgical systems. In powered orthoses or "exoskeletons" being developed for rehabilitation, humans are basically encapsulated in the device creating a potentially hazardous situation. Powered leg exoskeletons such as the the *Lokomat™ Gait Orthosis* are being used to train stroke and spinal cord injury patients how to walk again (Bernhardt et al., 2005). Arm exoskeletons such as *ARMOR* (Mayr et al., 2006), ARMin (Nef et al., 2006), RUPERT (He et al., 2005), and *UW Prototype III* (Rosen, 2005) are being developed for therapy of hemiparetic stroke patients. The MGA Exoskeleton is being used for shoulder rehabilitation and is comparable in strength to the average adult male (Carignan et al., 2005). While all of these systems have adequate sensors to control the robot, they are insufficient to enforce patient safety.

It is important to realize that safety is not an absolute concept – a system can only be built to reduce the risk of an accident to an acceptable level (Shaw, 1995; Dunn, 2003). Safety is also an attribute of the entire system and is not driven by only certain components of the system. This requires that safety analyses include all system components: software, hardware, and the operators (Anderson, 1993; Leveson, 1995; Sommerville, 1995).

This chapter will detail a system safety design process that can systematically evaluate the design of a rehabilitation robot against its project safety and failure rate criteria. When these criteria are not satisified, the process can identify system components or failure combinations that require additional design consideration, so that the project criteria might be satisfied. Modifications directed by this process can result in a sufficiently safe system design for safety-critical rehabilitation robot applications. The application of this process to two case studies will be presented. The first case study is the MGA Exoskeleton introduced above, which will be used as an illustrative example. The second case study is a multi-arm space robot experiment, to which this process was originally applied. This robot has several years of operational history against which this process can be evaluated.

Definitions

There are many different definitions of safety-related terms. For consistency, the definitions used in this chapter are taken from Vesely (1981) and Leveson (1995):

- A *failure* is an abnormal occurrence
- A *fault* is a higher-order event caused by one or more failures.
- A *hazard* is a system state and other environmental conditions that inevitably leads to an accident.
- An *accident* is an undesired and unplanned event that results in a level of loss, in this case, injury to the patient.
- *Safety* is freedom from accidents.

Fig. 1 depicts symbols used in this work to represent fault events and gates.

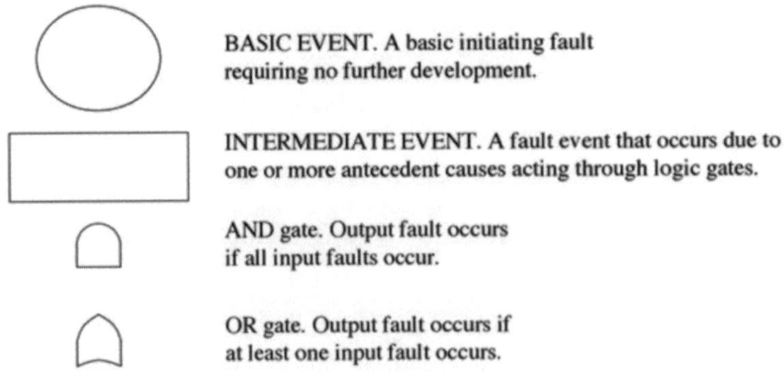

Fig. 1. Symbols used in fault trees.

2. Safety analysis techniques

Previous medical robotics have had to address the issue of patient safety (Varley, 1999; Taylor et al., 1991, Duchemin et al., 2004). One of the unique aspects of rehabilitation robots is that the human in-the-loop is the patient. With surgical or radiological systems such as *Da Vinci* and *Cyberknife*, a patient is being "operated" on by the robot; however, a clinician is directing the robot. With a rehabilitation robot, the subject may fill the role of both patient and operator. This introduces additional safety criteria over and above that used in more traditional medical robots.

Unfortunately, there is no industry-standard approach to designing these safety-critical robot systems. Despite this, numerous other fields have standard and accepted analytical methods used to design safety-critical systems (Weber et al., 2003). These methods come under the banner of "system safety engineering" (Stephenson, 1991; Blanchard, 1991), and have been used to develop safety-critical systems in domains ranging from aircraft flight management systems (Parnas et al., 1991) to nuclear power plants (Potocki de Montalk, 1991).

2.1 Current approaches

Some of the more common design techniques are described in the following sections and can be loosely categorized as either "top-down" or "bottom-up" techniques. Top-down techniques typically work from a high-level description, and attempt to identify combinations or sequences of components that contribute to system level events. Bottom-up techniques typically work from the component level outward and upward. Hybrid techniques combine both top-down and bottom-up approaches. A brief description is now given of the more standard techniques.

2.1.1 Top-down approaches

Preliminary hazard analysis (PHA) is an early phase of lifecycle-based hazard analysis, which also involves system and subsystem hazard analysis (Leveson, 1995). Its objective is to assess potential hazards caused by the system, to identify inherent hazards, and to assess the criticality of arising accidents (Vesely, 1981). The resultant hazards can be used as inputs to fault tree analysis or similar techniques.

Hazard operability is a qualitative, creative thinking technique developed by, and primarily used by, the chemical industry. It is simple, but very labor intensive, and is designed to identify and analyze hazards systematically (Stephenson 1991; Leveson, 1995). As with PHA, the results of a hazard operability study can be used as inputs to fault tree analysis or similar techniques.

Fault tree analysis (FTA) is a deductive technique to determine the sequence of faults that could cause a given top-level hazard (or *top event*). The resulting fault trees can be represented as boolean expressions and reduced to the minimum combination of failures that could cause the top-level hazard. The trees can also be quantitatively evaluated to provide estimates of the probability of the top event occurring, given the probabilities of the constituent failures. Fault trees can have trouble dealing with timing (Gorski et al., 1995), redundancy, and differing mission phases (Leveson, 1995). It is also a time-consuming, qualitative technique, although its absolute accuracy is usually secondary to identifying failure sequences (Ozog & Bendixen, 1987). The determination of the top-level event is critical; failure to determine a top-level event by a PHA, for example, results in the hazard not being examined and, consequently, the system may not cope with that hazard (Leveson, 1995; Vesely, 1981).

While typically applied to a system design, FTA has recently been applied to software to determine how failures in its implementation could cause a hazard (Leveson 1984; Knight & Nakano, 1997). It can be used to determine cases where the implemented design could cause a hazard, or show which modules are most critical to the safe operation of the system. Methods exist to potentially build the trees from a logical system model (Bruns & Anderson, 1993), or from a completed code base (Voas, 1995), though this may occur too late in the design cycle to be cost-efficient. It also difficult to evaluate such fault trees quantitatively, as there exist few methods to assign probabilities to failure of software logic.

2.1.2 Bottom-up approaches

Failure mode effects analysis (FMEA) is traditionally used to predict equipment reliability and emphasizes successful functioning of a component as opposed to the failure of the component. It is a systematic technique that is system-oriented, not hazard-oriented (Hope et al., 1983). It is more time-consuming than fault tree analysis and does not cope with multiple failures, timing, or redundancy (Ozog & Bendixen, 1987; Leveson, 1995).

Failure modes, effects, and criticality analysis (FMECA) is a very similar technique, that adds extra steps and data to an FMEA related to controls and control procedures.

Event tree analysis is an inductive method to identify outcomes of a given initiating event and can identify the components that most contribute to a failure. It is practical for independent events and a stable event chronology, and may provide top events for subsequent fault tree analysis. Event trees can become very large and suffer difficulties with timing data and more than two states. They may also require fault tree analysis to develop failure probabilities for branches, and analysts have to be able to define all initiating events (Ozog and Bendixen, 1987; Leveson, 1995).

2.1.3 Hybrid approaches

Cause-consequence techniques combine fault-trees and event-trees. They work by selecting a critical event and determining the contributing factors using fault tree analysis and the resulting consequences using event tree analysis. They can represent delays and event combinations, but they can become large and unwieldy. In addition, their outcome is only related to the cause being analyzed (Hope et al., 1983; Leveson, 1995).

2.1.4 Synthesized techniques

Applied in isolation, none of the above techniques can produce a system design that is sufficiently safe. Synthesizing combinations of these techniques can produce a system safety design process that utilizes the strengths of each technique, thereby providing a design methodology that not only identifies hazards and their contributing fault scenarios, but can also potentially evaluate the design qualititively and quantitatively. This synthesized technique may be used to determine the specific need of additional system components, required to enforce the project's safety critiera.

2.2 Previous synthesized safety analyses

Lankenau et al. (1998) combined FTA along with formal methods, to develop a safety layer for an autonomous wheelchair. They also applied a model checker over the fault trees, to attempt to verify that the system could never fail.

Combining FTA with an unspecified failure mode analysis technique, Cavallaro & Walker (1997) evaluated the safety and reliability of a manipulator system for hazardous material retrieval. They show results for only one hazard, and noted that some failure modes were not considered due to lack of details on software configuration and the operator interfaces.
Guiochet & Vilchis (2002) combined FMEA and FTA in a safety analysis of the design of an ultrasound robot for tele-echography. The two analyses were used in conjunction due to the complementary forward/backward approaches. While a hazard analysis is mentioned as part of their process, it is unclear where it fits into their process. They use FMEA to identify the failure leading to an accident, and use that failure as a top event for subsequent FTA. As some accidents require multiple failures either combinatorially or sequentially, these hazards will not be identified by the FMEA. However, results of the FMEA could be used to identify corrective measures for the system.

2.3 Chosen synthesized technique

For this work, a synthesized approach was chosen that combines PHA and FTA. This provides the means to enumerate the hazards a system presents, a method to determine the fault sequence and/or combinations that can cause the hazards, and both qualitative and quantitative metrics against which project safety and failure rate criteria can be compared. FTA was chosen over such techniques as FMEA, event trees or cause consequence trees since, in our experience, there are far fewer hazards than there are failure combinations leading to such hazards. Construction of fault trees requires less work than the other techniques in this scenario – however, the issues of timing and redundancy in a robot system must be explicitly addressed within the FTA.
For the two case studies presented here, the distributed, hard real-time nature of the robot is leveraged alongside safety checks to specifically target components that do not make their deadlines. It is considered a failure if a computing component does not make an internal processing deadline, or an external communication deadline. This is an FTA primitive event, allowing timing-related failures to be explicitly modelled in the fault trees.
Redundant components may be explicitly modelled within the fault trees. This leads to more work in the fault tree construction but ensures that the redundancy is dealt with directly. It is also possible to ignore redundancy under certain circumstances, where the modelling of additional components would only lead to decreased hazard probabilities. In this case, the resultant hazard probabilities will err on the conservative side.
The approach described here was initially developed for a dexterous robot designed to fly on NASA's space shuttle (Roderick et al., 2004). This system was the first (and to our knowledge, the only) American robotic system to be certified through three of the four phases of the NASA Space Shuttle Safety Review process. This pioneered a solely computer-based hazard control system for payloads operating on the shuttle, and demonstrated successful application of this technique to a safety-critical robot system.

3. System safety design process

The overall goal of this process is to evaluate a system design to determine whether it is "sufficiently safe". The concept of sufficiently safe is one that the specific project must establish, which forms the basis for the *project's safety criteria*. This will include factors such as regulatory standards as well as the potential consequences to the patient of an accident occurring. It is not possible to make a system absolutely safe; however, if the likelihood of an accident is small enough – or the consequences of an accident are negligible enough – the system may be considered sufficiently safe (Anderson, 1993; Shaw, 1995). At some point, continuing to modify a system design to cope with ever more incredible failures simply results in an excessively complex design, and a subsequent reduction in overall system reliability and/or safety (Duchemin et al., 2004). Notably, this concept of accepting some degree of risk is enshrined in UK law under the *principle of reducing risks as low as reasonably practicable* (McDermid, 2001).

3.1 Process description

A flow diagram illustrating the system safety design process is shown in Fig. 2. The basic inputs to this process are an initial system design description, the project safety criteria, and the project failure rate criteria. During a given iteration of the system design, the specific deliverables or outputs from this process are a list of hazards from the PHA, the fault trees from the FTA, and any qualitative and/or quantitative results from the FTA. These outputs also form the overall outputs of the process.

The initial system design is evaluated through a PHA, and the hazards identified by the PHA each constitute top events from which FTA can begin. Each top event is considered individually, and the immediate, necessary, and sufficient causes by which this event could occur are identified. These immediate events are summarily examined for their causal events, and this step-by-step analysis continues until individual component failures are reached. These component failures are the basic causes that, when combined in the manner indicated by the fault tree, guarantee that the top level hazard will occur. (See Leveson (1995) for further details of PHA, and Vesely (1981) for fault trees and their construction.)

The resulting fault trees can be qualitatively examined to determine if the project's safety criteria are being met, i.e., whether the system is sufficiently safe. If not, additional components may be added in an effort to deal with the specific safety issues raised by the FTA. The system design is then modified accordingly, and the process begins again. Once the FTA results show that the project's safety criteria are met, the system design can be considered sufficiently safe.

The qualitative analysis entails forming and evaluating the minimal cut sets for each fault tree. A minimal cut set is defined as *a smallest combination of component failures which, if they all occur, will cause the top level hazard to occur* (Vesely, 1981). The minimal cut sets can be ranked by size, providing a qualitative indication of failure importance and the ability to determine if the system meets its design criteria. If failure events are assumed to be independent, then the failure probabilities associated with minimal cut sets can decrease by several orders of magnitude as the size of the cut set increases. Hence ranking cut sets gives a gross indication of the importance of the cut set (Vesely, 1981).

Once the system design has satisfied the project's safety criteria, the fault trees can be quantitatively analyzed to determine an indicative system failure rate. An overall probability for each cut set is evaluated based upon the failure probabilities of its constituent events. The top-level hazard is then a function of the probabilities of each of its constituent cut sets. If the computed system failure rate is higher than desired, then sensitivity analysis of the input fault probabilities can indicate which components signficantly contribute to the overall rate. These specific components can be flagged for additional inspection or higher-tolerance part replacement, in an effort to reduce their failure probability. In addition, further iterations of the safety design process may occur with the aim of modifying the system design to reduce the system failure rate, while still satisfying the project's safety criteria. A more detailed description of the quantitative analysis is outlined in the next section.

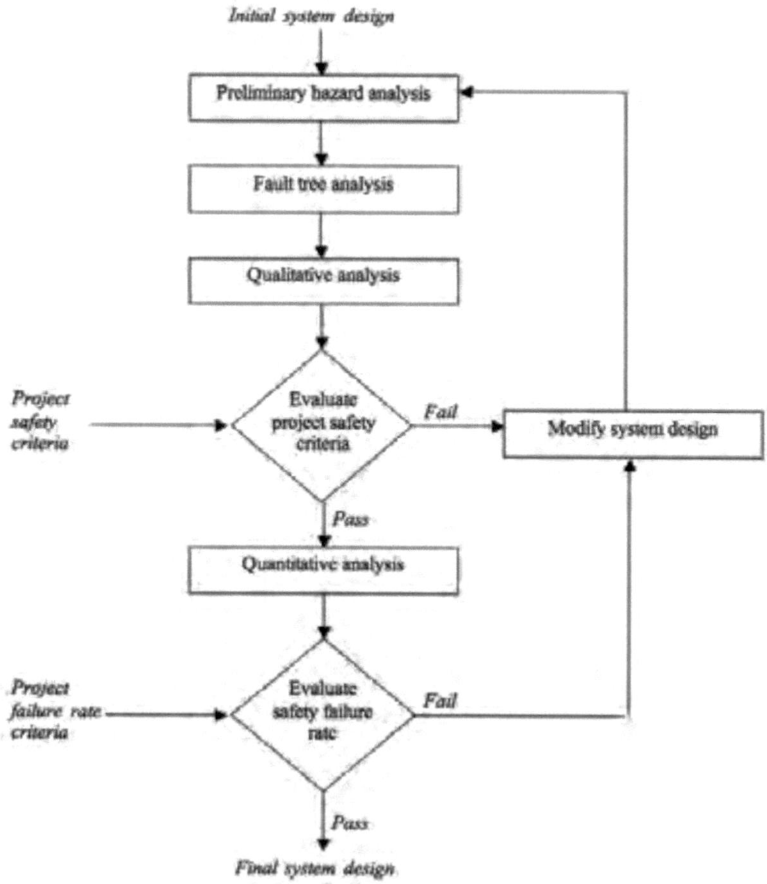

Fig. 2. Approach to system design for safety.

3.2 Quantitative Analysis

The *lambda-model* adopted for this analysis assumes that events are mutually independent and mutually exclusive, and requires knowledge of whether a failure is repairable or non-repairable (Vesely, 1981). The linear assumptions of this model will result in a conservative estimate of hazard probability, thus allowing only an order of magnitude accuracy. Given the additional imprecision in the input failure probability data, this allows only indicative quantitative evaluation. The following development is summarized from (Vesely, 1981).

The failure probability distributions are exponential as the model assumes that the failure probabilities are directly related to component operating times. Hence, the probability $F(t)$ that the component suffers its first failure within time period t, given it is initially working, is

$$F(t) = 1 - e^{-\lambda t} \tag{1}$$

which is accurate to within 5% for $F(t) < 0.1$ and can be approximated to first order by

$$F(t) \cong \lambda t \tag{2}$$

The derivative of $F(t)$, the probability density function $f(t)$, is

$$f(t) = \lambda e^{-\lambda t} \tag{3}$$

Let $q(t)$ be the component unavailability,

$$q(t) = F(t) \cong \lambda t \tag{4}$$

the probability that the component is down at time t and unable to operate if called upon.
Let $w(t)$ be the component failure occurrence rate

$$w(t) = f(t) = \lambda e^{-\lambda t} \tag{5}$$

where $w(t)\cdot\Delta t$ is the approximate probability that the component fails between time t and $t+\Delta t$. For time t small compared to $1/\lambda$, such that $\lambda t < 0.1$, $e^{-\lambda t} \cong 1$,

$$w(t) = f(t) \cong \lambda \tag{6}$$

Let $W_i(t)$, the minimal cut set occurrence rate for cut set i, be the probability per unit time of the minimal cut set i failure occurring

$$\begin{aligned} W_i(t) &= q_2(t)q_3(t) \ldots q_{n_i}(t)w_1(t) \\ &+ q_1(t)q_3(t) \ldots q_{n_i}(t)w_2(t) \\ &\ldots \\ &+ q_1(t)q_2(t) \ldots q_{n_{i-1}}(t)w_{n_i}(t) \end{aligned} \tag{7}$$

where n_i is the number of components in cut set i. The first term of $W_i(t)$ is the probability that all components except component 1 are down at time t and then component 1 fails, and similarly for the other terms. Substituting (4) and (6) into (7), $W_i(t)$ becomes

$$\begin{aligned} W_i(t) &= (\lambda_2 t)(\lambda_3 t) \ldots (\lambda_{n_i} t)\lambda_1 \\ &+ (\lambda_1 t)(\lambda_3 t) \ldots (\lambda_{n_i} t)\lambda_2 \\ &\ldots \\ &+ (\lambda_1 t)(\lambda_2 t) \ldots (\lambda_{n_{i-1}} t)\lambda_{n_i} \\ &= n_i \Sigma_{i=1,n_i} (\lambda_i) t^{n_{i-1}} \end{aligned} \tag{8}$$

The system failure occurrence rate, $W_s(t)$, is the probability per unit time that the top event occurs at time t

$$W_s(t) = \Sigma_{i=1,N} W_i(t) \tag{9}$$

where N is the number of minimal cut sets. For an operational system, the system failure rate, $W_s(t)$, is the probability of interest.

4. Case Study: The MGA Exoskeleton rehabilitation robot

The MGA Exoskeleton mentioned briefly in the introduction will be used as an illustrative example of how to conduct this design process. This arm exoskeleton was designed to treat shoulder pathologies such as rotator cuff tear and shoulder impingement syndrome. It has four shoulder degrees of freedom (three rotations and a scapula elevation), an elbow pitch joint, and a passive forearm pro/supination joint. It is capable of producing 134 N-m of torque at each shoulder joint and 64 N-m at the elbow, which is comparable to the output of the average adult male (Caldwell et al., 1998). The human interfaces consist of a torso mount for the scapula, an orthotic splint for the upper arm, and a hand grip. The system is fast and powerful, and because of the arm restraints, fast patient egress is not possible.

The project safety criteria specifies that no single failure can cause a hazard and the the system must be *fail-safe*. A fail-safe system is one that will achieve a safe state in the presence of a detected fault (Dunn, 2003; Roderick et al., 2004). When a fault is detected, the exoskeleton should either a) halt arm motion and hold the current position, or b) safe the arm by removing power to the motors. It is important to note here that fail-safe does not necessarily mean powering off the robot - that might actually endanger the patient more. For example, placing the exoskeleton in a passive, gravity-assist configuration might be the primary fail-safe state.

Conducting a fault tree analysis is a top-down process in which the operating modes and control system form an integral part. The procedure, illustrated in Fig. 3, begins with the task protocol such as enabling a resistive rotational movement about the shoulder. The task then determines the operating mode of the robot. For example, performing a shoulder abduction exercise would require that the resistance profile about a particular shoulder axis be controlled. The operating mode then determines what controller(s) needs to be activated to realize that particular protocol. Finally, the safety system must monitor and protect the patient from potential hazards during execution of the task.

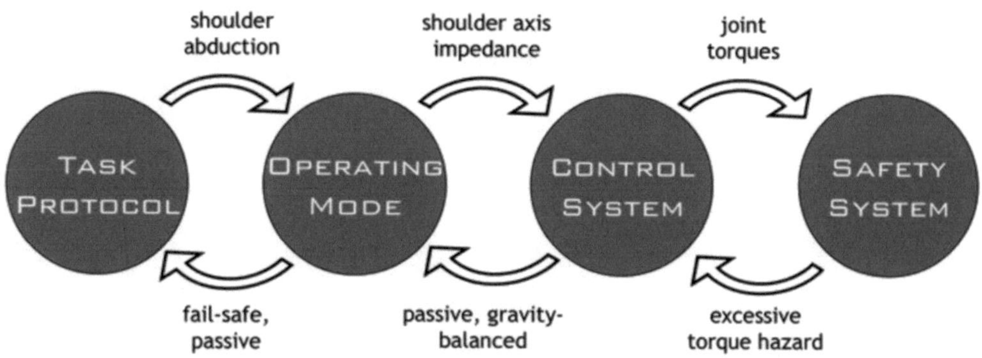

Fig. 3. The medical robot design begins with the task and loops to the safety system and back again.

4.1 Protocols and Operating Modes

There are basically two classes of shoulder therapy protocols currently being implemented on the exoskeleton: *iso-lateral exercise* and *functional training*. Iso-lateral exercises are those that occur around a single rotation axis of the shoulder or along a straight line path of the hand. Functional training involves more general movement of the hand through three-dimensional space which occurs in everyday tasks.

Iso-lateral exercises closely mimic those currently performed manually or with the assistance of exercise machines. Examples of shoulder rotation exercises include shoulder abduction/adduction and internal/external rotation as shown in Fig. 4 (Liszka, 2006). In rotational exercises, the motion of the shoulder joints is determined by the resistance about the desired shoulder axis of rotation. Examples of exercises involving straight line motion of the hand include upright rows and wall push-ups.

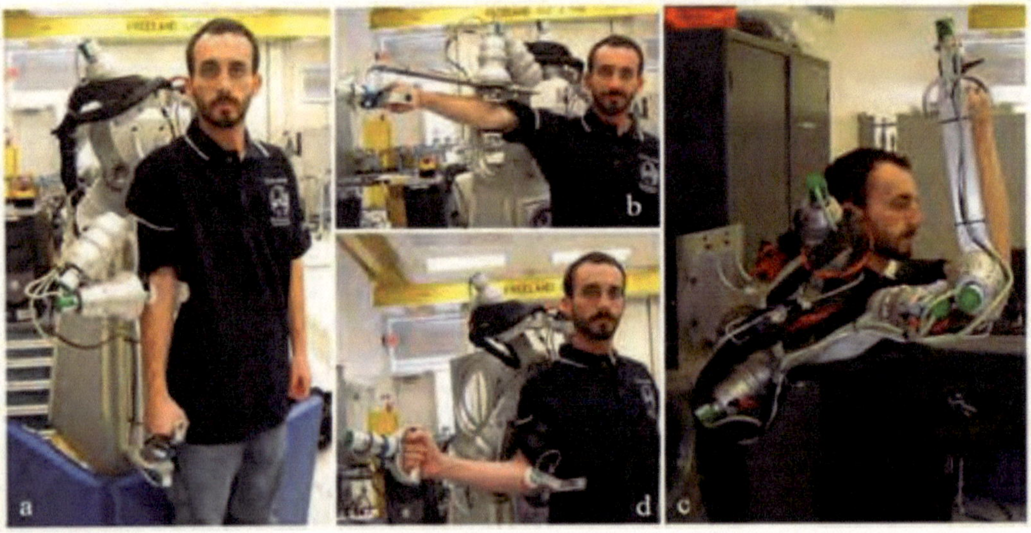

Fig. 4. Exoskeleton shown at (a) full shoulder adduction (b) 90 degree shoulder abduction, (c) mid-elbow flexion, and (d) near full lateral rotation.

During *functional training*, the patient views the simulated task and a representation of their arm through a head mounted display, while the exoskeleton provides haptic feedback to the patient. A force sensor located at the hand gripper senses the forces being exerted by the patient during "contact" with the virtual environment and relays them to the controller which commands the exoskeleton in response to the interaction. Examples of functional training are proprioceptive neuromuscular facilitation (PNF) patterns and simulations of activites of daily living.

4.2 Control System

The modular control architecture implemented on this system is shown in Fig. 5. The exercise protocol is first parsed into a control mode based on the desired activation of the arm joints. This code then determines which controller(s) should be activated for the possible combinations of arm groups: scapula, shoulder, elbow pitch, and elbow orbit. These groups can implement impedance (torque command) and admittance (position command) modes depending upon the availability of force sensing and the impedance settings. In the case where both modes are feasible, e.g. rowing, the level of impedance often determines which mode will be implemented.

As an example, the impedance control module used for controlling the resistance about an arbitrary shoulder axis is shown in Fig. 6. The stiffness and damping about the desired Cartesian axes of rotation are set using the desired impedance Z_d. The desired orientation of the glenhumeral (GH) joint is input to the controller and "differenced" with the sensed GH orientation computed from the forward kinematics of the shoulder joints to produce the angle-axis error. The GH angular velocity error is then multiplied by the desired impedance to produce the desired GH torque. This torque is then mapped to joint torques τ_d via the transpose-Jacobian, which is added to a feedforward compensation torque to produce the torque servo command τ_d.

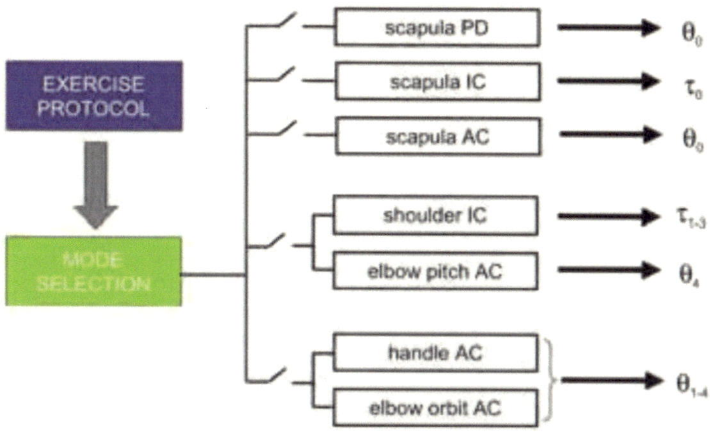

Fig. 5. Modular control architecture for the MGA Exoskeleton.

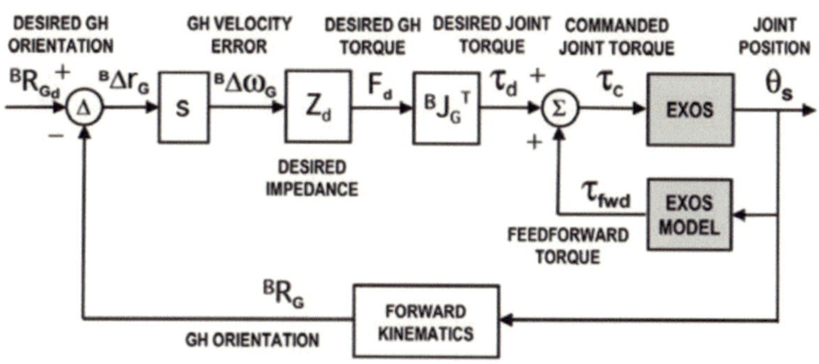

Fig. 6. Exoskeleton impedance controller for shoulder axis rotation.

4.3 Safety System

The above control modes and their associated control systems define the minimum suite of sensors and actuators that are required to carry out operations, a partial diagram of which is shown in Fig. 7. This constitutes the initial system design description, and must now be evaluated to determine whether it satisfies the safety criteria of the project.

The PHA for this project involved defining the system boundary, determining the types of possible accidents, and identifying hazards that may cause such accidents. The following were used to aid in identification of the hazards: lessons learned from previous robotic systems, historical operational data, and critical examination of the results of the PHA conducted on a previous robot with a similar architecture (the second case study in this work). Conducting a PHA is an iterative engineering task, and required several sessions.

Given the initial system design description (shown visually in Fig. 7), the PHA identified three potential hazards (in this context, "excessive" means an unhealthy level, leading to injury):

Hazard A: Moving the patient outside their safe position range.
Hazard B: Moving the patient at an excessive velocity.
Hazard C: Applying excessive torque to the patient or, conversely, allowing the patient to apply excessive torque against the robot.

Each of these hazards will be considered in turn, through the FTA and subsequent modifications to the system design.

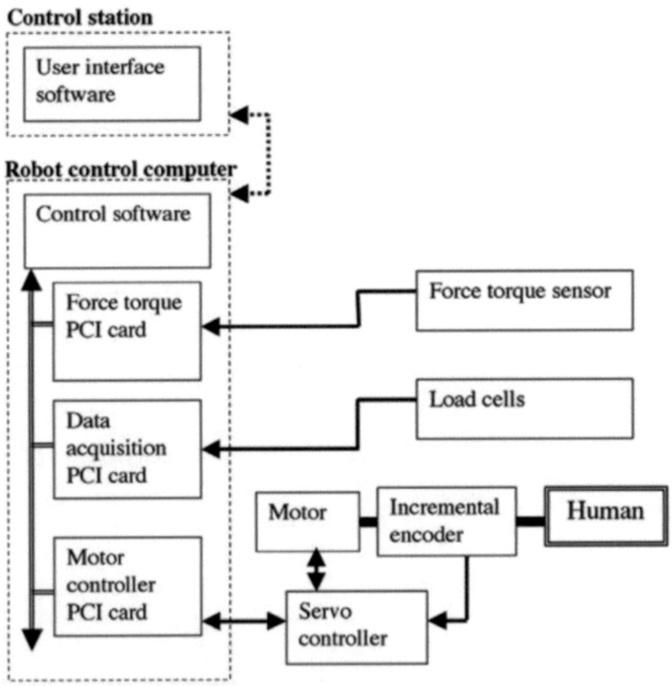

Fig. 7. Initial system design. This is the minimum suite of sensors and actuators required for operations. For clarity, only major system components are shown. Also, the set of sensors and actuators required for only one of the five degrees of freedom is shown.

4.3.1 Hazard A: Moving the patient outside their safe position range

A fault tree developed from the initial system design of Fig. 7, and the top event "Moving the patient outside their safe position range", is shown in Fig. 8. The top event can be caused by any one of numerous possible intermediate events, due to the OR gate attached to the top event (see definitions in Fig. 1). The intermediate event shown, "Uncommanded motion due to joint runaway", can be caused solely by a failure of the incremental encoder, which is a primary component of the control law used to drive the motor.

This scenario fails the project safety criteria, and so additional components were added to the system and the PHA and FTA were repeated. The modified system design is shown in Fig. 9, where the shaded components, an absolute encoder and a power amplifier, are additions over the initial system design (Roderick & Carignan, 2005).

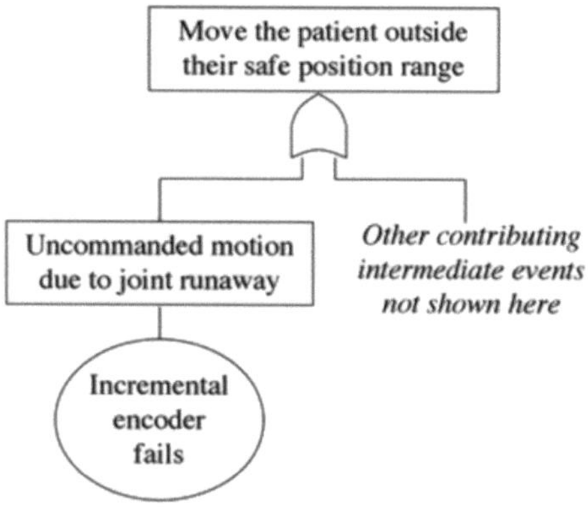

Fig. 8. Fault tree for the initial system design and the top event "Moving the patient outside their safe position range". This fault tree shows that a single fault, that of the incremental encoder, could cause the top event to occur.

The fault tree for this top event and the modified system design is shown in Fig. 10. This fault tree considers the addition of a second encoder and a software-based divergence check to the system design. The divergence check is designed to detect a failed encoder by comparing the values of the two encoders, and flagging a fault if they differ by more than a prescribed tolerance. This fault tree demonstrates that the addition of the second encoder and the encoder divergence check will satisfy the project safety criteria for this hazard: no one failure is capable of producing the hazard.

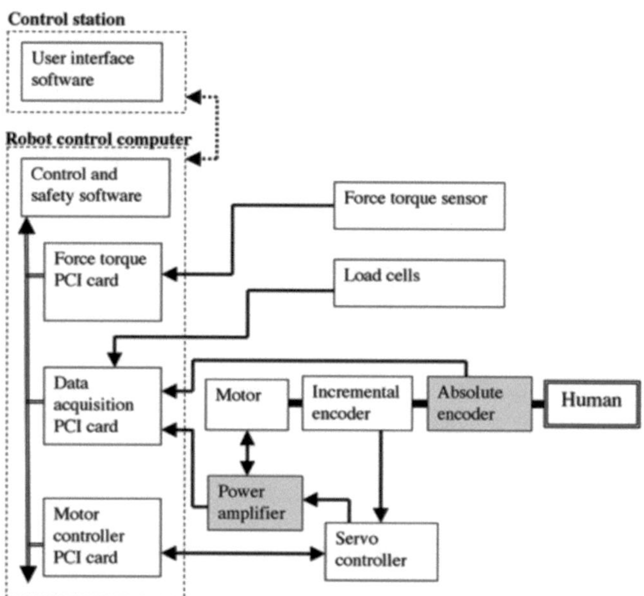

Fig. 9. Modified system design with additional components to satisfy project safety criteria. The additions over the initial system design of Fig. 7 are shaded. For clarity, only major system components of relevance are shown. Also, the set of sensors and actuators required for only one of the five degrees of freedom is shown.

While the modified system design does prevent a single failure from causing this hazard, closer examination of Fig. 10 shows that a double failure could still cause the hazard. If both encoders fail in such a way that they output almost the identical same value they would pass the encoder divergence check. While this failure combination is possible, particularly for certain values (depending on the encoders construction, 0 or -1 are likely candidates), it is highly unlikely to occur at the same time, and thus could be deemed an "incredible" failure and removed from further analysis. While further modifications to the system design, such as a third encoder, may enable detection of such situations, the additional system complexity may be unwarranted as well as potentially contributing to lower system reliability. The tradeoff between these measures is beyond the scope of this chapter.

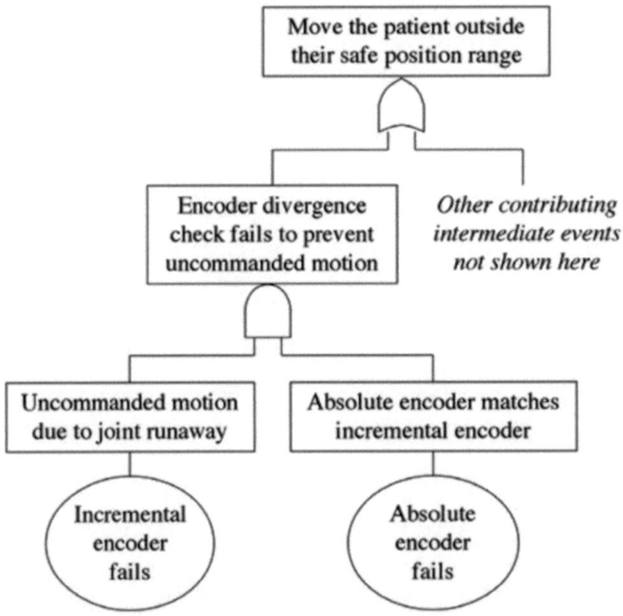

Fig. 10. Fault tree for the modified system design and the top event "Moving the patient outside their safe position range". This fault tree indicates that two simultaneous faults are required for the intermediate event shown to cause the top event to occur.

To help determine the overall likelihood of such incredible failures occurring, the fault trees may be quantitatively evaluated. As noted in Section 3.1, FTA is generally a qualitative technique, who's quantitative accuracy is indicative at best. Quantitative analysis may therefore simply be beneficial in ranking failures by probabilistic likelihood, versus using the output probabilities as absolute indications of safety (Roderick, 2000).

4.3.2 Hazard B: Moving the patient at an excessive velocity

The fault trees for this hazard are very similar in structure to those for the previous hazard. This is primarily due to the system computing velocity based on sequential encoder readings, and hence there are identical measures to sense excessive velocity or to detect a failed component that contributes to velocity sensing. Thus, this hazard is not considered any further here.

4.3.3 Hazard C: Applying excessive torque to the patient

A fault tree for the initial system design and the top event, "Applying excessive torque to the patient", is shown in Fig. 11. A single failure of the servo controller, which is responsible for providing power to the motor, is capable of producing uncommanded motion and hence, potentially, applying excessive torque to the patient. The fault tree of Fig. 12 is for the modified system design and shows the addition of a separate power amplifier with built-in motor current sensor, as well as a software-based motor power check (not shown). This power check compares the motor current draw with the requested output of the servo controller, to determine if either component is at fault. This fault tree indicates that the project safety criteria are satisfied by these additions.

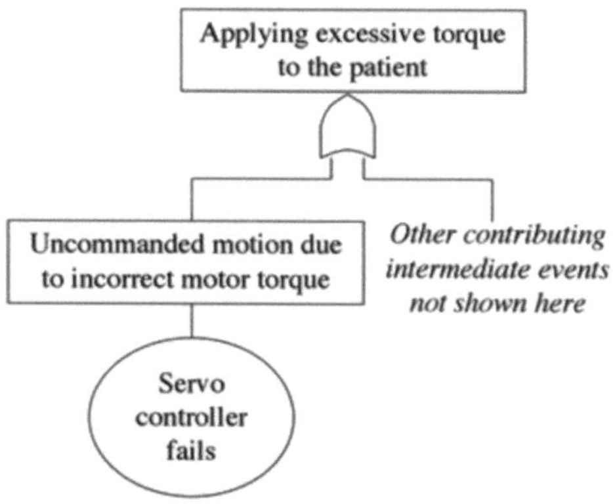

Fig. 11. Fault tree for the initial system design and the top event "Applying excessive torque to the patient". This fault tree shows that a single fault, that of the servo controller, could cause the top event to occur.

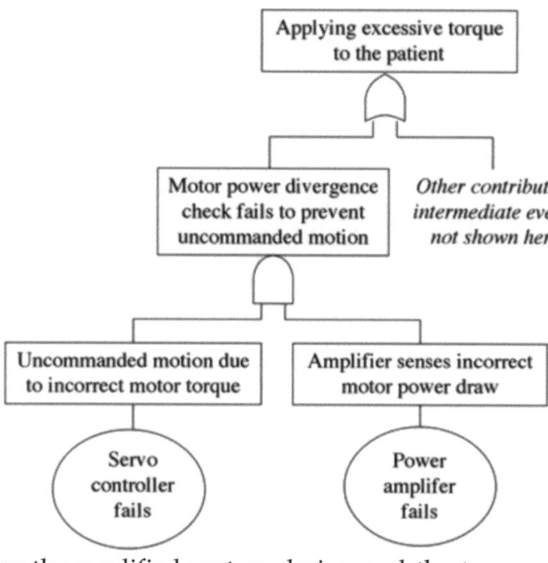

Fig. 12. Fault tree for the modified system design and the top event "Applying excessive torque to the patient". This fault tree indicates that two simultaneous faults are required for the intermediate event shown to cause the top event to occur.

4.4 Summary

Through several iterations of system safety engineering, the final system design of Fig. 13 was reached. Comparison with the initial system design of Fig. 7 shows the addition of extra sensors for each degree of freedom, as well as multiple emergency stop capabalities. Note that for brevity of explanation, only trivial examples of fault trees and their associated system design modifications have been shown. This project is also a work-in-progress, so little operational data exists at this time. Therefore, operational results from a similar robotic system with a substantial amount of operating time will now be considered.

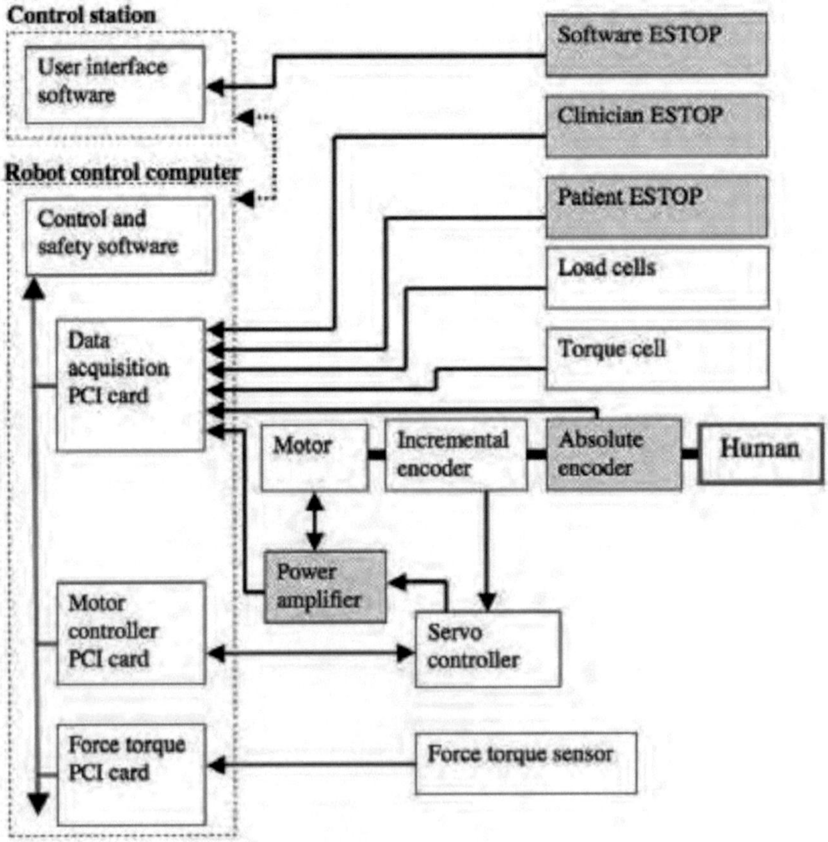

Fig. 13. Final system design showing the additional safety-related components (shaded), over those required solely to realize the system's control modes.

5. Case study: The Ranger Telerobotic Shuttle Experiment

The system safety design process described here was originally applied to the Ranger Telerobotic Shuttle Experiment (RTSX). This four-manipulator, 33 degree of freedom robot was designed and built to fly on NASA's space shuttle as a satellite servicing flight demonstration experiment. The robot has sufficient power, speed and reach, to potentially damage or destroy critical components necessary for the shuttle's operation and safe return to Earth. Non-flight versions of this robot have several hundred hours of lab and neutral

buoyancy operational time over the past five years. This provides long term data against which this system safety design process can be evaluated.
The MGA Exoskeleton in the previous case study and the RTSX robot have similar overall system architectures, and both use identical electromechanical actuator and sensor technology. They also use similar control software, with variations only in the specific control modes, device drivers, and the safety checks specific to each robot. Though the hazards listed for each system may appear different, the subtrees contributing to the individual hazards are nearly identical for each robot (e.g. encoders failing and causing uncommanded motion, distributed control components failing to meet their deadline). This strong similarity allows for direct application of the process to both robot systems.
The project safety critiera were driven by a NASA-defined "fail-safe" hazard control approach. This pioneering approach (for NASA) allowed a computer-based control system to have total control of a hazardous payload when traditional approaches are infeasible (Roderick et al., 2004). The fundamental precept of this fail-safe approach is that the control system must *reliably detect the first failure* and *transition the system to a safe state*. The system need not necessarily be one-fault tolerant, nor does it have to cope with failures subsequent to the first. It simply has to be able to reliably attain a safe state despite the presence of any one failure. This defined the project safety critiera. The project failure rate criteria were based on the intended 48-hour mission length.
Based on an initial system design, a PHA identified the following three hazards that Ranger presented to the shuttle and its crew:

Hazard A:	Manipulator motion physically damages the shuttle or prevents a safe return to Earth (e.g. by preventing the payload bay doors from closing)
Hazard B:	Releasing an untethered object (e.g. an orbital replacement unit) that damages the shuttle or becomes orbital debris
Hazard C:	An object (e.g. an item's restrainting bolt) breaks due to excessive force or torque, and the subsequent pieces damage the shuttle or become orbital debris

Applying FTA to the initial system design, given these three hazards, resulted in the addition of double and triple modular redundancy in certain critical computer components, software algorithms, and sensors. It also resulted in a complete partitioning of system wide safety protocols into an autonomous vehicle-based software safety system that was totally isolated from the rest of the system (Roderick, et al., 2004). This mechanism alleviated the need for safety certification and verification of operators, input devices, communication protocols, and the multitude of operator control stations. This dramatically reduced the complexity of the safety system, which in turn reduced development time, testing effort, and (hopefully) produced a more reliable and safer system.

5.1 Qualitative analysis

The distribution of minimal cut sets by size, for each hazard, is shown graphically in Fig. 14 for the final system design. There are over 3500 minimal cut sets in total, with the smallest minimal cut set size being 2, the maximum size 13, and the average size about 5. As there are no single-component minimal cut sets, this system design satisfies the project's safety criteria. Although there exist double component cut sets, the majority of failure scenarios leading to a hazard involve three or more events. Fig. 14 also shows that only Hazards A and C have double component cut sets, and Hazard B requires at least three failures before a hazard can occur. There is a significant difference in the number of minimal cut sets for each hazard, largely due to the varying number and size of subtrees for each individual hazard.

5.2 Quantitative analysis

A quantitative probabilistic analysis of RTSX's fault trees was conducted based on limited historical data available from a prototype robot. For this analysis, all RTSX failures were considered non-repairable, since during the mission neither hardware nor software could be repaired nor modified. In computing the hazard probabilities, the assumption of the λ-model that $\lambda t < 0.1$ (in order to simplify $F(t) = 1\text{-}e^{-\lambda t}$) was not valid for the two largest failure probabilities. This assumption was considered acceptable at that time, which has since been validated by operational results.

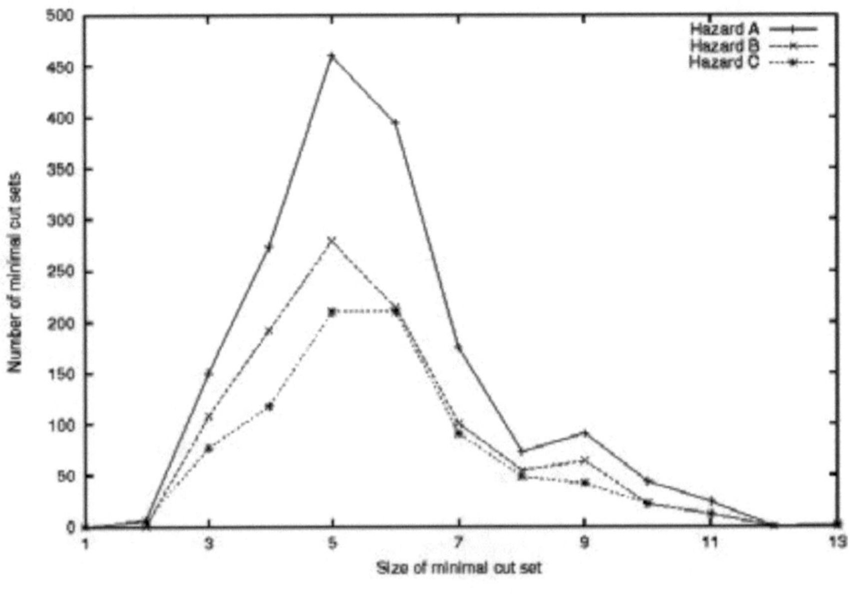

Fig. 14. Distribution of minimal cut set sizes, by hazard.

The estimated probabilities of the occurrence of Hazards A, B, and C for t=1 hour are 0.0464, 0.00182, and 0.00783, respectively. Though this type of probabilistic analysis is known to be conservative, these numbers are uncomfortably high. Examination of the individual subtrees showed that the top five subtrees are significantly more likely to occur then the remaining subtrees. The probabilities of these top five most likely subtrees, and their percentage contribution to their parent hazard's probability, are shown in Table 1. Note that the probability of occurrence in one hour of the remaining subtrees is 0.00005 or lower, or at least two orders of magnitude less likely than any of the top five most likely subtrees. Also note that Hazards B and C are both predominantly caused by one subtree each, i.e., one set of failure combinations. The components and failures making up these individual subtrees could be targetted for significant examination and validation, or potential redesign to reduce their overall probablity of occurence. Note once again that hazard probabilities

calculated from an FTA are only indicative, due to the inherent uncertainty in failure probabilities and the assumptions of the lamba-model.
Sensitivity analysis of the input failure probabilities was conducted on all subtrees, in an effort to identify the effect of their inherent uncertainty. This uncertainty occurs due to assumptions made by manufacturers when defining failure rates for individual commercial off-the-shelf components, as well as from the assumptions and estimates used to extrapolate data from the historical prototype system.

Subtree	**Type**	**Probability of occurrence in 1 hour**	**% of parent hazard's probability**
A3	Main DMU SW failure causes excess velocity	0.038	81.9
C2	FT sensor failure causes over-torque	0.00775	98.9
A4	Operator failure causes boundary crossing	0.00705	15.2
B1	Operator failure causes gripper open	0.00179	98.2
A2	LPU SW failure causes excess velocity	0.00122	2.6

Table 1. Estimated probabilities for top five most likely subtrees, and their percentage contribution to the parent hazard's probability.

This analysis individually varied the input failure probability of each failure contributing in a fault tree, and determined the subsequent variation in the parent hazard's probability. Each input failure probability was varied up and down by one order of magnitude. The variation in Hazard C's probability, as a function of the variation in input failure probability is shown in Fig. 15. As expected, the plots indicate a general exponentially increasing effect on the hazard probability as a function of increased individual failure probability. The graph dramatically illustrates that a small number of failure probabilities can significantly increase the overall hazard probability. These individual components could be targeted for additional testing to better determine their predicted failure rates, with a subsequent improvement in the accuracy of the overall hazard probabilities. The graphs for Hazards A and B show the same trends and are not presented here.

5.3 Summary

Despite having fairly high hazard probabilities, RTSX has operated well below these numbers indicating that the computed quantitative probabilities are indeed conservative. In several hundred hours of operation, only one accident has occurred, which was in the form of uncommanded motion. This failure was due to an improperly coded safety check on the bounds of a critical input parameter, and it occurred in the presence of an incomplete and more primitive safety system than was specified in the final system design. The rarity of these events is perhaps an indicator of the overly conservative nature of the probability analysis, as well as an outgrowth of the estimates used in extrapolating failure probabilities from a prototype historical system. The solid operational history may, in fact, validate the system design modifications indicated by this process, and demonstrate the success of the process when applied to a safety critical robot system.

6. Conclusion

A methodology has been presented that can qualitatively and quantitatively evaluate a system design against a set of project safety criteria. This methodology allows system designers to target individual components or failures, in an effort to make the system more safe. While this methodology cannot produce an absolutely safe system, it provides a mechanism by which a system design can be judged to be sufficiently safe. The methodology also provides for indicative quantitative analysis of a system, which evalutes the system's overall failure rate.

This methodology was applied to two example robotic systems: a shoulder rehabilitation exoskeleton and a multi-arm dexterous space robot. Qualitative analysis of each system allowed for targetted modifications to the system design, producing final systems that were sufficiently safe when judged against the project's safety criteria. Quantitative analysis of the second system indicated uncomfortably high failure probabilities, however, operational data to date indicates the very conservative nature of this analysis, and validates that it can only be used as an indicative evaluation.

Future work for the MGA exoskeleton involves full completion of the FTA, including enumeration of all cut sets, as well as completion of the quantitative analysis. A partial FMEA has already been performed on the MGA Exoskeleton. Completion of this FMEA and comparison to the PHA hazard list may indicate additional hazards, or subtrees of the FTA, that need to be considered. Also, a more comprehensive version of this process would include an FMEA as a useful component. Operational data will continue to be taken for RTSX, and for the exoskeleton once development is complete. Comprehensive comparison of the operational data with respect to the input failure proabilities may help identify certain failures or failure types, that untowardly affect the hazard probability. These variances in the input failure probabilities could be taken into account to improve the accuracy of future quantitative analyses.

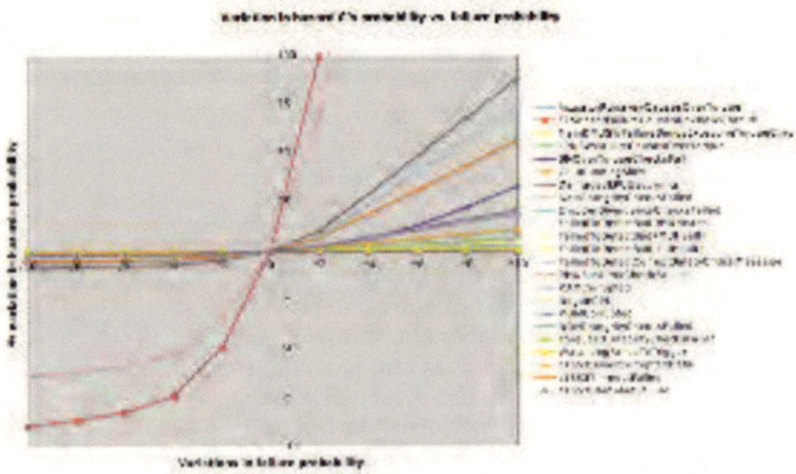

Fig. 15. Percent variation in Hazard C probability as a function of variation in failure probabilities.

7. References

Adler J.R. Jr.; Chang, S.; Murphy, M.; Doty, J.; Geis, P. & Hancock, S. (1997). The Cyberknife: a frameless robotic system for radiosurgery, *Stereotact Funct Neurosurg*, Vol. 69 (1-4 Pt 2), pp. 124-8.

Anderson, T. (1993). Safety-Status and Perspectives, *Proc. of the 12th Int. Conf. on Computer Safety, Reliability and Security*, Janusz Gorski eds., Poznan-Kierkz, Oct. 1993.

Bernhardt, M.; Frey, M.; Colombo, G. & Riener, R. (2005). Hybrid force-position control yields cooperative behaviour of the rehabilitation robot LOKOMAT, *9th Int. Conf. on Rehabilitation Robotics (ICORR)*, Chicago, pp. 536-539.

Blanchard, B. (1991). *Systems Engineering Management*, John Wiley & Sons, New York.

Borras. C. (2006). Overexposure of radiation therapy patients in panama: problem recognition and follow-up measures, *Rev Panam Salud Publica*, Vol. 20, No. 2/3, pp. 173–187.

Bruns, G. & Anderson, S. (1993). Vaildating Safety models with Fault Trees. *Proceedings of 12th International Conference on Computer Safety, Reliability and Security*, Ed. Janusz Gorski, Poznan-Kierkz, Oct. 1993.

Caldwell, D.; Favede, C. & Tsagarakis N (1998). Dextrous exploration of a virtual world for improved prototyping, *Proc. of the IEEE Int. Conf. on Robotics and Automation*, Leuven, Belgium, May 1998, pp. 298–303.

Carignan, C.; Liszka, M. & Roderick, S. (2005). Design of an Exoskeleton with Scapula Motion for Shoulder Rehabilitation, *Proc. IEEE Int. Conf. on Advanced Robotics (ICAR)*, Seattle, pp. 524-531, July 2005.

Cavallaro, J. R. & Walker, I. D. (1997). Failure Mode Analysis of a Proposed Manipulator-based Hazardous Material Retrieval System, *Proc. 7th American Nuclear Society Topical Meeting on Robotics and Remote Systems*, Vol. 2, pp. 1096-1102, Augusta, April 1997.

Duchemin, G.; Poignet, P.; Dombre, E. & Pierrot F. (2004). Medically Safe and Sound, *IEEE Robotics & Automation Magazine*, Vol. 11, No. 2, June 2004, pp. 46-55.

Dunn, W. (2003). Designing Safety-Critical Computer Systems, *Computer*, Nov. 2003, pp. 40-46.

Gorski, J.; Maggott, J. & Wardzinski, A. (1995). Modelling Fault Trees as Petri Nets, *Proc. of 14th Int. Conf. on Computer Safety, Reliability and Security*, Oct. 1995.

Guiochet, J. & Vilchis, A. (2002). Safety Analysis of a Medical Robot for Tele-Echography, *2nd IARP IEEE/RAS Joint Workshop on Technical Challenge for Dependable Robots in Human Environments*, Toulouse, pp. 217-227.

Guthart, G. & Salisbury, J. K. (2000). The intuitive telesurgery system: Overview and application, *Proc. of the IEEE Int. Conf. on Robotics and Automation*, pp. 618-622, San Fransisco, Apr. 2000.

He, J.; Koeneman, E.; Huang, H.; Herring, D.; Sugar, T.; Herman, R. & Koeneman, J. (2005). Design of a Robotic Upper Extremity Repetitive Therapy Device, *Proc. Int. Conf. on Rehabilitation Robotics (ICORR)*, Chicago, pp. 95-98.

Hope, S.; Bjordal, E.; Diack, H.; Eddershaw, B.; Joanny, L.; Ortone, G.; Payne, F.; Searson, A.; Sedlacek, K. & Strien, W. (1983). Methodologies for hazard analysis and risk assessment in the petroleum refining and storage industry. *Journal of Hazard Prevention*, Jul/Aug, 1983, pp 24-32.

Knight, J. & Nakano, L. (1997). Software test techniques for system fault-tree analysis, *Proc. of 16th International Conf. on Computer Safety, Reliability and Security*. Ed. Peter Daniel. York, Sept. 1997.

Krebs, H.I.; Volpe, B.T; Ferraro, M.; Fasoli, S.; Palazzolo, J.; Rohrer, B.; Edelstein, L. & Hogan, N. (2002). Robot Aided NeuroRehabilitation: From evidence based to science based rehabilitation, *Topics in Stroke Rehabilitation: Clinical Applications of New Technology*, Vol. 8, No. 4, 2002, pp. 54-70.

Lankenau, A.; Meyer, O. & Krieg-Bruckner, B. (1998). Safety in robotics: the Bremen Autonomous Wheelchair, in *Advanced Motion Control, 1998. AMC '98-Coimbra., 1998 5th International Workshop on*, 29 Jun-1 Jul 1998, pp 524-529.

Leveson, N. (1984). Software Safety in Computer-Controlled Systems, *Computer*, Vol. 17, No. 2, 1984, pp. 48-55

Leveson, N. & Turner, C. (1993). An Investigation of the Therac-25 Accidents, *Computer*, Vol. 26, No. 7, July 1993, pp. 18-41.

Leveson, N. (1995). *Safeware: System Safety and Computers*, Addison-Wesley, Reading, Mass.

Liszka, M. (2006). *Mechanical Design of a Robotic Exoskeleton for Shoulder Rehabilitation*, M.S. Thesis, Dept. of Aerospace Engineering, Univ. of Maryland, Dec. 2006.

Mayr, A.; Mina, S.; Köchln, G.; Kronreif, G. & Saltuari, L. (2006). A New Driven Orthosis for the Upper Extremity (ARMOR): Preliminary Results, *4th World Congress for NeuroRehabilitation, Neurorehabil Neural Repair* 2006, Vol. 20, No. 1.

McDermid, J. (2001). Software safety: Where's the evidence? *Aus Workshop on Industrial Experience with Safety Critical Systems and Software*, Brisbane, July 2001.

Nef, T.; Mihelj, M.; Colombo, G. & Riener R. (2006). Armin – robot for rehabilitation of the upper extremities, *Proc. IEEE Int. Conf. on Robotics and Automation*, Orlando, pp. 3152–3157.

Ozog, H. & Bendixen, L. (1987). Hazards identification and quantification. *Journal of Hazard Prevention*, Sep-Oct, 1987, pp 6-13.

Parnas, D.; Asmis, G. & Madey, J. (1991). Assessment of Safety-Critical Software in Nuclear Power Plants, *Nuclear Safety*, Vol. 32, No. 2, 1991, pp. 189-198.

Potocki de Montalk, J. (1991). Computer Software in Civil Aircraft, *Microprocessors & Microsystems*, Vol. 17, No. 1, 1991, pp. 17-23.

Roderick, S. (2000). *Validation of a Computer-Based Hazard Control System for a Robotic Payload on the Space Shuttle*, M.S. Thesis, Dept. of Aerospace Engineering, University of Maryland, College Park, MD.

Roderick, S.; Roberts, B.; Atkins, E.; Churchill, P. & Akin, D. (2004). An Autonomous Software Safety System for a Dexterous Space Robot, *Journal of Aerospace Computing, Information, and Communication*, AIAA, Dec. 2004.

Roderick, S. & Carignan, C. (2005). An Approach to Designing Software Safety Systems for Rehabilitation Robots, *Proc. of the Int. Conf. on Rehabilitation Robotics (ICORR)*, Chicago, pp. 252-257, June 2005.

Rosen, J.; Perry, J.C.; Manning, N.; Burns, S. & Hannaford, B. (2005). The human arm kinematics and dynamics during daily activities - toward a 7 DOF upper limb powered exoskeleton, *12th Int. Conf. on Advanced Robotics (ICAR)*, Seattle, 2005, pp. 532-539.

Salisbury, J. Kenneth, Jr. (1998). The Heart of Microsurgery, *Mechanical Engineering*, Dec. 1998, p. 46-51.

Shaw, R. (1995). Safety cases – How Did We Get Here? *12th Annual CSR Workshop Safety and Reliability of Software-Based Systems*, Roger Shaw ed., Bruges, Sept. 1995.

Sommerville, I. (1995). *Software Engineering*, 5th ed., Addison-Wesley.

Stephenson, J. (1991). *System Safety 2000*, Von Nostrand Reinhold.

Taylor, R.; Paul, H.; Kazanzides, P.; Mittelstadt, B.; Hanson, W.; Zuhars, J.; Williamson, B.; Musits, B.; Glassman, E. & Bargar, W. (1991). Taming the Bull: Safety in a Precise Surgical Robot, *Proc. of the 5th Int. Conf. on Advanced Robotics: Robots in Unstructured Environments*, Vol. 1, June 1991, pp. 865-870.

Varley, P. (1999). Techniques for Development of Safety-Related Software for Surgical Robots, *IEEE Trans. on Information Technology in Biomedicine*, Vol. 3, No. 4, Dec. 1999, pp. 261-267.

Vesely, W. (1981). *Fault Tree Handbook*, U.S. Nuclear Regulatory Commission.

Voas, J. M. (1995). A Statistial and Automated Code-Based Fault Tree Mitigation Framework for C++, *Safety and Reliabilty of Software-Based Systems, 12th Annual CSR Workshop*, ed. Roger Shaw, Bruges, Sept. 1995.

Weber, W.; Tondok, H. & Bachmayer, M. (2003). Enhancing Software Safety by Fault Trees: Experiences from an Application to Flight Critical SW, *Proc. of the 22nd Int. Conf. on Computer Safety, Reliability and Security*, Edinburgh, Sept. 2003.

5

Work Assistive Mobile Robot for the Disabled in a Real Work Environment

Hyun Seok Hong, Jung Won Kang and Myung Jin Chung
KAIST
Republic of Korea

1. Introduction

Previous works related to welfare service robotics have mainly focused on assisting the disabled in their daily life. Robot systems such as the Intelligent Bed-Robot System (Kim et al. 2002) and Care Robot System (Yoo, 2003a) are designed to help the disabled in performing daily activities in specialized indoor environments. Human-machine interfaces such as Eye Gaze Estimation System (Yoo, 2003b) have been developed to facilitate easy control of the robot system. FRIEND (Martens, 2001) and KARES II (Bien, 2003) are wheelchair-based rehabilitation robotic systems equipped with a robot arm and are designed to help the disabled manipulate small objects such as food, drink, books, etc.
It is important that human beings have the opportunity to feel self-worth and happiness by living productive lives through their own vocation. Therefore, the development of a vocational robotic system has important implications with respect to welfare. Although some vocational assistive robots have been developed, they are limited to office environments. The robot RAID (Eftring, 1993), which was developed at the Rehabilitation Engineering Research Center in Sweden, assists in removing books from a bookshelf, bringing documents, and serving drinks in a office environment. The robot known as WALKY (Neveryd, 1994) can avoid obstacles while it maneuvers to deliver objects in a laboratory environment. The robot ProVAR (Van der Loos, 1999) receives orders via a speech recognition system and helps to process office tasks such as serving drinks and delivering documents, diskettes, video tapes, etc. In addition, the current status of the robot is displayed through a monitor.
Due to regional differences in industrial structures, the types of tasks that the disabled can perform differ from country to country. As a result, robots assisting the disabled in a real manufacturing environment can be more useful than robots providing assistance in office environments in some countries.
However, there has been relatively little research reported on the development of vocational robotic systems in real manufacturing environments. The objective of the present work is to develop mobile robot systems that assist the disabled to work in real manufacturing factories. Specifically, the assistive robot is targeted for the disabled in Korea, where the authors dwell. In this research, to clearly determine the objectives of developing assistive mobile robots, a mission statement is addressed based on statistical data. Furthermore, the target manufacturing environment is surveyed to specify the dimensions and working algorithm of the work assistive mobile robot. Two work assistive mobile robots are

proposed and developed according to slightly different function definitions. User trials are performed for the two work assistive mobile systems. The robot systems are expected to provide practical assistance to disabled workers and help satisfy their desires and fulfill their capabilities so that they can become productive members of society. We expect that this will result in an increase in the working population of the disabled.

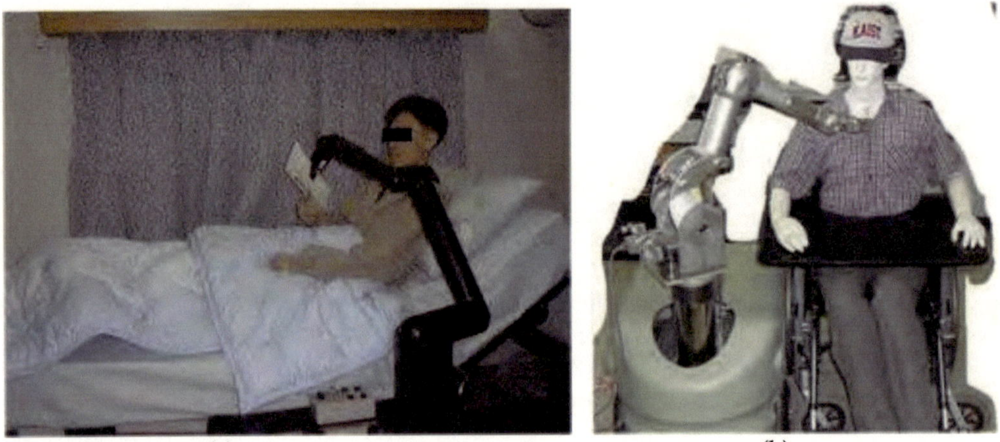

(a) (b)

Fig. 1. Examples of robots for daily activities of the disabled; (a) Intelligent bed-robot system, (b) KARES II.

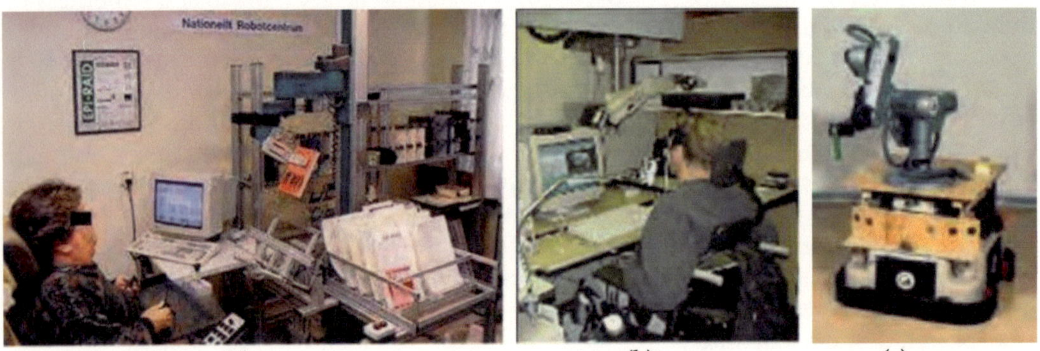

(a) (b) (c)

Fig. 2. Examples of robots for desktop vocational activities of the disabled; (a) RAID, (b) ProVAR, (c) WALKY.

2. Derivation of Mission Statements

Our objective in developing the present robot systems is to assist the disabled as much as possible in real employment situations. For determining our specific mission, we surveyed an abundance of data pertaining to people with disabilities in real employment situations. We categorized the survey results into three criteria, 'A. to assist the disabled as much as possible,' 'B. to consider the real situation of employment for the disabled and 'C. to provide assistance for the most necessary tasks for the disabled in the work space'.

2.1 Survey based on Criterion A

In order to assist the disabled as much as possible, we investigated disability types and the type of work presently being performed in Korea by workers with disabilities. To this end, we surveyed data[1] on the disabled in Korea. Among people with disabilities, 55.1%suffer from limb impairment, 8.7% cerebral paralysis, 10.5% visual disorder, 8.8% hearing disorder, and 0.8% speech disorder. On the other hand, there were relatively few people with internal organ impediments or cognitive disabilities.

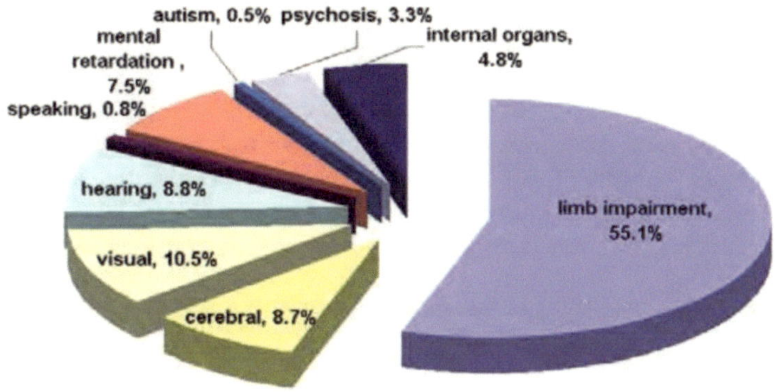

Fig. 3 Distribution of the disabled

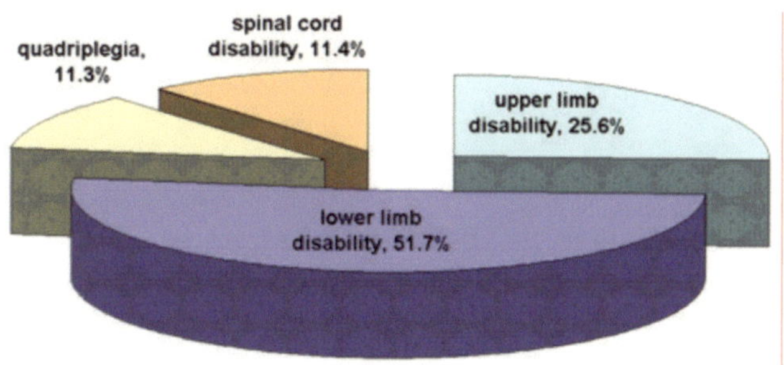

Fig. 4 Distribution of limb impairment and cerebral paralysis

Types of disorder	Large workshop	Small workshop
Limb impairment	82.0%	81.0%
Cerebral paralysis	0.2%	0.2%
Visual disorder	4.4%	3.1%
Hearing disorder	9.8%	6.2%
Speech disorder	1.2%	1.1%
Other	2.4%	8.4%

Table 1. Distribution of actual employment for the disabled. Companies with more than 300 employees are classified as a large workshop.

[1] Statistical data from reports (written in Korean): "The present condition of registered disable people," published by the Korea Ministry of Health and Welfare, Sep. 2004, "Research on the actual conditions of the disabled in 2000," published by the Korea Institute for Health and Social Affairs, 2000, "Research on the actual conditions of disabled workers in 2000," published by the Korea Employment Promotion Agency for the Disabled, 2000.

Fig. 3 shows the distribution of the disabled, and Fig. 4 describes the disability distribution of people who suffer from limb impairment or cerebral paralysis. From the distributions, it is noted that the percentage of disabled having leg impediments is large. Table 1 shows that most people with disabilities who have entered the workforce have limb impairment regardless of the scale of the workshop. Therefore, it is desirable to develop a robot system that assists workers who suffer from limb impairment.

2.2 Survey based on Criterion B

In order to assess the real employment situation of the disabled, we visited vocational education facilities[2] and companies[3] that hire disabled workers. As shown in Fig. 5, our survey results show that the physically disabled tend to prefer computer-oriented jobs, as there are numerous occupations in this field and these jobs require little spatial movement. According to the results, they are also interested in mechanical jobs, primarily because there is huge industrial demand for labor and the other is that they can gain expertise in performing these jobs.

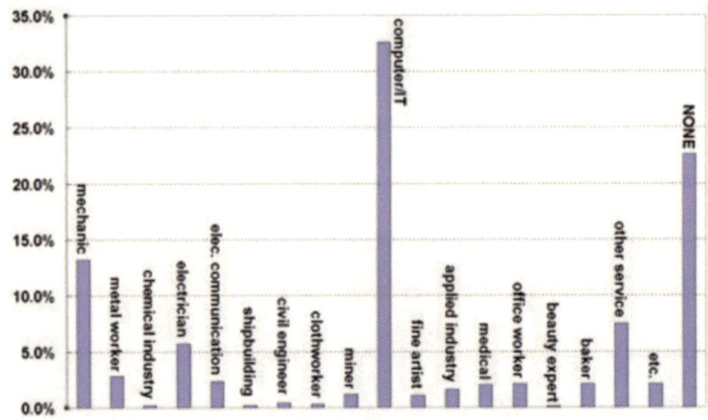

Fig. 5. Vocational fields in which the disabled desire training.

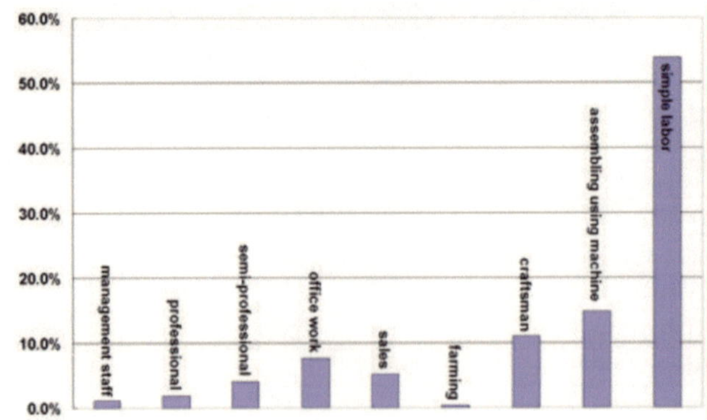

Fig. 6. Vocational fields for which the employers seek workers; 'simple labor' and 'assembling using a machine' include assembling and classifying circuit parts, moving boxes, packing, delivering, and cleaning up.

[2] Bundang branch of the Korea Employment Promotion Agency for the disabled and vocational schools in Daejeon and Ilsan.

[3] Eleven factories including Mugunghwa Electronics and Immanuel Electronics, which mainly make electronic products, and Boram-Dongsan, which mainly assembles mechanical parts.

However, vocational fields[4] for which employers wish to hire disabled workers mainly involve simple labor, as shown in Fig. 6. According to these investigations, there are huge gaps between occupations that people with disabilities want and occupations that companies need to fill. As a result, although many social organizations provide vocational education to the disabled, due to the actual employment situation the disabled mainly perform simple labor. Therefore, it is desirable to develop an assistive robot system that can help the disabled work in performing physical and simple labor such as assembling and classifying circuit parts, moving boxes, and packing and delivering goods.

2.3 Survey based on Criterion C

According to the survey results shown in Table 2, disabled laborers experience difficulties when they should carry heavy materials.

Situations	Large workshop	Small workshop
Transferring goods	55.4%	33.8%
Moving around the workshop	14.5%	31.5%
Operating machines	27.9%	20.0%
Difficulty to understand instructions	24.4%	22.3%
Operating speed	20.0%	31.5%

Table 2. Situations where a disabled worker requires help. Duplicated answers are permitted. Companies with more than 300 employees are classified as a large workshop.

Survey results also show that those who have upper limb impediments desire a robot system that can help perform movements normally performed by the arms (fixing, loading, fine motion, etc). Those with leg impediments meanwhile require a system to substitute the functions of the leg (movement, loading, etc) and those who have both impediments would like a system that would provide assistance when they should carry heavy materials. Target objects for transferring goods are divided into heavy and light objects[5]. In the case of fine motion tasks, the assistive robot system cooperates with the human and supports roller inserting and PCB inspection tasks. Therefore, it is necessary to design a work assistive robot that can transfer goods, perform dexterous tasks, and move around freely.

From the above survey results, our mission has been determined. The following is our mission statement: to develop a work assistive mobile robot to help the disabled who have lower limb(s) or upper limb disabilities, or lower limb(s) and upper limb disabilities obtain employment in manufacturing factories involving the performance of simple physical labor.

3. Work Space Environment of Real Manufacturing Factories

3.1 Work Space Environment of Real Manufacturing Factories

As described earlier, our work assistive robot helps the disabled person to work in a real manufacturing factory. Before designing this assistive robot, the environments of real

[4] Statistical data from the report (written in Korean): "Classified statistics on the disabled in the first quarter of 2002," published by the Korea Employment Promotion Agency for the Disabled, 2002.

[5] Boxes used in a real factory are investigated and classified into two groups: heavy boxes (maximum size: 65×35×40cm, shape: box, maximum weight: 30kg), and light boxes (maximum size: 30×25×10cm, shape: box or bag, maximum weight: 3kg).

manufacturing factories should be known. We surveyed several manufacturing factories that employ workers with disabilities. Through the survey, we defined the general environment to help the disabled. Manufacturing factory environment survey results are described in Fig. 7 ~ Fig. 10.

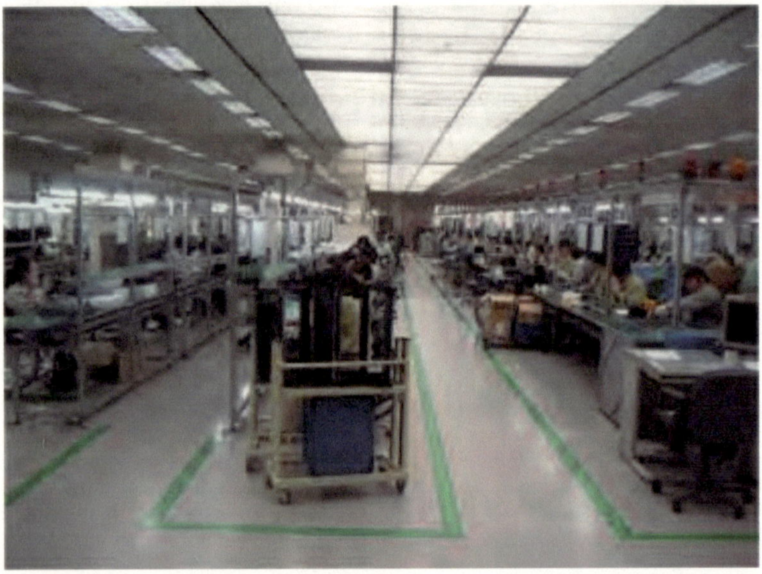

Fig. 7. Whole view of general environment of manufacturing factory. Safety lines are painted around work tables.

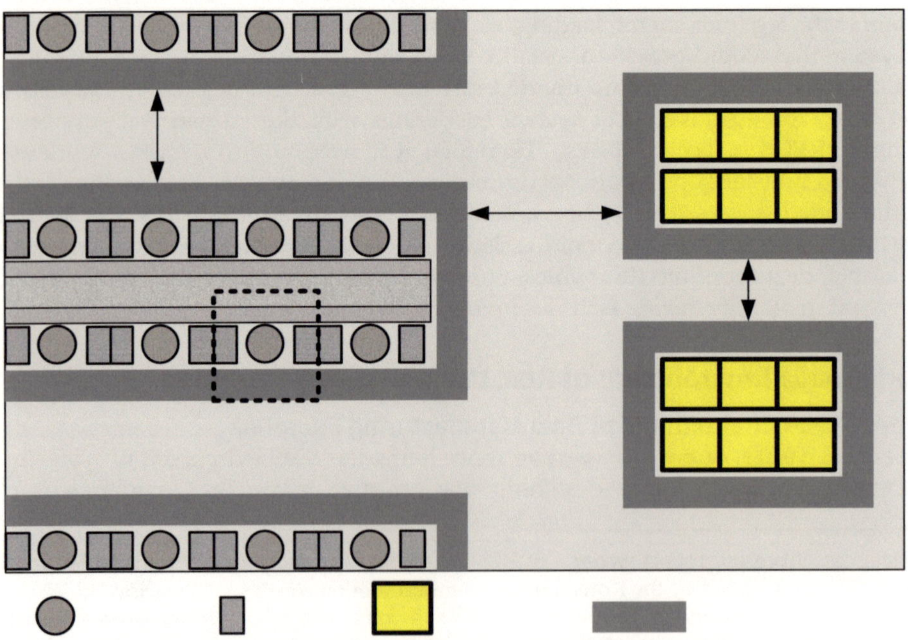

Fig. 8. Top view of general environment of manufacturing factory (dimensions in [cm]).

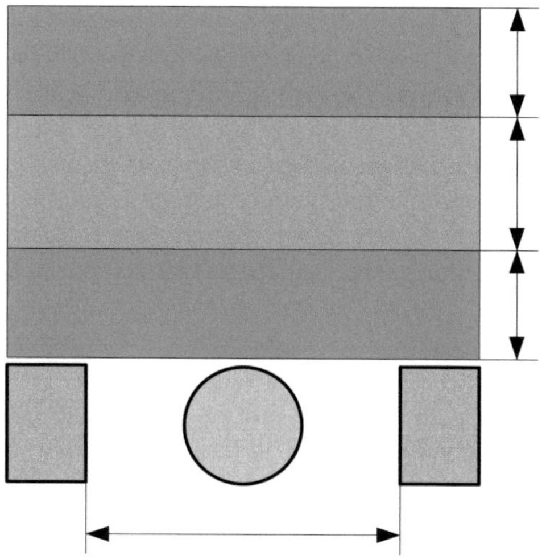

Fig. 9. Top view of space allocated for an employee working at worktable in manufacturing factories (dimensions in [cm]).

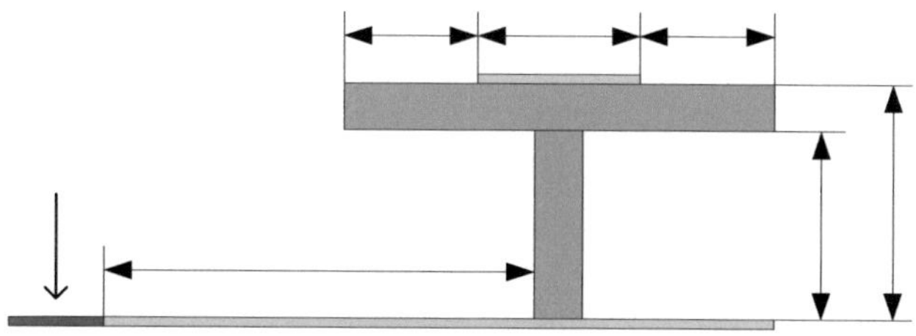

Fig. 10. Side view of space allocated for an employee working at worktable in manufacturing factories (dimensions in [cm]).

The major work in the factories is making electronic products such as battery chargers, vacuum cleaners and circuits that require soldering, and assembling task. For the tasks, as described in Fig. 8, most manufacturing factories are composed of long tables equipped with a conveyor, a warehouse containing parts in boxes on palettes, safety lines around these elements, and aisles between tables and storage areas. There are aisles with various widths, excluding the safety line width (10cm):

-between tables: min. 120cm, max. 140cm

-between storage areas: min. 80cm, max. 120cm

-between tables and storage areas: 210cm

Allocated space for a worker who works at a worktable is expressed in the dotted box in Fig. 8 while Fig. 9 and Fig. 10 show top and side views of the space, respectively. For each worker doing table tasks, boxes containing parts are stacked at the left and right sides, and the width between the boxes is 75cm at the minimum and 90cm at the maximum. The table height of the lower side is 70cm and the width between the safety line and table is about 100cm.

In the environment, workers perform dexterous tasks such as soldering and assembling at the work table. When workers do not have enough parts, they move to the warehouse, and pick up boxes that contain parts. After returning to the work table, they resume working.

3.2 Required Specification of Work Assistive Mobile Robot System

The purpose of our robot system is to help the disabled to work in a factory environment. Therefore, the robot should have function on behalf of the legs and arms of the disabled worker. In a factory, workers carry boxes including assembled parts, load and unload boxes from a warehouse, and perform dexterous tasks. In order to help the disabled worker, we adopted a mobile platform with four wheels and equipped it with a forklift and a robot arm. The forklift helps to load and unload the boxes that contain parts to be assembled. Also, the robot arm helps to move light parts and to perform dexterous jobs such as providing aid when soldering.

From the environment survey results and task analysis, the required specifications for the mobile robot system are determined. The robot arm should be able to perform various dexterous tasks such as soldering, assembling, and moving light goods. The forklift should be able to lift up boxes that are more than 30kg. The mobile platform should be small enough to move through narrow aisles between tables in factories. The size of the robot system should be less than 1500mm in length and 700mm in width. The robot should be able to carry a payload of 120kg, including 80kg for the worker's weight and 30~40kg for a box.

By using this robot, the worker can easily move around, even in a confined area. The worker can also load, unload, and transfer boxes without difficulty. The robot arm also helps in performing dexterous tasks.

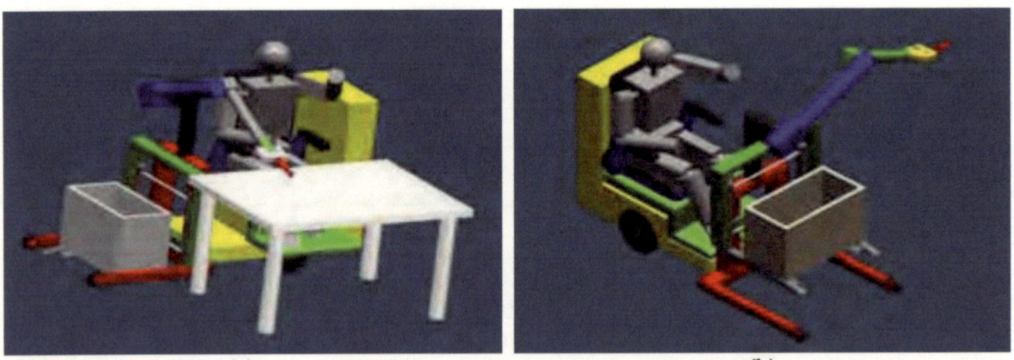

(a) (b)

Fig. 11. Basic concept of work assistive mobile robot system type I; (a) assisting table tasks, (b) moving objects.

4. Development of Work Assistive Robot Systems

After a survey of general factories environments, we developed two work assistive robot systems. Work assistive mobile robot system type I is focused on versatility and work assistive robot system type II is mainly focused on mobility. Each robot system was developed after defining tasks and functions. We also conducted user-trials with the robot systems in a real factory to obtain feedback from real workers.

4.1 Work Assistive Mobile Robot System Type I

4.1.1 Design of Work Assistive Mobile Robot System Type I

We assume that the disabled user works sitting on the chair of the work assistive mobile robot. Therefore, the height of the robot chair should be designed to be lower than that of

a desk. Furthermore, the chair should be designed to rotate up to a right angle to work at a desk. When parts to be assembled are needed or it is necessary to transfer goods, the person moves the robot and picks up and puts down the objects. Therefore, a fork-lift system is adopted in the robot system. When the robot moves, obstacle avoidance is employed and a related alarm is used for safety. The basic concept of the work assistive mobile robot system is described in Fig. 11. Fig. 11 describes a scenario to help the disabled person to work at their table tasks (soldering, assembling, etc.) and to move boxes containing parts. To support table tasks, the mobile robot is parked parallel with the table, and the chair of the robot is rotated toward the table. This setting makes it easy to use the robot arm to perform a task, and the fork-lift can be employed to load the box at the proper height.
The driving mechanism for the work assistive mobile robot is an important issue because the fork-lift must move heavy boxes. We considered two driving mechanisms: forward wheel steering/backward wheel driving and forward wheel driving/backward wheel steering. A forward wheel steering/backward wheel driving mechanism is a popular mechanism for three or four wheel scooters. However, this mechanism is not appropriate for a work assistive robot that has a fork-lift at its front area, especially with regard to steering. A forward wheel driving/backward wheel steering mechanism is also a popular mechanism for commercial forklift trucks, and is more appropriate. Therefore, we adopted a forward wheel driving/backward wheel steering mechanism.

4.1.2 Development of Work Assistive Mobile Robot Type I

Based on the design result of the robot, we developed work assistive mobile robot type I, as shown in Fig. 12. As noted earlier, the work assistive mobile robot type I is based on a forward wheel driving/backward wheel steering mechanism. For this mechanism, the robot has two motors, one for driving and another for steering. The mobile platform is basically controlled by a DSP controller and several peripherals. It also has four limit switches for emergency stopping, and ten ultrasonic sensors to detect obstacles to the rear for collision avoidance. Additionally, a camera is set up in the rear area and a monitor connected with it displays rear objects. The fork-lift system has two actuators to place and lift objects. A MANUS arm is equipped in front of the mobile platform. All components are controlled and communicated through the main system, which is run by a personal computer. Each component of work assistive mobile robot type I such as the robot arm, mobile platform, and fork lift is controlled by a 2-axis joystick, with several operation modes for controlling each component.

Size	650×1400× 550[mm] (width×length×height)
Speed	12[km/h]
Max. Load (Robot)	200 kg
Max. Load (Lift)	60 kg

Table 3. Specifications of work assistive mobile robot type I

From a structural point of view, we divided the work assistive mobile robot system into one main system and three subsystems according to their functions. Fig. 13 shows each module configuration of the robot system.

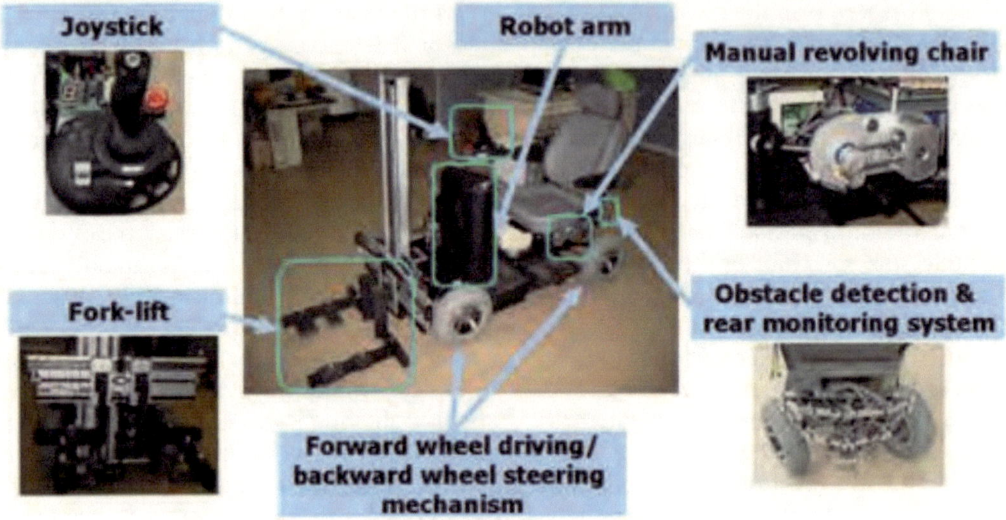

Fig. 12. Developed work assistive mobile robot type I.

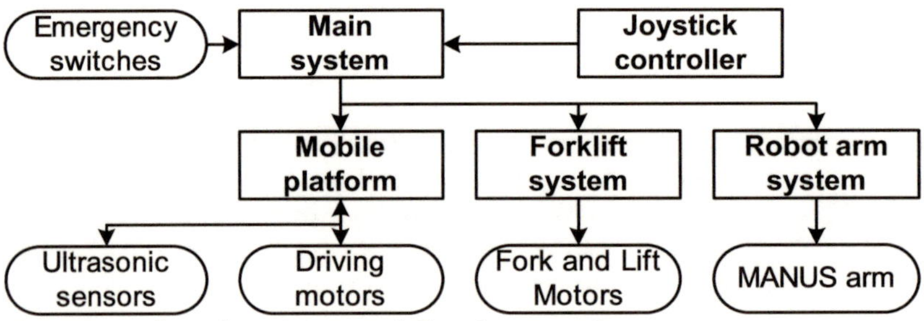

Fig. 13. Architecture of work assistive mobile robot type I.

The main system is a PC that runs RTAI-linux for real-time control. It is connected to subsystems, i.e., the mobile platform, fork-lift system, robot arm system, and the joystick controller. The joystick connection uses a USB communication port of the main computer, whereas others connections are through the RS232 port. Command data is composed of a start byte, data bytes, and an end byte. The number of data bytes corresponds with the number of actuators in each subsystem. For example, a command data from the main system to the mobile platform has one start byte (eight bits), two data bytes, and one end byte. Each data byte has a value between -125 and 125. The start byte value is 126, and the value of the end byte is 127. This short data length speeds up communication.

4.1.3 User-trials

We conducted a series of user-trials of the developed work assistive mobile robot system with the participation of disabled persons who work in actual manufacturing factories, Boram-Dongsan and Mugungwha Electronics in Korea. We gathered their feedback about the robot. The participants were randomly selected among factory workers who have lower-limb or upper-limb impairments or lower-limb and upper-limb impairments. Fig. 14 shows pictures describing the user-trials of work assistive mobile robot system type I.

After conducting the user-trials of work assistive mobile robot system type I, we asked the subjects questions pertaining to the velocities of driving and steering, the convenience of the joystick interface, ease of riding, the risk during driving, and the need for the rear camera. The velocities of moving forward and reversing were confirmed by the respondents as being appropriate. However, they pointed out that the steering speed was slightly slow. This problem was caused by a high reduction ratio gearbox to generate high torque, and was fixed by using a gearbox with a lower gear ratio and a motor with higher torque. The respondents also said the joystick interface was very easy to use. They also reported that they felt safe while moving. This is due to the intuitive joystick control method and the ultrasonic sensor system to avoid collision with obstacles. However, they habitually did not use the rear monitoring system.
Additionally, we identified some shortcomings: (1) the robot arm system is hard to control, and should be smaller or be installed on a work desk; (2) the mobile base and the radius of turning of the robot need to be smaller and the chair needs to be rotated electrically and its should be height lower; and (3) the fork of the fork-lift system should smaller or capable of being folded electrically. We considered these problems for developing the next version, type II.

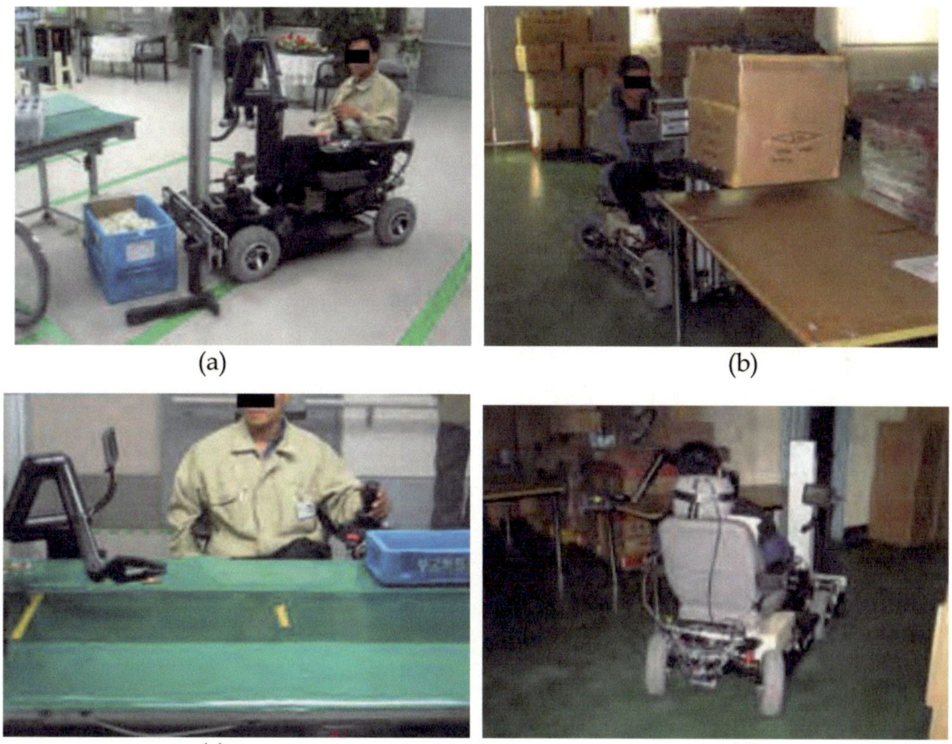

(a) (b)

(c) (d)

Fig. 14. User trials for Work Assistive Mobile Robot System Type I; (a) Moving objects - lifting up, (b) Moving objects - lowering, (c) Working at a desk, (d) Moving around.

4.2 Work Assistive Mobile Robot System Type II

Based on the results of the user-trials of work assistive mobile robot system type I, we developed work assistive mobile robot system type II. The basic function, control system architecture, and the method of user-trials are basically the same as those of type I.

4.2.1 Design of Work Assistive Mobile Robot System Type II

Since a robot arm is chiefly used in table tasks and is not used when the robot moves around, the robot arm is installed on the table, and a foldable fork-lift is incorporated in order to reduce the size of the robot. One very important issue is the driving mechanism. The robot should be capable of moving in a confined space. For this, we adopted an omni-directional wheel driving mechanism. Among the available omni-directional wheels, we use four omni-directional wheels called 'mecanum wheels'. A mecanum wheel consists of one active main wheel and several passive rollers around the main wheel. When the main wheel rotates, a force vector along the wheel and a force vector perpendicular to the wheel are created. The net force, which determines the moving direction of the robot, is created by combining each force vector of the four wheels. By simply controlling the rotation of each wheel without steering them, the robot can move in any direction. Although the power efficiency of the omni-directional mechanism is relatively low and it is difficult to fabricate mecanum wheels, we choose this mechanism since the use of four wheels will guarantee stability. By using the omni-directional wheel driving mechanism, positioning tasks become much easier, especially in narrow aisles, for upper limb impaired workers.

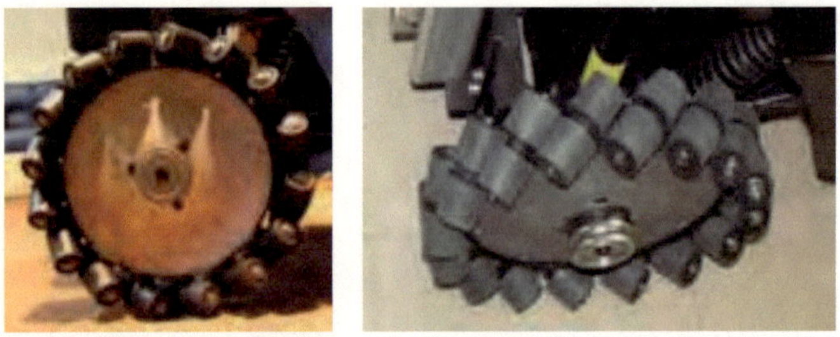

Fig. 15. Mecanum wheel for omni-directional movement.

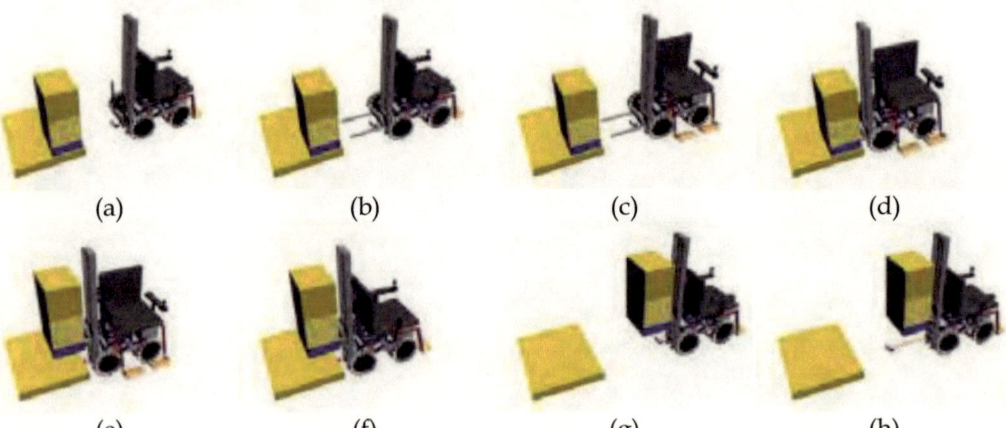

Fig. 16. Scenario of work assistive mobile robot type II; (a) robot moves to the warehouse and orients the rear side to a box on a pallet in the warehouse; (b) the user unfolds the fork using switch; (c) the user rotates the chair using a switch and prepares to extract the box; (d) the robot moves toward the box, and grips the pallet; (e) the user makes the robot raise the fork using a switch; (f) the user rotates the chair using the switch toward forward; (g) the robot moves toward the table; (h) when moving boxes, two sonar sensors are stretched out by DC motors so as not to interfere with boxes on the fork-lift.

Fig. 16 describes the task of moving a box from a warehouse to a work table. When the user simply moves around, the fork is folded, and thus the actual size of the robot is relatively small. When the user picks up boxes, he/she unfolds the fork. While lifting objects, the user can vary the rotation angle to see and check the objects of interest by revolving the chair electrically.

During the transfer of objects, the robot can be used in a confined environment since its steering radius is actually zero. When the user works at a table, the chair can be rotated toward the table.

4.2.2 Development of Work Assistive Mobile Robot System Type II

Fig. 17 shows the developed work assistive mobile robot type II. As noted earlier, for in order to realize a robot with a smaller size and smaller turning radius, we used an omni-directional driving mechanism at the cost of efficiency and excluded the robot arm subsystem. We adopted a foldable fork controlled by motors and equipped the fork-lift system at the rear side. We also adopted an electrically revolving chair so that the user can face the forklift when operating it. Two sonar sensors are used to detect obstacles in the rear. All these components are controlled by a 3-axis joystick and several switches and buttons.

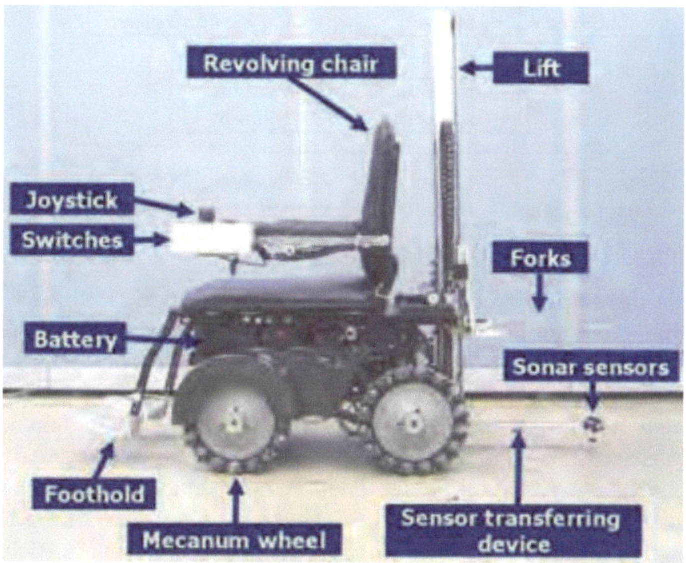

Fig. 17. Developed work assistive mobile robot type II.

Size	760 x 1140 x 510[mm](WxLxH)		
Speed(Robot)	Translation	Slow Mode	2.5 ~ 3[km/h]
		Fast Mode	5[km/h]
	Rotation	45 [deg/s]	
Speed(Chair)	Rotation	18.4 [deg/s]	
Max. Load(Robot)	120 kg		
Max. Load(Lift)	35 kg		

Table 4. Specifications of work assistive mobile robot type II.

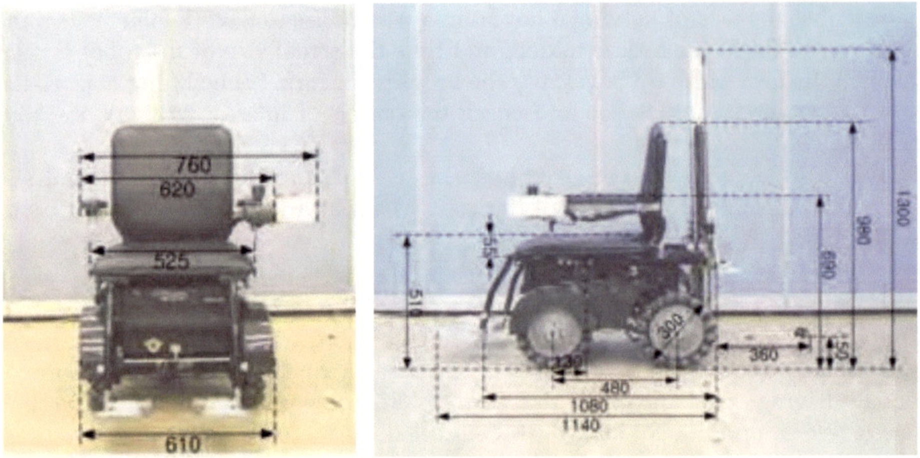

Fig. 18. Developed work assistive mobile robot type II (dimensions in [mm]).

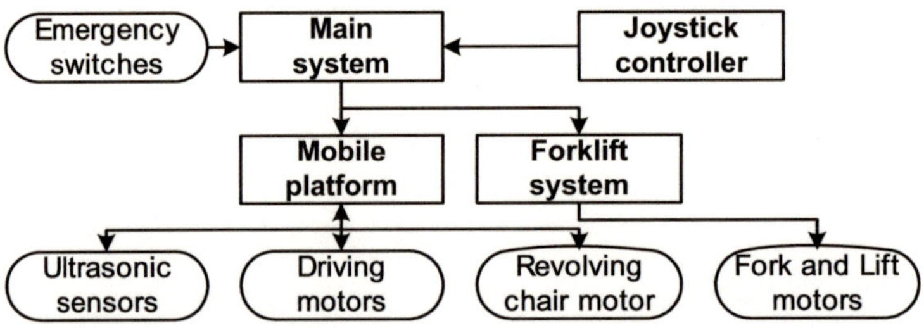

Fig. 19. Architecture of work assistive mobile robot type II.

Fig. 18 shows the developed work assistive mobile robot type II along with its size. The developed robot is small enough to assist in the performance of table tasks. Furthermore, the robot can be parked parallel with the table, and the chair can be rotated to face the table. In addition, the fork is foldable, and the fork-lift can be used as a box feeding device.

The work assistive mobile robot system type II consists of one main system and two subsystems, a mobile platform and a fork lift system. Fig. 19 shows each module configuration. The main system, which is based on FPGA (Field Programmable Gate Array) circuit, receives user input from the joystick controller and emergency switches. According to the user input, the main system gives commands to the mobile platform components such as four driving motors, the revolving chair motor, ultrasonic sensors, and the fork lift system components.

4.2.3 User-trials

Among the enhancements of the work assistive mobile robot system type II, many users applauded the omni-directional mechanism because of its ease of control. Fig. 20 shows pictures of the user-trials.

The participants commented that, "it is very good idea to move boxes when moving around", "the robot is small enough, having a similar size to an electrical wheelchair", "due to the small size, table work is possible without transferring to the table chair", "due to the omni-directional wheel driving mechanism and joystick, it is very easy to control the mobile robot", and "the collision avoidance device helps avoid collisions". However, some participants said, "to avoid collisions in the rear, a rear monitoring system may be needed". This is because the work assistive mobile robot type II does not adopt a rear monitoring system.

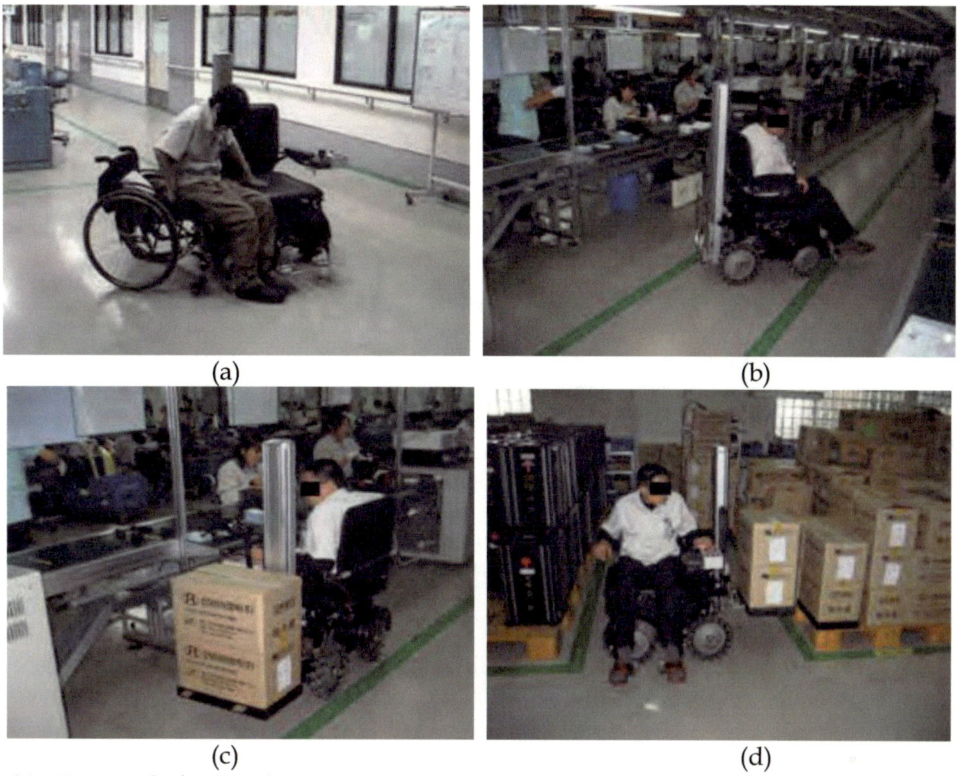

Fig. 20. User trials for Work Assistive Mobile Robot System Type II; (a) Transferring boxes, (b) Moving around, (c) Working at a desk, (d) Moving boxes.

5. Conclusion

Considering the real employment situation of the disabled, it was concluded that there is demand for a robot system that can be used in a real manufacturing environment. To derive our mission statement, we conducted a survey with three criteria: 'A. to assist the disabled as much as possible'; 'B. to consider the real situation of employment for the disabled'; and 'C. to provide assistance for the most necessary tasks for the disabled in the work space'. Based on the survey results, our goal can be stated as follows: To develop work assistive mobile robots to help persons with limb disabilities obtain jobs in manufacturing environments where they can perform simple manual labor. Here, simple labor includes such tasks as circuit inspection and moving boxes.

For our goal, we developed two types of work assistive mobile robots, which are small enough to work in the confined environments of real factories. Work assistive mobile robot type I is equipped with a forklift to move boxes and a robotic arm to help with jobs requiring more dexterity. Robot type II is compact in size, adopting an omni-wheel driving mechanism, and is equipped with a lift having a foldable fork. We gathered feedback from empirical work done on the two robots.

It has been verified by user-trials and feedback that the proposed work assistive robot is capable of assisting a person with a disability to work in a manufacturing environment and perform the same tasks as a normally-abled worker. Further study should be carried out to make the proposed robot more convenient to operate and smaller in size.

6. Acknowledgment

This work was supported by the SRC/ERC program of MOST/KOSEF (grant #R11- 1999-008).

7. References

Bien, Z.; Kim, D. J.; Chung, M. J.; Kwon, D. S. & Chang, P. H. (2003). Development of a wheelchair-based rehab robotic system(KARES II) with various human-robot interaction interfaces for the disabled, *Proceedings of the 2003 IEEE/ASME International Conference on Advanced Intelligent Mechatronics (AIM2003)*, ISBN 0-7803-7759-1, Kobe, Japan, Jul. 2003.

Chang, P. H.; Park , S. R.; Cho, G. R.; Jung, J. H. & Park, S. H. (2005). Development of a robot arm assisting people with disabilities at working place using task-oriented design, *Proceedings of the 9th International Conference on Rehabilitation Robotics (ICORR 2005)*, pp. 482–487, ISBN 0-7803-9004-0, Chicago, IL, USA, Jun. 28 - Jul 1, 2005.

Eftring, H. & Bolmsjö, G. (1993). RAID - A robotic workstation for the disabled, *Proceedings of the 2nd European Conference on the Advancement of Rehabilitation Technology*, pp 24.3, ISBN 91-88336-19-0, Stockholm, Sweden, May 1993.

Hong, H. S.; Jung, S. Y.; Jung, J. H.; Lee, B. G.; Kang, J. W.; Park, D. J. & Chung, M. J. (2005). Development of work assistive mobile robot system for the handicapped in a real manufacturing environment, *Proceedings of the 9th International Conference on Rehabilitation Robotics (ICORR 2005)*, pp. 197–200, ISBN 0-7803-9004-0, Chicago, IL, USA, Jun. 28 - Jul 1, 2005.

Kim, Y.; Park, K. H.; Bang, W. C.; Kim, M. J.; Han, J. S. & Bien, Z. (2002). Development of intelligent bed-robot system for the elderly or the disabled, *Proceedings of 3rd International Workshop on Human-friendly Welfare Robotic Systems(HWRS 2002)*, pp. 94-98, Daejeon, Korea, Jan. 20-22, 2002.

Martens, C.; Ruchel, N.; Lang, O.; Ivlev, O. & Graser, A. (2001). A FRIEND for assisting handicapped people, *Robotics & Automation Magazine*, Vol. 8, issue 1, Mar. 2001, pp. 57-65, ISSN 1070-9932.

Neveryd, H. & Bolmsjö, G. (1994). WALKY, a mobile robot system for the disabled, *Proceedings of the Fourth International Conference on Rehabilitation Robotics (ICORR 1994)*, pp. 137-141, Wilmington, Delaware, USA, Jun. 1994.

Van der Loos, H. F. M.; Wagner, J. J.; Smaby, N.; Chang, K.; Madrigal, O.; Leifer, L. J. & Khatib, O. (1999). ProVAR assistive robot system architecture, *Proceedings of the 1999 IEEE International Conference on Robotics and Automation (ICRA 1999)*, Detroit, pp. 741–746, ISBN 0-7803-5180-0, Michigan, USA, May 1999.

Yoo, D. H.; Hong, H. S.; Kwon, H. J. & Chung, M. J. (2003). Human-friendly care robot system for the elderly, *Proceedings of the 8th International Conference on Rehabilitation Robotics (ICORR 2003)*, pp. 188-191, ISBN 89-88366-09-3, Daejeon, Korea, Apr. 2003.

Yoo, D. H. & Chung, M. J. (2003). Non-contact eye gaze estimation system using robust feature extraction and mapping of corneal reflections, *Proceedings of International Conference of Advanced Robotics (ICAR 2003)*, pp. 911-913, ISBN 972-96889-8-2, Coimbra, Portugal, Jun. 2003.

6

The Evolution and Ergonomics of Robotic-Assisted Surgical Systems

Oussama Elhage, Ben Challacombe, Declan Murphy, Mohammed S Khan, Prokar Dasgupta
Guy's and St Thomas Hospitals NHS Foundation Trust
King's College London, School of Medicine
United Kingdom

1. Introduction

A surgical robot has been defined as "a computer-controlled manipulator with artificial sensing that can be reprogrammed to move and position tools to carry out a range of surgical tasks" (Dasgupta et al, 2005). The first fully automated surgical device used in clinical practice was developed by Wickham (Harris et al, 1997) to resect prostates in the 1980's at Guy's Hospital in London. Currently, robotic devices are available in many surgical specialities fulfilling an increasing number of roles. The most commonly used is the da Vinci™ master-slave system (Intuitive Surgical, Ca, USA). The da Vinci™ system is widely available commercially. It is composed of three components: surgeon console, patient-side cart and image-processing/insufflation stack. Its stereoscopic vision, motion scaling and EndoWrist™ technology with seven degrees of freedom (DOF) are major advancements. By far the most common procedure performed with the assistance of the da Vinci™ system is laparoscopic radical prostatectomy. Other urological procedures performed using robotic assistance include cystectomy, nephrectomy, partial nephrectomy, pyelolithotomy and pyeloplasty. Other specialities adopting this technology include cardiothoracic surgery, gynaecology, and general surgery. Ergonomically ineffectual instruments and monophasic monitors in laparoscopy are linked to surgeon's musculoskeletal injuries and fatigue (Van Der Zee et al, 1997). Robotic surgery offers a different approach for the surgeon's position, with added visual benefits and increased dexterity. Research in the 'dry lab' environment has shown that the robotic techniques, though somewhat slower, offered more precision than conventional laparoscopy (Nio et al, 2002). Laparoscopy naïve surgeons have a shorter learning curve with robotic-assisted techniques compared with equivalent laparoscopic tasks. Research is ongoing in the assessment of fatigue when using robotic-assisted, laparoscopic and open techniques (Elhage et al, 2007). It is suggested that the improved ergonomic conditions offered by robotic systems may allow surgeons to operate more efficiently and with greater precision. As a result patients may have less morbidity and a shorter recovery time.

2. The Evolution of robotics in surgery

2.1 History of surgical robots

Leonardo Da Vinci designed the first robot. It was an automated knight capable of performing basic movements to entertain his patrons (Rosheim, 2006). However, it was not until late in the 20th century that robotic technology became widely available for medical applications. In the 1980's researchers explored the potential of robotics in surgery. Several investigative projects started in the United States (US) and Europe, some independently and some as collaborative work.

2.1.1 Neurosurgery and orthopaedic systems

Initially the greatest potential for robotics was anticipated to be in the fields of neurosurgery and orthopaedics due to their defined parameters and devices such as the ROBODOC (Integrated Surgical Systems, CA, USA) were developed. The hypothesized advantages were: an increase in the three-dimensional (3D) accuracy, increased reproducibility of repeated procedures, increased precision of movements by scaling the motion of the surgeon several times and the ability to perform surgery from a distance (telesurgery). Neurosurgery became a suitable platform for testing early robotic systems because the cranium is a rigid container with fixed landmarks that can be used as data points. Thus stereotactic frames were developed in the late 1980's for the purposes of cranial biopsy and were combined with robots such as the Unimate Puma (Programmable Universal Machine for Assembly, CT, USA) and neuronavigator wand (ISG Technologies, ON, Canada). These consist of robotic arms moved by a surgeon combined with a computer capable of 3D imaging.

A number of robotic frames exist that can assist with surgical procedures. The PUMA 200 robot has been used in the resection of mid-brain tumours in children (Drake et al, 1991), while the Minerva device allows neurosurgical needle placement whilst the patient is within a Computerised Tomography (CT) scanner (Glauser et al, 1995). A frameless image-guided computer controlled system has been launched, the Neuromate (Integrated Surgical Systems), which includes a pre-surgical planning workstation which subsequently interacts with the surgeon during surgery. In orthopaedics, where the bones allow fixed device positioning due to their rigidity, several robots have been developed to perform accurate reaming and cutting of bones to facilitate the insertion of prostheses. By combining increased precision with a digitally stored osseous image, bones can be reamed to provide optimal contact with prosthetic stems such as in uncemented total hip replacements, e.g. ROBODOC (Integrated Surgical Systems) (Cain et al, 1993). This robot, first produced in 1992, is designed for use in primary and revision total hip replacement as well as in total knee replacement. It consists of a preoperative planning workstation (Orthodoc) and a five-axis robotic arm with a high-speed burr as an end effector, which mills the femoral canal for the selected implant chosen beforehand. Orthodoc is used to precisely plan surgery by integrating CT scans of the patient to allow accurate pre-operative implant selection. Clinical studies in the USA using ROBODOC with 65 patients, and with 900 patients in a German study show that the robotic system produces a radiographically better fit and positioning of the implant, and eliminates intra-operative femoral fractures (Bargar et al, 1998). It is vital that this generation of orthopaedic robots are built with safety constraints, as seen with the Acrobot, which allows motion in pre-programmed regions, by the surgeon back-driving the robot motors, while preventing motion in prohibited areas. This active constraint robot (or Acrobot) is programmable and has potential for minimally invasive procedures such as unicompartmental knee replacement (The Acrobot company, 2007).

2.1.2 Automated surgical robotic system

One of the pioneers of robotic surgery was John Wickham, a urologist from Guy's Hospital. He developed the first clinical robot in urology, the PROBOT in 1989. Wickham worked on a transurethral resection of prostate (TURP) robotic frame in a joint project with the mechanical engineering department at Imperial College, Guy's Hospital and the Institute of Urology in London (Harris et al, 1997). The device attempted to perform robotic TURP. As the prostate gland is a relatively fixed organ and the procedure requires repeated similar movements TURP is suited for total robotic control. The frame is constructed to support a six-axis Unimate Puma robot combined with a Wickham Endoscope Liquidizer and Aspirator. The liquidiser blade rotates at 40,000 rpm and initial clinical trials in patients, following successful tests on prostate-shaped potatoes, showed that the PROBOT assisted TURP to be safe, feasible and rapid. Further trials using the PROBOT for TURP resulted in an improvement in patients' symptoms (Harris et al, 1997). One important concept in the design was that the tool could cut only within an ultrasound guided, physically restricted volume, making the device intrinsically safe. Although never mass produced, this was the first truly automated robotic device used clinically, as opposed to the subsequent master-slave devices which were developed in the United Sates.

2.1.3 Master-Slave systems

These devices started in the 1980's as the telepresence system and were collaborative efforts between the National Aeronautics and Space Administration (NASA), which had the expertise in virtual reality, and Stanford Research Institute headed by Philip Green (Satava, 2002). Several years passed before the next generation of robotic devices became available. Computer Motion (Berkeley, CA, USA) first introduced the Automated Endoscopic System for Optimal Positioning (AESOP™) in the mid-1990's. AESOP controls an endoscope in response to the surgeon's commands, using either voice, foot or hand control. By imitating the form and function of a human arm, it eliminates the need for a member of the surgical team to manually control a laparoscopic camera. With precise and consistent movements, AESOP gives the surgeon direct control over a steadier operative field of view. AESOP responds to a vocabulary of 23 commands and was the world's first US Food and Drug Administration (FDA) -cleared surgical robot capable of assisting in minimally invasive procedures (FDA, 1999). Since its introduction, AESOP has assisted in more than 45,000 minimally invasive surgical procedures in more than 350 hospitals internationally. It is now regarded as a standard tool in performing laparoscopic radical prostatectomy and enables independent operating. Laparoscopic images with the AESOP are steadier with less camera changes and inadvertent instrument collisions compared with an inexperienced human assistant (Kavoussi et al, 1995). Another development was the EndoAssist (Armstrong Healthcare, High Wycombe, UK) a free-standing laparoscopic camera manipulator, controlled by infrared signals from a headset worn by the surgeon. It was also introduced in the 1990s (Finlay, 1996). It is considerably less expensive than the AESOP but takes up more space in the operating room.

The first master-slave system was also developed by Computer Motion, the ZEUS Robotic Surgical System, which allowed the surgeon to control laparoscopic instruments at a console remote from the operating table. It was first used on humans in 1998 and in 2001 it allowed a surgeon in New York to perform a laparoscopic cholecystectomy on a patient in Strasbourg, the first reported transatlantic telesurgery (Marescaux et al, 2001). The ZEUS system has now been phased out as a result of the merger of Computer Motion with Intuitive Surgical (Sunnyvale, California, USA) in 2003 paving the way for the development of da Vinci master-slave systems which now dominate the field of robotic-assisted surgery.

2.1.4 Telerobotic surgery and telementoring

An Italian group led by Professor Rovetta performed a number of experiments investigating the possible applications of telerobotics and reported to have carried out the first telerobotic surgery in 1995; a prostate biopsy (Rovetta & Sala, 1995). The field of telerobotics in urology, in particular percutaneous nephrolithotomy (PCNL), has been led by L.R. Kavoussi, D. Stoianovici and the Urobotics team at Baltimore. The percutaneous access robot (PAKY-RCM) was initially developed in 1996 and was superseded by the production of the Tracker in 2003. This can be mounted on the operating table. It has six DOF and can be used with fluoroscopy or CT guidance to improve the accuracy of needle placement. This can provide a precise and reliable method of routinely performing the preliminary step in PCNL or tissue biopsy and can be controlled remotely. The Baltimore group has also telementored several procedures around the world including laparoscopic adrenalectomy, radical nephrectomy, varicocelectomy and renal cyst ablation (Janetschek et al, 1998), (Lee et al, 2000), (Frimberger et al, 2002). The first randomised controlled trial of trans-Atlantic telerobotics was performed between Guy's and Johns Hopkins Hospitals with robotic needle punctures during PCNL into a kidney model controlled remotely. The robot took longer to perform the procedure but was significantly more accurate than a human. There was no difference between trans-Atlantic and local needle insertions with regard to either time or accuracy (Challacombe, et al, 2003)

3 Technology of robotic surgery

3.1 The da Vinci systems

The daVinci is the most advanced master–slave system developed until now. It is not an autonomous robot. The surgeon sits remote from the patient and controls three or four da Vinci robotic arms which are docked through laparoscopic ports at the patient side. The system has three components: (a) a surgeon console, (b) a patient-side cart and (c) an image-processing or insufflation stack. The three-dimensional view from the endoscope is projected in the console at 6-10 magnification. The surgeon's thumb and forefinger control the movements of the robotic arms. Foot pedals allow control of diathermy and other energy sources. Motion scaling enhances the elimination of tremor, allowing very smooth and precise movements. The robotic arms are mounted on the patient-side cart, one of which holds the high-resolution three-dimensional endoscope. Specialised EndoWrist™ (Intuitive Surgical, California, USA) instruments are mounted on the remaining arms. The image-processing/insufflation stack contains the camera-control units for the three-dimensional imaging system, image-recording devices, a laparoscopic insufflator and a monitor allowing two-dimensional vision for the assistants. The three-dimensional vision, enhanced magnification, motion scaling and most importantly the endowrist technology makes easier for the operating surgeon to perform complex laparoscopic procedures (Murphy et al, 2006).

3.2 Current application

Since it became commercially available, the da Vinci system has been used to perform procedures in several surgical specialties including urology, abdominal, thoracic, cardiac, and gynaecological surgery, ranging from complex cancer operations to organ transplantation. However the most commonly performed procedure using the da Vinci systems is radical prostatectomy for localised prostate cancers. Robotic radical prostatectomy was first described by Menon and five years after the introduction of da Vinci system it is expected to be used to perform 48000 cases or 63% of all radical prostatectomies in USA by the end of 2007 (Menon, 2001, 2007). The risks and complications of radical prostatectomy on patients are well recognised and include bleeding and the need for blood transfusion, impotence, urinary incontinence and incomplete clearence of cancer. The early reports on the clinical and functional outcomes suggest that the new technique is as good as the standard open surgical technique in terms of cancer clearance, and may be better in terms of need for transfusion, recovery time, sexual potency and urinary continence (Ficarra et al, 2007). Another operation that is increasingly gaining acceptance in clinical practice is the robotic radical cystectomy; a new technique has been described by Dasgupta (Raychaudhuri et al, 2006). However the lack of randomisation and long term outcome does not allow definite conclusions regarding the superiority or otherwise of the new robotic technology. Other procedures performed using the da Vinci robot are still evolving and results are still scarce.

4. Ergonomics and robotic assisted surgery

4.1 Basics of ergonomics in modern surgery

Ergonomics is derived from the Greek ergon (work) and nomos (laws). Definitions vary, Oxford dictionaries define it as 'the study of people's efficiency in their working environment' (Oxford English Dictionary, 1998). The international ergonomics association (IEA) has a more specific approach and defines it as 'the scientific discipline concerned with the understanding of interactions among humans and other elements of a system, and the profession that applies theory, principles, data and methods to design in order to optimize human well-being and overall system performance'. (IEA website, 2007). IEA divides ergonomics into domains of specialisations. Organisational ergonomics deals with human interaction with work systems and policies. Cognitive ergonomics concentrates on the human mental ability to cope and interact with various work conditions. Physical ergonomics is the study of the effect of working conditions on human body. Interest in ergonomics in surgery has become more important following the introduction of minimal access surgical instruments and systems. Factors affecting efficiency of surgery include access, vision, manoeuvrability and the ease of using instruments. Open surgery provides the surgeon with excellent exposure, direct vision of the operative field and user-friendly instruments. Minimally-invasive surgical techniques including laparoscopic surgery offer significant advantages for patients in terms of lower morbidity and reduced recovery times. Factors affecting efficiency of surgery include access, vision, manoeuvrability and the ease of using instruments. But these instruments are not always as easy to manoeuvre as open surgical tools. Minimally-invasive surgical techniques offer significant advantages for patients in terms of lower morbidity and reduced recovery times. By contrast to open surgery, the technical challenges to laparoscopic surgery may lead cumulatively to specific ergonomic problems for the surgeon. Laparoscopic surgeon has to learn to adapt to monoscopic vision in 2 dimensions (2D). Tendick et al found that 2D monoscopic display decrease operator accuracy and increase movement time. Manipulation of long laparoscopic instruments causes a number of problems. There is a fulcrum effect at the point of trocar insertion through the abdominal wall, where hand movement to the right produces a movement to the left at the tip of the instrument at the operative field. Instruments are long and move in a cone-shaped way with the tip of the cone at the trocar's insertion point of the abdominal wall. Arc-like movements of the upper extremity are necessary to produce small movements of the end effector. Laparoscopic surgery allows 4 DOF at the operative site restricting manoeuvrability to great extent. During laparoscopic surgery the majority of the surgeon's movements are at the level of the hands, wrists and, to a lesser degree, the shoulders. The rest of the body is in an upright position which may be responsible for the neck and back discomfort associated with laparoscopy. A team from Sacramento video taped laparoscopic surgeons while operating and noted the awkward upper extremity movements of the surgeon and a static trunk and neck position (Nguyen et al, 2001), Berguer et al studied various types of laparoscopic handles. They recorded the positions and the electromyographic (EMG) signals of the wrists and forearms of surgeons using the instruments and found that higher degree of muscles contractions are required compared to open surgery and with laparoscopic handles often extreme positions of flexion and ulnar deviation at the wrist are required to perform a task (Berguer et al, 1998). Hemal et al reported many musculoskeletal injuries associated with laparoscopic surgery. When asking 131 laparoscopic surgeons 22% complained of eye strains, 18% of arm, shoulder, and finger numbness. Neck, back and forearm pain were among the common complaints (Hemal et al, 2001). These problems increase the overall fatigue of the surgeon and restrict the number of minimally invasive procedures that can be done by single surgeon in a given operative session.

The master-slave robotic surgical systems may help resolve some of the ergonomic problems described above. The surgeon is seated at a console remote from the patient, providing a much more ergonomic posture than that of the traditional patient-side surgeon. The finger-tip controls allow "intuitive" rather than "fulcrum"-type control over the laparoscopic instruments, thereby reducing fatigue in the upper extremity and neck. The complex surgical tasks e.g. (suturing) are made easier by the EndoWrist technology which allows an overall 7 DOF as compared to 4 DOF for laparoscopy. Another advantage is the 3D stereoscopic vision with enhanced magnifications and motion scaling of surgeon's hand movements down to the site of operation. This allows the surgeon to feel almost immersed in the operative field. Jourdan et al conducted a study where they compared tasks performed under either monoscopic or stereoscopic vision and found that stereoscopic vision provides a significant advantage (Jourdan et al, 2004). Another aspect of robotic assisted surgery was studied by a team from Amsterdam; they compared laparoscopy and robotic assisted surgery by asking expert laparoscopists and medical students to complete validated tasks. The students who were laparoscopy and robotics naïve required more time to perform equally accurate tasks compared with experienced laparoscopic surgeons (Nio et al, 2001). In a more recent study, Berguer and Smith studied the physical and mental workload of laparoscopic and robotic assisted surgery during a surgical conference. Surgeons performed simulated tasks while the investigators recorded errors and EMG

signals for physical workload, and assessed skin conductance for mental workload. They found that robotic assisted technique was slower and less precise than laparoscopic for simple tasks; however they were equally fast for complex techniques and possibly less stressful (Berguer & Smith, 2006).
We are currently comparing the impact of physical activity of both techniques on surgeons in a dry lab setting. Standard tasks are performed using open, laparoscopic and robotically assisted techniques. EMG sensors record muscular activity; motion capture cameras capture postural variation. An analysis of the obtained data will allow objective comparison of these techniques and will help to understand the impact on surgeons. (Figure 1)

4.2 Advantages and disadvantages

As we have seen in previous sections, robotic surgery offers accurate dissections, less blood loss, quick recovery of patient; it probably is more ergonomically effective compared to other minimally invasive techniques. However this technology is still out of the reach of many healthcare institutions, especially the public sector due to the high initial costs (£750,000), maintenance (£70,000/year) and the cost of consumables. An important disadvantage is the lack of tactic feedback. The surgeon is not able to feel for the tissue however surgeons learn to adapt to visual feedback to compensate. Research in this field is still inconclusive and bridging this problem would take robotic surgery to a higher level. Other disadvantages are summarised in table 1 below.

4.3 Future

Recently Intuitive Surgical introduced the da Vinci S which has improved maneuveriblilty, faster set up time, and improved video display. The next generation of da Vinci is expected to have a smaller console and surgical cart, and possibly haptic feedback technology. Preoperative imaging e.g. CT, Magnetic Resonance Imaging (MRI) may be integrated in the system to help the surgeon plan surgery. A new concept of robot built with non-magnetic or dielectric materials is being developed by the team from Baltimore led by Stoianovici. This development will allow the compatibility of robotics with MR imaging, thus allowing MRI guided robotic procedures (Muntener, 2006). However the most exciting next generation of robots are nanorobots which are micron small robots which could be able to deliver targeted gene therapy (Murphy et al, 2006). Robotic surgery is in its infancy and certainly is growing fast.

Advantages	Three-dimensional visualisation Enhanced degrees of freedom No fulcrum effect Motion scaling Elimination of tremor Reduced fatigue Ergonomic positioning
Disadvantages	Expensive capital and running costs No tactile feedback Reduced trainee experience Set-up times lengthy

Table 1. Advantages and disadvantages of robotic surgery (Murphy et al, 2006).

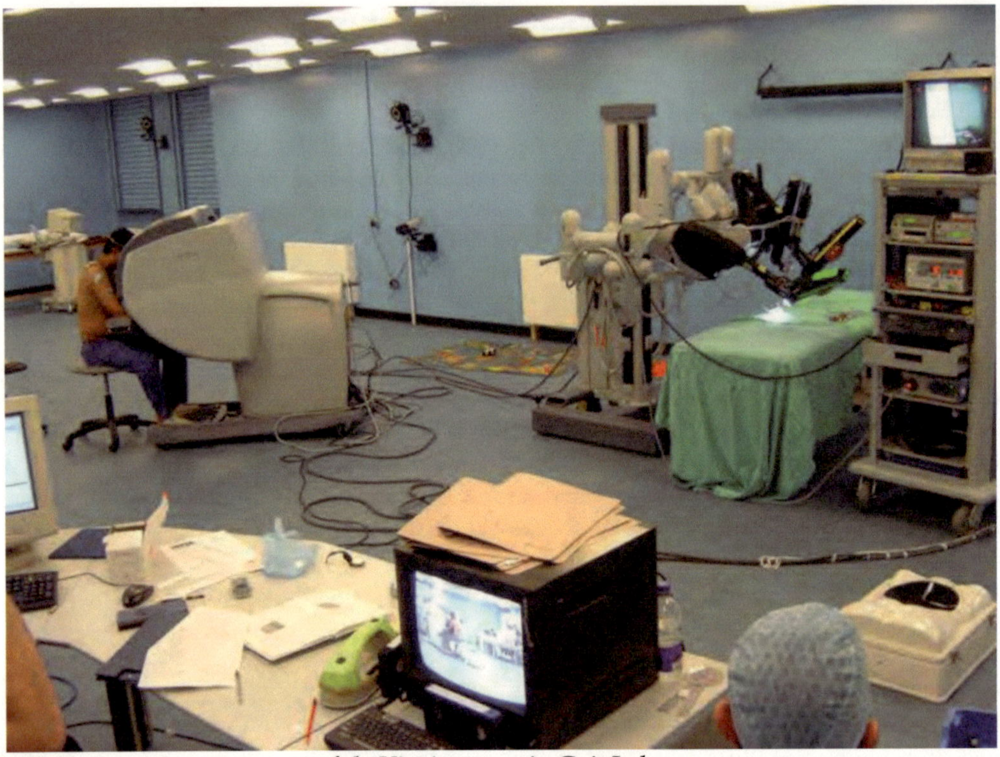

Fig. 1. Ergonomic assessment of da Vinci system in Gait Lab.

Acknowledgement to Dr Adam Shortland, Clinical Scientist and Manager of One Small Step Gait Laboratory, Guy's Hospital, London

5. References

Acrobot. The Acrobot Company Limited , www.acrobot.co.uk. Accessed on: 26-3-2007. Ref Type: Electronic Citation

Bargar, W. L., Bauer, A., & Borner, M. (1998). "Primary and revision total hip replacement using the Robodoc system", *Clin.Orthop.Relat Res.* no. 354, pp. 82-91.

Berguer, R., Gerber, S., Kilpatrick, G., & Beckley, D. (1998) "An ergonomic comparison of in-line vs pistol-grip handle configuration in a laparoscopic grasper", *Surg Endosc.*, vol. 12, no. 6, pp. 805-808.

Berguer, R. & Smith, W. (2006). "An ergonomic comparison of robotic and laparoscopic technique: the influence of surgeon experience and task complexity", *J Surg Res.*, vol. 134, no. 1, pp. 87-92.

Cain, P., Kazanzides, P., Zuhars, J., Mittelstadt, B., & Paul, H. (1993). "Safety considerations in a surgical robot", *Biomed.Sci.Instrum.*, vol. 29, pp. 291-294.

Challacombe, B. J., Kavoussi, L. R., & Dasgupta, P. (2003). "Trans-oceanic telerobotic surgery", *BJU Int*, vol. 92, no. 7, pp. 678-680.

Dasgupta, P., Jones, A., & Gill, I. S. (2005). "Robotic urological surgery: a perspective", *BJU Int*, vol. 95, no. 1, pp. 20-23.

Drake, J. M., Joy, M., Goldenberg, A., & Kreindler, D. (1991). "Computer- and robot-assisted resection of thalamic astrocytomas in children", *Neurosurgery*, vol. 29, no. 1, pp. 27-33.
Elhage, O., Challacombe, B., Murphy, D., & Dasgupta, P. (2007). "Ergonomics in minimally invasive surgery", *Int J Clin.Pract.*
Ergonomics definition (1998). *The New Oxford Dictionary of English*, Pearsall J., ed., Oxford University Press, p. 624.
Ergonomics definition (2007). *The International Ergonomics Association website* , http://www.iea.cc/ergonomics/, accessed: 26/03/2007,Ref Type: Electronic Citation
Ficarra, V., Cavalleri, S., Novara, G., Aragona, M., & Artibani, W. (2007). "Evidence from robot-assisted laparoscopic radical prostatectomy: a systematic review", *Eur Urol*, vol. 51, no. 1, pp. 45-56.
Finlay P.A. (1996). "Clinical experience with a goniometric head-controlled laparoscopic manipulator", in *IARP Workshop on Medical Robotics*. October 1996, Vienna.
Frimberger, D., Kavoussi, L., Stoianovici, D., Adam, C., Zaak, D., Corvin, S., Hofstetter, A., & Oberneder, R. (2002). "[Telerobotic surgery between Baltimore and Munich]", *Urologe A*, vol. 41, no. 5, pp. 489-492.
Glauser, D., Fankhauser, H., Epitaux, M., Hefti, J. L., & Jaccottet, A. (1995). "Neurosurgical robot Minerva: first results and current developments", *J Image Guid.Surg*, vol. 1, no. 5, pp. 266-272.
Harris, S. J., Arambula-Cosio F., Mei, Q., Nathan, M. S., Hibberd, R. D., & Wickham, J. E. (1997). "The Probot-an active robot for prostate resection.", *Proc Inst Mech Eng*, vol. 211, pp. 317-325.
Hemal, A. K., Srinivas, M., & Charles, A. R. (2001). "Ergonomic problems associated with laparoscopy", *J Endourol.*, vol. 15, no. 5, pp. 499-503.
Janetschek, G., Bartsch, G., & Kavoussi, L. R. (1998). "Transcontinental interactive laparoscopic telesurgery between the United States and Europe", *J Urol.*, vol. 160, no. 4, p. 1413.
Jourdan, I. C., Dutson, E., Garcia, A., Vleugels, T., Leroy, J., Mutter, D., & Marescaux, J. (2004). "Stereoscopic vision provides a significant advantage for precision robotic laparoscopy", *Br.J Surg*, vol. 91, no. 7, pp. 879-885.
Kavoussi, L. R., Moore, R. G., Adams, J. B., & Partin, A. W. (1995). "Comparison of robotic versus human laparoscopic camera control", *J Urol*, vol. 154, no. 6, pp. 2134-2136.
Lee, B. R., Png, D. J., Liew, L., Fabrizio, M., Li, M. K., Jarrett, J. W., & Kavoussi, L. R. (2000). "Laparoscopic telesurgery between the United States and Singapore", *Ann.Acad.Med.Singapore*, vol. 29, no. 5, pp. 665-668.
Marescaux J, L. J. G. M. e. al. (2001). "Transatlantic robot-assisted telesurgery.", *Nature*, vol. 413, pp. 379-380.
Menon, M. (2007). "The future of robotics in urology", in *Eurpean Association of Urology*. March, 2007, Berlin.
Muntener, M., Patriciu, A., Petrisor, D., Mazilu, D., Bagga, H., Kavoussi, L., Cleary, K., & Stoianovici, D. (2006). "Magnetic resonance imaging compatible robotic system for fully automated brachytherapy seed placement", *Urology*, vol. 68, no. 6, pp. 1313-1317.
Murphy, D., Challacombe, B., Khan, M. S., & Dasgupta, P. (2006). "Robotic technology in urology", *Postgraduate Medical Journal*, vol. 82, no. 973, pp. 743-747.

Nguyen, N. T., Ho, H. S., Smith, W. D., Philipps, C., Lewis, C., De Vera, R. M., & Berguer, R. (2001). "An ergonomic evaluation of surgeons' axial skeletal and upper extremity movements during laparoscopic and open surgery", *Am.J Surg*, vol. 182, no. 6, pp. 720-724.

Nio, D., Bemelman, W. A., Den Boer, K. T., Dunker, M. S., Gouma, D. J., & van Gulik, T. M. (2002). "Efficiency of manual vs robotical (Zeus) assisted laparoscopic surgery in the performance of standardized tasks", *Surg Endosc.*, vol. 16, pp. 412-415.

Raychaudhuri B., Khan M. S., Challacombe B., Rimington P., Dasgupta P. (2006). Minimally invasive radical cystectomy. *BJU Int.* vol. 98, no. 5, pp. 1064-7.

Rosheim, M. E. (2006). *Leonardo's lost robots* Springer, Berlin.

Rovetta A, Sala. R. (1995). "Robotics and telerobotics applied to a prostate biopsy on a human patient.". proceedings of: *Second Symposium on Medical Robotics and Computer Assisted Surgery*. Baltimore.

Satava, R. M. (2002). "Surgical robotics: the early chronicles: a personal historical perspective", *Surg Laparosc.Endosc.Percutan.Tech.*, vol. 12, no. 1, pp. 6-16.

Tendick F. & Cavusoglu M.C. (1997). "Human-Machine interfaces for minimally invasive surgery", in *19th Annual International Conference of the IEEE Engineering in Medicine and Biology Society*, Chicago, pp. 2771-2776.

Tewari, A., Peabody, J., Sarle, R., Balakrishnan, G., Hemal, A., Shrivastava, A., & Menon, M. (2002). "Technique of da Vinci robot-assisted anatomic radical prostatectomy", *Urology*, vol. 60, no. 4, pp. 569-572.

Van Der Zee, D. C. & Bax, N. M. A. (1995). "Digital nerve compression due to laparoscopic surgery", *Surg Endosc.*, vol. 9, no. 740.

7

Design and Implementation of a Control Architecture for Rehabilitation Robotic Systems

Duygun Erol & Nilanjan Sarkar
Vanderbilt University
USA

1. Introduction

Stroke is a highly prevalent condition especially among the elderly that results in high costs to the individual and society (Matchar & Duncan, 1994). According to the American Heart Association, in the U.S., approximately 700,000 people suffer a first or recurrent stroke each year (American Heart Association, 2006). It is a leading cause of disability, commonly involving deficits of motor function.

Recent clinical results have indicated that movement assisted therapy can have a significant beneficial impact on a large segment of the population affected by stroke or other motor deficit disorders. Experimental evidence suggests that intensive movement training of new motor tasks is required to induce long-term brain plasticity. The availability of movement training techniques, however, is limited by the amount of costly therapist's time they involve and the ability of the therapist to provide controlled, quantifiable and repeatable assistance to arm movement. Consequently, robot assisted rehabilitation that can quantitatively monitor and adapt to patient's progress, ensure consistency during rehabilitation may provide a solution to these problems.

In the last few years, robot-assisted rehabilitation for physical rehabilitation of the stroke patients has been an active research area to assist, monitor, and quantify rehabilitation therapies (Krebs et al., 2004, Lum et al., 2006, Kahn et al., 2006a, Kahn et al., 2006b, Loureiro et al., 2003). These robotic devices are used to recover arm movement after stroke, which provide opportunities for repetitive movement exercise and more standardized delivery of therapy with the potential of enhancing quantification of the therapeutic process. The first robotic assistive device used as a therapeutic tool, the MIT Manus (Krebs et al., 2003, Krebs et al., 2004) uses impedance controller to provide assistance to move patient's arm to the target position in an active assisted mode, where patients can visually see their movement and target location. In (Krebs et al., 2004) they expand the capabilities of MIT Manus to include motion in a three-dimensional workspace to rehabilitate other muscle groups and limb segments than shoulder and elbow. The Mirror Image Movement Enabler (MIME) and the Assisted Rehabilitation and Measurement (ARM) Guide, expanded the investigations of therapeutic applications of robots into the chronic stroke population. MIME uses a PUMA 560 manipulator to provide assistance to move the participant's arm with a pre-programmed position trajectory using Proportional-Integral-Derivative (PID) controller (Lum et al., 2006). ARM Guide is capable of generating both horizontal and vertical motion, and giving resistance and support to the patient (Kahn et al., 2006a, Kahn et al., 2006b). The

GENTLE/s (Loureiro et al., 2003) is a haptic robot used to provide assistance to patients to move to the target positions along with a predefined path using admittance control. The participant's movement trajectory is represented in the virtual environment.

The promising results of the above-mentioned rehabilitation robotic systems indicate that robots could be used as effective rehabilitation tools. Current theories of stroke rehabilitation point towards paradigms of intense and repetitive use of the affected limb as a means for motor program reorganization. However, it has also been demonstrated in (Carey et al., 2005) that repetitive execution of simple motor tasks may not be as effective as execution of more complex motor tasks that involve in-depth cognitive processing. Precision-demanding tasks that challenge motor learning processes create richer conditions for change in the brain reorganization on rats (Black et al., 1990, Kleim et al., 2002), primates (Plautz et al., 2000, Nudo et al., 1996) and human (Pascual-Leone et al., 1995). It was shown that movement tracking training that requires cognitive processing achieved greater gains in performance than that of movement training that did not require cognitive processing (Carey et al., 2005). Additionally, it was shown that finger movement tracking training produced greater gains in the range of motion and tracking accuracy compared to finger movement training that required no temporospatial processing (Carey et al., 2006). Thus, it would be useful if a tracking movement training method can be developed, where the patients not only make repetitive movement but also pay attention to tracking accuracy. However, in such a tracking task, patients may not be able to track the desired motion because of their impairments. Thus, a low-level controller can be designed to provide assistance to the patient to track the desired motion accurately based on his/her performance.

The existing robotic rehabilitation systems primarily use low-level assistive controllers to assist the movement of patients' arms. For example, MIT Manus uses an impedance controller, MIME uses a PID controller and GENTLE/s uses an admittance controller for movement assistance. In some cases, the rehabilitation system keeps track of the status of the task (e.g., AutoCITE (Taub et al., 2005)). However, to our knowledge, none of these systems has a dedicated high-level controller that can comprehensively monitor the task, provide assessment of the progress, and alter the task parameters to impart effective therapy based on patient's performance in an automated manner. Instead, in these existing robotic rehabilitation systems, a therapist administers the therapy where he/she monitors the progress of the tasks, patient's safety, and assess whether the task needs to be updated based on current condition of the therapy. As a result, it is likely to consume more time of the therapist, increase workload of the therapist, and consequently, increase the cost of treatment. In the current work, we present the design and development of a high-level controller that work in conjunction with the low-level controllers such that it can determine the task updates dynamically based on patients' performance; and monitor the safety related events in an automated manner and generate an accommodating plan of action.

In this chapter, we present a new control architecture which consists of a low-level controller and a high-level controller. The low-level controller is used to provide robotic assistance as and when needed to the participants to complete an upper arm rehabilitation task. This task is designed to impart movement training that requires cognitive processing. The high-level controller is used to monitor the progress of the rehabilitation task and make decisions on the modification of the task that might be needed for the therapy. In order to demonstrate the efficacy of the proposed control architecture, we needed to develop a rehabilitation robotic system, which is also presented in this chapter.

This chapter is organized as follows. It first presents the overall control architecture in Section 2. Then the rehabilitation robotic system is presented in Section 3. The low-level controller and the high-level controller have been described in Section 4 and Section 5, respectively. Results of the experiments are presented in Section 6 to demonstrate the efficacy of the low-level controller and the high-level controller on unimpaired participants. Section 7 discusses potential contributions of this work and possible directions for future work.

2. Control Architecture

The patients are asked to perform a rehabilitation task. However, the patients may not be able to complete the rehabilitation task because of their motor impairment. A low-level controller could be used to provide robotic assistance to participants' arm movement as and when needed to help them to complete the reaching task. Note that various robot, human and general task related information, called events, could affect the reaching task. For example, if the robot joint motor develops any fault; or if the patient feels uncomfortable he/she might want to stop the task; or the patient is more than capable of performing the current task and he/she needs more challenging task etc. These set of information may require some adjustments of the planning of the task. As a result, the low-level controller also needs to be aware of these adjustments of the task to accomplish the therapy requirements.

In order to provide therapy that can accommodate the above requirements, a high-level controller could be used in conjunction with the low-level controller that monitors the task and patient's safety and informs the low-level controller about the task updates. The high-level controller in here plays the role of a human supervisor (therapist) who would otherwise monitor the task and assess whether the task needs to be updated. However, in general, the high-level controller and the low-level controller cannot communicate directly because each may require different types of inputs and outputs. For example, a high-level controller may operate in the discrete domain whereas a low-level controller may operate in the continuous domain. Thus an interface is required which can convert continuous-time signals to sequences of discrete values and vice versa. Hybrid system theory provides mathematical tools that can accommodate both continuous and discrete system in a unified manner. As a result, in this work, we take the advantage of using a hybrid system model to design our control architecture. A hybrid system model has three parts, a "Plant", a "Controller" (supervisor) and an Interface (Koutsoukos et al., 2000, Antsaklis & Koutsoukos, 2003). In order to avoid confusion about terminology, we call the "Controller" in hybrid system model a high-level controller. The continuous part, identified as the "Plant" is the low-level controller. Fig. 1 presents the proposed control architecture. There has been no work to our knowledge on designing such a hybrid system for rehabilitation purposes. However, in this chapter, we argue that such a hybrid system framework could be useful in automating robotic rehabilitation and providing important aid to the therapist. Hybrid control framework has been effectively used in other fields, such as industrial robotics, medicine, and manufacturing (Antsaklis & Koutsoukos, 2003).

In this architecture (Fig. 1), the state information from the robot and the human is monitored by the process-monitoring module through the interface to trigger the relevant events. Each event is represented as a plant symbol so that the high-level controller can recognize the event. Once the high-level controller receives the event through a plant symbol, the decision making module of the high-level controller generates sequences of control actions using its decision rules. The high-level controller is designed considering the need of the therapist and the patient and it can be easily modified and extended for new task requirements. The decision of the high-level controller is sent to the low-level controller through the interface using the control symbols. Interface converts the control symbols to the plant inputs which are used to update the task. The updated task is then executed by the low-level controller. This cycle continues to complete the therapy.

The proposed control architecture is flexible and extendible in the sense that new events can be included and detected by simply monitoring the additional state information from the human and the robot, and accommodated by introducing new decision rules and new low-level controllers.

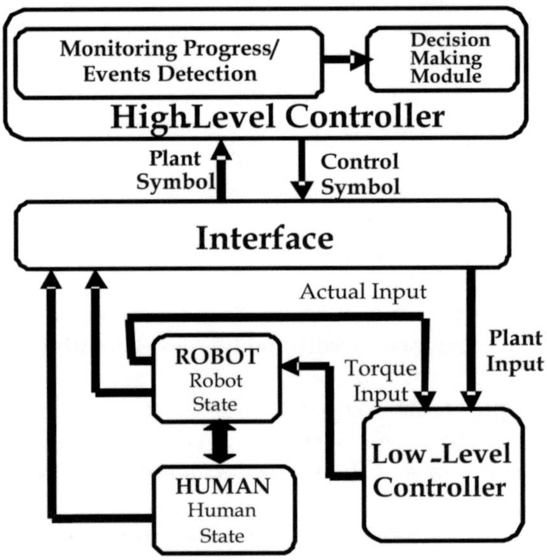

Fig. 1. Control Architecture.

3. The Rehabilitation Robotic System

A PUMA 560 robotic manipulator is used as the main hardware platform in this work. The manipulator is augmented with a force-torque sensor and a hand attachment device (Fig. 2).

3.1 Hardware

The PUMA 560 is a 6 degrees-of-freedom (DOF) device consisting of six revolute joints (PUMA web site). In order to record the force and torque applied by the human, an ATI Gamma force/torque sensor is used. The robot is interfaced with Matlab/Real-time Workshop to allow fast and easy system development. The force values recorded from the force/torque sensor are obtained using a National Instruments PCI-6031E data acquisition card with a sampling time of 0.001 seconds. The joint angles of the robot are measured using encoder with a sample time of 0.001 seconds from a Measurement Computing PCI-QUAD04 card. The torque output to the robot is provided by a Measurement Computing PCIM-DDA06/16 card with the same sample time. A computer monitor is placed in front of the participant to provide visual feedback about his/her motion trajectory during the execution of the task.

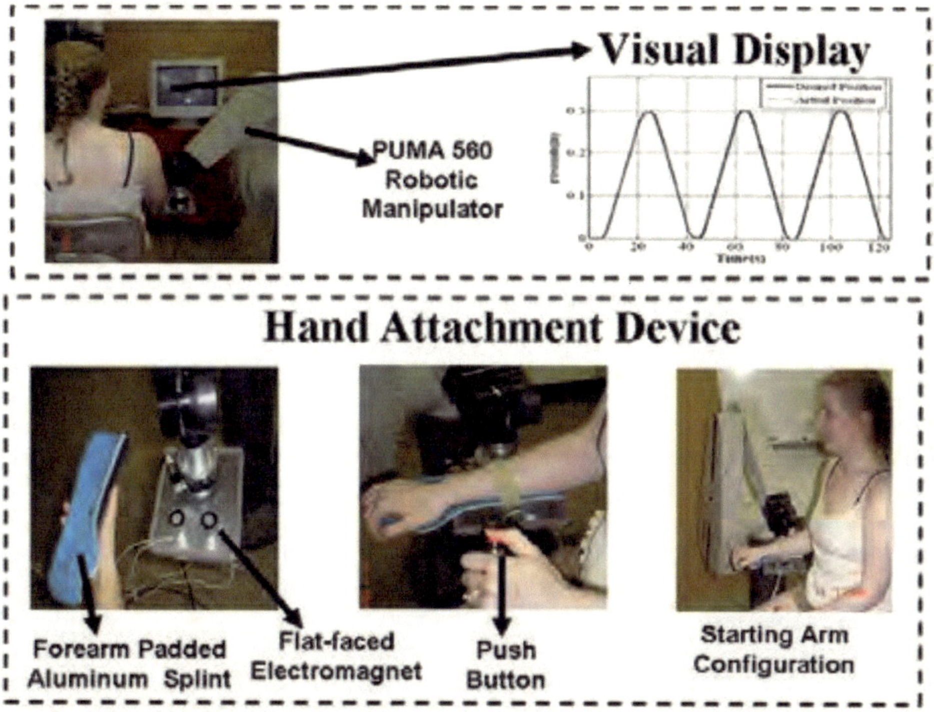

Fig. 2. Participant Arm Attached to Robot.

3.2 Hand Attachment Device

Since in this work we are primarily interested in effecting assistance to the upper arm, we design a hand attachment device where the participant's arm is strapped into a splint that restricts wrist and hand movement. The PUMA 560 is attached to that splint to provide assistance to the upper arm movement using the low-level controller (Fig. 2). Forearm padded aluminum splint (from MooreMedical), which ensures the participant's comfort, is used as a splint in this device. We further design a steel plate with proper grooves that hold two small flat-faced electromagnets (from Magnetool Inc.) that are screwed on it. This plate is also screwed with the force-torque sensor, which provides a rigid connection with the robot. We attach a light-weight steel plate under the splint, which is then attached to the electromagnets of the plate. These electromagnets are rated for continuous duty cycle (100% duty cycle), i.e., they can run continuously at normal room temperature. Pull ratings of these magnets are 40lb. We have used two electromagnets to have a larger pulling force to keep the splint attached to the hand attachment device. An automatic release (AU) rectifier controller (Magnetool Inc.) has been used to provide a quick, clean release of these electromagnets. A push button, which has been connected to the AU Rectifier Controller, is used to magnetize and demagnetize the electromagnets when the participant wants to remove the hand attachment device from the robotic manipulator in a safe and quick manner.

3.3 Discussion on Safety of the Rehabilitation Robotic System

Ensuring safety of the participant is a very important issue when designing a rehabilitation robotic system. Thus, in case of emergency situations, therapist can press emergency button. The patient and/or the therapist can quickly release the patient's arm from the PUMA 560 by using the quick-release hand attachment device (as described above) to deal with any physical safety related events. In order to release the participant's arm from the robot, the push button is used. When the push button is pressed electromagnets are demagnetized instantaneously and the participant is free to remove the splint from the robot. This push button can also be operated by a therapist. Additionally, we have covered the corner of the arm device with a foam self stick tape in order to avoid sharp surface.

4. Low-Level Controller

The objectives of the current work is to: i) design an upper arm movement rehabilitation task that requires cognitive processing as well as could contribute to a variety of functional daily living activities, and ii) design a controller to provide robotic assistance to help participants to perform the above movement rehabilitation task. In what follows we present the basic design of the task and the low-level controller.

4.1. Task Design

Let us first briefly review the task design of some well-known robotic rehabilitation systems. MIT Manus uses impedance controller to provide assistance to move patient's arm to the target position in an active assisted mode, where patients can visually see their movement and target location (Krebs et al., 2003, et al., 2004). MIME provides assistance to move the participant's arm with a pre-programmed position trajectory using proportional-integral-derivative (PID) controller (Lum et al., 2006). The participant is asked to maintain a specified off-axis force while they are trying to reach toward a goal position using ARM Guide (Kahn et al., 2006a, Kahn et al., 2006b). The GENTLE/s provides assistance to patients to move to the target positions along with a predefined path using admittance control. The participant's movement trajectory is represented in the virtual environment in (Loureiro et al., 2003). The therapy tasks designed for the rehabilitation robotic devices require predominantly shoulder motion or elbow motion, or some of them require the combination of both shoulder and elbow motion.

We choose a reaching task that is commonly used for rehabilitation of upper extremity after stroke. In this task, the participants are asked to move their arms in the forward direction to reach a desired point in space and then bring it back to the starting position repeatedly within a specified time. In other words, they have to follow a desired position trajectory. The reaching task designed in here requires combination of the shoulder and elbow movement which could increase the active range of motion (AROM) in shoulder and elbow in preparation of later functional reaching activities in rehabilitation. The allowable motion is restricted only to the direction of the task. For example, if the task requires the participants to move their arms in the Y-direction, then they will not be able to move their arms in X or Z directions. However, they can move their arms in the Y-direction at a velocity that could be the same, higher or lower than the desired velocity. The idea here is to improve the ability of participant's arm movement in one direction at a time by helping them to improve their speed of movement. Improving the speed of movement for such tasks is an important criterion to measure the success of a therapy. For example, in Constraint Induced Movement Therapy (CIMT) (Taub et al., 1999) during the performance of the wipe table task, participants are required to complete as many back and forth motion as possible in a certain amount of time across the table and back between the two targets. The number of times of the completed movement in a certain amount of time is used as a metric to evaluate the participants' progress. If participants can improve their speed of movement, the metric described above will capture this progress. In this work, we constrain the motion of the arm in the horizontal plane and in one direction (along the Y-axis). Although, in this work the motion of the arm is constrained in the horizontal plane in one direction (along the Y-axis), it could also be designed for other directions (e.g., X-axis) or combination of directions (e.g., XY-axes) based on task requirements (only shoulder or elbow motion or the combination of shoulder and elbow motion).

In order to include cognitive processing within this reaching task, we ask the participants to follow a visually presented desired motion trajectory that is likely to command their concentration. The participants receive visual feedback of both their actual position and the desired position trajectories on a computer screen, which is placed in front of them. They are asked to pay attention to tracking the desired position trajectory as accurately as possible, which keeps them focused on the task. The visual feedback is used not only to inform the participants of how closely they are tracking the desired motion but also as a motivational factor to keep them focused on the task. The tip of the position trajectory that the participant is required to follow represents the velocity of the task trajectory.

The task presented here incorporates cognitive processing by asking the participants to follow the tip of the visually presented trajectory. The tip of the trajectory represents the current desired velocity. By asking the participant to follow the tip makes him/her focused on the task. This task is different from other tasks that have been used in the context of robotic rehabilitation in that here we are interested in improving the speed of motion in one direction at a time using visual feedback, which could be useful in a number of therapy tasks.

4.2. Controller Design

The controller designed in this work is responsible for providing robotic assistance to a participant to complete the movement tracking task in an accurate manner. The existing robotic rehabilitation systems operate in robot task-space to provide robotic assistance to the patients to follow a desired trajectory to complete a rehabilitation task (Krebs et al., 2004, Lum et al., 2006, Kahn et al., 2006a, Kahn et al., 2006b). Recently, a human-arm joint impedance controller is proposed, which operates in joint-space, to provide assistance to participants to follow desired joint angle trajectory (Culmer et al., 2005) specified for each individual joint (e.g., elbow joint). It is still not clear, however, whether the assistance in the task-space or in the joint-space will likely to have the best results for rehabilitation purposes. In this work, we design a controller that is responsible for providing the robotic assistance to participants to complete a rehabilitation task in task-space (Erol & Sarkar, 2007). In this controller, an outer force feedback loop is designed around an inner position loop (Fig. 3). The tracking of the reference trajectory is guaranteed by the inner motion control (Sciavicco & Siciliano, 1996). The desired force, which is given as a force reference to the controller, is computed by a planner. The proposed controller is similar to an impedance controller; however it allows specifying the reference time varying force directly. The equations of motion for the robot are given by:

$$\Gamma = M(q)\ddot{q} + Co(q)(q,\dot{q}) + Ce(q)\left|\dot{q}^2\right| + G(q) \tag{1}$$
$$u - J^T(q)F = M(q)\ddot{q} + V(q,\dot{q}) + G(q)$$

where $M(q)$ represents the inertia matrix, $V(q,\dot{q})$ is the summation of the matrix of coriolis torques $Co(q)(q,\dot{q})$ and centrifugal torques $Ce(q)\left|\dot{q}^2\right|$, $G(q)$ is the vector of gravity torques. Γ is the generalized joint force torque which is calculated using $u - J^T(q)F$, where u is the input to the manipulator, $J(q)$ is the Jacobian matrix and F is the contact force exerted by the manipulator. Using inverse dynamics control, manipulator dynamics are linearized and decoupled via a feedback. The dynamic equation of the robotic manipulator was given in (1). Control input u to the manipulator is designed as follows:

$$u = M(q)y + V(q,\dot{q}) + G(q) + J^T F \tag{2}$$

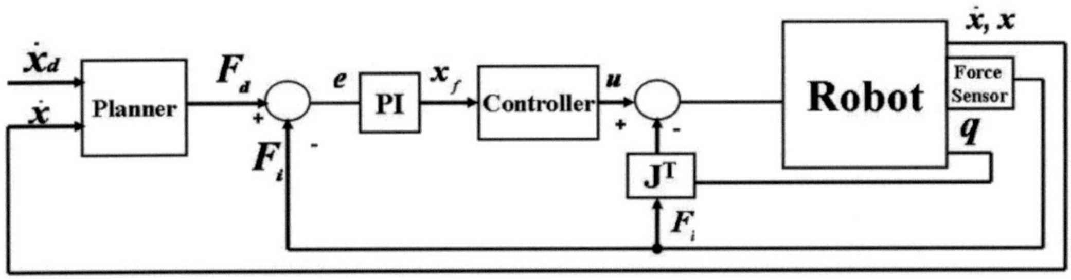

Fig. 3. Low-Level Controller.

which leads to the system of double integrators

$$\ddot{q} = y \tag{3}$$

In (3), y represents a new input. The new control input y is designed so as to allow tracking of the desired force F_d. To this purpose, the control law is selected as follows:

$$y = J(q)^{-1} M_d^{-1}(-K_d\dot{x} + K_p(x_f - x) - M_d\dot{J}(q,\dot{q})\dot{q}) \tag{4}$$

where x_f is a suitable reference to be related to force error. M_d (mass), K_d (damping) and K_p (stiffness) matrices specify the target impedance of the robot. x and $\dot{x}$ are the position and velocity of the end-effector in the Cartesian coordinates, respectively. The relationship between the joint space and the Cartesian space acceleration is used to determine position control equation.

$$\ddot{x} = J(q)\ddot{q} + \dot{J}(q,\dot{q})\dot{q} \quad and \quad \ddot{x} = J(q)y + \dot{J}(q,\dot{q})\dot{q} \tag{5}$$

By substituting (4) into (5), we obtain

$$\ddot{x} = J(q)(J(q)^{-1} M_d^{-1}(-K_d\dot{x} + K_p(x_f - x) - M_d\dot{J}(q,\dot{q})\dot{q})) + \dot{J}(q,\dot{q})\dot{q}$$
$$\ddot{x} = -M_d^{-1}K_d\dot{x} + M_d^{-1}K_p(x_f - x) \tag{6}$$
$$M_d\ddot{x} + K_d\dot{x} + K_p x = K_p x_f$$

Equation (6) shows the position control tracking of x with dynamics specified by the choices of K_d, K_p and M_d matrices. Impedance is attributed to a mechanical system characterized by these matrices that allows specifying the dynamic behavior. Let F_d be the desired force reference, which is computed using a PID velocity loop:

$$F_d = P_d(\dot{x}_d - \dot{x}) + I_d \int(\dot{x}_d - \dot{x})dt + D_d \frac{d(\dot{x}_d - \dot{x})}{dt} \tag{7}$$

where $\dot{x}_d$, $\dot{x}$, P_d, I_d and D_d are the desired velocity, actual velocity, the proportional, integral and derivative gains of the PID velocity loop, respectively. The relationship between x_f and the force error is expressed in (8) as:

$$x_f = P(F_d - F_i) + I\int(F_d - F_i)dt \tag{8}$$

where P and I are the proportional and integral gains, respectively, and F_i is the force applied by the human. Equations (6) and (8) are combined to obtain below equation:

$$M_d\ddot{x} + K_d\dot{x} + K_p x = K_p(P(F_d - F_i) + I\int(F_d - F_i)dt) \tag{9}$$

We can observe from (9) that the desired force response is achieved by controlling the position of the manipulator.

4.3. Decision of Robotic Assistance during Task Execution

During the tracking task, the activation of the low-level controller to provide robotic assistance is decided based on the participant's actual velocity ($\dot{x}$). If the actual velocity lies within an acceptable band, then it is understood that the participant is able to track the trajectory without robotic assistance. The acceptable band consists of upper and lower bounds on velocity, which are defined as:

$$\dot{x}_{upper} = \dot{x}_d + \left(\dot{x}_d * \frac{percentage}{100}\right), \quad \dot{x}_{lower} = \dot{x}_d - \left(\dot{x}_d * \frac{percentage}{100}\right) \tag{10}$$

where *percentage* is the value used to increment and decrement the desired velocity to define the upper and lower velocities for the selected $\dot{x}_d$. If the $\dot{x}$ is not between $\dot{x}_{upper}$ and $\dot{x}_{lower}$, then the low-level controller is activated to provide assistance to keep the participant's motion in the desired velocity range. However, note that any participant will require a finite amount of time to generate the desired motion. The controller should not be activated until it is determined that the participant is not able to generate the required motion by his/her own effort. Thus, initially a desired $\dot{x}_d$ is decided and it's upper ($\dot{x}_{upper}$) and lower ($\dot{x}_{lower}$) bound is calculated using (10). In order to determine the velocity trajectories $\dot{x}_d(t)$, $\dot{x}_{upper}(t)$ and $\dot{x}_{lower}(t)$, we use a generator block to generate smooth velocity trajectories within a specified distance using a skew-sine function. As a result, we define an algorithm to determine the average velocity of the participant $\dot{x}_{ave}$ (as opposed to instantaneous velocity) and average value of the upper $\dot{x}_{upperave}$ and lower $\dot{x}_{lowerave}$ velocity bounds for a given period of time, which are used to decide if the robotic assistance is needed. $\dot{x}_{ave}$, $\dot{x}_{upperave}$ and $\dot{x}_{lowerave}$ are calculated using the equations:

$$\dot{x}_{ave} = \frac{1}{\left(\frac{tf-ti}{ts}\right)} \sum_{t=ti}^{tf} (\dot{x}(t)), \dot{x}_{lowerave} = \frac{1}{\left(\frac{tf-ti}{ts}\right)} \sum_{t=ti}^{tf} (\dot{x}_{lower}(t)), \dot{x}_{upperave} = \frac{1}{\left(\frac{tf-ti}{ts}\right)} \sum_{t=ti}^{tf} (\dot{x}_{upper}(t)) \quad (11)$$

where tf, ti and ts are the final time, starting time and sampling time, respectively. $\dot{x}(t)$ is the participant's actual velocity at time t . If $\dot{x}_{lowerave} < \dot{x}_{ave} < \dot{x}_{upperave}$ is satisfied, then the low-level controller is not activated and participant continue tracking task without robotic assistance. If $\dot{x}_{lowerave} < \dot{x}_{ave} < \dot{x}_{upperave}$ is not satisfied then the controller is activated to provide robotic assistance to the participant to track the desired motion.

4.4. Switching Mechanism

Note that the controller will be switching in and out to provide robotic assistance. In order to ensure smooth switching, a switching mechanism that we have previously shown to guarantee bumpless switching for satisfactory force response (Mallapragada et al., 2006) is used in this work. This mechanism modifies the position reference, which is the input for the inner loop of the force controller, at the time of the switching in such a way that it is equal to the position reference at the time before switching occurred. The control action in (8) can be modified as below:

$$x_{fp}(t) = x(t) \quad and \quad x_{ff}(t) = Pe(t) + I(X_i(t) + X_{io})dt \quad (12)$$

Here $x_{fp}(t)$ is the position reference when the controller is not active, which is equal to the position of the human/robot $x(t)$. $x_{ff}(t)$ is the position reference determined using the P and I gains when the controller is active. $X_i(t)$ represents the integral action and X_{io} is the initial condition of the error integrator. $e(t)$ is defined as the $F_d - F_i$. If t_s is the time of switching, then equation (12) can be used to find the position reference just before the time of switching.

$$x_{fp}(t_s^-) = x(t_s^-) \quad (13)$$

where $x(t_s^-)$ represents the position of the human/robot right before the switching occurred. The position reference just after the switching is given as:

$$x_{ff}(t_s^+) = Pe(t_s^+) + I(X_i(t_s^+) + X_{io})dt \quad (14)$$

The integral action associated with the controller is reset during the switching so that:

$$X_i(t_s^+) = 0 \quad (15)$$

The force error defined as $F_d - F_i$ is set to zero just after the time of the switching for a small period of time. Hence:

$$Pe(t_s^+) = 0 \quad (16)$$

After the time of the switching F_d which is calculated using (7), and F_i, which is recorded from the force sensor are provided to the controller. The initial condition X_{io} is defined as:

$$X_{io} = x(t_s^-)/I \tag{17}$$

Then, substituting (15)-(17) into (14) we can observe that

$$x_{ff}(t_s^+) = x_{fp}(t_s^-) \tag{18}$$

This relation ensures that the position reference is indeed continuous during switching which guarantees bumpless activation and deactivation of the low-level controller.

5. The High-Level Controller

The high-level controller monitors the progress of the task, the status of the plant, and makes decision on the modification of the task that might be needed for the therapy. The high-level controller decisions are executed by the low-level controller to accomplish the task requirements. In this section, we first present the theory of the high-level controller, followed by the design rationale and details of the high-level controller.

5.1. Model

The high-level controller is a discrete-event system (DES) deterministic finite automaton, which is specified by $D=(\tilde{P},\tilde{X},\tilde{R},\psi,\lambda)$ (Koutsoukos et al., 2000, Antsaklis & Koutsoukos, 2003). Here $\tilde{P}$ is the set of discrete states. Each event is represented as a plant symbol, where $\tilde{X}$ is the set of such symbols, for all discrete states. The next discrete state is activated based on the current discrete state and the associated plant symbol using the following transition function: $\psi : \tilde{P} \times \tilde{X} \rightarrow \tilde{P}$. In order to notify the low-level controller the next course of action in the new discrete state, the controller generates a set of symbols, called control symbols, denoted by $\tilde{R}$, using an output function: $\lambda : \tilde{P} \rightarrow \tilde{R}$. The action of the high-level controller is described by the following equations:

$$\tilde{p}_j[n] = \psi(\tilde{p}_i[n-1], \tilde{x}_k[n]) \tag{19}$$

$$\tilde{r}_c[n] = \lambda(\tilde{p}_j[n]) \tag{20}$$

where $\tilde{p}_i, \tilde{p}_j \in \tilde{P}$, $\tilde{x}_k \in \tilde{X}$ and $\tilde{r}_c \in \tilde{R}$. i and j represent the index of discrete states. k and c represent the index of plant symbols and control symbols, respectively. n is the time index that specifies the order of the symbols in the sequence.

5.2. Design Rationale for the High-Level Controller

Let us explain the role of each element of the automaton $D=(\tilde{P},\tilde{X},\tilde{R},\psi,\lambda)$ in the context of rehabilitation tasks. $\tilde{P}$ is the set of discrete states. A rehabilitation therapy may consist of several actions and each discrete state may capture one of these actions. The action that takes place in each discrete state could be used to update the rehabilitation task. For example, if improving the speed of motion is the objective, then each category of speed (e.g., slow, medium, fast etc.) could be chosen as discrete states. When new actions are required for a rehabilitation task, new states can easily be included in the set of the states, $\tilde{P}$. Once the set $\tilde{P}$ is chosen, the next design parameters are what are called "events" that could affect the rehabilitation task. Events are various robot, human and general task related information that provide the current status of the task.

The set of events are not unique and are decided considering the need of the therapy, and the capabilities of the rehabilitation robotic systems. Generally the available sensory information from the robotic systems and the input from the therapist and the participant provide the core of the set of the events. When these events occur it may require some adjustments of the planning of the rehabilitation task. As discussed earlier, this sensory information may not be directly interpreted by the high-level controller. As a result, each event is represented as a plant symbol so that the high-level controller can recognize the events. $\tilde{X}$ is the set of the plant symbols, which is designed based on the set of events. The transition function $\psi : \tilde{P} \times \tilde{X} \rightarrow \tilde{P}$ uses the current state and the plant symbol to determine the next action that is required to update the rehabilitation task. For example, when the participant is performing the rehabilitation task and an event that requires the task to be stopped occurs, then the transition function is used to transit from one active state, which executes the task as required, to another one, which stops the task execution, based on the event. The high-level controller generates a control symbol, which is unique for each state, using the output function λ. $\tilde{R}$ is the set of the control symbols. The output of the control symbols are plant inputs which is in charge of the modification of the rehabilitation task. The control symbols and its outputs are decided based on the task requirements and the abilities of the low-level controller. For example, if the objective of the rehabilitation task is to increase the participant's range of motion, then the control symbol generates plant inputs to the low-level controller to change the desired goal position of the task in order to make the task more/less challenging for the participant. It is clear from the above discussion that the design of the various elements of the automaton $D=(\tilde{P},\tilde{X},\tilde{R},\psi,\lambda)$ is not unique and is dependent on the task at hand, and sensory information available from the robotic system. In what follows we present the design of these elements with regard to the objective of the rehabilitation task we present in this chapter.

The design of the elements of $D=(\tilde{P},\tilde{X},\tilde{R},\psi,\lambda)$ for the reaching task that has been described in Section 4.1 is motivated by the specific objective of the task. In here, the objective of the reaching task is to improve the participant's speed of movement while considering the current movement ability of the participant and the safety of the task. The participant is required to complete the movement in a certain amount of time, which represents the velocity of the task trajectory. The desired velocity trajectory could be updated to improve the participant's speed of movement and to ensure the safety of the participant. Thus the discrete states could be the level of speed at which the therapy is imparted to the participant. In order to decide the set of events, all sensory information that the current rehabilitation robotic systems can generate is analyzed. The rehabilitation robotic system used in this work has a force sensor to record the applied force of the participant, a PCI card to record the robot joint angles, and pause, stop and restart buttons for task execution. A counter is also used to record the number of times participant needed robotic assistance to determine the improvement of participant's movement ability. This set of information is used to define several events in our work. Once the discrete states and the events are determined, the necessary plant and control symbols are designed based on the structure of the high-level and low-level controllers, and the objectives of the task (e.g., when should discrete states be changed, how to increase or decrease speed etc.). The design details of the high-level controller for the reaching task are given in the next section.

5.3. Design Details of the High-Level Controller

We initially define the following discrete states $\tilde{p}$: stay, difficult, easy, stop and pause. Stay ($\tilde{p}_1$) implies the participant needs to continue the task at the same difficulty level by keeping the desired velocity same. Difficult ($\tilde{p}_2$) means the participant has improved his/her task performance and task need to be more challenging by increasing the desired velocity. Similarly, easy ($\tilde{p}_3$) implies changing the task parameters to make the task easier by decreasing the desired velocity. Stop ($\tilde{p}_4$) and pause ($\tilde{p}_5$) are defined in their usual ways. New discrete states can easily be included in the design of the high-level controller when new control actions are needed to modify the task parameters.

The state information from the robot and the human is detected to define the events. The state information from the robot and the human can be a continuous signal or a discrete value. Let S_{Rn} and S_{Hn} represent the sets of robot and human state information, respectively. In this research, the continuous signals that are detected from the robot are: i) robot's joint angles (S_{R1}), ii) the force reference calculated using (7) (S_{R2}), iii) the participant's velocity, which is measured from the tool frame velocity (S_{R3}). The discrete value detected from the robot is the participant's progress during the tracking task (S_{R4}). In order to find S_{R4}, the number of times participant needed robotic assistance at 10th trial (n_{10}) and at 50th trial (n_{50}) were recorded. Decision logic is defined to determine the value of S_{R4} using (21). Δp is the percentage value that is used to detect the improvement of the participant's movement ability in terms of the number of times he/she needs assistance from the robotic device, which is likely to be specified by the therapist based on individual progress.

$$\begin{aligned}
&\textit{if} \quad n_{50} < \left(n10 - \left(n10 * \frac{\Delta p}{100} \right) \right) \quad \textit{then} \quad \{S_{R4}=1\} \\
&\textit{elseif} \quad n_{50} > \left(n10 + \left(n10 * \frac{\Delta p}{100} \right) \right) \quad \textit{then} \quad \{S_{R4}=-1\} \\
&\textit{else} \quad \{S_{R4}=0\}
\end{aligned} \tag{21}$$

Robot and human state information is monitored to trigger relevant events to modify the task. When these events are triggered, the interface provides the necessary plant symbol ($\tilde{x}$) to the high-level controller. Currently we have defined nine events for the proposed high-level controller. However, the number of events can be easily extended. Five of these (E1, E2, E3, E4 and E5) are robot generated, and three of these (E6, E7 and E8) are human generated events. The other event, which is a secondary event, is called SE1. This is used to detect the previous state when the participant wants to continue with the task after he/she stops. The high-level controller needs to know which state was active before the pause or stop button was pressed in order to provide the same task parameters to the participant when he/she resumes the task. For example, when the participant presses pause button, a value is assigned to SE1. This value is retrieved when the participant resumes the task so that he or she can continue the therapy with the same task requirements. Events are reset at the beginning of task execution. Additionally, the triggered event is reset when a new event occurs. When the participant requires less, more or same level of robotic assistance to track the desired trajectory, E1, E2 and E3 is triggered, respectively. E4 occurs when the robot's joint angles are out of range. If the force reference (calculated by (7)) provided to the low-level controller to assist the participant and the participant's velocity ($\dot{x}$) are above predefined threshold values, then E5 and E6 are triggered, respectively. E7 occurs when the participant presses the pause or the stop button. In order to continue with the task, the participant resets the pause button and E8 event is triggered. Plant symbols ($\tilde{x}$) are designed based on the events as shown in Table 1. The *joint_limits* are known from the robot's specifications. $F_{dthreshold}$ and $\dot{x}_{threshold}$ are determined by the therapist at the beginning of the task execution. Note that if any of E4, E5, E6, and E7 or their combinations occurs then the state stop ($\tilde{p}_4$) is activated. Thus we assign the same plant symbol, $\tilde{x}_4$ for these events.

The secondary event, SE1, is defined as follows: if the state is difficult and E7=1, then SE1=1. We assign a corresponding plant symbol $\tilde{x}_6$. Similarly, if the state is easy and E7=1, then SE1=2, and the plant symbol $\tilde{x}_7$ is assigned. If the state is stay and E7=1, then SE1=3. We assign a corresponding plant symbol $\tilde{x}_8$. SE1 releases state information when E7=0 and E8=1.

Table 1. Plant Symbols for the High-Level Controller.

Signals from Human and Robot	Event Triggered	Plant Symbol
$S_{R4}=1$	$E1=1$	$\tilde{x}_1$
$S_{R4}=-1$	$E2=1$	$\tilde{x}_2$
$S_{R4}=0$	$E3=1$	$\tilde{x}_3$
S_{R1}>*joint_limits or*	$E4=1$	$\tilde{x}_4$
$S_{R2}> F_{dthreshold}$ *or*	$E5=1$	
$S_{R3}> \dot{x}_{threshold}$ *or*	$E6=1$	
$S_{H1}=1$	$E7=1$	
$S_{H2}=1$	$E8=1$	$\tilde{x}_5$

When any of these events is triggered, the high-level controller decides the next plan of action to modify the task. When an event is triggered, the corresponding plant symbol ($\tilde{x}$) is generated by the interface. The current state ($\tilde{p}$) and the plant symbol ($\tilde{x}$) are used by the high-level controller to determine the next state. Then the high-level controller generates the corresponding control symbol ($\tilde{r}$) for this new state and provides it to the interface. The add feasible paths in the proposed high-level controller is shown in Fig. 4 (left). In this figure, $\tilde{r}_c$ s are corresponding control symbols for each plant symbol $\tilde{x}_k$, where *c=1,2,…5* and *k=1,2,…8*. Any event that generates corresponding plant symbols $\tilde{x}_k$ along with the current state information $\tilde{p}_i$ determines the next $\tilde{p}_j$ and as a result, $\tilde{r}_c$, where *i=1,2,…5* and *j=1,2,…5*. In our application only one state is active at any given time, and therefore we

uniquely assign a control symbol $\tilde{r}_i$ for each discrete state $\tilde{p}_i$. Since the low-level controller cannot interpret the control symbols, the interface converts them to the appropriate values for α and β for (22) to execute the task. The available control symbols $\tilde{r}_i$ and their corresponding α and β values for the plant input are defined in a table in Fig. 4 (right).
The plant equation which determines the desired velocity for the low-level controller is defined as:

$$\dot{x}_{dm} = \beta(\dot{x}_d + (\alpha * delta)) \tag{22}$$

where $delta$ is selected as a constant value to increase and decrease the $\dot{x}_d$, which makes the task more or less challenging. $\dot{x}_{dm}$ is the new desired velocity value used to determine the new $\dot{x}_{upper}$ and $\dot{x}_{lower}$. Then the reference generator block is used to determine velocity trajectories $\dot{x}_d(t)$, $\dot{x}_{upper}(t)$ and $\dot{x}_{lower}(t)$ using new $\dot{x}_{dm}$, $\dot{x}_{upper}$ and $\dot{x}_{lower}$. The $\dot{x}_{ave}$, $\dot{x}_{upperave}$ and $\dot{x}_{lowerave}$ are calculated using (11). If $\dot{x}_{lowerave} < \dot{x}_{ave} < \dot{x}_{upperave}$ is not satisfied then the low-level controller is activated to provide assistance to complement participant's effort to complete the task in a precise manner. The Matlab/Simulink/Stateflow software is used to implement the proposed high-level controller (Stateflow/Matlab).

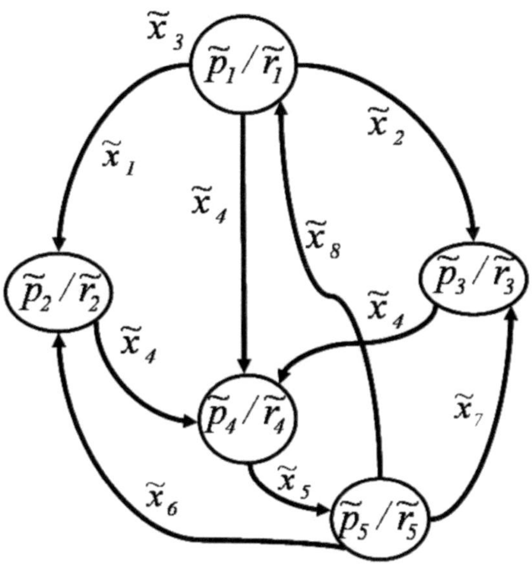

Control Symbol	Constant Value
$\tilde{r}_1$	$\alpha=0,\beta=1$
$\tilde{r}_2$	$\alpha=1,\beta=1$
$\tilde{r}_3$	$\alpha=-1,\beta=1$
$\tilde{r}_4$	$\beta=0$
$\tilde{r}_5$	$\beta=0$

Fig. 4. Feasible Paths in the High-Level Controller.

6. Results

In this section we present the experimental results on unimpaired participants to demonstrate the efficacy of both the low-level and high-level controller.

6.1. Experiment Procedure

Participants are seated in a height adjusted chair as shown in Fig. 2 (top left). The height of the PUMA 560 robotic manipulator has been adjusted for each participant to start the tracking task in the same arm configuration. The starting arm configuration is selected as shoulder at neutral 0° position and elbow at 90° flexion position. The task requires moving the arm in forward flexion to approximately 60° in conjunction with elbow extension to approximately 0°. Participants are asked to place their forearm on the hand attachment device as shown in Fig. 2 (bottom left) when the starting arm configuration is fixed. The push button has been given to the participants that can be used during the task execution in case of emergency situations (Fig. 2- bottom middle). The participants receive visual feedback of their position on a computer monitor on top of the desired position trajectory (Fig. 2-top right). Participants were asked to execute the tracking task 50 times.

6.2. Low-Level Controller Evaluation

We had conducted two experiments to evaluate the proposed low-level controller. In the first experiment, the participants were required to perform the tracking task without any external resistance applied to his/her upper arm. Participants were asked to track the position trajectory displayed on the computer screen. The participant's $\dot{x}_{ave}$ was calculated using (11) and if it was in between $\dot{x}_{upperave}$ and $\dot{x}_{lowerave}$ then robot did not need to provide any assistance. However, friction and gravity compensation were always activated in order for the participant to move the robot along with his/her arm in an effortless way. If the $\dot{x}_{ave}$ was not between $\dot{x}_{upperave}$ and $\dot{x}_{lowerave}$, then low-level controller was activated to provide robotic assistance to complement participant's effort to complete the task in a precise manner. During these two experiments, the number of trials and the number of times participant needed robotic assistance were recorded to observe the improvement of participant's movement ability.

In the second experiment, we asked the participant to perform the same task as in Experiment 1; however, in this case, the participant's arm movement ability was constrained with a resistive band (Thera-bands). This was done to simulate the movement of a stroke patient who may experience variable stiffness during the course of motion. In order to apply resistance to participant's upperarm, a mechanism was designed as shown in Fig. 5. Thera-bands are color-coded into many levels of resistance, thus different color resistive bands can be selected in order to simulate different stiffness of the stroke patient's arm. We selected the green (heavy) color resistive band for our experiment, because it provided sufficient resistance to participant's movement while not inhibiting their ability to complete the task. The mechanism has a rod which can slide right or left to change the position of the attachment and can be used for both right-handed and left-handed participants. The rod has holes on it to adjust the location of the resistive band on the upper arm that may vary among participants. The resistive band is connected to the participant's upper arm through a soft strapped attachment to prevent the participant's arm from the irritation that may be caused when the band is stretched. A seat-belt mechanism that connects the rod to the resistive band attachment can be used to release the rod from the resistive band quickly.

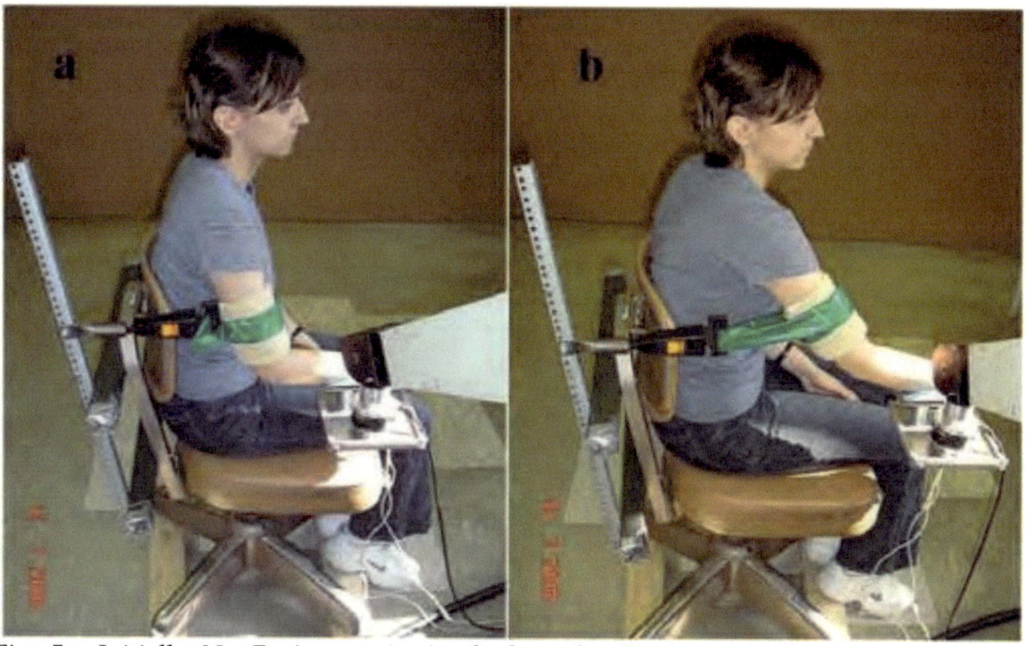

Fig. 5a. Initially No Resistance is Applied to the Participant's Upper Arm, Fig. 5b. Resistance is Applied to the Participant's Upper Arm in the Direction of Motion as the Task Begins.

Three female and one male participants within the age range of 25-30 years took part in the experiments that were described in above. All participants were right-handed. In these experiments (i.e., Experiments 1 and 2 as described in above), the participant tried to track the desired position trajectory by visually looking at the computer screen. Each participant performed the task 50 times for each experiment. $\dot{x}$ was selected as $0.02m/s$, which was chosen in consultation with a physical therapist who works with stroke patients at the Vanderbilt Stallworth Rehabilitation Hospital. The $\dot{x}_{upper}$ and $\dot{x}_{lower}$ were selected as 25% more and less of $\dot{x}$, which were $0.025m/s$ and $0.015m/s$, respectively. The range could be increased or decreased based on participant's movement ability. Then, $\dot{x}_d(t)$, $\dot{x}_{upper}(t)$ and $\dot{x}_{lower}(t)$ velocity trajectories were generated using the reference block. The $\dot{x}_{ave}$, $\dot{x}_{upperave}$ and $\dot{x}_{lowerave}$ were calculated using (11) at every 5 seconds. 5 seconds were sufficient to estimate the progress of the participant. If $\dot{x}_{lowerave} < \dot{x}_{ave} < \dot{x}_{upperave}$ was not satisfied then the controller was activated for the next 5 seconds to provide robotic assistance to the participant to track the desired motion within the desired velocity range.

In the first experiment, each participant performed the tracking task without any external resistance applied to his/her upper arm. The idea was to assist the participants as and when they were out of the velocity band. It was noticed that the participants needed less assistance from the robot as they practiced more (Table 2). This result implies that the participants learned how to accomplish the task with practice.

Table 2. Number of Times Robot Assisted for Experiment 1.

Trial Range / Number of Assistance for	1-10	11-20	21-30	31-40	41-50
P1	8	6	5	4	3
P2	14	13	13	12	11
P3	13	11	9	8	7
P4	12	12	11	10	9

Now we present the detailed analysis of the data for one participant (P1) as an example to demonstrate the effectiveness of the low-level controller. This data represented P1's 50th trial. It could be observed from Fig. 6 that the participant's average velocity (stars), which was calculated every 5 seconds using (11), was out of range at A, B and C points. The controller was activated for the next 5 seconds to provide robotic assistance in order to take participant's velocity inside the velocity boundary, thus the controller was active between A-A′, B-B′ and C-C′ (Fig. 6). It could be seen that the participant's velocity was brought inside the desired range at A′, B′ and C′ points, which verified that the assistive ability of the proposed low-level controller.

We further analysed the amount of time taken by the low-level controller (t_S, in seconds) to take $\dot{x}$ into the desired velocity range. Here t_S is defined as the settling time, which is the time taken between the moment the low-level controller was activated and the actual velocity reached the boundary of the desired velocity range. The mean and standard deviation of t_S for all participants' data for Experiment 1 are presented in Table 3.

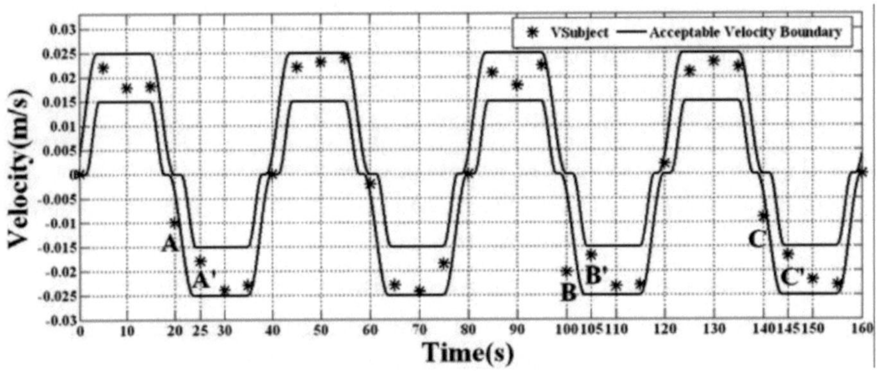

Fig. 6. Calculated Average Velocities for Experiment 1.

Table 3. Settling Time for Experiment 1.

Participant	Mean	Standard Deviation
P1	0.4723	0.1502
P2	0.5801	0.1937
P3	0.4929	0.1272
P4	0.545	0.232

Thus it can be observed from the above set of results that the proposed low-level controller could assist as and when needed and the provided robotic assistance could quickly (i.e., in approximately *0.55* seconds) bring the participant's velocity in the desired range.
In the second experiment, the participant's arm movement ability was constrained with a resistive band as shown in Fig. 5. The participants were asked to track the desired motion by visually looking at the screen as before. It was observed that the participants needed more robotic assistance when their motion was constrained. It could also be observed from Table 4, participants learned how to accomplish the task with practice.

Table 4. Number of Times Robot Assisted for Experiment 2.

Trial Range / Number of Assistance for	1-10	11-20	21-30	31-40	41-50
P1	13	12	12	11	9
P2	16	16	14	13	13
P3	14	13	13	12	12
P4	15	15	14	13	13

We present the mean and standard deviation of the settling time of the low-level controller in Table 5 for all participants' data when they performed Experiment 2. The second experiment was conducted to observe the performance of the controller in an artificially constrained motion scenario, which might provide insight about applying the system to stroke patients whose movement could be naturally constrained. It can be observed that the controller was able to assist as and when needed and could bring the actual velocity of the participant's arm within the desired range in about *0.65* seconds.

Table 5. Settling Time for Experiment 2.

Participant	Mean	Standard Deviation
P1	0.6317	0.232
P2	0.6274	0.2677
P3	0.6438	0.2674
P4	0.6985	0.248

6.3. High-Level Controller Evaluation

In order to demonstrate the efficacy of the proposed high-level controller, we had designed two experiments. In the first experiment, we had demonstrated the efficacy the proposed high-level controller to modify the task when the participant improved his/her movement ability to track the desired trajectory. In the second experiment, we had demonstrated the efficacy of the high-level controller to modify the task in order to ensure the safety of the participants.
In the first experiment, we had used P1's low-level controller results. Δp, was selected as *30*, which could be varied based on participant's progress and the therapist's choice. It was observed from Table 2 that n_{10}=8 and n_{50}=3 and the first criteria in (21) was satisfied, thus E1

was triggered and the plant symbol $\tilde{x}_1$ was generated from the interface difficult ($\tilde{p}_2$) state became active and the control symbol $\tilde{r}_2$ was generated. The interface converted this control symbol to α=1 and β=1. Amount of the increment ($delta$) to increase the difficulty level of the task was an important issue that needed to be decided. In rehabilitation therapies, increasing $\dot{x}_d$ with a small increment would be more desirable especially for low-functioning stroke patients. In this experiment, we had incremented $\dot{x}_d$ by 20%, where $delta = 0.004$. New desired velocity was calculated using (22), which was *0.024m/s*. The velocity boundaries were calculated using (11) as *0.03m/s* and *0.018m/s* for $\dot{x}_{upper}$ and $\dot{x}_{lower}$, respectively. We had asked P1 to perform the tracking task 50 times with this new velocity boundary. Low-level controller provided robotic assistance to the participant as and when they were out of the new velocity band. It was observed that the P1 needed more robotic assistance when the desired velocity to complete the task was increased. It could be seen that P1 learned how to accomplish the task with practice (Table 6).

Table 6. Number of Times Robot Assisted for P1 with New Velocity Boundary.

Trial Range / Number of Assistance for	1-10	11-20	21-30	31-40	41-50
P1	11	10	9	8	7

In the second experiment, we had assumed a safety event had occurred when P1 was performing the task with new increased velocity band. In this experiment, at some point of time during the task P1 wanted to pause for a while and then reset the pause button when she was ready to complete the rest of the task. This scenario might represent when a stroke patient want to pause for a while due to some discomfort. When the task had initially started, E1 was triggered and the plant symbol $\tilde{x}_1$ was generated from the interface. difficult ($\tilde{p}_2$) state became active and the control symbol $\tilde{r}_2$ was given to the interface. The interface converted this control symbol to constant values α=1 and β=1. The plant equation (22) was used to calculate $\dot{x}_{dm}$ (the desired velocity), which was *0.024m/s*. The reaching task required participant to move *0.3m*, thus, the initial position (*0*), desired position (*0.3*) and desired $\dot{x}_{dm}$ (*0.024m/s*) was provided to the reference block to generate the smooth desired velocity trajectory from A to B (Fig.7-left-solid line).

When P1 pressed the pause button at B, E7 was triggered. When E7 was triggered, plant symbol $\tilde{x}_4$ was generated from the interface and stop ($\tilde{p}_4$) state became active. When stop state was active, the high-level controller provided the control symbol $\tilde{r}_4$ and β=0 was given to (22) and $\dot{x}_{dm}$ was determined as zero. The zero velocity could cause a sudden stop. In order to prevent P1 from suddenly stopping, the reference generator block was used to provide a smooth velocity trajectory to bring the motion to stop. In this case, the velocity was detected when E7 was triggered and the desired velocity was given

as zero and using the reference generator block, the smooth desired velocity was given to the low-level controller from B to C (Fig.7-left-solid line). It could be seen that P1's position (Fig. 7 - right) did not change after the velocity became zero until P1 reset the pause button. SE1 was set to 1 because the state was difficult and E7=1. When the participant reset the pause button, E8 was triggered and $\tilde{x}_5$ plant symbol was given to the interface, and pause ($\tilde{p}_5$) state became active and the high-level controller provided $\tilde{r}_5$. Then $\tilde{x}_6$ was given to the interface because SE=1. The corresponding control symbol $\tilde{r}_2$ was generated, and α=1 and β=1 values were given to (22) for calculation of $\dot{x}_{dm}$, which was *0.024m/s*. It could be seen that the high-level controller resumed the task in such a manner that the participant could continue with the therapy with the same task parameters. The participant's position at the time of the triggering of E8 was automatically detected and was given as an initial position to the reference generator block and the desired position was set to *0.3*. The velocity trajectory from C to D was generated and given to the low-level controller (Fig.7-left-solid line). On the other hand, if we did not use this high-level controller, the desired velocity trajectory would not have been automatically modified to register the intention of the participant to pause the task. As a result, the velocity trajectory would have followed the dashed line in Fig. 7-left. In such a case, when P1 wanted to start the task again, the desired velocity trajectory would start at point C′ with non-zero velocity (Fig. 7-left-dashed line). This could create unsafe operating condition. In addition, since the desired velocity computation would not have included the pause action, restarting the task at point C′ would not allow the completion of the task as desired. For example, in this case, if P1 had used the dashed velocity trajectory, she would start moving in the opposite direction at point C′. It could be possible to pre-program all types of desired velocity trajectories beforehand and retrieve them as needed. However, for non-trivial tasks such a mechanism might be too difficult to manage and extend as needed. The presented high-level controller provides a systematic mechanism to tackle such issues. It could also be seen that new velocity trajectories could be created dynamically using the generator block. In order to generate the required trajectories, the task parameters were needed. High-level controller monitored the progress of the task and made decision on the modification of the task parameters.
When the participant reached the desired position, which was *0.3m*, then the velocity trajectory from D to E was generated and given to the low-level controller (Fig.7-left-solid line) so that P1 moved back to the starting position (Fig.7-right).

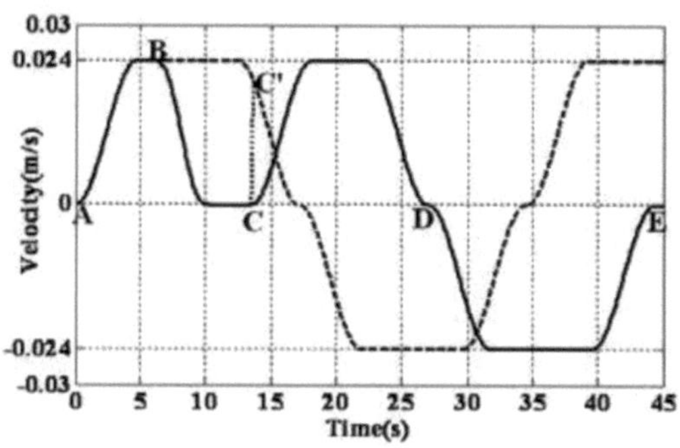

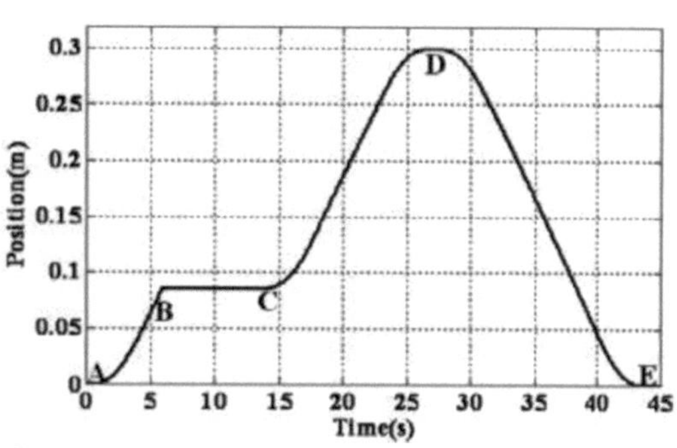

Fig. 7. Motion Trajectories When Task is Paused.

As could be seen from the results, the high-level controller determined the task parameters dynamically based on participant's performance and monitored the safety related events to generate the necessary motion trajectories at the required time.

7. Conclusions and Future Work

In this work we present a new control approach to offer robotic assistance for stroke patients that include the coordination between a high-level controller and a low-level controller. The control architecture presented here is an example of a hybrid control system. There has been no work to our knowledge on designing similar type of control architecture for rehabilitation purposes.

We have initially designed a movement tracking task where the participants not only make repetitive movement but also pay attention to the desired speed of motion from visual feedback. The task was designed in such a manner that it required cognitive processing. Including cognitive processing in the task design is an important criterion because it had been previously shown that the movement tracking task that requires cognitive processing achieved greater gains for brain reorganization of stroke patients than that of movement task that does not require cognitive processing (Carey et al., 2005, Carey et al., 2006).

We have presented a low-level controller to provide robotic assistance to participants to complete the movement tracking task. The high-level controller coordinates with the low-level controller to improve the robotic assistance with the following objectives: 1) to monitor the upper arm rehabilitation task; and ii) to make necessary decisions to address the status of the task. We present a systematic design procedure for the high-level controller to accomplish the above objectives. Note that the proposed high-level controller can be integrated with other low-level controllers with minor modifications. We have conducted experiments with unimpaired participants and demonstrated the usefulness of the high-level and low-level controllers. The results of the use of the low-level controller have demonstrated that the participants needed less assistance from the robot as they practiced more, which implies that the participant's ability to complete the desired motion within a defined velocity range have been improved. Improving the velocity of patient's movement could be an important criterion to measure the success of a rehabilitation therapy. We have also demonstrated that the low-level controller provides assistance to the participants as and when needed and quickly brought the participant's velocity in the desired range. The results of the use of the high-level controller have demonstrated that the task parameters could be determined dynamically based on participant's performance and monitored for safety related events to generate the necessary motion trajectories at the required time. The speed of motion is used as the task parameter in this work. However, the high-level controller can determine other task parameters such as desired reaching position. In some of the rehabilitation tasks, the reaching task is shaped by defining the target position closer to or away from the patient to change the difficulty level of the task. In such a case, for example, the high-level controller can determine the target position based on the participant's progress while monitoring the safety related events.

We are aware that a PUMA 560 robot might not be ideal for rehabilitation applications. However the use of the hand attachment device, which has been described in Section 3, provided a quick release mechanism to protect the participant's arm from injuries. Note that the presented control framework is not specific to the proposed rehabilitation robotic system but can be integrated with any previously proposed rehabilitation robotic system.

An important direction for future development involves testing the usability of the proposed control architecture with stroke patients. Functional magnetic resonance imaging (fMRI) procedure can be used to investigate whether the presented task that included cognitive processing result in long-term brain reorganization. New methods to detect human state information can be integrated into the control architecture such as ECG signals can be used to monitor patients' heart rate to detect their exhaustion and a voice recognition system can be integrated to examine the patient's verbal commands. The proposed control architecture is flexible and extendible in the sense that new events can be included and detected by simply monitoring the additional state information from the human and the robot. In this regard, we are currently working with Vanderbilt University's Stallworth Rehabilitation Hospital to include additional human and robot information.

8. Acknowledgments

We gratefully acknowledge the help of Dr. Thomas E. Groomes who is the Medical Director of Spinal Cord and Traumatic Brain Injury Program, and therapist Sheila Davy of Vanderbilt University's Stallworth Rehabilitation Hospital for their feedback about experimental setup and task design during this work. The work was supported by Vanderbilt University Discovery grant.

9. References

Antsaklis, P.J. & Koutsoukos, X.D. (2003) Hybrid Systems: Review and Recent Progress. In: *Software-Enabled Control: Information Technologies for Dynamical Systems,* T. Samad and G. Balas, (Ed.), IEEE Press, pp. 1-29.

American Heart Association: Heart and Stroke Statistical Update (2006). Available from: http://www.Americanheart.org/statistics/stroke.htm.

Black, J.E.; Isaacs, K.R.; Anderson, B.J.; Alcantara, A.A. & Greenough, W. T. (1990). Learning causes synaptogenesis, whereas motor activity causes angiogenesis, in cerebellar cortex of adult rats. *Proceedings of National Academy of Science,* Vol. 87, No. 15, pp. 5568-5572.

Carey, J.R.; Bhatt, E. & Nagpal, A. (2005). Neuroplasticity Promoted by Task Complexity. *Exercise and Sport Science Review,* Vol. 33, pp. 24-31.

Carey J.; Durfee, W.; Bhatt, E. ; Nagpal, A.; Weinstein, S.;Anderson, K. & Lewis, S. (2006). Tracking vs. Movement Telerehabilitation Training to Change Hand Function and Brain Reorganization in Stroke. *Submitted to Neurorehabilitation and Neural Repair.*

Culmer, P. ; Jackson, A. ; Richardson, R. ; Bhakta, B. ; Levesley, M. & Cozens, A. (2005). An admittance control scheme for a robotic upper-limb stroke rehabilitation system. *International Conference on Engineering in Medicine and Biology Society,* pp. 5081 - 5084.

Erol, D. & Sarkar N. (2007). Design and Implementation of an Assistive Controller for Rehabilitation Robotic Systems. *International Journal of Advanced Robotics Systems,* Vol. 4, No. 3.

Kahn, L.E.; Zygman, M.L; Rymer, W.Z. & Reinkensmeyer, D.J. (2006a). Robot-assisted reaching exercise promotes arm movement recovery in chronic hemiparetic stroke: a randomized controlled pilot study. *Journal of NeuroEngineering and Rehabilitation,* Vol. 3, No.12, pp. 1-13.

Kahn L.E; Lum P.S.; Rymer W.Z. & Reinkensmeyer D.J. (2006b). Robot-assisted movement training for the stroke-impaired arm: Does it matter what the robot does? *Journal of Rehabilitation Research & Development*, Vo. 43, No. 5, pp. 619-630.

Kleim, J. A.; Barbay, S. & Cooper, N.R. (2002). Motor learning-dependent synaptogenesis is localized to functionally reorganized motor cortex. *Neurobiology Learning and Memory*, Vol. 77, pp. 63-77.

Koutsoukos, X.D.; Antsaklis, P.J.; Stiver, J.A. & Lemmon, M.D. (2000). Supervisory control of hybrid systems. *Proceedings of the IEEE on Special Issue on Hybrid Systems: Theory and Applications*, Vol. 88, No. 7, pp. 1026 – 1049.

Krebs, H.I.; Palazzolo, J.J.; Dipietro, L.; Ferraro, M.; Krol J.; Rannekleiv, K.; Volpe, B.T. & Hogan N. (2003). Rehabilitation Robotics: Performance-Based Progressive Robot-Assisted Therapy. *Autonomous Robots*, Vol. 15, No. 1, pp. 7-20.

Krebs, H. I.; Ferraro, M., Buerger, S.P., Newbery, M. J., Makiyama, A., Sandmann, M.; Lynch, D.; Volpe, B. T. & Hogan, N. (2004). Rehabilitation robotics: pilot trial of a spatial extension for MIT-Manus. *Journal of NeuroEngineering and Rehabilitation*, Vol. 1, No. 5, pp. 1-15.

Loureiro, R.; Amirabdollahian, F.; Topping, M.; Driessen, B. & Harwin, W. (2003). Upper limb mediated stroke therapy - GENTLE/s approach. *Autonomous Robots*, Vol.15, pp. 35-51.

Lum, P.S.; Burgar, C.G.; Van der Loos, H.F.M.; Shor, P.C.; Majmundar M. & Yap R. (2006). MIME robotic device for upper-limb neurorehabilitation in subacute stroke subjects: A follow-up study. *Journal of Rehabilitation Research & Development*, Vol. 43, No. 5, pp. 631-642.

Mallapragada, V.; Erol, D. & Sarkar, N. (2006). A New Method for Force Control for Unknown Environments. *Proceedings of the International Conference On Intelligent Robots and Systems*, pp. 4509 - 4514.

Matchar, D.B. & Duncan, P.W. (1994). Cost of stroke, *Stroke Clinical Updates*, Vol. 5, pp. 9-12.

Nudo, R.; Milliken, G.; Jenkins, W. & Merzenich M. (1996). Use-dependent alterations of movement representations in primary motor cortex of adult squirrel monkeys. *The Journal of Neuroscience*, Vol. 16, No. 2, pp. 785-807.

Pascual-Leone, A.; Nguyen, K.T.; Kohen, A.D.; Brasil-Neto, J.; Cammarota, A. & Hallett M. (1995). Modulation of muscle responses evoked by transcranial magnetic stimulation during the acquisition of new fine motor skills. *Journal of Neurophysiology*, Vol. 74, pp. 1037-1045.

Plautz, E.J.; Milliken, G. W. & Nudo, R J. (2000). Effects of repetitive motor training on movement representations in adult squirrel monkeys: role of use versus learning. *Neurobiology of Learning and Memory*, Vol. 74, pp. 27-55.

PUMA 560 Related Sites on the Internet, Available from: www.ee.ualberta.ca/~jasmith/puma/pumasites.html.

Sciavicco, L. & Siciliano, B. (1996). *Modeling and Control of Robot Manipulators*, McGrawHill, ISBN-1852332212, Great Britain.

Stateflow, Mathworks Inc, http://www.mathworks.com/products/stateflow/?BB=1

Taub, E.; Uswatte, G. & Pidikiti, R. (1999). Constraint-Induced Movement Therapy: A New family of techniques with broad application to physical rehabilitation – a clinical review. *Journal of Rehabilitation Research and Development,* Vol. 36, pp. 237-251.

Taub, E.; Lum, P.S.; Hardin, P.; Mark V.W. & Uswatte, G. (2005). AutoCITE: Automated Delivery of CI Therapy With Reduced Effort by Therapists. *Stroke*, Vol. 36, pp. 1301-1304.

8

A 3-D Rehabilitation System for Upper Limbs "EMUL", and a 6-DOF Rehabilitation System "Robotherapist", and Other Rehabilitation Systems with High Safety

Junji Furusho & Takehito Kikuchi
Osaka University
Japan

1. Introduction

Movements of upper limbs are indispensable for daily activities. For the aged or disabled persons, it is especially important to exercise for the maintenance or recovery of upper limb function. There are many patients of paralysis caused by stroke. For example, in Japan more than two hundred and fifty thousand people have stroke every year, and many of them are paralyzed. The human brain is capable of an extraordinary degree of plasticity (self-organization), enabling learning, and leaving open the possibility for motor recovery (Janet & Shepherd, 1998). Therefore, neuro-rehabilitation for stroke-patients is effective. Using apparatus that applies robotic technology and virtual reality makes new training methods and exercises in rehabilitation possible (Krebs, Volpe et al., 2000), (Burgar, Lum et al., 2000), (Charles, Krebs et al., 2005).

Force display systems are expected as effective and advantageous interfaces for some scenes, for example computer-assisted-surgery, kinds of rehabilitation methods and so on. In this technology, some kinds of feedback force are generated with mechanical actuators. And such a virtual force is computed in real time by simulating a physical phenomenon of the virtual world in which the operator exists.

Feeding back the quantitative evaluations to the training by a computer can enhance the qualitative effect of training. Therefore, some rehabilitation systems using these technologies for upper limbs have been developed. However, most of them apply training within a two-dimensional horizontal plane. Many movements, however, in daily activities need to move arms in a vertical direction. A system therefore that enables exercise in three-dimensions would seem to be more effective for such training. Although the MIME system (Burgar, Lum et al., 2000) using PUMA-560 by VA and Stanford Univ. can give training in three-dimensions, the PUMA-560 is a robot originally developed for industrial use and may not be sufficiently safe to train the aged and/or disabled.

We have developed innovative rehabilitation supporting robots; "EMUL" and "Robotherapist." The EMUL has performed well in clinical studies, and Robotherapist was exhibited at the Prototype Robot Festival at the 2005 International Exposition held in Aichi Prefecture, Japan.

"EMUL", short for "Exercise Machine for Upper Limbs", was developed through robotic and virtual reality technology in a 5-year NEDO (New-Energy and Industrial Technology Development Organization of Japanese Government) project (Furusho, Koyanagi, Imada et al., 2005), (Furusho, Koyanagi, Kataoka et al., 2005). It enables new training methods and exercises for use in the field of rehabilitation. The EMUL has 3-DOF (degrees of freedom) for shoulder and elbow training, and this satisfies many of the movements involved in daily activities. Another important feature is safety. In EMUL, ER (electro-rheological) fluid actuators ensure mechanical safety. "Robotherapist" is a 6-DOF rehabilitation robot based on EMUL which has a 3-DOF controllability added at wrist rotations (Furusho, Hu, Kikuchi et al., 2006). In this chapter, we describe mechanism and software of EMUL, Robotherapist and other rehabilitation systems using functional fluids with high safety.

Furusho Laboratory of Osaka University developed 2-D rehabilitation system for upper limbs "NIOH-1" using ER fluid actuators in 1997 (Furusho, Wei, Koga, 1995), (Furusho & Sakaguchi, 1999). EMUL and Robotherapist were developed on the basis of the technology of NIOH. Recently we have developed a upper-limb-rehabilitation system "PLEMO" using ER fluid brakes which could be used in facilities for elderly people and so on (Kikuchi, Furusho et al., 2007), (Kikuchi, Hu et al., 2007).

Furusho Laboratory studied biped locomotion robots during the 1980s and the beginning of 1990s, and realized the human-like biped locomotion with kick action [Furusho & Masubuchi, 1987], [Furusho & Sano 1990]. On the basis of this biped locomotion technology and the technology about functional fluids, we developed the first intelligent prosthetic ankle. Moreover we are developing intelligent ankle-foot orthoses using MR (Magnetorheological) fluid in a 3-year NEDO project. These systems are also introduced in this chapter.

2. 2-D Rehabilitation System "NIOH"

2.1 ER Actuaor

ER fluid is a fluid whose rheological properties can be changed by applying an electrical field (Bossis, 2002). Figure 1 shows the conceptual illustration of an ER fluid actuator. The ER actuator is composed of an ER clutch and its drive mechanism consisting of a motor and a reduction-gear-unit. The rotational speed of the motor is kept constant. The output torque of ER actuator is controlled by the applied electric field (Furusho, 2001), (Furusho & Kikuchi, 2006).

The input torque is transferred to the rotating cylindrical section of the output axis via the particle-type ER fluid filled in the rotating cylinder. Both the input axis cylinders and the output axis cylinder serve as electrodes, and output torque is controlled by the electric field applied between the electrodes. The output cylinder is made of aluminum alloy in order to reduce the moment of inertia of the output axis.

An actuator using ER fluid is effective for human-coexistent mechatronics systems like rehabilitation systems for upper limbs. Figure 2 shows a conceptual illustration of Human-Machine-Coexistent-Mechatronics (HMCM) System using ER Actuators. Merits of ER actuators in applications to HMCM system are as follows:

A: From the Viewpoints of the Characteristics of Operation

(a) Since ER actuators have good back-drivability, the operator can easily operate HMCM system from its end-effector.

(b) When HMCM system is driven by the operator from its end-effector, HMCM system can be moved quickly over the rotational speed of the input cylinder of the ER clutch.

B: From the Viewpoints of Performances in Force Display System:

(a) Quick force response property originated from the low inertia property of ER actuator and the rapid response of ER fluid make the force presentation with high fidelity possible.

(b) Force display systems with large-force presentation ability can be realized safely.

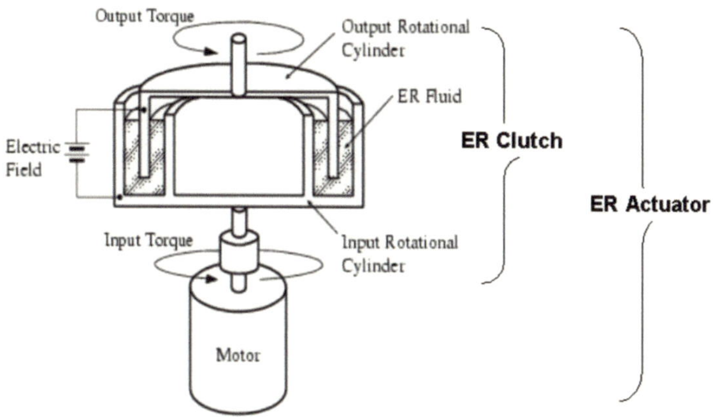

Fig. 1. Conceptual illustration of ER actuator

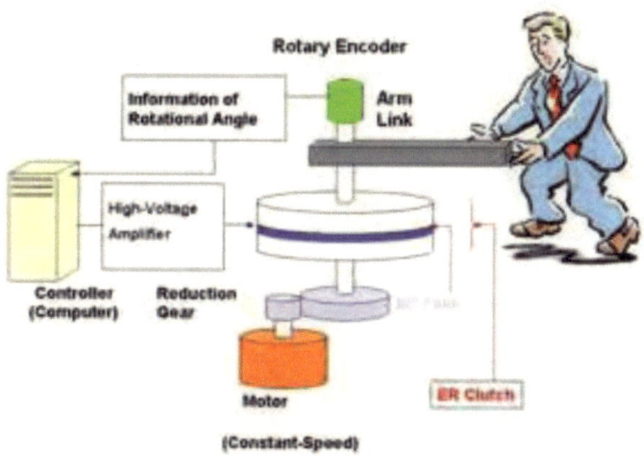

Fig. 2. Conceptual illustration of Human-Machine-Coexistent-Mechatronics (HMCM) Systems using ER actuators.

2.2 Consideration about Safety

A rehabilitation system for upper limbs which has large working area can be regarded as a kind of robots. In such a human-coexistent robot system where an operator must be in contact with or close to the robot, the safety-securing system is necessary in order that an operator can use the robot safely (ISO10218). In industrial robots, an operator cannot access a robot except for teaching in order to avoid hazardous conditions. Figure 3 shows the structure of safety in human-coexistent robots.

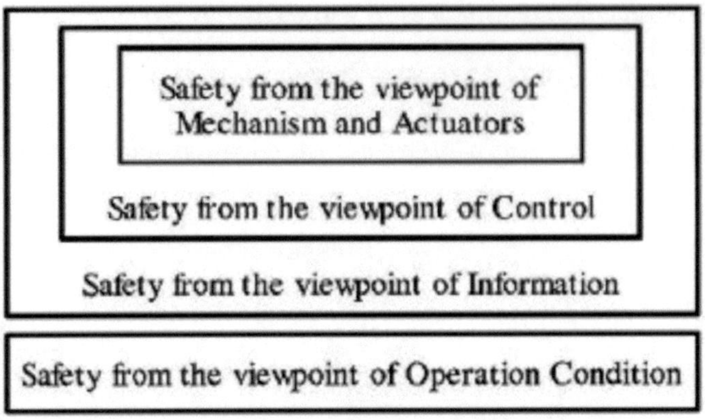

Fig. 3. Structure for securing safety in Human-Coexistent Robots.

ER actuators have the following merits from the viewpoint of safety.

(1) The maximum driving speed of the output shaft of the ER actuator is restricted by the rotational speed of the input shaft of the ER clutch. Therefore, when the rotational speed of the input shaft is set slow, HMCM systems using ER actuators are safe for operators.

(2) The inertia of the output part can be made very small. So, in the case of unexpected accidents, the impact force caused by the inertia of the actuator can be reduced.

Since International Safety Standards for human-coexistent robots have not been established yet, we have no other choice but to use the ISO and domestic standards for machines working close to human beings (see Table 1). The developed rehabilitation system can assure these standards of Table 1 by the usage of ER actuators and the mechanical design as follows:

(1) The items (a) and (b) of Table 1 are satisfied by setting the rotational speed of the input cylinder slow.

(2) The item (c) is satisfied by using a 60-watt motor for the drive of the input rotational cylinder.

(3) Risk Reduction by Design (item (d)) is realized by mechanical limitation of each joint, mechanical gravity-compensation and the usage of ER actuators.

(a) End-effector Speed is less than 0.25 [m/s]	ISO10218: Manipulating industrial robots--Safety
(b) Low Energy Property	ISO14121: Safety of machinery--Principles of risk assessment
(c) Actuator Power is less than 80 [W]	JAPAN, JIS B 8433, 1983: General Code for Safety of Industrial Robots
(d) Risk Reduction by Design	ISO12100: Safety of machinery--Basic concepts□ general principles for design

Table 1. International and Domestic Safety Standards.

2.3 Rehabilitation and Force Display Systems Using ER Fluids

Furusho Lab. of Osaka University has been developing rehabilitation systems and force display systems using ER fluids since 1993 (Furusho, Wei et al., 1995).

Figure 4 shows the 2-DOF rehabilitation systems "NIHO-1" using ER actuators (Furusho & Sakaguchi, 1999). The rehabilitation training system was installed in a hospital for testing purpose. 13 patients volunteered to participate in several experiments for evaluation of upper limb's physical capability and for rehabilitation training. The patients suffered from arm paralysis due to a damaged spinal cord or clogged brain artery. Figure 5 shows the 2-DOF rehabilitation system "NIHO-2" using ER actuators (Ishikawa, 2000).

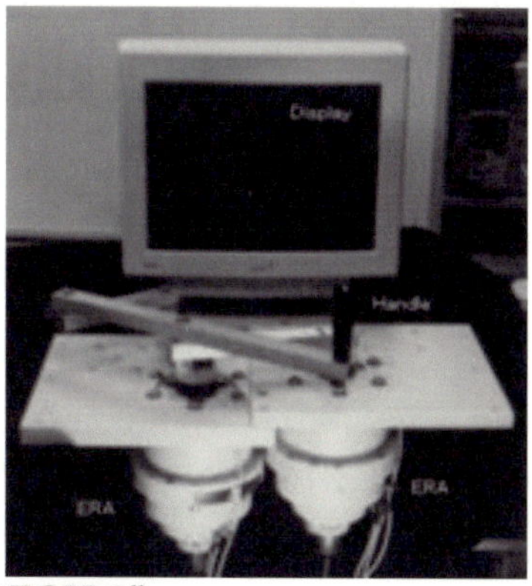

Fig. 4. Rehabilitation system "NIOH-1".

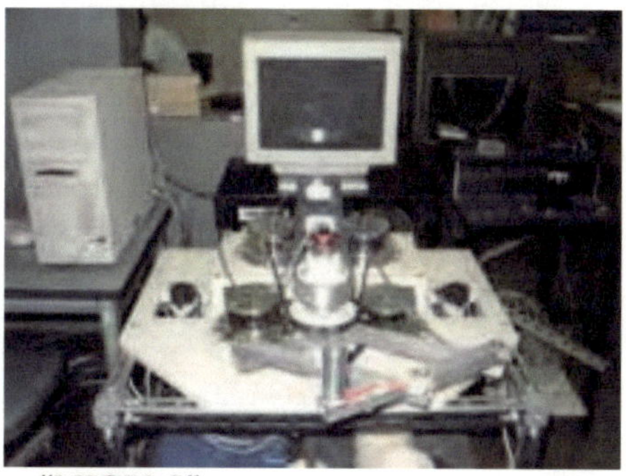

Fig. 5. Rehabilitation system "NIOH-2".

3. A 3-D Rehabilitation System for Upper Limbs Developed in a 5-year NEDO Project "EMUL"

3.1 Introduction

The percentage of aged persons in society and their number are increasing, and their physical deterioration has become a social problem in many countries. Early detection of function deterioration and sufficient rehabilitation training are necessary, not only to decrease the numbers of aged who are bedridden or need nursing care, but also to enable the aged to take an active part in society.

This research has been conducted as a part of the NEDO (New Energy and Industrial Technology Development Organization) 5-year Project, "Rehabilitation System for the Upper Limbs and Lower Limbs" since 1999 . Furusho Laboratory of Osaka University and Asahi-kasei Group developed a 3-D rehabilitation system for upper limbs "EMUL". Hyogo Medical College took part in the project in the final year.

3.2 3-DOF Rehabilitation Training System

We have developed a 3-D rehabilitation system that has a performance suitable for rehabilitation for upper limbs and can display force senses in three-dimensional space (Furusho, Koyanagi, Imada et al., 2005), (Furusho, Koyanagi, Kataoka et al., 2005). Figure 6 shows the whole rehabilitation system. The maximum output torque of the ER actuator is about 3.0 [Nm]. As shown in Fig. 6, a patient can get exercise, sitting on a chair by gripping the handle of the upper limb exercise machine. The major targets in this study are hemiplegic patients who were paralyzed by stroke. The training is thought to include physical therapeutic exercises, such as passive and active exercises, and occupational therapeutic exercise like eating movement.

EMUL has the following specifications.

1) EMUL has 2 DOF for horizontal rotation and 1 DOF for vertical rotation.
2) The length of each link is 0.45 [m] and the height of the whole machine is about 1 [m].
3) All the actuators are set on the base of EMUL.
4) The vertical rotation part adopts a parallel link mechanism. This makes the gravity-effect compensation by counterbalance-weight in all posture possible.
5) The 3rd link is driven by spatial parallel link mechanism instead of belt-pulley and gear transmission system.
6) The motion range is about 0.90[m] (W) * 0.54[m] (D) * 0.50[m] (H).
7) The generative force at the end-effector is about 23 [N] in the horizontal plane and about 60 [N] in the vertical direction.

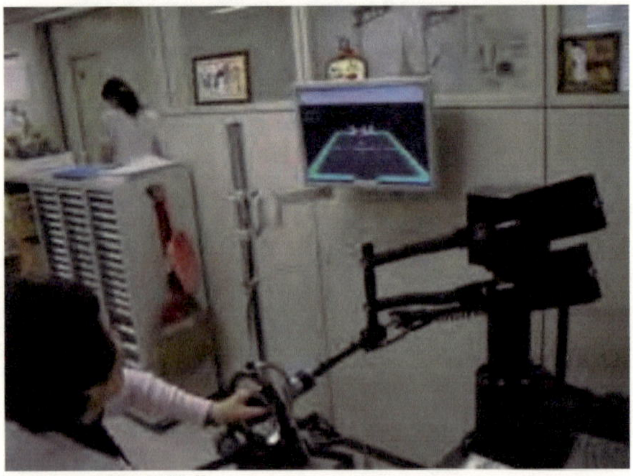

Fig. 6. Rehabilitation system "EMUL".

3.3 Software for Training

We show some examples of the training software.

A: Picture-Mask Erasing

As shown in Fig. 7, a semitransparent mask of a picture of 0.40 [m] * 0.40 [m] is erased by a virtual eraser which is operated by a patient. The patient can sense a reaction force from the picture surface through the gripper of 3-D rehabilitation system. For example, when 80 percent of the mask is erased, this picture vanishes and then the next new picture appears 0.05 [m] behind the vanished picture. The pictures are changed one after another until the

6th picture. This software has the effect of improvement about the dexterity and the movable range of limbs.

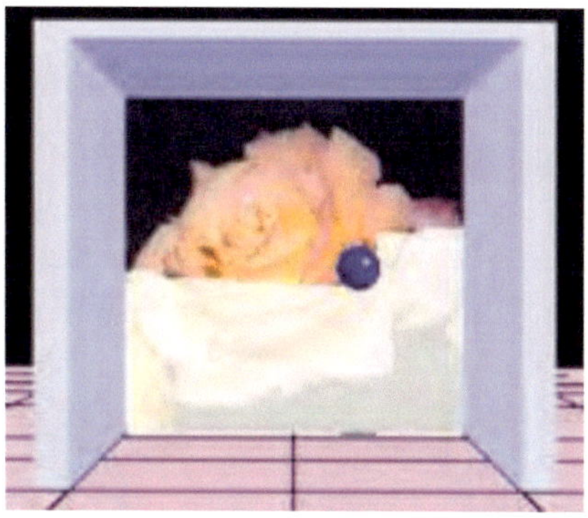

Fig. 7. Picure-mask erasing.

B: Virtual Maze & Virtual Hockey

Figure 8 shows a virtual maze of 0.40 [m] * 0.30 [m].When a virtual maze is completed, this maze disappears and then the next new maze appears 0.05 [m] behind the disappeared maze. The mazes are changed one after another until the 6th maze. This software has the effect of improvement about the dexterity and the movable range of limbs.

Figure 9 shows a virtual hockey game with impact-force-sense. Virtual hockey has the training effect about dexterity and agility.

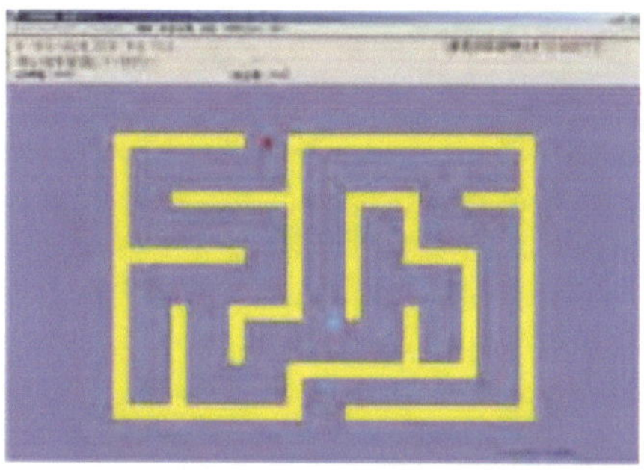

Fig. 8. Virtual maze.

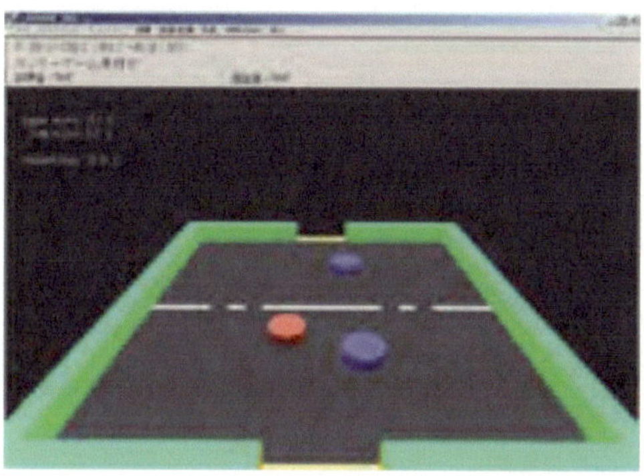

Fig. 9. Virtual hockey.

3.4 Clinical Testing

We conducted clinical testing for six patients. Each patient trained three times a week for six weeks. They all are patients of hemiparesis caused by stroke. The good results were obtained for all patients.

Figure 10 shows the shape of movable range in Picture-Mask-Erasing training of Patient A (67 years old male; 8 months after stroke; Left-side hemiplegia). As seen from this figure, the movable volume is expanded by the training.

Many evaluation methods (Fugl-Meyer Evaluation, Brunnstrom Stage, etc.) have been proposed in rehabilitation (Fugel-Meyer, 1975), (Demeurisse, 1980). The training using the developed system improved Fugl-Meyer Evaluation and Brunnstrom Stage (Furusho, Koyanagi, Imada et al., 2005).

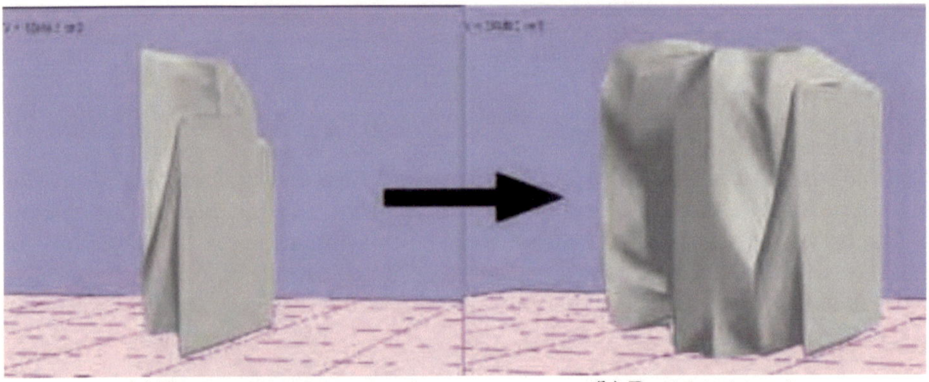

(a) Pre-treatment (b) Post-treatment

Fig. 10. Movable Range in Picture-Mask-Erasing.

At present we have started to evaluate the relationship between some kinds of training using EMUL and cortical activation during operation in joint research with Dr. Ichiro Miyai, Morinomiya Hosipital in in Osaka (Jin, Kikuchi, Haraguchi, Miyai et al., 2007). Figure 11 shows an experimental scene in which a subject operates EMUL and his cortical activation are measured using Near-infrared spectroscopic (NIRS) topography.

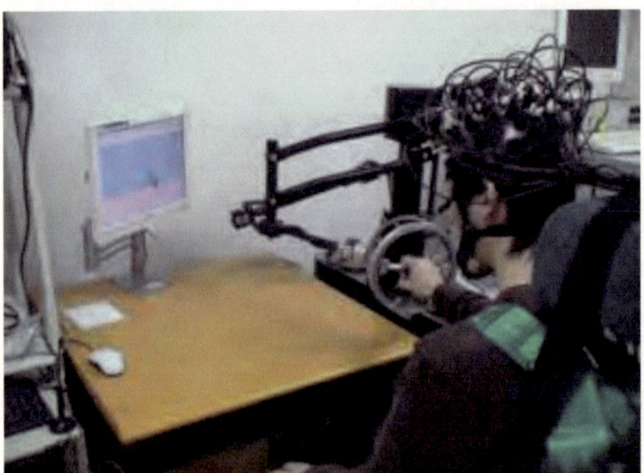

Fig. 11. EMUL and NIRS.

4. 6-DOF Rehabilitation System for Upper Limbs including Wrists "Robotherapist"

4.1 Introduction

We have developed Robotherapist, which is a 6-DOF force display system for upper limbs including wrists (Furusho, Hu, Kikuchi et al., 2006). The system can measure positions and postures of an operator's hand, and generate a large force sense including the wrist torque to the operator. This system enables efficient rehabilitation trainings, which focus on the harmonic movement of the whole upper limb. Robotherapist was exhibited at ``The Prototype Robot Festival at the 2005 International Exposition held in Aichi Prefecture, Japan'' (See Fig. 12).

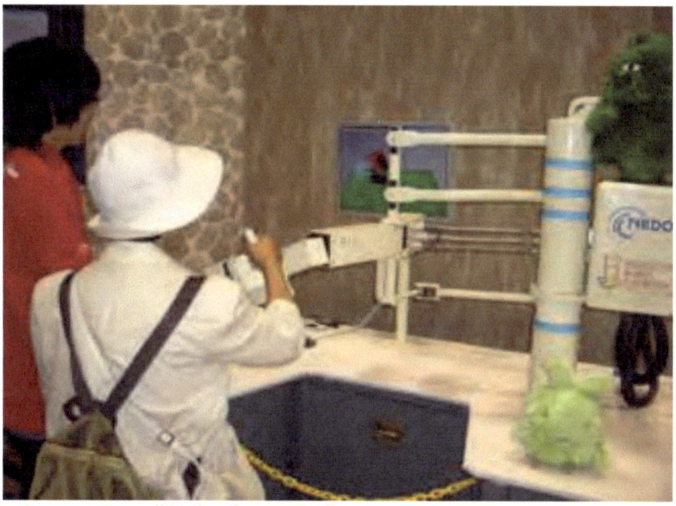

Fig. 12. Rehabilitation system "Robotherapist".

4.2 Mechanism of Robotherapist

A structure of Robotherapist can be divided into two mechanism groups: one is for positioning of an operating part (3-DOF) and another is for posturing of it (3-DOF). ER actuators drive all of 6-DOF.

A: Mechanism for positioning of an operating part

Figure 13 shows the mechanism for the positioning. As seen from this figure, Robotherapist has 2-DOF for a horizontal rotation and 1-DOF for a vertical movement in arm parts. Actuators for arm motions are set on a base in order to reduce the inertia of the moving parts. Link2 is a parallel link mechanism. A counter-balance weight compensates a gravity-effect of these links in all posture.

B: Mechanism for posturing of an operating part

The mechanism for posturing has 3-DOF; that is, roll, pitch and yaw rotation. Generally, a heavy weight of an end-effecter impairs smooth acceleration of operation. Additionally, such a weight is very risky when the end-effecter collides with the operator. Therefore, the operating part was designed as light as possible. Actuators for the operating part are placed near Link1, and a torque of each actuator is transmitted to it by driving shafts and wire-pulleys systems.

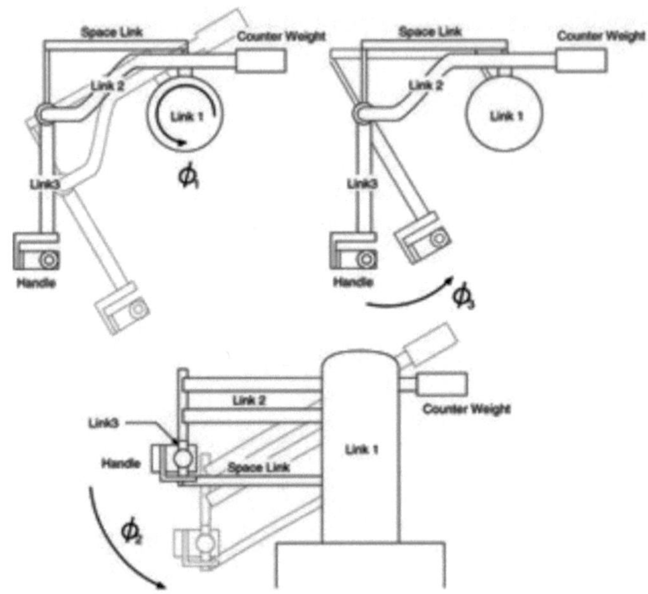

Fig. 13. Configuration of Robotherapist.

4.3 Application Software of Robotherapist

We have also developed application software of Robotherapist for upper limb rehabilitation that includes upper limb's harmonic movements. Important viewpoints for the rehabilitation training software are as follows;

1. Many movements using the shoulder, the elbow, and the wrist harmonically are included.
2. The sense of amusement is needed for long-term training.
3. The recovery degree of upper limbs function can be evaluated properly.

The developed applications are the following four kinds.

A: Water Supply (see Fig. 14)

The operator grasps a handgrip of a watering pod and gives water to the ground. The amount of the water, which comes out of the pod is calculated according as a tilt of the pod, and flower blooms gradually grow up according to the quantity of the given water. The goal of this game is making flower blooms on the whole ground. The system gives the operator a force depending on the tilt and the weight of residual water in the pod. The operator has to cooperate his shoulder, elbow, and wrist, in order to control the position and the tilt of the pod.

B: Window Sweep (see Fig. 15)

At first whole area of the window is masked in white. The operator grasps a wiper and removes the white mask. If the mask is removed, a picture appears in the window. When the wiper is pressed on the window, the reaction force from the window is given to the operator. In order to remove the white mask efficiently, it is necessary to control not only the position but also the posture of the wiper. Therefore, the operator should move his shoulder, elbow, and wrist harmonically.

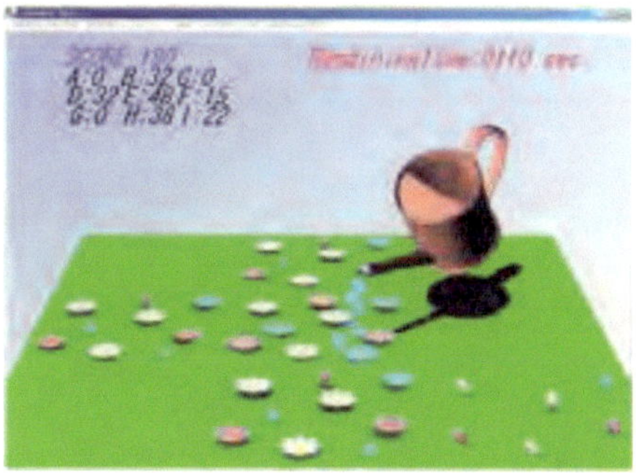

Fig. 14. Water supply.

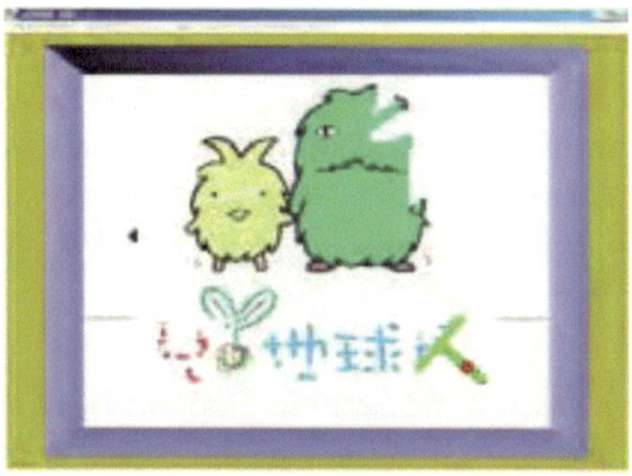

Fig. 15. Window sweep.

C: Squash & Block Break (see Fig. 16 & Fig. 17)

These two games have a same concept. The operator strikes back a ball with a racket, and make the ball hit targets. Breaking all targets is the goal of these games. When the ball hits the racket, a sense of impulse is given to the operator. In Squash, the targets are panels. If the ball hits a panel several times, the panel will disappear and the picture over the panel appears. In Block Break, the targets are spherical blocks. When a block is hit the ball or other blocks, the block vibrates. If the ball hits a block several times, the block will disappear like the case of Squash.

In these games, the operator is required controlling the posture of the racket in order to strike back the ball well. Moreover, it is required to move a whole upper limb quickly, and much amusement nature is included.

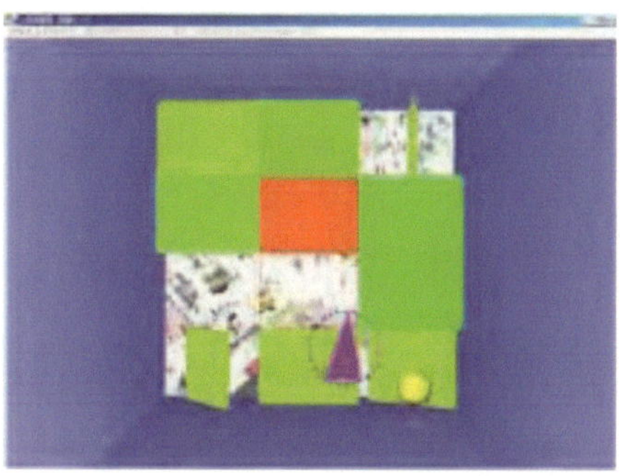

Fig. 16. Squash.

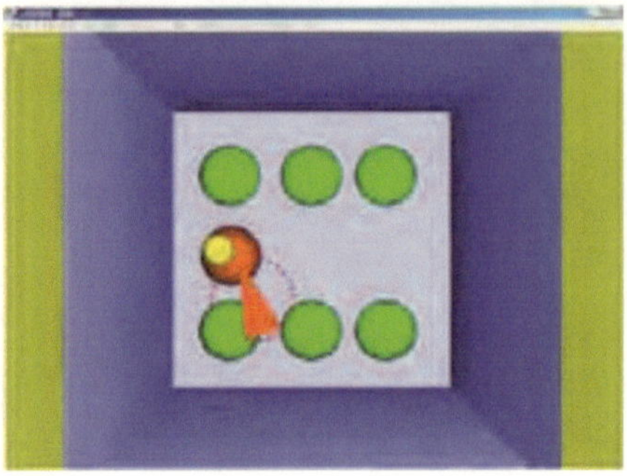

Fig. 17. Block break.

4.4 Application Software of Robotherapist Based on PNF Techniques

Furusho Laboratory of Osaka Univ. and Prof. Kunihiko Oda of Osaka Electro-Communication Univ., Dept. of Physical Therapy are developing the evaluating software developed for the rehabilitation of patients suffered from cerebellum malfunction based on Proprioceptive Neuromuscular Facilitation (PNF) techniques (Furusho, Kikuchi, Oda et al., 2007), (Kikuchi, Furusho, Oda et al., 2007).

A: Rhythmic Stabilization

Figure 18 shows the image of Rhythmic Stabilization, and Figure 19 shows the graphics of Rhythmic Stabilization. As shown in Fig. 18 and Fig. 19, a therapist gives each force from random directions quickly to the hand of a patient. And then the patient is instructed to maintain the position of his/her hand. In Rhythmic Stabilization, therapist want to know whether a patient can maintain the position of his/her hand, and how strong the force is, and which direction he is weak in.

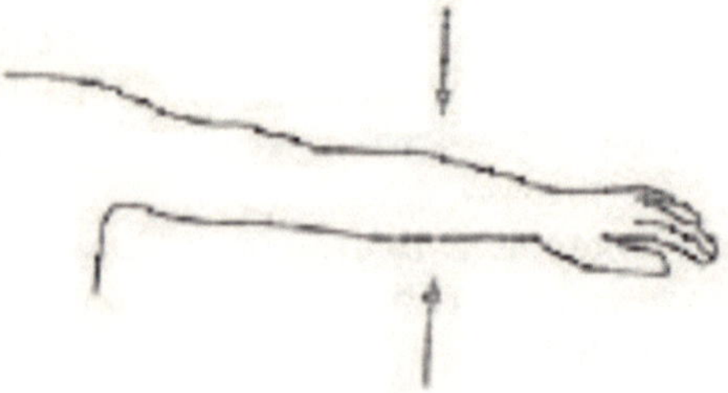

Fig. 18. Image of rhythmic stabilization.

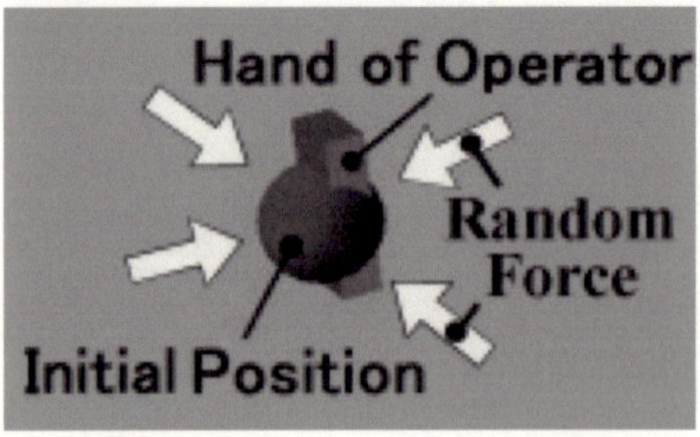

Fig. 19. Display of rhythmic stabilization.

B: Finger Nose Finger (FNF)

As shown in Fig. 20 and Fig. 21, a patient repeats the movement between therapist's finger and his/her nose under the expected orbit. In FNF, therapist would judge recovery degree of patient by his/her movement.

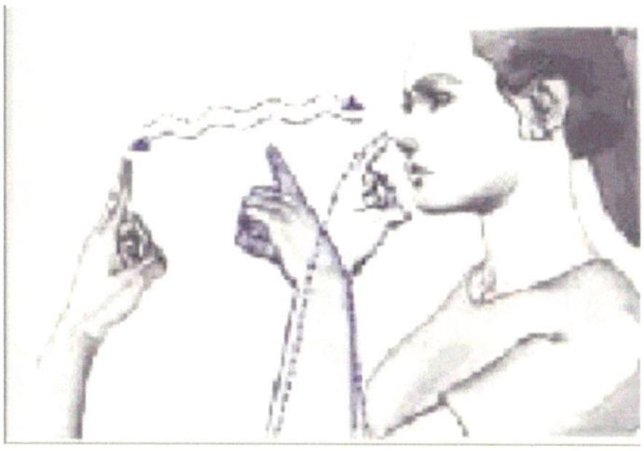

Fig. 20. Image of FNF.

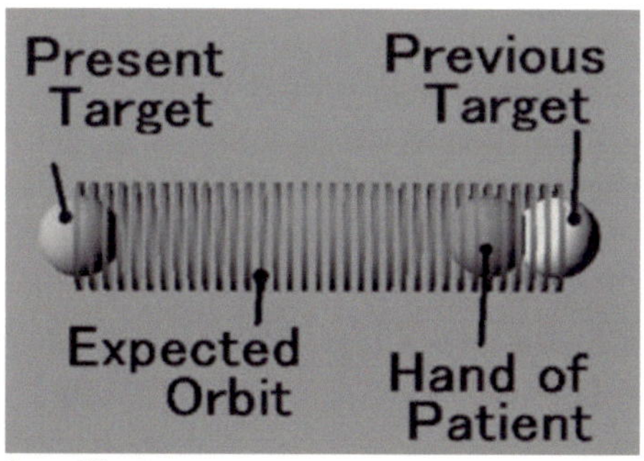

Fig. 21. Display of Finger Nose Finger.

C: Arc Exercise with GUR

In PNF, a therapist gives opposite force to patient in order to guide patient's hand in the desired direction. Then the patient resists the force from the therapist and knows which the desired direction is. We name this technique "Guidance Utilizing Reaction". As shown in Fig. 22, a patient extends his/her arm and moves his/her handle just on the arc orbit. When he moves it along the orbit, there is no force. Otherwise when the handle is away from the given orbit, the patient can sense force to his/her body.

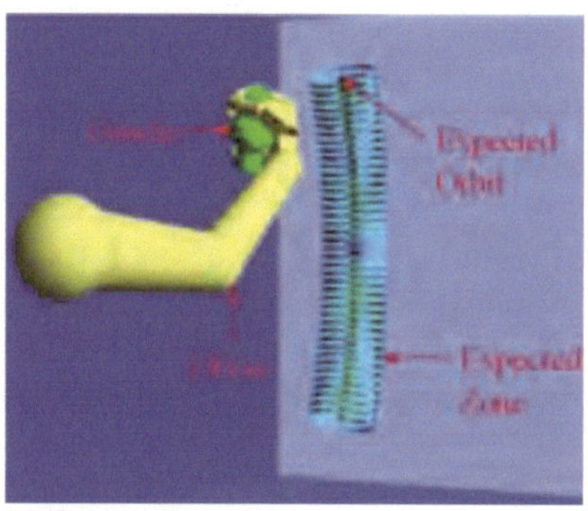

Fig. 22. Display of Guidance Utilizing Reaction.

5. Quasi-3-DOF rehabilitation System "PLEMO"

5.1 Introduction

In general, therapists make the rehabilitation program based on an inspection and a measurement of each patient. However, it is difficult to adopt appropriate rehabilitation programs for all patients, because the evaluation method is based on experiences of each therapist. Recently, Evidence Based Medicine (EBM) is required strongly in the field of rehabilitation. Therefore robot-aided rehabilitation is expected to quantify the effect of rehabilitative activities.

As shown in section 3 and 4 of this chapter, we developed 3-D rehabilitation system for upper limb "EMUL" and 6-DOF rehabilitation system "Robotherapist", and conducted clinical test. EMUL and Robotherapist adopted to use ER actuators and clutch mechanism for its actuation part. This mechanism makes these systems so safe and back-drivable. However, they have disadvantages in cost, because this system became enlarged to realize the force-feedback in large 3-D space. A system which is more compact and better for maintenance should be required for practical use.

To meet the demands above, we developed new haptic device which has 2-DOF force-feedback function in working plane but its working plane can be adjusted by the inclination of the table. We named this system "Quasi-3-DOF Rehabilitation System for Upper Limbs" or "PLEMO" (shown in Fig. 23) (Kikuchi, Furusho, Jin et al., 2007) (Kikuchi, Hu et al., 2007). PLEMO was developed to realize quantitative evaluation of the rehabilitation training for patients with spasticity after stroke. In this section, we describe the mechanism of PLEMO and its software for upper limb rehabilitation.

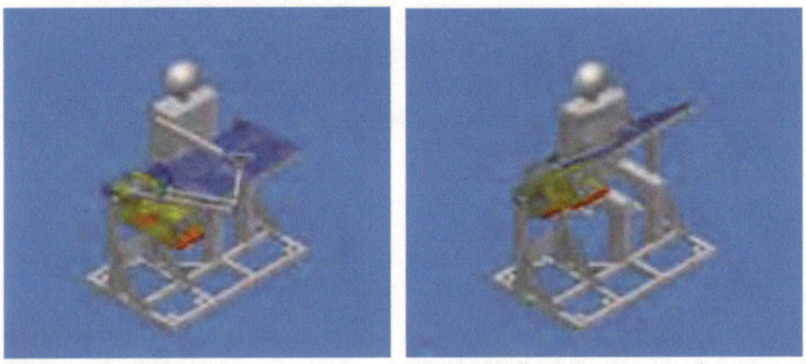

Fig. 23. Quasi-3-DOF rehabilitation system "PLEMO": Horizontal state (left) and slanted state (right).

5.2 ER Brake

Using ER fluid as working fluid, we construct electrically controllable brake (ER brake) with high-performance (good rapidity and repeatability of brake torque) (Kikuchi, Furusho et al., 2003). We use this brake for the force generators of new rehabilitation system (force-feedback system).

Figure 24 show the sectional view and appearance of the brake. As shown in the left drawing of Fig. 4, this brake consists of multi-layered disks. ER fluid is filled between the rotor-disks and stator-disks. As a result, six layers of ER fluid generate brake torque with the change of the fluid. Piston mechanism works for the prevention of liquid spill with the expansion of the fluid. We can control the brake torque form 0.1 [Nm] to 4.0 [Nm] with applied electric field from 0.0 [kV/mm] to 3.0 [kV/mm]. Additionally, response time of torque is several milliseconds.

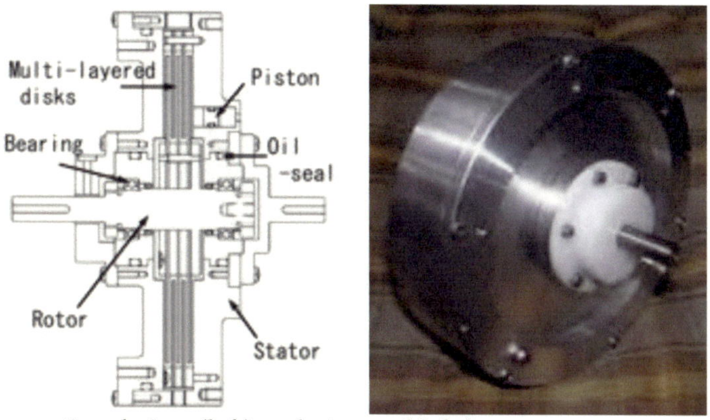

Fig. 24. ER Brake: sectional view (left) and picture (right).

Figure 25 shows a passive force display using ER brakes (IEEE Virtual Reality 2001) in previous research (Furusho, Sakaguchi et al., 2002). In the research, we established control methods with a passive force display system on 2-D space. On the basis of this technology, we developed basic structure and control method of PLEMO.

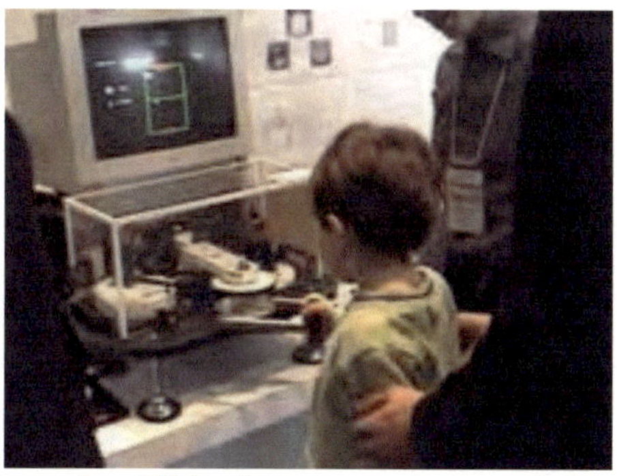
Fig. 25. Passive force display using ER brakes

5.3 Quasi-3-DOF Rehabilitation System for Upper Limbs, "PLEMO"

We developed a new haptic device with the two ER brakes shown in Fig. 26. This is a passive-type force display which can output several kinds of virtual force, for example resistance, viscosity, vibration etc.

This machine has two active degrees of freedom (DOF) in a working plane and one passive DOF of the inclination of the working plane. We named this system "Quasi-3-DOF Rehabilitation System for Upper Limb" or "PLEMO". PLEMO is a combination of "pleasant" and "motivation". This word includes our hope that this system gives patents a pleasant experience of recovery and motivation for rehabilitation trainings. This system is safe for human because it uses only brakes. Force control unit consist of the two ER brakes and the brake torque generates output-force on a handle through a parallel linkage.

Figure 27 is a structure and signal flow chart of this system. Working area of PLEMO is 0.6 [m] (W) * 0.5 [m] (D). Adjustable angle of the inclination is from -30 to 90 degrees. Plemo-P1 realizes from vertical training to horizontal training by only one system. Total size of the system is 1.0 [m] (W) * 0.6 [m] (D) * 0.7 [m] (H), except for the display. This is similar to the size of general desks. Not to use any actuator contributes to make this system more compact, simple, and reasonable for cost.

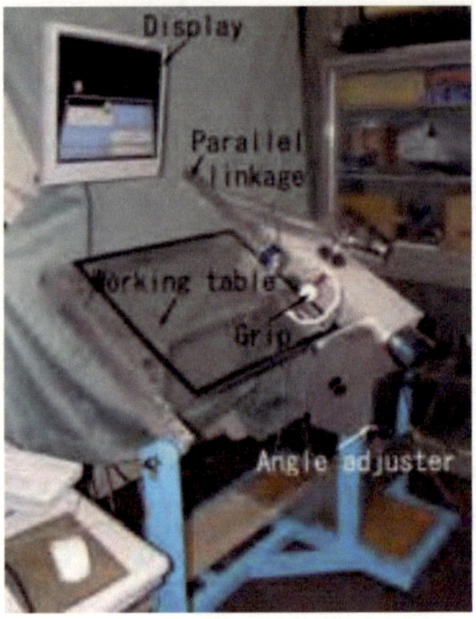

Fig. 26. PLEMO.

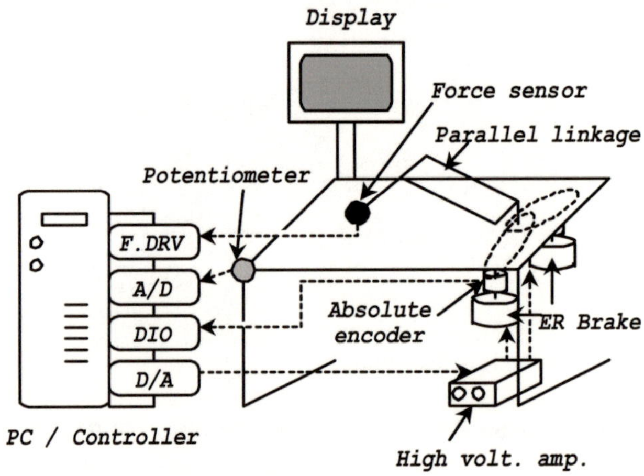

Fig. 27. Structure and signal flow of PLEMO.

5.4 Software of PLEMO

We develop a rehabilitation software shown in Figure 28. This is a tracking test program. An operator grips the handle and moves it to track a target ball. The position of operating handle is displayed as red sphere. The target ball is moving along the target track. White zone in this figure means smooth area without any force-feedback. Blue zone means sticky area; operator feels virtual force like moving his hand in the viscous fluid. It is easy to change kinds of the virtual forces and its area.

Data of position, velocity and operating force are saved in the output files and we can evaluate accuracy of poison and velocity, range of motion, cognitive faculty and so on. We should make decision of the training protocol and evaluating method depending on the symptom of patient individually.

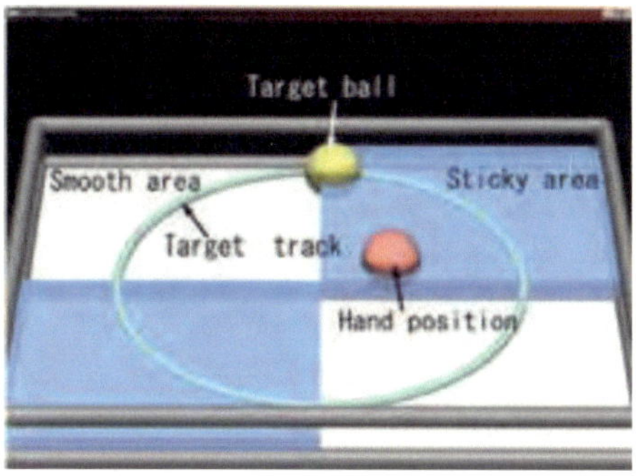

Fig. 28. View of tracking test.

6. Intelligently-Controlled Prosthetic Ankle Joint Using MR Fluid

MR fluid is the non-colloidal solution mixed with ferromagnetic metal particles whose diameter is several millimetres. It is a kind of functional fluid changing viscosity (about several milliseconds in response) of its appearance according to the magnitude of the magnetic field.
All prosthesis users need "foot" part. This part moves so frequently and widely that it needs to be as light as possible. It also must be silent and strong because it is used in daily life. If stiffness or spring characteristics of prosthesises can be changed according to the timing of walking and dorsiflection can be kept adequately, it will be much easier for users to walk and run.
A lot of intelligent prosthetic knees have been developed and are sold on the market. But none of prosthesis that can control the ankle was on the market.
Figure 29 shows an example of a prosthetic "foot" part. It is composed of a prosthetic ankle joint and a foot-ankle unit. Energy of movement stored at the elastic part (rubber) of the prosthetic ankle joint is relieved when kicking, producing driving force. This rubber can also absorb shocks when the heel hits on the ground, and changing the angle smoothly.
After kicking back, a leg leaves from the ground and swings forward during swing phase. Then the rubber goes back to its balanced midpoint, which makes the ankle turns from the dorsal direction instantly (deflecting a tiptoe upward, as shown in Fig. 29 (a)) to the plantar direction (swaging a tiptoe underneath, as shown in Fig. 29 (c)).

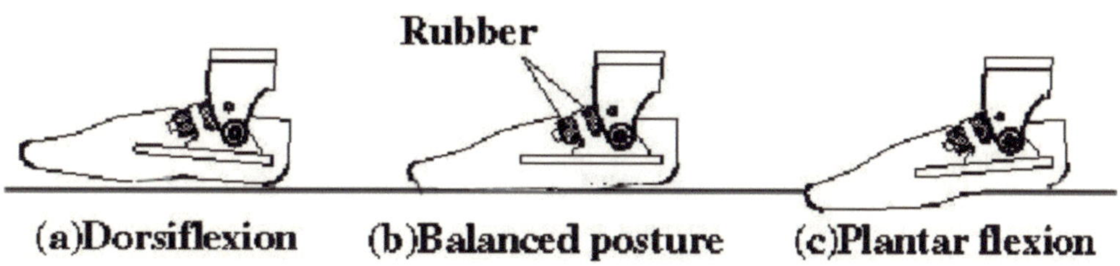

Fig. 29. Prosthetic foot.

Since there is a problem that the tiptoe of the prosthesis tends to collide on the ground (see Fig. 30), users have to walk paying attention to lifting legs in order not to tumble. This is why users walk unnaturally causing to use unnecessary energy. To solve this problem, we suggest setting a linear brake at "foot" part.

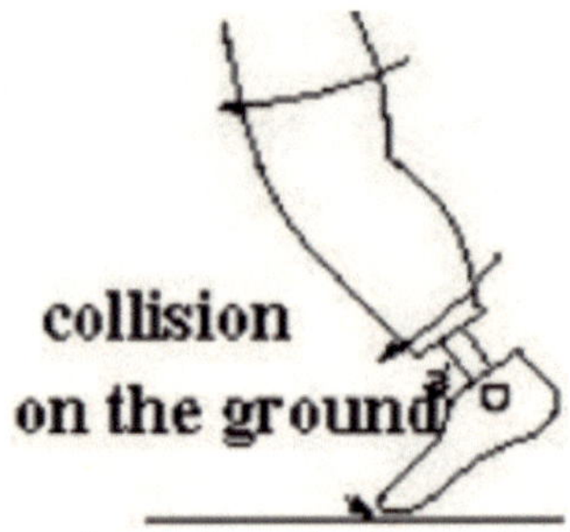

Fig. 30. Walking appearance of prosthetic foot during swing phase.

The MR (Magnetorheological) fluid has been used for the linear brakes. Figure 31 shows a schematic of MR Linear Brake (MRLB). MRLB consists of a piston composed of two rods, a bobbin sandwiched by the rods on both sides, and MR fluid inside a cylinder. When electric current is applied to the coil which rolls the bobbin, magnetic field is generated in loops as follows; Bobbin→MR fluid→Cylinder→MR fluid →Bobbin.

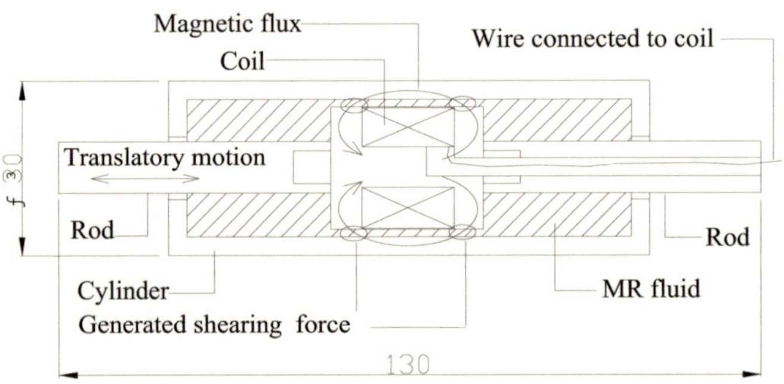

Fig. 31. Construction of MR Linear Brake.

We developed two prototypes of the intelligent prosthetic ankle joint using MR brakes (Furusho, Takesue et al., 2004), (Li, Furusho et al., 2006), (Li, Tokuda, Furusho et al., 2006). Figure 32 shows the 2nd prototypes. Figure 33 and Figure 34 show the series of static images extracted from moving images of the walking experiments. Circles around the ankle in these figures show the test subject's left leg (a swinging leg).

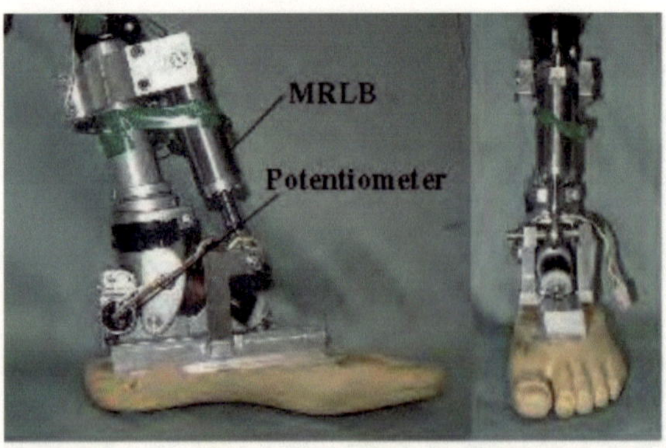

Fig. 32. 2nd prototype.

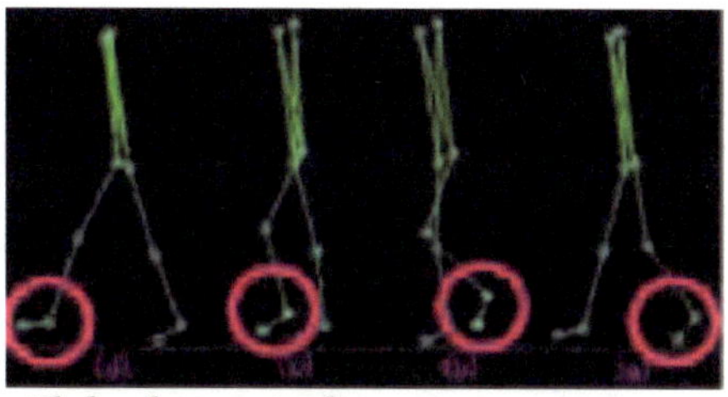

Fig. 33. Walking positions with brake control.

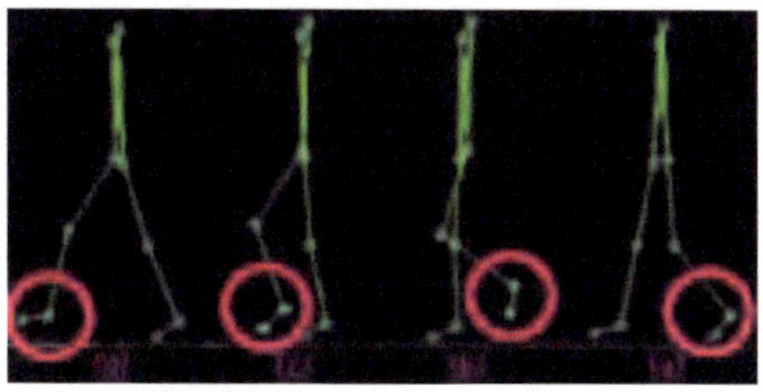

Fig. 34. Walking positions without brake control.

The subject's impressions of experiments with 2nd prototype are as follows: "I felt easier to walk by keeping dorsiflexion. I didn't care the total weight only for some hours, but if I use it in my daily life all day, it will be a load for me ".

7. Intelligent Ankle-Foot Orthosis with Shear-type MR Fluid Brake

Recently, as habits of people has changed, stroke patients tend to increase. There are many cases of the hemiplegia as aftereffects of a stroke. Stroke patient with hemiplegia show difference in the degree by a part and a range of a lesion caused by a disease, however rehabilitation is indispensable to restore functional disorder of lower limbs. We are developing intelligent ankle-foot orthoses using shear-type MR fluid brakes in a 3-year NEDO project (2006~2008)(Furusho, Li et al., 2007), (Furusho, Kikuchi et al., 2007).

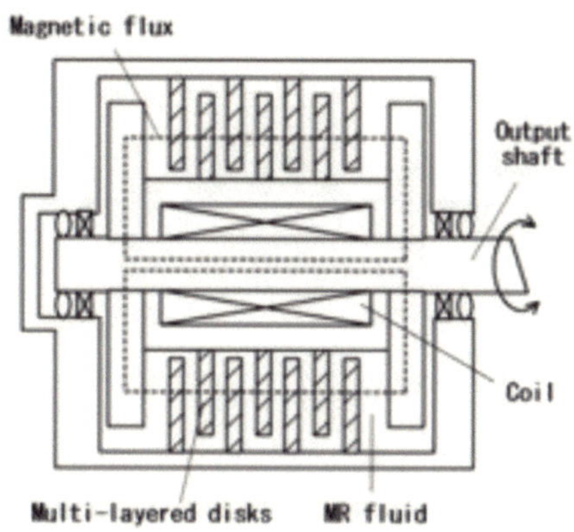

Fig. 35. Structure of MRB.

Figure 35 shows a conceptual illustration of shear-type MR fluid brakes. A coil rolled round a shaft give an MR fluid a magnetic field. Scroll number of coils and spindle diameter are decided by performing magnetic field analysis. As for materials of each part, magnetism materials are used in a magnetic circuit part. In addition, a housing is made of a nonmagnetic body, to avoid the magnetic flux from leaking.

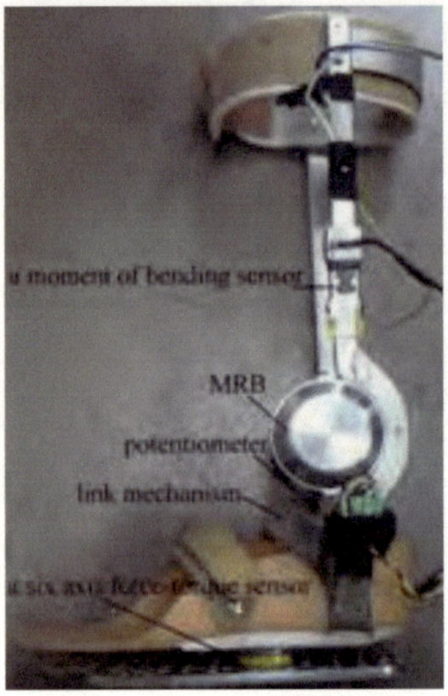

Fig. 36. Ankle-Foot Orthosis.

Figure 36 shows the second Prototype of intelligent ankle-foot orthosis using the shear-type MR fluid brake. We obtain the maximum torque of 24 [Nm] with the idling torque of 0.1[Nm]. We use four sensors: potentiometer on the ankle, 6-axis force-torque sensor at the center of a foot bottom, a moment of bending sensor and an acceleration sensor on the prop part of an orthosis side.
We divide a walking step into four; into heel reaching the ground, tiptoe reaching the ground, heel leaving ground, tiptoe leaving ground (see Fig. 37). These states are detected by using the above sensors, and then the brake torque is controlled in accordance with each state.

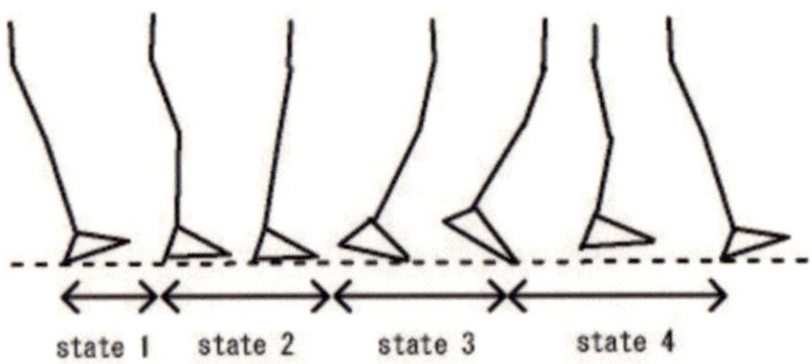

Fig. 37. Walking State.

8. Conclusion

High safety rehabilitation systems using functional fluid were introduced. Two units of EMUL were made in the 5-year NEDO project, and they were transferred from NEDO to Furusho Laboratory of Osaka University. We continue clinical evaluation of 3-D rehabilitation system and quasi-3-DOF rehabilitation system by using EMUL, Robotherapist and PLEMO.
We have been studying rehabilitation robotics mainly from the standpoint of mechatronics and virtual reality. Now, we started to study it also from the standpoint of physical therapy and motion control of human beings.

9. References

Bossis, G. (2002). Ed., *Proceedings of the eighth International conference on Electrorheological fluids and Magnetorheological Suspensions.* World Scientific

Burgar, C. G. ; Lum, P.S. ; Shor, P. C. & der Loos, H. M. V. (2000). Development of robots for rehabilitation therapy : The palo alto va/stanford experience, *Jurnal of Rehabilitation Reseach and Development*, Vol. 37, No.6, 663-673

Charles, S. ; Krebs, H. I. ; Volpe, B. T. ; Lynch, D. & Hogan, N. (2005). Wrist rehabilitation following stroke:Initial clinical results, *Proceedings of the 2005 IEEE 9th International Conference on Rehabilitation Robotics*, 13-16

Demeurisse, G. et al. (1980). Motor evaluation in vascular hemiplegia, *Eur, Neurol.*, Vol.19, 382-389

Fugel-Meyer A. R. et al. (1975). The post-stroke hemiplegic patient1, a method for evaluation of physical perpormance, *Scand. J. Rahabil. Med.*, Vol.7, 13-31

Furusho, J.; Li, C.; Morimoto, S.; Tokuda, M.; Kikuchi, T. & Hashimoto, Y. (2007). Development of Shear-type MR Brakes and their Application to Ankle-Foot Orthoses, *Proceedings of the International Conference on Complex Medical Engineering* (CD-ROM), 1283-1287

Furusho, J.; Kikuchi, T., Tokuda .M.; Kakehashi, T.; Ikeda, K.; Morimoto, S.; Hashimoto,Y.; Tomiyama, H.; Nakagawa, A. & Akazawa, Y.(2007). Development of Shear Type Compact MR Brake for the Intelligent Ankle-Foot Orthosis and Its Control (Research and Development in NEDO for Practical Application of Human Support Robot), *Proceedings of IEEE International Conference on Rehabilitation Robotics*, 89-94

Furusho, J.; Kikuchi, T.; Oda, K.; Ohyama, Y.; Morita, T.; Shichi, N.; Jin, Y. & Inoue, A.(2007). A 6-DOF Rehabilitation Support System for Upper Limbs including Wrists "Robotherapist" with Physical Therapy, *Proceedings of IEEE International Conference on Rehabilitation Robotics*, 304-309

Furusho, J.; Hu, X.; Kikuchi, T.; Nakayama, K.; Yamaguchi, Y.; Li, C.; Shichi, N.; Inoue, A. & Ryu, U. (2006). Development of a 6-DOF force display system using ER actuator with high-safety, *Proceedings of the ACM International Conference on Virtual Reality Continuum and Its Applications 2006* (CD-ROM), 405-408

Furusho, J. & Kikuchi, T. (2006). Collaboration of medical engineering and fluid power (Review paper), Journal of the Japan Fluid Power System Society, Vol.37, No.5, 272-276 (In Japanese)

Furusho, J.; Koyanagi, K.; Imada, Y.; Fujii, Y.; Nakanishi, K.; Domen, K.; Miyakoshi, K. U. Ryu, S. Takenaka, A, Inoue. (2005). A 3-D Rehabilitation system for Upper Limbs Developed in a 5-year NEDO Project and its Clinical Testing, *Proceedings of the 2005 IEEE 9th International Conference on Rehabilitation Robotics* , 53-56

Furusho, J.; Koyanagi, K.; Kataoka, J. Ryu, U.; Inoue, A. & Takenaka, S. (2005). Development of 3-D rehabilitation system for upper limb -1st report: development of mechanism including ER actuators and whole system -, *Journal of the Robotics Society of Japan*, Vol.23, No.5, 629-636 (In Japanese)

Furusho, J. & Takesue, N. et al. (2004). Development of intelligent prosthetic ankle joint (1st report, development of linear-type MR-fluid brake), *Transactions of the Japan Society of Mechanical Engineers (C)*, Vol.70, No.695, 275-282

Furusho, J.; Sakaguchi, M.; Takesue, N. & Koyanagi, K. (2002). Development of ER brake and its application to passive force display, *Journal of Intelligent Material Systems and Structures*, Vol. 13, No. 7/8, 425-429

Furusho, J. (2001). Mechatronics system using ER fluids (review paper), Journal of Japan Hydraulics and Pneumatic Society, Vol. 32, No .6, 390-395 (In Japanese)

Furusho, J. & Sakaguchi, M. (1999). New actuators using ER fluid and their applications to force display devices in virtual reality and medical treatments, *International Journal of Modern Physics B*, Vol.13, No.14, 15 & 16, 2151-2159

Furusho, J.; Wei, Z. & Koga, S. (1995). Development of an actuator with low inertia using electro-rheological fluid and its application to virtual reality, *Proceeding of the 72nd JSME Spring Annual Meeting*, Vol.4, 265-266

Furusho, J. & Sano, A. (1990). Sensor-based control of a nine-link biped, The International Journal of Robotics Research, Vol.9, No.2, 83-98

Furusho, J. & Masubuchi, M. (1987). A theoretically motivated reduced order model for the control of biped locomotion, *Trans. ASME, Journal of Dynamic Systems, Measurement and Control*, Vol.109, 155-163

Ishikawa, T. (2000). Basic Study on the Development of a Rehabilitation Training System, *Master's Thesis of Osaka Univesity.*

ISO10218 (1992). *Manipulating industrial robots-safty.*

Janet, C. & Shepherd, R. (1998). *Neurological Rehabilitation: Optimizing Motor Performance*, Butterworth-Heinemann, Boston

Kikuchi, T.; Furusho, J.; Oda, K.; Jin, Y.; Li, C.; Morita, T.; Shichi, N.; Ohyama, Y. & Inoue, A. (2007). Development of a 6-DOF rehabilitation robot and its software for clinical evaluation based on virtual reality, *Proceedings of the International Conference on Complex Medical Engineering*, (CD-ROM), 1306-1309

Kikuchi, T.; Hu, X.; Fukushima, K.; Oda, K. Furusho J. & Inoue, A. (2007). Quasi-3-DOF Rehabilitation System for Upper Limbs: Its Force-Feedback Mechanism and Software for Rehabilitation, *Proceedings of IEEE International Conference on Rehabilitation Robotics*, 24-27

Kikuchi, T.; Furusho, J.; Jin, Y.; Hu, X.; Fukushima, K. & Inoue, A. (2007). Development of the quasi-3-DOF rehabilitation system for upper limbs, "PLEMO", The Japanese Journal for Medical Virtual Reality, Vol.5, No.1, 24-31

Kikuchi, T.; Furusho, J. & Oda, K. (2003). Development of isokinetic exercise machine using ER brake, *Proceedings of 2003 IEEE International Conference on Robotics and Automation* (CD-ROM), 214-219

Krebs, H. I. ; Volpe, B. T. ; Aisen, M. L. & Hogan, N. (2000). Increasing productivity and quality of care : Robot-aided neuro rehabilitation, *Jurnal of Rehabilitation Research and Development*, Vol. 37, No.6, 639-652

Li C. & Furusho, J. et al. (2006) Developement of intelligent prosthetic ankle joint (2nd report, development of the 1st prototype with intelligent prosthetic ankle joint), *Transactions of the Japan Society of Mechanical Engineers (C)*, Vol.72, No.714, 493-498

Li, C.; Miwa, T.; Furusho, J.; Morimoto, S.; Koyanagi, K.; Nakagawa, A.; Akazawa, Y. & Hashimoto, Y. (2006). Research and developement of the intelligently-controlled prosthetic ankle joint, *Proceedings of 2006 IEEE International Conference on Mechatronics and Automation*, 1114-1119

Jin, Y.; Kikuchi, T.; Haraguchi, M.; Miyai, I.; Mihara, M.; Hatakenaka, M. & Furusho, J. (2007). Basic Study for Development of Evaluation System for Upper Limb's Rehabilitation System with 3-DOF Rehabilitation Robot "EMUL" and Near-infrared Spectroscopic (NIRS), *Proceedings of the 2007 JSME Conference on Robotics and Mechatronics*, (CD-ROM), 1A1-K03 (In Japanese)

9

The Rehabilitation Robots FRIEND-I & II: Daily Life Independency through Semi-Autonomous Task-Execution

Christian Martens*, Oliver Prenzel** & Axel Gräser**
*University of Bremen, Institute of Automation***
*Rheinmetall Defence Electronics**
Germany

1. Introduction

The rehabilitation robotic systems FRIEND[1]-I (Martens et al., 2001) and its successor FRIEND-II have been developing at the Institute of Automation (IAT), University of Bremen, Germany, since 1997 and 2003 respectively. The systems belong to the category "intelligent wheelchair mounted manipulators". They focus on users with high spinal cord injury, or with similar handicaps, who are unable to control the manipulator by means of a keyboard or joystick. The systems offer support during daily life activities and at professional life. The strategic objective of the FRIEND as well as the succeeding AMaRob[2] project, which focuses on the usage of FRIEND-II within the context of an intelligent environment, is to research into new methods to control the robotic system in such a way that their users become independent for at least 1.5 hours without support by nursing staff. Beside the aspect that this is one of the main requirements expressed by potential users, the fulfillment of this objective would have a strong impact on the commercialization of the rehabilitation robotic system itself.

This article gives an overview of the FRIEND project and the robotic systems there from evolved. It is divided into a practical part, which presents the systems from a user oriented perspective, and into a theoretical part, which satisfies the system-engineer's point of view. The user oriented part outlines the different development steps, functional improvements, hardware setups and lessons learned since 1997. Here, the facilities of the FRIEND-I system as well as a description of the innovations of the FRIEND-II system, currently under development, are described with specific emphasis of the AMaRob project. The reader becomes aware of the functionalities and services offered by the FRIEND rehabilitation robot and of the challenging technical complexity with which the development has to deal. The theoretical part is focused on the concept of semi-autonomous task-execution as a means of reasonable complexity reduction. Due to the consequent application of this concept a technically manageable robotic system emerges, which is able to execute tasks on a high level of abstraction in a reliable and robust manner. Within this context semi-autonomous task-

[1] FRIEND - Functional robot arm with user-friendly interface for disabled people
[2] AMaRob - Autonomous manipulator control for rehabilitation robots

execution is used as a synonym for system initiated and controlled user involvement during task-execution. For the realization of this approach the control architecture MASSiVE[3] has been designed and implemented. It supports task-execution on the basis of a priori defined and formally verified task-knowledge. This task-knowledge contains all possible sequences of operations as well as the symbolic representation of objects required for the execution of a specific task. The seamless integration of user interactions into this task-knowledge, in combination with MASSiVE's user-adapted human-machine interface (HMI) layer, enables the system to deliberately interact with the user during run-time. It is shown how MASSiVE's application within the FRIEND-II system supports the future development of new services that increase autonomy of the users.

2. Evolution of Rehabilitation Robots

The development of rehabilitation robots started at the end of the 80ies in the last century. It was driven by the intention to support elderly and disabled people during daily life activities, making them more independent from care personnel or relatives. Additionally, the promising concept of an artificial assistant should be improved and technologically explored. This explains the chronological order of the appearance of different kinds of rehabilitation robots as they are presented in the following.

The first step in the evolution of rehabilitation robots was the development of fixed workstation systems that could execute pre-programmed tasks, like picking up paper from a printer or taking a book from a bookshelf. Quite popular systems of this category are DeVAR (Van der Loos, 1995; Mokhtari & Amni, 2001), ProVAR (Wagner et al., 1998; Van der Loos et al., 1999), RAID (Dallaway & Jackson , 1993; Eftring, 1994), MASTER-RAID II (Dallaway et al., 1995; Busnel et al., 1999; Mokhtari & Amni, 2001) or CAPDI (Casals et al., 1999). All these systems have in common that they consist of an industrial robot that is mounted at a workstation. Furthermore, they possess HMIs that are adapted to their users' special needs resulting from his or her disability.

Due to their structured and well known environment, fixed workstation systems could process complex task efficiently. Because this ability is limited to these predefined tasks, it turned out that these systems were too restrictive for a flexible use, e.g. in the domestic environment. This was the main motivation for the development of special purpose wheelchair mounted manipulators, like MANUS (Mokhtari & Amni, 2001), Wessex/Weston robot arm (Hillman et al., 1999) or RAPTOR (Mahoney, 2001). By means of different HMIs, e.g. joystick, keyboard or space-mouse, the user can control the gripper of the arm with respect to a Cartesian coordinate system or control each joint of the arm directly. In contradiction to industrial robots the main goal for the development of these manipulators was to create lightweight robot arms that satisfy special security requirements resulting from the direct human-machine interaction. This comes along with a loss of positioning accuracy, so that the pre-programming of complex action sequences, even in structured environments, was no longer possible. This is the reason why the control of these systems can only be performed on a low level of abstraction. For example, the user can command the direction for the arm movement or open and close the gripper. Even though this kind of control offers a great flexibility in use, it puts a high cognitive load on its users. Especially for complex tasks

[3] MASSiVE - Multilayer Control Architecture for Semi-autonomous Service Robots with Verified Task Execution

this is tiresome and comes along with a loss of concentration (Kawamura et al., 1995). Additionally, the kinds of HMIs which come along with these manipulators exclude tetraplegic (spinal cord injuries above vertebrae C5) or persons with a similar clinical picture.
A possible approach to encounter the above mentioned problems is to develop fully autonomous and mobile assistants, which are able to execute tasks on a high level of abstraction. Example systems of this category are MOVAR (Van der Loos, 1995), URMAD (Innocenti et al., 1994), MOVAID (Dallaway et al., 1995), WALKY (Bolmsjö & Neveryd, 1995) or Care-O-Bot (May & Schäffer, 1999). All these systems consist of a mobile platform with a manipulator mounted on it. In order to act in an unknown environment they are equipped with different kinds of sensors, like ultra-sonic or laser-beam distance sensor, cameras etc. All sensors as well as the platform and the manipulator itself are connected to a computer system that processes the user commands and controls all peripheral components. At this point it has to be mentioned that, even though the above introduced idea of an autonomous robotic is as old as the history of robotics itself (Engelberger, 1989), its consequent realization has to be stated as unrealistic at the moment: Assuming that solutions for currently unsolved technical problems, like the real-time interpretation of camera images, are at hand, a fully autonomous system is cost-intensive and performs tasks with poor efficiency and reliability (Dario et al., 2004). This is because of its inherent high technical complexity. A manageable system with predictable behavior is required. With respect to the current state of science and technology, this requirement can be fulfilled only if the user's cognitive capabilities are taken into account, i.e. the robot executes the tasks semi-autonomously (Laschi et al., 2001; Martens et al., 2002; Colle et al., 2002).
Semi-autonomy takes the users' cognitive capabilities into account whenever a complex decision or environmental identification has to be made. Example systems of this category are the workstation mounted systems ISAC (Kawamura et al., 1995) and MUSIIC (Kazi, 1996; Kazi et al., 1997) as well as the wheelchair based systems KARES (Bien et al., 2001). The main principle is to offer simple but fully autonomous skills that can be activated by the user if necessary. Examples are the visually controlled grasping of objects (Lang et al., 2000), force-torque controlled drink serving (She et al., 2003b) or weight controlled pouring of a drink (She et al., 2003a). Because these skills are realized by sensor-based closed loop control processes, their execution becomes robust against dynamic environmental changes, even in unknown environments.
Even though offering autonomous executable skills reduces the amount of necessary user interactions during task-execution, a high cognitive load for the user still remains. He or she still has to remember the preconditions that have to be satisfied prior to the skill activation. For example, if a glass has to be grasped in a visually controlled manner, whereas the camera is mounted on top of the gripper (Lang et al., 2000), the user first has to move the gripper into the vicinity of the object to be grasped. Only if the underlying image processing system is able to extract significant features, the execution of the reactive grasping skill will be successful. Here, the approach of semi-autonomous task-execution, as it has been developed for the FRIEND-II robotic systems since 2003, will reduce the users' cognitive load. In the following, the rehabilitation robotic systems FRIEND-I & II are presented in general. Afterwards, the realization of the latter mentioned concept is described in detail.

3. Rehabilitation Robots FRIEND-I & II

This section gives an overview of the development steps of the FRIEND-I and FRIEND-II system as they have been undertaken since 1997. It is shown that the evolution of FRIEND-I closely correlates to the general evolution of rehabilitation robots as it has been described in the previous section. With the realization of an autonomously executed "serve-drink task" its full potential was tapped, so that the development of FRIEND-II started. FRIEND-II comes up of with a multitude of new hardware as well as software features that simplify the realization of flexible and robust task-execution. First, the new hardware setup is introduced in detail, before FRIEND-II's role as a subsystem embedded in an intelligent environment within the context of AMaRob is described.

3.1 FRIEND-I

FRIEND-I consists of an electric wheelchair and a MANUS (Exact Dynamics, Netherlands) robot arm. The robot arm is controlled by a PC, which is mounted on the backside of the wheelchair. For user interaction an LC-display is used. In order to execute different tasks autonomously, FRIEND-I is equipped with a stereo pan-tilt-zoom camera system, mounted on the back of the wheelchair, and a "smart tray". The tray is mounted at the front side of the wheelchair. It is characterized as "smart" due to its ability to locate object positions as well as to measure object weights, as described later in this section. A picture as well as a diagram of FRIEND-I is given in Fig. 1.
The first approach, to make the robot arm controllable for people with insufficient flexibility in their hands and arms for using a joystick or keyboard, was to equip the system with a speech control interface (Borgerding et al., 1999). By means of simple commands the robot can be operated with respect to different coordinate systems. The user can enter naturally spoken commands that are transformed into direct robot control actions. For example, if the user wants to pick up an object placed on the tray, a possible command sequence might be "Hand forward", "Hand down", "Stop", "Gripper open", "Hand forward", "Stop", "Gripper close". Because the user observes the actions of the robot arm continuously, he or she might interrupt the actions in erroneous situations.

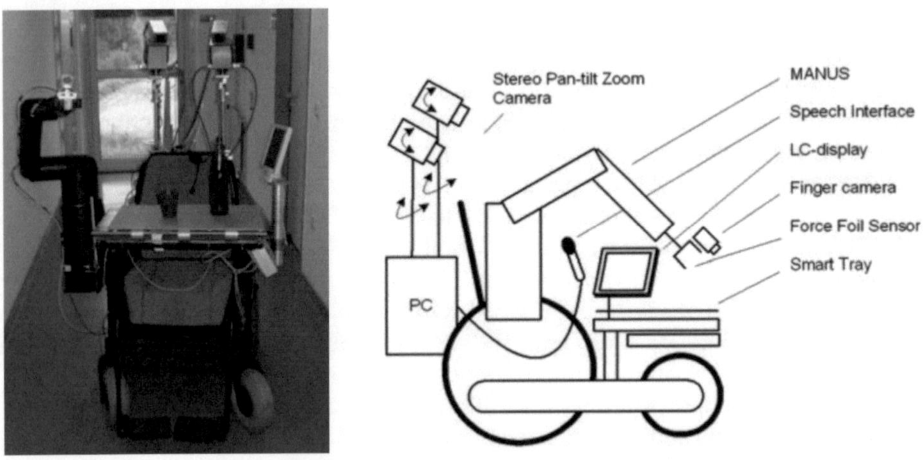

Fig. 1. Front view of FRIEND-I in summer 2003 (left) and schematic drawing (right).

By means of the speech interface it is possible even for a completely paralyzed user to command complicated tasks like grasping a bottle, pouring a drink in a glass and serve it to him- or herself. The drawback of this approach is that it requires high concentration over a long period of time. Therefore, in analogy to the robotic systems listed within the introduction, the succeeding approach in the FRIEND project was to pre-program often repeated tasks, like pouring and serving a drink or to put down objects on the tray. Even though it was convenient to activate the execution of these tasks by a single command, their application was too inflexible for the treatment of daily life activities.

A promising alternative was to increase the abstraction level of the commands by offering autonomously executable sensor-based skills[4]. The first implemented skill of this category was the camera controlled grasping of arbitrary objects. For its realization a finger camera was mounted on top of the robot gripper (Lang et al., 2000). If the user wants to grasp an object he or she moves the gripper into the neighborhood of the object to be grasped, until it can be seen by the finger camera. Starting from this position a visually controlled grasping action can be started with the command "grasp object". During the execution of the autonomous grasping action an underlying visual servoing algorithm continuously interprets image features that are assigned to natural or artificial markers on the objects.

The implemented grasping skill turned out to be robust during execution. Even under changing illumination conditions or with changes in the position of the target object the grasping tasks could be finished successfully without human intervention. It was possible to grasp an object placed in the workspace of the robot arm by means of three to five simple commands in comparison with 15-20 commands as necessary with direct voice control. Besides the reduction of necessary commands the whole execution time was reduced up to three times in average. This was the motivation to enhance the level of abstraction for task-execution again. The representative task of filling a glass with a drink and serve it to the user, short: the "serve-drink task" was chosen. The realization of this task unveils a number of challenging technical problems to be solved, which are also representative for further tasks. Therefore, the investigation and realization of the "serve-drink task" has the potential to develop a general method for robust high-level task-execution in rehabilitation robotic systems.

The underlying scenario of the task can be described as follows: A glass and an open bottle, filled with an unknown amount of drink, are arbitrarily placed on FRIEND-I's tray. After the user has entered the command "serve drink", the system has to fill the glass with the drink and move it to the mouth of the user. After the user finished drinking, the glass has to be put back on the tray. At the first sight the "serve drink task" seems to be trivial and restricted, but it deserves closer attention. First, the system has to locate the glass and bottle on the tray, grasp the bottle and move it close to the glass. Afterwards, the glass has to be filled and the bottle has to be placed back on the tray. Then the glass has to be grasped and moved close to the user's mouth. Finally, the glass has to be put back on the tray, ready for a succeeding pouring action. The execution of this scenario solely on the basis of image processing and visual servoing is very ambitious, especially if a robust behavior under all possible environmental conditions is requested. Additionally, unreliable behavior may cause dangerous situations for the user. To prevent such situations and to increase the system's reliability a "smart tray" was developed that is used in combination with the vision sensors (Volosyak et al., 2003).

The tray can be divided into two subsystems: A scale for the measurement of weight changes of objects placed on the tray and a touchpad for the detection of their positions. The

[4] These operations are characterized as skills, since they represent indivisible atomic functionalities of the system that execute autonomously sub-tasks by means of continuously processing sensor information. Examples are grasping an object or pouring a drink.

scale consists of an off-the-shelf digital scale with a measuring precision of ±1g that is connected to the main system PC. The position detection is realized by a touchpad sensor that was developed at the IAT. The touchpad consists of a 48x30 matrix, where each matrix element has binary output. Binary 1 denotes the presence of a weight greater then 3g per element, 0 indicates that there is no load on the corresponding matrix element. Hence, the result can be treated as a binary image and known image processing methods can be used for object localization. Fig. 2 (right) depicts the raw binary touchpad image resulting from a cup and a bottle that are placed on the tray. The outputs of the touchpad are processed by a microcontroller and send to the main PC. It is obvious that the positions of object segments can be easily determined on the basis of the binary touchpad image. But it is also evident that the amount of information from these images is insufficient for object identification. Here, additional sensor data is required that is fused with the touchpad information. By means of the information coming from the smart tray in combination with image processing results provided by the stereo-camera system, an autonomously executable "serve-drink task" was realized (Radchenko et al., 2004). The objective was to demonstrate that care personnel could place the involved objects, i.e. the glass and the bottle, on arbitrary positions on the tray and the system is able to execute the rest of the task autonomously. Even though this approach was independent of calibration, as it was for the pre-programmed tasks described before, the realization was fixed in the manner that the system could not be used for the processing of varying task scenarios. With the introduction of a flexible software-architecture this problem is solved within FRIEND-II, as described in the following.

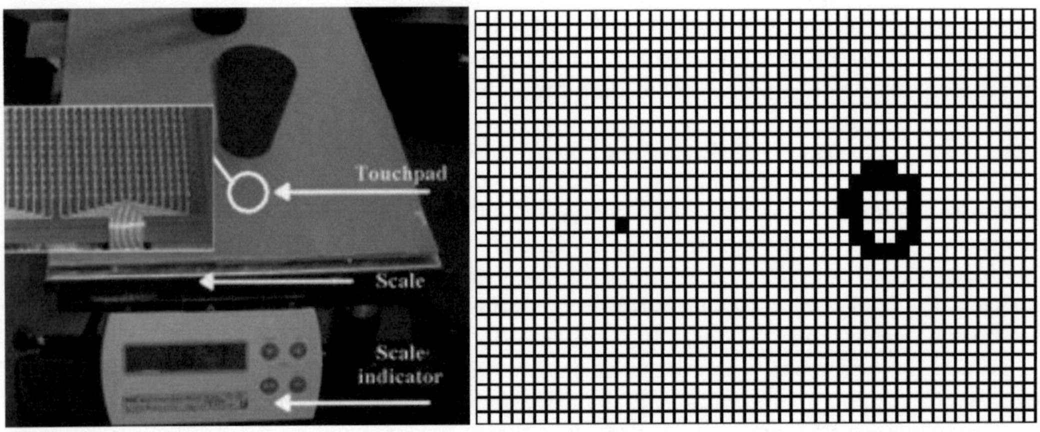

Fig. 2. Top view of the smart tray (left) and binary image of the sensor matrix (right).

3.2 FRIEND-II

The development of the FRIEND-II system started in 2003 with the objective to improve the FRIEND-I system and to benefit from the lessons learned so far. On the one hand, there were different shortcomings in FRIEND-I's hardware setup. On the other hand the flexibility of the control concept and the software-architecture in FRIEND-I was a rather basic approach that aimed to demonstrate the feasibility of rehabilitation robotic support scenarios. This section discusses the different extensions of FRIEND-II with respect to the hardware configuration, whereas the control concept MASSiVE is discussed in detail in the succeeding section.

Hardware Setup for Dexterous Manipulation in Clustered Environments

The MANUS robotic arm, which has been used in FRIEND-I, corresponds with its 6-joints kinematical structure to industrial robots. Such a structure turned out not to be suitable for dexterous manipulations. The ability to master manipulations with obstacle avoidance in clustered and mainly non-structured home environments is mandatory for the application in rehabilitation robotic scenarios.

Within FRIEND-II a dexterous 7 degrees-of-freedom robotic arm, which has been developed by Amtec Robotics (Berlin, Germany) under functional specifications by IAT, is used. It has a humanlike kinematical structure: The arm is composed of a series of turn- and pan-joints with perpendicular axes respectively. The arm is mounted on a linear axis which allows it to drive in a specific home position and reduce visibility if not in use (Fig. 3). At the wrist a multi-axis force/torque sensor, model Gamma, from ATI-Industrial Automation (NC, USA) is integrated. This compact, light and robust monolithic transducer uses silicon strain gauges, providing high noise immunity, to sense forces and torques from all three directions of the tool frame. To process the strain gauge information into CAN-Bus information a compact wrist mounted electronics unit has been developed. The robot arm is equipped with an Otto Bock SensorHand[5] as a gripper. The necessary mechanical as well as electrical adaptations were made in agreement with Otto Bock Health Care (Duderstadt, Germany). A gripper force and a slip control mode, which will be activated from the FRIEND-II system, are integrated in the SensorHand. As it has proven to be a benefit for the realization of robust operations, FRIEND-II is, like its predecessor, equipped with a smart tray for determination of object positions and weight changes. The camera Sony EVI-D70P was selected for the FRIEND-II image acquisition system. The selection was made on the basis of requirements for minimal lighting of the scene and particularly on the basis of a cost-effective connection of the camera with a pan-tilt head. The chosen pan-tilt zoom video camera system is mounted on the frame-rack behind the user.

With the help of the described improved hardware setup and the implementation of the new software control concept MASSiVE, the first successfully implemented scenario was an extended drink serving scenario, since this could serve as reference scenario for comparison with FRIEND-I. This scenario was presented at the Hannover-Fair 2005 and it turned out that during the whole week a robust execution, in the sense of the following explanation, took place. Independent of the initial configuration of bottle and glass (sometimes placed by fair visitors) the pouring action was executed as pre-determined. Beside the statement that a stable accuracy from different initial conditions is related to the improved manipulative capabilities of the new robotic arm, two other hardware components contributed also to the enhanced overall performance: The Otto-Bock gripper with its integrated intelligent force-control guaranteed a firm grip even on a slightly wet bottle. Furthermore, the force-torque-sensor enabled to implement a more flexible placing of objects even on non-tactile surfaces like an ordinary table. All in all the improved hardware setup of FRIEND-II is the basis for currently ongoing implementation of further scenarios. The well focused development of different representative and complete rehabilitation robotic scenarios on the basis of the experiences gathered with the FRIEND systems is the objective of the AMaRob project, which will be discussed in the following.

---

[5] http://www.ottobockus.com/products/upper_limb_prosthetics/myoelectric_hands_sensorhand.asp

AMaRob Project: Support Scenarios for Daily Life Autonomy

The project AMaRob is funded within the BMBF[6]-program "Leitinnovation Servicerobotik" (IAT, 2007; DLR, 2007). The overall objective is to demonstrate that 1.5 hours of complete autonomy from care personnel or nursing staff can be realized for tetraplegic people, solely supported by a rehabilitation robot. The suitability for daily use as well as efficiency from the economical viewpoint in one ADL (activities of daily living) and two working scenarios is to be examined. An important aspect with respect to the successful project process is the interdisciplinary cooperation. From the beginning on, therapists (Neurological Rehabilitation Center Friedehorst, Bremen, Germany), designers (i/i/d - Institute of Integrated Design, Bremen, Germany) and various experts for the different technological components (Meyra, Kalletal-Kalldorf; Otto-Bock, Duderstadt; Amtec Robotics, Berlin; IGEL GmbH, Bremen; all from Germany) are cooperation partners in the AMaRob project.

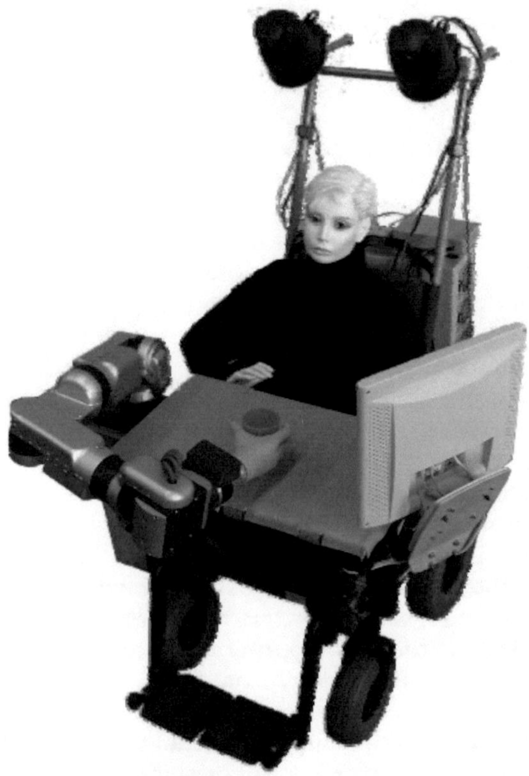

Fig. 3. Rehabilitation robotic system FRIEND-II.

The main development goal in the ADL scenario is the complete process of preparing and eating a meal. This starts with the retrieval of the desired meal from the storage, the proper heating procedure with respect to the contents of the meal, the eating and drinking procedure and finally the clearance of the dishes. In the first working scenario different electronic

[6] BMBF - German Federal Ministry of Education and Research ("Bundesministerium für Bildung und Forschung")

components are tested on the basis of manual inspection as well as functional tests. These tests are common tasks that are often accomplished by disabled people with remaining manual capabilities in the workshops at Friedehorst. The second working scenario deals with a service desk in a library, where books are rented or returned, and dues are paid, reservations are handled, etc.

During the AMaRob project, a redesign of FRIEND-II will take place. Development goals are an improved design for daily use, a smoother integration of sensors and actuators, including the new generation of Amtec Robotics manipulators. Another aspect that is valid for the development of all three scenarios is the investigation of methods to integrate distributed smart components, also known as ambient intelligence or ubiquitous computing (Korondi & Hashimoto, 2003). Its objective is to support the process of task-execution and to lower the technical complexity of the rehabilitation robotic system itself. Based on the experiences gathered with the smart tray within the FRIEND projects, it will be considered to place tactile skins on certain platforms that are in the center of manipulation, e.g. parts of the worktop in the kitchen or the desk in the workshop or library. Furthermore, RFID[7]-tags attached to objects will enable the decentralized storage of object relevant information, e.g. cooking instructions for a meal placed in a smart fridge that is equipped with RFID antenna. Fig. 4 illustrates an exemplary setup of an "intelligent" kitchen environment. With such an intelligent environment, a distributed system evolves with hardware that is distributed physically and that is managed by different processors. In Fig. 4 on the right side, a prototypic installation of an intelligent kitchen environment is depicted. Instead of using a real fridge, the first setup includes a cupboard, representing the fridge. This cupboard is equipped with two tactile layers, which consist of the same tactile skins as that one used for the smart tray component of the FRIEND-II system. Thus, less technical complexity of the rehabilitation robot itself is necessary with respect to required sensors and algorithms to retrieve location information about the meals in the smart fridge. Under the upper cupboard layer an RFID antenna is installed which covers the space above the two layers. The meal to be prepared for the disabled user is arranged on a special meal tray, which fulfils the following conditions:

- It is graspable by the robotic gripper
- The material is suitable for the heating in a microwave oven, is food safe and can be easily cleaned after usage
- The lid is equipped with RFID tags. This lid is also manageable by the robot and can be removed before heating to avoid damage of the RFID tag in the microwave oven.

Once care personnel inserts a meal in this kind of smart fridge, meal specific information will be stored on the RFID tag. This includes a description of the meal, cooking instructions and minimum durability. During the process of meal preparation, the locally stored meal information directly drives the heating procedure in the microwave oven. This oven is also part of the intelligent environment, since it is directly controllable from the system without manipulative interaction and consequently also reduces the technical complexity of FRIEND-II.

Besides the ongoing improvements on the hardware level and the application and enhancement of an overall software control concept, other key developments will be undertaken within AMaRob. This includes fast motion planning for collision free, intelligent and

[7] RFID – radio frequency identification

smooth manipulation in clustered environments (Ojdanic et al., 2006) or the realization of improved machine vision concepts respectively.

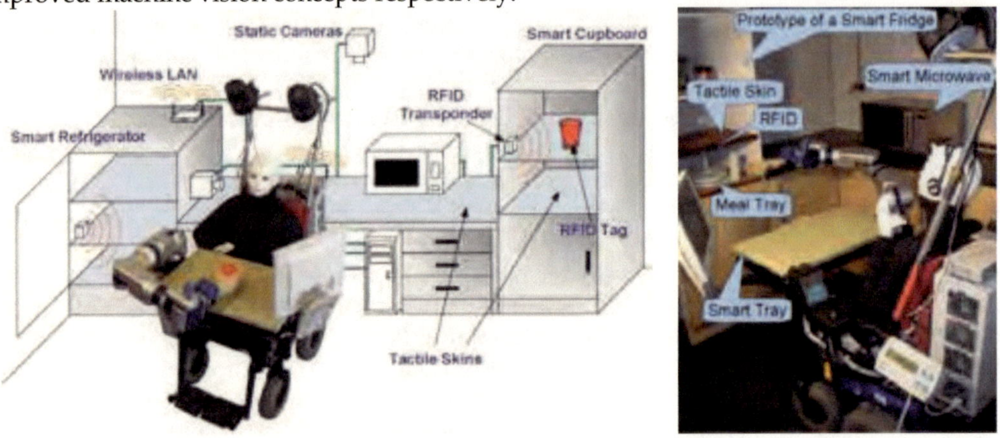

Fig. 4. FRIEND-II in intelligent environment, schematic version (left), first prototypic installation (right).

4. Semi-Autonomous Task-Execution

The preceding sections concentrated on the functional aspects of the FRIEND systems. This section is focused on the application of software-technical methods that help to cope with the inherent complexity of the robotic system and its environment. First, the design and implementation of an appropriate software-architecture is described. Afterwards, within the context of this architecture, task-knowledge data-structures, suitable for the inclusion of the user, as required for semi-autonomous task-execution, are introduced. It is shown how the consequent application of these concepts leads to a robotic system, which is able to execute tasks robustly on a high level of abstraction.

4.1 The Software-Architecture MASSiVE

From the software-technical point of view the realization of a service robot comes up with a multitude of challenging tasks to be solved within the context of an architecture: Distributed calculation, reactions to environmental changes and control of electro-mechanical devices under hard real-time requirements, processing of complex algorithms, adaptation to heterogeneous hardware interfaces, ergonomic human-machine interaction and autonomous planning of action sequences. The preceding enumeration doesn't claim to be exhaustive.

It turned out that hybrid multi-layer architectures, like TCA (Coste-Maniere & Simmons, 2000) or 3T (Bonasso et al., 1998), are predominating in the field of fully autonomous systems, since they provide a combination of deliberative and reactive behavior. A deliberative component is necessary for the creation of a high-level plan, i.e. for having a system that is able to receive task requests and to define a mission goal. The inclusion of reactivity has proven to be a suitable mean to achieve robustness with respect to environmental disturbances, comparable to the reflex system of living organisms. Therefore, a typical hybrid multi-layer architecture consists of three layers:

- Deliberator: Plans operations on a high level of abstraction, i.e. with the help of a symbolic planning strategy.

- Reactive Layer: Has access to the actuators and sensors of the system and offers reactive operations in the form of closed control-loops (i.e. coupling of sensors and actuators).
- Sequencer: Is responsible for the activation and deactivation of operations in the reactive layer according to the plan generated by the deliberator. Therefore, it plays the role of a mediator between deliberator and reactive layer.

Besides these layers a world model is included that contains the current system's perspective on the world according to the task to be executed. Due to the hybrid approach a separation of world-model data into two categories is mandatory: The deliberator operates with symbolic object representations (e.g. *C* for the representation of a cup), while the reactive layer deals with the sensor data taken from these objects, so-called sub-symbolic information. Examples are the color, size, shape, location or weight of an object.
To fulfill the requirements in the field of rehabilitation robotics, the software control architecture MASSiVE has been developed at the IAT. This control architecture is derived from the generally successfully applied architectures of autonomous systems as introduced before. However, in the field of rehabilitation, the user can be included in to the process of task execution, which leads to modifications towards a semi-autonomous system. Furthermore, the analysis of typical rehabilitation robotic support scenarios revealed the fact that these scenarios are mostly composed of a finite set of reusable basic operations (Martens, 2003b).
Fig. 5 depicts the emerging scheme of the modified control architecture. With respect to the semi-autonomous task-execution, the deliberator component of traditional hybrid control architectures has been replaced by an HMI, whereas symbolic planning is performed within the sequencer. The evident role of the HMI is the translation of high abstraction level task requests from the user (e.g. "Fetch cup", "Pour in a drink", etc.) into commands that are forwarded to the sequencer for further processing. Additionally, the HMI provides a complete infrastructure for task related user interactions. This includes the direct control of actuators within context-based constraints given by the sequencer. Within MASSiVE, the role of the sequencer is to act as a global control unit that coordinates the cooperation between all levels of the architecture (Martens et al., 2002). It is designed as a discrete-event-controller that operates on the basis of predefined task-knowledge, so-called process-structures, and generates task related action sequences.

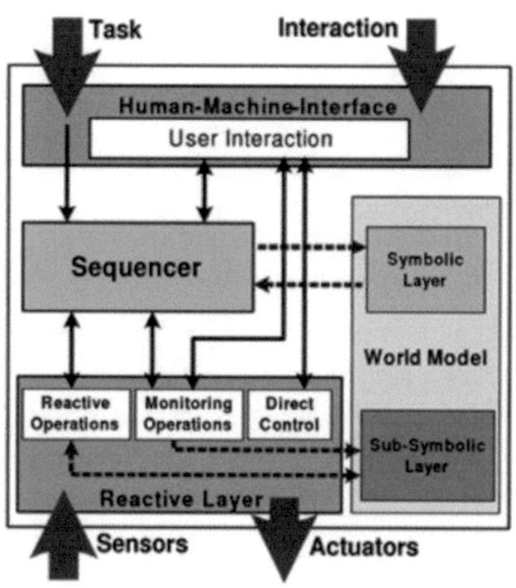

Fig. 5. Schematic overview of the control-architecture MASSiVE.

These process-structures are the basis of the principle to pre-structure the support scenarios. Despite their a-priori definition, they are still flexible enough to process a requested task under varying initial conditions, i.e. they can handle different initial situations and varying kinds of task participating objects. Due to the implicit restriction to task relevant information, this approach guarantees, in contradiction to classical AI-based task planning, a finite and, in the meaning of real-time suitability, reasonable size of the planning search space. Additionally, the formal verification of the task-knowledge with respect to reachability of situations or the correctness of its execution becomes possible. Even though this has no impact on the offered functionality of the robotic system, it is evident that the latter aspect plays a vital role for the commercialization of rehabilitation robots in general.

A planned action sequence consists of operations that are elementary from the sequencer's viewpoint. This motivates the term elementary executable operations (*EEOPs*). *EEOPs* include user interactions (e.g. identification of an object), direct control of actuators (e.g. movement of the camera system), monitoring operations (e.g. visual feature extraction of already identified object) and reactive operations (e.g. visually controlled object grasping). Thus, the basic operations already implemented for the FRIEND-I system are realized within this context as *EEOPs*. Due to the uniform software interface of *EEOPs*, the sequencer can generate action sequences independently of the kind of operation that has to be taken into account. After the generation of an *EEOP*-sequence is finished, the sequencer maps the *EEOPs* to skills that are executed asynchronously on distributed software-servers. These servers are part of the reactive layer or the HMI, respectively. In the reactive layer, a network of servers offers basic system skills that are grouped within the servers according to functional cohesion, as described in the following.

Infrastructure for Semi-Autonomous Task-Execution within Distributed Systems

The sequencer of the MASSiVE architecture (Fig. 6) consists of two modules that are designed as active objects: The *Task Planner* and the *Task Executer*. Active objects are a software design pattern to separate the execution of a method from its calling context with the help of threads, whereas the method's implementation is independent of any threading details (Gamma et al., 1995). Thus, the planner and executer are able to act independently. This enables the control of skill execution in the reactive layer as well as reactions in the planning layer like interruption of ongoing task execution or re-planning of required operation sequences.

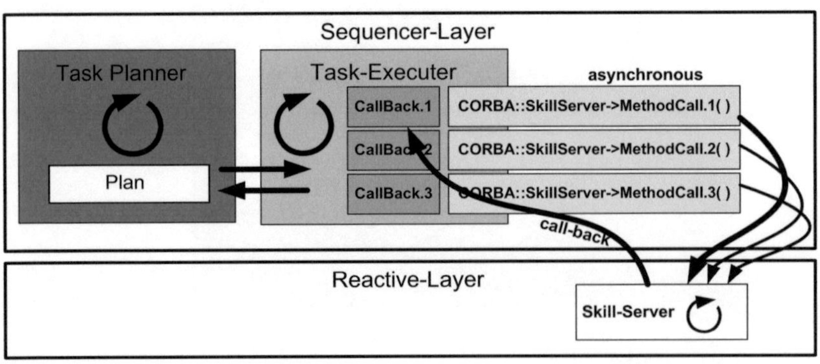

Fig. 6. Communication from sequencer layer.

To be able to execute several operations simultaneously, asynchronous calls of skill-methods are necessary. Furthermore, the operations may run on different processors, e.g. because of system-hardware that is distributed physically as it is the case for remote smart devices. The distribution of skill execution capabilities should be adaptable in a flexible manner, i.e. without changing the system structure or extensive re-implementations, to have the opportunity at hand to scale the computing power available for a single skill. All these demands are fulfilled entirely with the help of standardized and platform-independent communication infrastructures based on CORBA (Common Object Request Broker Architecture, (Gamma et al., 1995)). The following section describes the design and realization of the CORBA based reactive layer.

Reactive Layer

The name reactive layer resides from its purpose to provide reactive behavior. This means to directly couple sensorial input with the control of an actuator (i.e. to design a control loop) to establish autonomous behavior that is robust against dynamic environmental changes. As depicted in Fig. 5 the reactive layer is furthermore responsible for offering monitoring operations (based on input from the sensors) as well as direct control of the actuator (manipulative skills). The latter aspect is important for example when user interaction in the form of direct actuator-control becomes necessary. Due to this, several skill servers provide the necessary basic operations, i.e. skills, of the robotic system by accessing the sensors and actuators of the system or remote smart devices. This means, a skill layer has access to a hardware layer, whereas different hardware servers encapsulate basic hardware functionalities.

Skills have to operate on the already mentioned sub-symbolic environmental information. As shown in Fig. 5, the sequencer including the symbolic planning engine accesses the symbolic layer of the world model. Thus, the sequencer (on the basis of high-level process-structures and symbolic descriptions) is responsible for the correct abstract modeling of that segment of the environment that is relevant to the current task-execution. To administrate all sub-symbolic information in a structured manner, a sub-symbolic world model server is introduced within the reactive layer. Here, sub-symbolic information is stored with reference to symbolic information from the upper layer of the world model and consequently a connection between both layers of the world model (and therefore also between these both information layers) is established.

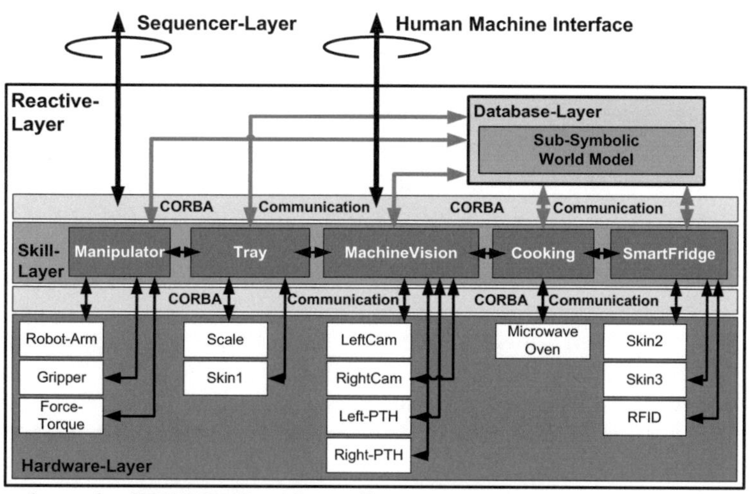

Fig. 7. Reactive layer for FRIEND-II with intelligent environment.

Skill Server

The criterion for separation into several skill servers is derived from the functional entities of the system. That means, one skill server offers all the system operations that have to be assigned basically to one certain entity. In case of scenarios that take place in an intelligent environment as introduced in Chapter 3.2, the necessary skill-servers are the *Manipulator-*, *Tray-*, *MachineVision-*, *Cooking-* and *SmartFridge-Skill-Server*, with their assigned hardware-servers as depicted in Fig. 7. Here, for instance, the Cooking-Skill-Server provides skills to access the hardware-server *MicrowaveOven* and thus to control this remote device or to extract data from it.

From the software-technical point of view, skills are methods of a skill server that are executed asynchronously. This means skill-methods are non-blocking and will return immediately after their activation. The problem of asynchronous execution is that no values or parameters can be returned. Therefore, sub-symbolic data that is generated during skill execution is stored within the world model. The information on the status of skill execution (e.g. successful execution) has to be transmitted via another communication way. For this issue call-back objects are introduced, which can be accessed by the skill caller and the skill method itself. Call-backs are also used for sending information from the skill caller to the skill while it is executing. This could be for example the command to stop the skill or to re-parameterize it. Fig. 6 already showed how the task executer within the sequencer maps call-back objects to asynchronously invoked methods and Fig. 8 demonstrates the communication mechanisms between sequencer- and skill-layer in more detail.

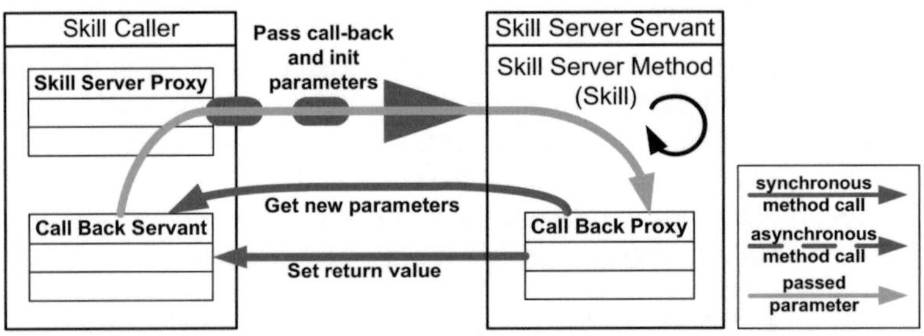

Fig. 8. CORBA-based asynchronous communication.

Hardware Server

For each hardware component, like the robot arm, a hardware server is implemented (see Fig. 7), which itself is connected to a certain skill server. The design principle is that only methods of this skill server can access the hardware directly. This decouples the upper layers of the software structure from the hardware. In case a hardware component is replaced, only the implementations of the hardware server methods have to be adapted, whereas the parameters of each method remain.

If for a hardware-component/-server a fast communication is required, i.e. the communication offset of CORBA cannot be accepted, a local instance of the hardware server implementation class can be used and the communication can be carried out via shared memory. Also the combination of client and servant in one process is possible. All three possibilities of using a hardware server are fully exchangeable and no re-design or new implementation is necessary.

Human-Machine-Interface

For the realization of the user involvement, which is initiated and controlled by the system, the HMI offers an interface that enables the sequencing layer to initiate user assistance via user interaction skills. From the user-centered viewpoint, the overall objective is to offer an intuitively controllable interaction skill, which hides all technical details, like the selection of necessary hardware resources or the control of the data flow. The connection between the HMI and MASSiVE is established by a software component that uses the interface of the sequencer to start and stop system tasks and offers a software-server to enable the sequencer initiating user interactions. From the sequencer perspective, the invocation of a user interaction is thus handled exactly like a skill activation within the reactive layer.
So far, the architectural concept designed for semi-autonomous task-execution has been discussed. In the following, process-structures as a substantial aspect for the control of user interactions and autonomous system operations within MASSiVE are presented.

4.2 Task-Knowledge Driven User-Interaction

According to the structure of the control architecture, process-structures come in two levels of abstraction: Abstract process-structures (PS_A) are associated with the abstract (symbolic) layer of task-knowledge representation and describe tasks in a user-oriented and non-technical way. This level of abstraction is suitable for task-oriented programming purposes (Martens, 2005). Elementary process-structures (PS_E) represent the part of the task-knowledge that is required within the environmental-related (sub-symbolic) level. The information on this level of abstraction subsumes necessary hardware resources, like sensors and actuators, as well as *EEOPs*. In the following, the different steps of task processing on the basis of abstract as well as elementary process-structures will be discussed. The activity diagram depicted in Fig. 9 gives a conceptual overview on the steps that are undertaken to process a task request in MASSiVE.

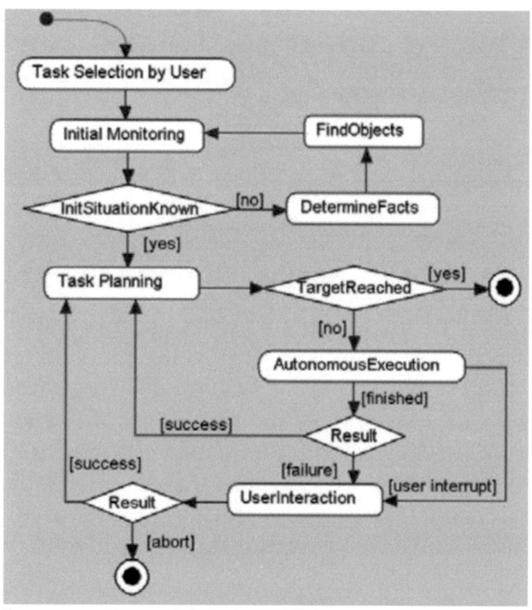

Fig. 9. Overview on task processing within MASSiVE.

Task Request

First, with respect to the task request from the HMI, the sequencer selects and loads an abstract process-structure. Abstract process-structures are derived from data-structures typically used in assembly planning, namely AND-OR-nets (Cao & Sanderson, 1998). Within the context of MASSiVE they have been enhanced with first-order predicate logic facts that assign, in a STRIPS[8]-like manner, pre- and post-conditions to the operations contained in the net. Aditionally, facts are used for the description of object states and relationships.
Fig. 10 depicts an iconic model of a possible PS_A that is assigned to the task request "Fetch cup". The iconic PS_A contains all object-constellations (*OC*s), i.e. objects in physical contact, which might appear during the execution of this task, as well as all possible operations performed by the system. Within this context *all* has to be interpreted as from an application programmer's viewpoint. The operations are called composed operators (*COP*), since they represent a composition of *EEOP*s and their decomposition takes place on the level of PS_E. They interconnect the different *OCs* of the PS_A, meaning that the system transforms the constellations of objects by executing a sub-task. Due to their derivation of AND-OR-nets, there are three different kinds of *COP*s: Assembly and disassembly operations as well as internal state transitions. The semantics of the first two types is self explaining, whereas the latter version is used to represent internal changes within a single *OC* without changing the components being in physical contact (e.g. moving a book on a table).

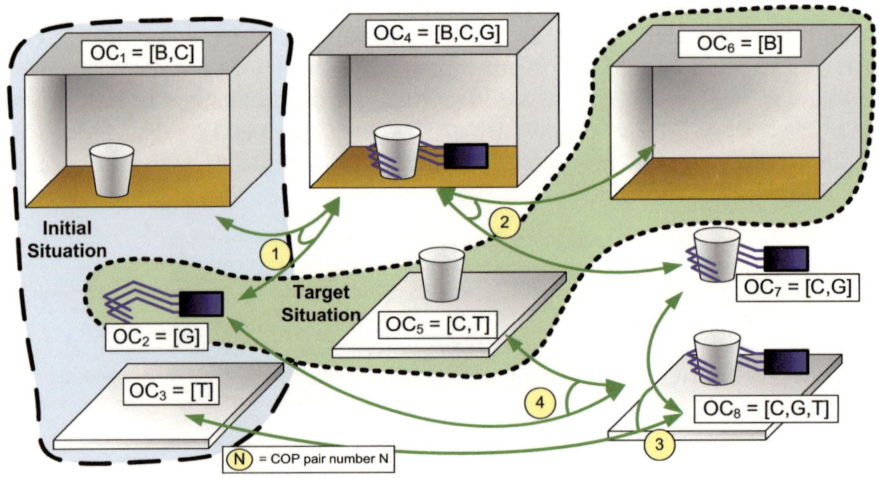

Fig. 10. Abstract process-structure (PS_A) for the task request "Fetch cup".

As listed in Table 1, the "Fetch cup" scenario solely consists of *COP*s of the first two categories. The numbers of each pair of operations refer to the numbers given in Fig. 10. The objects involved in the task scenario are a box *B* (e.g. an abstract representation of an already opened cupboard), a cup *C*, the gripper of the service robot *G* and a table *T*. Some exemplary *OC*s of Fig. 10 are: OC_1 = "the cup is located inside the box", OC_4 = "the grasped cup is located inside the box" or OC_5 = "the cup is located on top of the table". Beside the enumeration of contained objects, each *OC* possesses a set of first order predicate logics facts, which represent the object states as well as their relationship respectively.

[8] STRIPS: Stanford Research Institute Problem Solver (Fikes, 1971)

No.	**List of COPs used in Fig. 10:** (AOP - assembly operation, DOP - disassembly operation)
1	AOP: GraspObjectInContainer(G, C, B) DOP: DepartFromContainer(G, C, B)
2	AOP: PlaceObjectInside(G, C, B) DOP: GetObjectOutside(G, C, B)
3	AOP: PutDownObject(G, C, T, FreePlacePos) DOP: MoveObject(G, C, T, FreePlacePos)
4	AOP: GraspObject(G, C, T) DOP: Depart(G, C, T)

Table 1. Composed operators of the "Fetch Cup" scenario.

On the basis of *OC*s a situation S_k is described as follows: S_k is a set of *OC*s that contains all objects of the PS_A exactly once and is part of the situation-graph (Prenzel, 2005), which interconnects all valid situations via the operations defined within the PS_A. Assuming the correctness of the PS_A, which is verified automatically off-line, a target situation S_T can be reached from any situation S of the situation-graph via the application of a finite number of operations. This circumstance is the basis of the planning concept applied in MASSiVE, which is explained in more detail below. S_T has a fix association with the task to be solved according to the given task request. For the example task depicted in Fig. 10 the target state is defined as: $S_T = \{OC_2, OC_5, OC_6\}$, i.e. the task request "Fetch cup" is associated with the target situation where the cup has finally been placed on the table and the empty gripper as well as the empty cupboard remain.

So far, the explanations concentrated on the design of a PS_A. Its information is used to drive the planning process of a task request. Here, according to the conceptual sequence of activities depicted in Fig. 9, the task related PS_A is loaded first. Afterwards, the so-called process of initial monitoring is started. This process determines the initial situation S_I of the chosen PS_A that corresponds to the current environmental situation. From out this situation a path to the target situation can be processed.

Initial Monitoring

The situation monitoring process is controlled by the information contained within the set of situations associated with a PS_A and is executed in a semi-autonomous manner also (Prenzel, 2005). As illustrated in Fig. 9, the monitoring process consists of the determination of the first order logic facts that are assigned to the different *OC*s. Within the given process-structure, the set of facts listed in Table 2 has to be determined during initial monitoring.

To give an illustration of the monitoring approach in MASSiVE, the example of finding the cup to be retrieved from the cupboard will be taken into account. Fig. 11 shows a respective setup of a user interaction that will occur in this case. Here, the FRIEND-II system has been moved in front of a cupboard in which several cups are placed. During this user interaction the user is requested by the system to control the pan-tilt head devices (and thus move the cameras), so that the object of interest is in their sight (the left camera image is displayed to the user). During the movement of the cameras, the image processing system segments objects positioned in the middle of the camera image in real-time. The segmentation result is overlaid to the image, so that the user is able to decide whether the desired object is highlighted or not.

Fact	Description
HoldsNothing(G)	The gripper G holds nothing.
IsInFreePos(G)	The gripper G is in a free position.
IsInsideContainer(C, B)	The cup C in inside the container B (box).
HasFreeStoringSpace(B, C)	The box B has enough free space for the cup C.
IsGripped(G, C)	The cup C is gripped by the gripper G.
IsPlacedOn(C, T)	The cup C in place on top of the table T.

Table 2. Set of facts in "Fetch Cup" scenario.

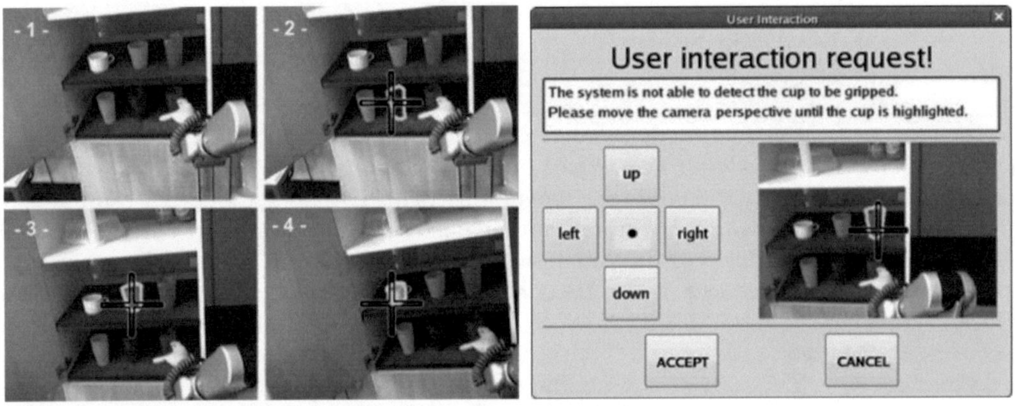

Fig. 11. Experimental setup for finding a cup in a cupboard.

With respect to finish the initial monitoring, the determination of other task relevant objects is performed analogously within a user interaction in case the autonomous object detection fails (or is not unique). After the initial object detection is completed, additional object specific sub-symbolic information is extracted according to the concept of object-anchoring (Prenzel, 2005). This information is stored in the sub-symbolic layer of the system's world model (Fig. 5), to be accessible for all skills that are executed within the reactive layer. Thus, during further task processing steps the degree of the system's autonomy increases with the increasing amount of acquired environmental information.

Task Planning and Execution

According to Fig. 9 task planning and execution takes place, after the initial situation S_I is monitored successfully. Planning is necessary in order to determine a sequence of operations that is adapted to the current environmental situation. The applied planning method is equivalent on both levels of process-structures, i.e. PS_A and PS_E, as exemplified in the following: In the scenario of Fig. 10 with its assigned PS_A it shall be assumed that the initial situation has been determined during initial monitoring. Thus, the task planning objective is to transform this initial situation $S_I = \{OC_1, OC_2, OC_3\}$ into the target situation $S_T = \{OC_2, OC_5, OC_6\}$. Since the transformation of situations is realized by means of the execution of operations, the generation of action sequences is reduced to a graph search problem. Here, the search is realized by means of the Dijkstra algorithm (Martens, 2003a). According to the assumed initial situation S_I, the first *COP* in the sequence of planned *COPs* is *GraspObjectInContainer*. Because this *COP* cannot be executed directly within the architecture, it has to be decomposed to a level of abstraction that deals with *EEOPs*.

The result of the *COP* decomposition, i.e. its assigned elementary process-structure (PS_E), is depicted in Fig. 12. Here, to reduce the complexity of the illustration, only a segment of the complete PS_E is shown – the upper part, as indicated by the dashed box, has been left out. However, the principle of a PS_E can be clarified as follows: The flow of control is modeled on the basis of a Petri-net. As depicted, transitions of this Petri-net are arranged in pairs (or tuples), which represent the execution of an *EEOP*. Each transition of a pair (or tuple) represents the execution of an *EEOP* with different execution results. This is denoted by the different return values. The different nature of *EEOPs*, as introduced in Chapter 4.1, is specified with the help of the prefix in the transition name: *DC* stands for "direct control" of an actuator, *USER* for "user interaction and *REAC* for "reactive operation", i.e. an *EEOP*, which is in fact a closed control loop that couples sensors and actuators. *EEOPs* of the fourth category, the "monitoring operations", with the prefix *MON*, are not part of the depicted segment of PS_E.

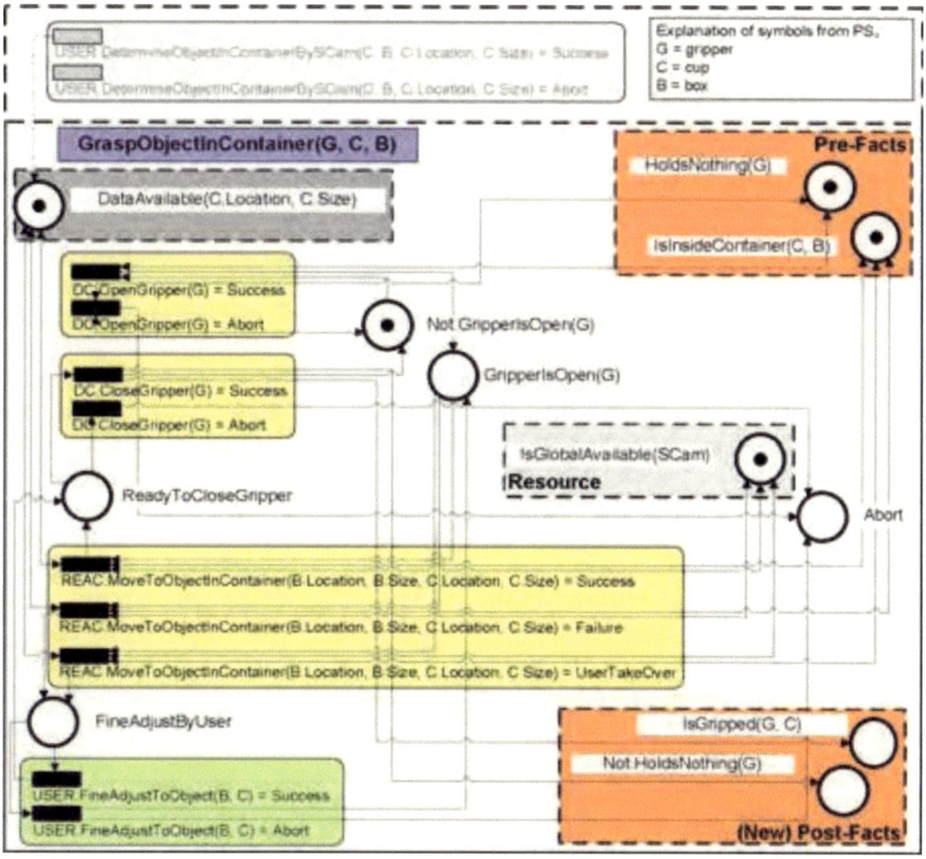

Fig. 12. Section of elementary process-structure (PS_E) representing the *COP "GraspObjectInContainer"* (upper part is left out).

Task planning on the basis of the Petri-net is equivalent to the planning process performed on the basis of the PS_A. Starting from an initial situation (initial marking with tokens in the Petri-net) the shortest sequence of operations (fired transitions) is calculated by means of the

Dijkstra algorithm. During task execution, a single transition from out a pair (or tuple respectively) is fired according to the actual return value of the respective *EEOP*. If the return value fits to the pre-planned one, the next *EEOP* of the plan is chosen. Otherwise, a re-planning step has to be performed. Because decomposition has the meaning of replacing the formal parameters of a PS_E with the actual parameters determined by the PS_A, the resulting sequence of *EEOPs* considers the objects that have been localized during the initial monitoring process.

The elementary process-structures in the form of a Petri-net include different modeling aspects and represent the following:

- Control flow (e.g. controlled involvement of the user into data monitoring or direct actuator control)
- Resource usage (e.g. *IsGlobalAvailable(SCam*[9]*)*)
- Data flow and data availability (e.g. *DataAvailable(C.Location, C.Size)*)
- Interconnection to abstract layer and to the world model via facts (e.g. *HoldsNothing(G)*)

The advantage of using Petri-nets as a modeling tool is the availability of mathematical methods for the structural analysis of PS_E. Due to the illustrated stringent and application specific syntax within a PS_E, offline verification becomes possible. This includes the verification with respect to dead-locks, resource-conflicts, modeling errors, state-reachability, availability of sub-symbolic data and the direction of data flow (Martens, 2003b).

During runtime, the initial marking in a PS_E is set according to the current status of task execution. For the example depicted in Fig. 12, since the task participating object *B* (box) and *C* (cup) have already been identified during the initial monitoring process, a new acquisition of the data is not required. Thus, the token in the place "*DataAvailable(C.Location, C.Size)*" will be part of the initial marking. In any other case, where this information which is required for the subsequent manipulative operation *REAC.MoveToObjectInContainer* is not yet available, it will be generated within the upper part (not depicted) of the PS_E via monitoring *EEOPs* or user interactions respectively. The target marking in a PS_E, which is required to apply planning by graph search, is specified during the definition of a PS_E. One rule with respect to the target marking specification is that it has to include the post-facts associated with the *COP* assigned to a certain PS_E. Post facts in Fig. 12 are *IsInsideContainer(C, B)* (also pre-fact), *IsGripped(C, G)* and *Not.HoldsNothing(G)*. With the help of post- and pre-facts, the connection and consistency between the sub-symbolic control level (PS_E) and the abstract level (PS_A) are guaranteed.

Here, according to the given state of the Petri-net, the manipulative *EEOPs DC.OpenGripper, REAC.MoveToObjectInContainer* and *DC.CloseGripper* will be executed. Within the reactive manipulation *EEOP*, a motion planning algorithm is started, which retrieves and operates on the previously (during initial monitoring) generated environmental information from the world model (Prenzel et al., 2006; Ojdanic et al., 2006). Due to the structure of the task-knowledge contained within the PS_E and the usage of the Dijkstra algorithm, the result of the planning process is that autonomous *EEOPs* are executed first and user interaction *EEOPs* follow in case the system fails (this general idea is also illustrated in Fig. 9). Furthermore, manipulative *EEOPs* can be interrupted by the user, e.g. in case he can already foresee a possible collision. This is indicated by the "[user interrupt]" transition in Fig. 9 or the third

[9] SCam = Stereo-camera system

transition of the reactive *EEOP* in Fig. 12 respectively. The concrete and more detailed description of this kind of interaction enforced by the user is discussed in (Lüth et al., 2007). The complete planning and execution cycle is continued until the given task is completed or has been aborted, e.g. according to the user's intention or due to a critical and irresolvable system status.

The described approach leads to a system that is able to operate robustly, even if it is not able to execute all steps fully autonomously. Moreover, it supports the evolutionary development of the system with increasing autonomy. This means, it is possible to initially realize a rehabilitation robotic support scenario with a low level of autonomy and to replace missing autonomous functionality with user interactions. Subsequently and in an evolutionary manner, more and more user interactions are replaced by autonomous operations by developing more intelligent skill algorithms or using additional sensors and actuators.

For recapitulating this section it is referred to Fig. 9. After the user's initial task selection, the first system controlled user interaction takes places within the initial monitoring. Initial identification tasks that cannot be solved fully autonomously without unreasonable increase of technical complexity are given back to the user to be solved by him. The same approach is taken into account within the ongoing process of task-execution.

5. Conclusion

This paper gives an overview of the functional capabilities of the rehabilitation robotics systems FRIEND-I and FRIEND-II as well as an introspective view of the used underlying control principles and applied software techniques. It is shown that during the different development steps of FRIEND-I the control of the system evolved from out direct speech control of the manipulator up the fully autonomous execution of a "serve-drink task". It turned out that the control of a rehabilitation robot like FRIEND-I becomes possible for a person without manipulative capabilities in his or her arms and hands. But there is still the need for more robustness and reliability in execution, flexibility in usage and relief for its users, if the overall objective of 1.5 hours of autonomy for daily life activities has to be reached. The most important lesson learned within the FRIEND-I project is the application of the semi-autonomous task execution principle. The motivation is that the involvement of the user's cognitive capabilities has the potential of reducing the system's complexity dramatically, so that a technical manageable system emerges.

The consequent implementation of this principle has been realized within the successor system FRIEND-II. On the one hand FRIEND-II comes up with new sophisticated hardware components like a 7 DOF manipulator or a force-torque controlled gripper. It is evident that the usage of these hardware components leads to more robustness in execution. On the other hand FRIEND-II has been software-technically designed for its application within an intelligent environment, where different daily life as well as working scenarios, as specified within the AMaRob project, will be managed. It is shown that the beforehand mentioned requirements of user involvement and distributed execution, as necessary for its application within the intelligent environment, are satisfied by the multi-layer architecture MASSiVE. For user involvement, MASSiVE offers an infrastructure for task-knowledge driven task planning, whereas the user interaction is an integral part within this knowledge. During task execution the system requests the user whenever it has to come to a decision on a cognitive level and the algorithmic realization of this process it too complex and error prone. But even though the user is requested, he or she is relived from tiresome and complicated tasks like remembering the necessary sequence of actions that have to be fulfilled before the execution of the next steps becomes possible. Within MASSiVE's HMI-level the current task context is known, so that a specific and efficient request limited to the current context can be initiated. This has been demonstrated by the detection of a certain cup in a cupboard full of cups, where the application of a well known image segmentation algorithm leads to the same results, from the user's point of view, as a complex image analysis.

The requirement for reactive and distributed execution is satisfied by MASSiVE's reactive layer, which is controlled by the intermediating sequencer. From the sequencer's point of view the reactive layer is as a pool of skills, from which some have to be selected and combined according to a task plan in order to reach the goal of a requested task. Within this context the reactive layer encapsulates the underlying hardware and offers environmental information on a pre-processed symbolic level. Because each hardware component is managed by a separate software server, which itself is managed within the reactive layer according to a well defined server interface concept, the inclusion of new components, like the smart devices within the intelligent environment, has no design consequences for the superior levels like the HMI-layer or the sequencer respectively.

The first task scenario which has been managed with FRIEND-II on basis of MASSiVE is the "serve-drink task" also. Even though the functional improvement with respect to FRIEND-I is not evident, its execution is more flexible from the viewpoint of software technique. Within FRIEND-I subtasks of the "serve-drink task", like grasping, replacing or putting down objects, were programmed in a pre-determined sequence. Within FRIEND-II these subtasks evolve from out a planning process performed on basis of task-knowledge. Due to this flexibility the next development steps concentrate on the implementation of new subtasks, i.e. skills that will be integrated into the already existing task-knowledge data-basis. On the basis of this extended task-knowledge new tasks, as specified within the AMaRob project, will be managed within the next two years.

Another area of active research, which is also important with respect to further improvements of rehabilitation robots, is the system control via non-invasive brain-computer interfaces (BCIs). In (Lüth et al., 2007) first results are presented that show the feasibility of user interactions in MASSiVE solely on the basis of brain signal interpretation. The applied principle is the detection of either the characteristic P300 waveform or steady state visual evoked potentials (SSVEP) in the visual cortex of the user, who is concentrating on a continuously blinking light source. The bandwidth of this kind of input media is still very low and also it is currently not yet possible to realize user interactions with fast reaction times. However, due to ongoing improvements of this technique, a very promising opportunity to command a robotic system arises for highly handicapped users.

6. References

Bien, Z. Z.; Song, W.-K; Kwon, D.-S.; Chung, M.-J.; Park, H.-S.; Kim, D.-J.; Kim, J.-H. & Lee, K. (2001). A Wheelchair Robot System and its Various Interface Methods for the Disabled Persons, *Proceedings of the 1st Workshop on Technical Challenge for Dependable Robots in Human Environments,* Seoul, Korea, May 21-22, 2001

Bolmsjö, G. & Neveryd, H. (1995). WALKY, an Ultrasonic Navigating Mobile Robot for the Disabled, *Proceedings of the 2nd TIDE Congress*, pp. 366-370, ISBN 978-90-5199-220-5, Paris, France, April 1995, IOS Press, Amsterdam

Bonasso, R.; Kortenkamp, D.; Schreckenghost, D. & Ryan, D. (1998). Three tier architecture for controlling space life support systems, *Proceedings of IEEE International Joint Symposium on Intelligence and Systems (SIS) 1998,* pp. 195-201, ISBN 0-8186-8548-4, Rockville, MD, USA, May 1998

Borgerding, B.; Ivlev, O.; Martens, C.; Ruchel, N. & Gräser, A. (1999). FRIEND - Functional Robot Arm with User Friendly Interface for Disabled People, In:, *Assistive Technology on the Threshold of the New Millennium: AAATE'99, Proceedings of the 5th European Conference for the Advancement of Assistive Technology,* C. Bühler, H. Knops (Ed.), pp. 286-290, , IOS Press, ISBN 1-58603-001-9, 1st-4th November 1999, Amsterdam

Busnel, M.; Coulon-Lauture, F.; Détriché, J.-M.; Le Claire, G. & Lesigne, B. (1999). The robotized workstation -MASTER- for users with tetraplegia: Description and evaluation. *Journal of Rehabilitation Research and Development,* Vol. 36, No. 3, July 1999, pp. 217-229, ISSN 0748-7711

Cao, T. & Sanderson, A. C. (1998). AND/OR net representation for robotic task sequence planning, *IEEE Transactions on Systems, Man and Cybernetics,* Vol. 28, Issue 2, May 1998, pp. 204–218, ISSN 1094-6977

Casals, A.; Merchan, R.; Portell, E.; Cufi; X. & Contijoch, J. (1999). CAPDI: A Robotized Kitchen for the Disabled and Elderly, *Proceedings of the 5th European Conference for the Advancement of Assistive Technology (AAATE),* pp. 346-351, ISBN 1-58603-001-9, Düsseldorf, Germany, November 1-4, 1999, IOS Press, Amsterdam

Colle, E.; Rybawzyk, Y. & Hoppenot, P. (2002). Arph: an assistant robot for disabled people, *Proceedings of IEEE International Conference on Systems, Man and Cybernetics,* pp. 176–181, ISBN 0-7803-7437-1, Yasmine Hammamet, Tunisia., 6-9 October 2002unKhoc cho nho thuong voi trong long, khoc cho noi sau nhe nhu khong. Bao nhieu yeu thuong nhung ngay qua da tan theo khoi may bay that xa... http://nhatquanglan1.0catch.com

Coste-Maniere, E. & Simmons, R. (2000). Architecture, the backbone of robotic systems, *Proceedings of International Conference on Robotics and Automation,* pp. 67–72, ISBN 0-7803-5886-4, San Francisco, CA, USA, April 2000

Dallaway, J.L. & Jackson, R.D. (1993). CURL - today and tomorrow, *Proceedings of the 2nd Nordic Workshop on Rehabilitation Robotics,* Orup Rehab Center, Sweden (HADAR, Malmö),, September 1993

Dallaway, J. L.; Jackson, R. D. & Timmer, P.H.A. (1995). Rehabilitation Robotics in Europe. *IEEE Transactions on Rehabilitation Engineering 1995,* Vol. 3, No. 1, March, 1995 pp. 33-45, ISSN 1063-6528

Dario, P.; Dillman, R. & Christensen, H. I. (2004). EURON research roadmaps, *Key Area 1 on Research Coordination,* http://www.euron.org

DLR. (2007). Key research program "Leitinnovation Servicereobotik", *www.service-robotik.de,* DLR - Project executing organization for German Federal Ministry of Education and Research ("Bundesministerium für Bildung und Forschung")

Eftring, H. (1994). Robot control methods and results from user trials on the RAID workstation, *Proceedings of the 4th International Conference on Rehabilitation Robotics (ICORR),* pp. 97-101, Wilmington, Delaware, USA, June 1994

Engelberger, J. F. (1989). *Robotics in Service,* MIT Press, ISBN 0-2620-5042-0, Cambridge, MA, USA

Fikes, R. & Nilsson, N. (1971). STRIPS: A new approach to the application of theorem proving to problem solving, *Artificial Intelligence, Vol. 2,* pp. 189-208. Reprinted in Readings in Planning, J. Allen, J. Hendler, and A. Tate (Ed.), 1990, Morgan Kaufmann Publishers, San Mateo, California

Gamma, E.; Helm, R.; Johnson, R. & Vlissides, J. (1995). *Design Patterns: Elements of Reusable Object-Oriented Software,* Addison-Wesley Professional, 1st edition ed., 1995, ISBN 0-2016-3361-2

Hillman, M. R. et al. (1999). Design of a Wheelchair Mounted Robot, *Proceedings of the 5th European Conference for the Advancement of Assistive Technology (AAATE)*, pp. 316-321, ISBN 1-58603-001-9, Düsseldorf, Germany, November 1-4, 1999, IOS Press, Amsterdam

IAT. (2007). AMaRob - Autonomous Manipulator Control for Rehabilitation Robots, *Project-webpage, www.amarob.de*

Innocenti, C.; Mondino, G.; Regis, P. & Sandini, G. (1994). Trajectory Planning and Real-time Control of an Autonomous Mobile Robot Equipped with Vision and Ultrasonic Sensors, *Proceedings of the International Conference on Intelligent Robots and Systems (IROS) 1994*, pp. 1861-1866, ISBN 0-7803-1933-8, Munich, Germany, September 12th-16th, 1994

Kawamura, K.; Bagchi, S.; Iskarous, M. & Bishay, M. (1995). Intelligent robotic systems in service of the disabled, *IEEE Transactions on Rehabilitation Engineering*, Vol. 3, No. 1 , Mar 1995, pp. 14 -21

Kazi, Z. (1996). Multimodally Controlled Intelligent Assistive Robot, *Proceedings of 16th Annual RESNA Conference*, pp. 348-350 Salt Palace Convention Center, Salt Lake City, Utah, USA, June 1996

Kazi, Z.; Chen, S.; Beitler, M.; Chester, D. & Foulds, R. (1997). Grasping at Straws: An Intelligent Multimodal Assistive Robot, *Proceedings of the 5th ICORR'97*, pp. 87-90, Bath Institute of Medical Engineering, University of Bath, UK, April 1997

Korondi, P. & Hashimoto, H. (2003). Intelligent Space as an Integrated Intelligent System, *Keynote Paper in Proceedings of the International Conference on Electrical Drives and Power Electronics,* pp. 24-31, 2003

Lang, O.; Martens, C & Gräser, A. (2000). Realisation of a Semiautonomous Grippingskill for the Support of Disabled People, *Proceedings of Robotik 2000*, pp. 273-278, ISBN 3-18-091552-8, Berlin, 29./30. June 2000, VDI Berichte 1552, VDI Verlag GmbH, Düsseldorf

Laschi, C.; Teti, G.; Tamburrini, G.; Datteri, E. & Dario, P. (2001). Adaptable semi-autonomy in personal robots, *Proceedings of IEEE International Workshop on Robot and Human Interactive Communication,* pp. 152–157, ISBN 0-7803-7222-0, Bordeaux, Paris, France, September 2001

Lüth, T.; Ojdanić, D.; Friman, O.; Prenzel, O. & Gräser, A. (2007). Direct control in a rehabilitation robotic system via a Brain-Computer Interface, Proceedings of the International Conference on Rehabilitation Robotics ICORR, Noordwijk, Netherlands, 13-15 June 2007

Mahoney, R. M. (2001). The Raptor Wheelchair Robot System, *Proceedings of the 7th International Conference on Rehabilitation Robotics (ICORR) 2001*, Mokhtari, M. (Ed.) Integration of Assistive Technology in the Information Age, pp. 135-141, ISBN 1-58603-171-6, Evry, France, IOS Press, Amsterdam

Martens, C.; Lang, O.; Ruchel, N.; Ivlev, O. & Gräser, A. (2001). A FRIEND for Assisting Handicapped People. *IEEE Robotics and Automation Magazine,* Vol. 7, No. 1, March 2001, pp. 57-65, ISSN 1070-9932

Martens, C.; Kim, D.-J.; Han, J.-S.; Gräser, A. & Bien, Z. Z. (2002). Concept for a modified hybrid multi-layer control-architecture for rehabilitation robots, *Proceedings of the*

3rd International Workshop on Human-friendly Robotic Systems, pp. 49-54 Daejeon, Korea , January 21-22, 2002

Martens, C. (2003a). Generation of parallel executable control sequences for rehabilitation robotic systems on the basis of hierachical petri-net based task representation, In: *Methods and Applications in Automation,* B. Lohmann, A. Gräser, (Ed.), pp. 73–85, Shaker Verlag, ISBN 3-8322-4502-2, Aachen

Martens, C. (2003b). *Teilautonome Aufgabenbearbeitung bei Rehabilitationsrobotern mit Manipulator,* Ph.D. thesis University of Bremen, Shaker-Verlag, ISBN 3-8322-2400-9, Aachen

Martens, C. (2005). Task oriented programming of service-robots on the basis of process-structures, In: *Methods and Applications in Automation,* B. Lohmann, A. Gräser, (Ed.), pp. 45–56, Shaker Verlag, ISBN 3-8322-4502-2, Aachen

May, T. & Schäffer, C. (1999). Care-O-bot: A System for Assisting Elderly and Disabled Persons in Home Environments, *Proceedings of the 5th European Conference for the Advancement of Assistive Technology (AAATE),* pp. 340-345, ISBN 1-58603-001-9, Düsseldorf, Germany, November 1-4, 1999, IOS Press, Amsterdam

Mokhtari, M. & Amni, C. (2001). Assistive Technology for the Disabled People: Should it Work? The French Approach, *Proceedings of the 2nd International Workshop on Human-friendly Welfare Robotic Systems,* pp. 134-136, KAIST, Daejeon, Korea January 2001, HWRS-ERC, Daejeon

Ojdanic, D.; Ivlev, O. & Gräser, A. (2006). A new fast motion planning approach for dexterous manipulators in 3D-Cartesian space, *Proceedings of ISR-Robotik Joint Conference on Robotics,* p. 49, ISBN 3-18-091956-6, International Congress Centre Munich, Germany, May 15-17 2006, VDI Wissensforum IWB GmbH, Düsseldorf, Germany

Prenzel, O. (2005). Semi-autonomous object anchoring for service-robots, In: *Methods and Applications in Automation,* B. Lohmann, A. Gräser, (Ed.), pp. 57–68, Shaker Verlag, ISBN 3-8322-4502-2, Aachen

Prenzel, O.; Ojdanic, D. & Gräser, A. (2006). Manipulative Robotic Tasks in Smart Home Environments, *Proceedings of 4th International Conference On Smart Homes and Health Telematics (ICOST),* pp. 172-179, ISBN 1-58603-623-8, ISSN 1383-813X, Belfast, Northern-Ireland, UK, June 26-28, 2006, Series: Assistive Techology Research Series, IOS Press, (Ed.) C. Nugent, J.C. Augusto, Vol. 19

Radchenko, O.; Martens, C.; Pape, A.; She, H.; Volosyak, I. & Gräser, A. (2004). FRIEND – An Intelligent Assistant in Daily Life, In: *Advances in Rehabilitation Robotics: Human-friendly Technologies on Movement Assistance and Restoration for People with Disabilities - Part II Rehabilitation Robots for Assistance of Human Movements, II.1 Conceptions and Experimental Design,* Ed.: Z. Zenn Bien, Dimitar Stefanov, pp. 95–126, Springer-Verlag, ISBN 3-540-21986-2, Heidelberg, Germany

She, H.; Martens, C. & Gräser, A. (2003a). Application of Programming by Demonstration in the Rehabilitation Robotic System FRIEND, *Proceedings of the 8th International Conference on Rehabilitation Robotics (ICORR) 2003,* pp. 39-42, ISBN 89-88366-09-3, Daejeon, Korea, 23-25 April 2003, HWRS-ERC

She, H.; Martens, C.; Gräser, A.; Kim, D.-J.; Lee, H.-E. & Bien, Z. Z. (2003b). Soft Computing-based Robust Contact/Non-contact Detection during Serving a Beverage Task, *Proceedings of the IEEE International Conference on Fuzzy Systems (FUZZ-IEEE 2003),* pp. 613-617, Marriott Pavilion Downtown Hotel, St. Louis, MO, May 25-28, 2003

Van der Loos, H.F.M. (1995). Lessons Learned in the Application of Robotics Technology to Field of Rehabilitation. *IEEE Transactions on Rehabilitation Engineering*, Vol. 3, No. 1, March 1995, pp. 46-55, ISSN 1063-6528

Van der Loos, H.F.M.; Wagner, J.J.; Smaby, N.; Chang, K.-S.; Madrigal, O.; Leifer, L.J.; Khatib, O. (1999). ProVAR assistive robot system architecture, *Proceedings of International Conference on Robotics and Automation (ICRA) 1999*, pp. 741-746, ISBN 0-7803-5180-0, Marriott Hotel, Renaissance Center, Detroit, Michigan, May 10-15, 1999, IEEE Robotics and Automation Society

Volosyak, I.; Radchenko, O.; Pape, A., Martens, C.; She, H.; Wendland, E. & Gräser, A. (2003). Smart tray for the support of a wheelchair mounted manipulator, *Proceedings of the International Conference on Economic, Engineering and Manufacturing Systems ICEEMS 2003*, ISBN 973-635-215-3, Brasov, Romania, 23-24 October, 2003

Wagner, J.J; Van der Loos, H.F.M; Leifer, L.J. (1998). Dual-Agent User Interface for an Assistive Robot, *Proceedings of the 21st Annual RESNA Conference*, pp. 286-288, ISSN 0883-4741, ISBN 0-932101-4-2, Minneapolis, MN. Washington DC, June 1998, RESNA Press

10

Functional Rehabilitation: Coordination of Artificial and Natural Controllers

Rodolphe Héliot[1,2], Christine Azevedo[3], & Bernard Espiau[1]
[1] *INRIA Rhône Alpes, France*
[2] *CEA-LETI, France*
[3] *INRIA Sophia Antipolis / DEMAR – LIRMM, France*

1. Introduction

Walking and standing abilities, though important for quality of life and participation in social and economic activities, can be adversely affected by central nervous system (CNS) disorders such as spinal cord injury, stroke or traumatic brain injury. One characteristic of motor deficiencies which affect lower extremities is their impact on both static and dynamic postural equilibrium. Depending on the impairment level, functional rehabilitation techniques may be needed for a patient to stand up and walk (Popovic and Sinkjær, 2003). Functional electrical stimulation (FES) can induce contraction of skeletal muscles by applying electrical stimuli to sensory-motor system via electrodes which can be placed on the skin (Kralj et al., 1983), or implanted (Guiraud et al., 2006). FES applications applied to lower limbs include foot drop correction, single joint control, cycling, standing up, walking… (Zhang and Zhu, 2007).

Two distinct objectives may be targeted when using those techniques, depending on the type of disorder: chronic assistance or acute training.

FES can be applied for **standing and gait restoration in paraplegic patients**. Paraplegia is a condition where both legs are paretic (incomplete paraplegia) or paralyzed (complete paraplegia). Physiological effects of FES-assisted verticalization in paraplegic patients include: prevention of muscle atrophy, promotion of renal functions, improvement of joint range of motion, well being, improved digestion, bowel and bladder functions, retardation of bone-density loss, decreased spasticity, reduced risks of pressure sores, improved cardiovascular health, improved skin and muscle tone (Cybulski and Jaegger, 1986). In theory, FES-assisted ambulation can give to the user greater access to locations inaccessible to wheelchairs, assist transfers, and facilitate face-to-face interaction with others. In addition to the physical effects of exercise, FES for standing, transfer, and ambulation applications can offer functional and psychological benefits. Today, all FES standing or ambulation systems use walkers, parallel bars, or elbow canes for balance and support. FES systems for standing and ambulation can be strictly FES, or combine FES with various types of braces (hybrid systems) like orthoses and exoskeletons (Kobetic et al., 2003).

FES can also be applied for **walking assistance and training in hemiplegic patients**. Hemiplegia is a condition where one side of the body is paretic or paralyzed; it is usually the consequence of a cerebro-vascular accident. Both sensory and motor functions can be more or less affected. One of the main consequences of hemiplegia is the drop-foot syndrome. Due to lack of controllability of muscles involved in flexing the ankle and toes, the foot drops downward and impedes the normal walking motion. Most hemiplegic patients recover their walking, but often this walking is not functional (foot-drop, stability on the paretic leg, fast fatigue, etc.). Today, there are commercially available assistive systems that use surface electrodes and prevent drop-foot. Providing ability to walk in stroke patients (Mauritz, 2002) has been demonstrated to help in recovering and results in better walking. The classical methods to provide walking are: therapist assisted walking, treadmill walking with reduced body weight by means of harness, use of robotic mechanisms (Lunenburger et al., 2007). Current results suggest that the repeatability and reproducibility of the movement are essential within this context for an optimal recovery. The FES used in the framework of exercise was termed Functional Electrical Therapy (FET). When the spinal cord lesion is incomplete, paraplegic patients can also benefit from adapted training in order to recover mobility (Barbeau et al., 1999).

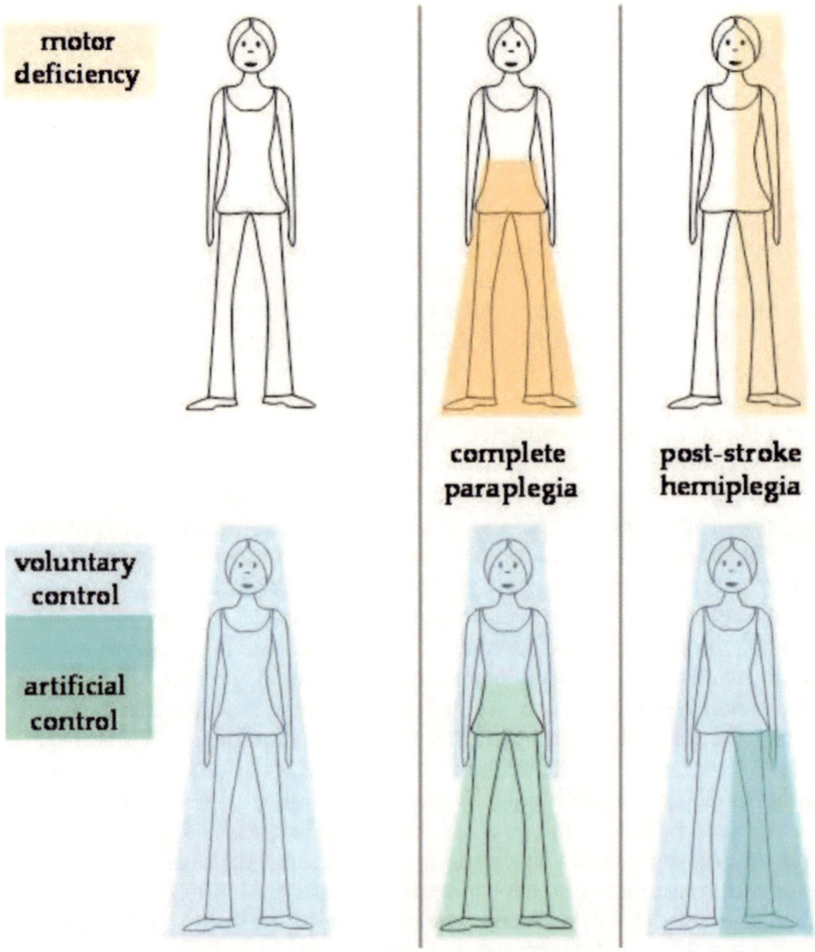

Fig. 1. Application and characteristics of FES assistive systems to rehabilitation of spinal cord injured paraplegic and post-stroke hemiplegic patients.

In paraplegia and hemiplegia, it is important to notice that the upper extremities (trunk and arms) remain functional as well as one of the legs in the cases of hemiplegia (figure 1) (Azevedo and Héliot, 2005). Therefore, when attempting to control posture and locomotion through FES, an important issue is the enhancement of the interaction between: a) the artificial FES-system controlling the deficient body segments and b) the natural system represented by the patient voluntary actions through his valid limb motion. In most of FES-systems, voluntary movements of valid limbs are usually considered as perturbations. As an example, the trunk represents 60% of the total body mass and is positioned relatively high with respect to the base of support. Therefore, trunk movements strongly influence the equilibrium control whereas legs have an adaptive role to ensure an adequate support base for the centre of mass projection. Collaboration between trunk and legs sounds therefore indispensable to ensure postural balance, and should be taken in account in a FES-based control system. In a similar way, when one leg functions normally, like in hemiplegia, it would be suitable to use information from this leg to inform the artificial controller about the contralateral leg state. This approach is also a way to give the patient an active role in the control of his/her movements. The FES-assistance system should adapt to patient behaviour and intentions expressed through his valid limbs motions, instead of imposing an arbitrary motion on the deficient limbs.

This consideration (need for collaboration between healthy and deficient limbs) led us to the idea that valid limbs should be observed in order to improve the artificial control. Developing sensory based FES assistive-systems implies to use sensors to measure the voluntary actions of the patient.

Our approach consists of placing sensors on subject's healthy limbs (trunk, intact leg...) in order to optimize the interaction at two levels:

- **Strategic level**: identifying the postural action the patient intends to execute, as soon as possible, in order to allow for optimal posture preparation and execution
- **Tactic level**: monitoring the ongoing action relatively to a reference pattern in order to generate an adapted and optimized command for the deficient limbs

Therefore, our approach requires the specification of two classes of functions, which use sensor measurements from valid limbs as inputs (see section 2 for a description of the used sensors). Transitions functions S_{ij} which correspond to detection of intention, will be detailed in section 3, and illustrated with a sit-to-stand transfer action for paraplegic patients under FES. Then, for each identified action, control functions C_i have to be defined, which monitor the ongoing movement and provide with the adapted command; this part will be presented in section 4, and illustrated with a walking action for stroke patients using FES. In both cases, after theoretical considerations followed by some simulation results, real-time experiments are presented in order to validate the developed methods.

One can notice that the framework presented in Figure 2 mixes discrete (action to action transitions) and continuous (control functions within an action) behaviors; this duality raises some integration issues that will be addressed in section 5.

2. Sensors

Our approach aims at observing valid limbs to help the control of deficient limbs. One important constraint is to minimize the number and size of sensors involved in movement observation to propose realistic solutions for rehabilitation applications to be used by physiotherapist and/or the patient himself.

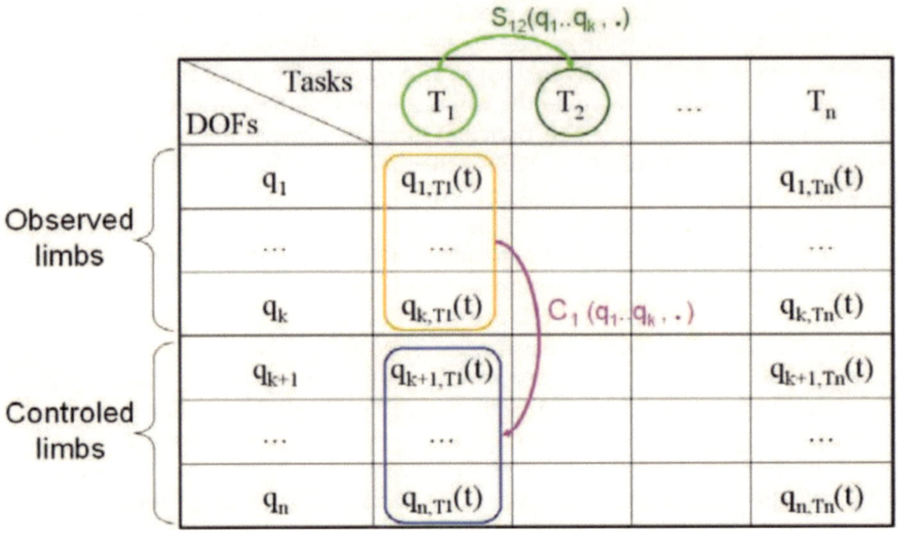

Fig. 2. This table sums up the two envisioned cooperation levels between valid and deficient limbs. The strategic levels, i.e. transitions from a task to another, are represented by transitions functions S_{ij} from a task to another. Tactic level is represented by control functions C_i which role is to provide an adapted command to the controlled limbs. Both of these processings are based on measurements from sensors placed on valid limbs.

Different types of sensors may be used to achieve motion identification and monitoring. Although EMG (Electro-Myo-Graphic), ENG (Electro-Neuro-Graphic) or even EEG (Electro-Encephalo-Graphic) measurements could possibly provide with early information about the intention of action, they suffer from important drawbacks (reliability and robustness) which prevent from their use as embedded on a patient. Foot switches are easy to use and reliable, but provide with very weak information about the movement. Flexible goniometers can measure joint angles, but are difficult and time demanding to mount on the subject, and can be easily broken.

We therefore preferred movement sensors which can provide us with some extrinsic information, such as the dynamics of the movement itself. We found that this kind of information was well-suited for a further adaptation of the artificially generated movements with respect to the natural ones. Such embedded systems of motion capture, like accelerometers, or gyrometers, are today widely used for movement analysis purposes, and find lots of applications in medical or rehabilitation systems (Luinge and Veltink, 2004; Pappas et al., 2002).

Since size and cost of those systems are important issues in our application, we selected a set of micro-sensors minimizing these parameters. The movement sensor we use is a micro-sensor developed by CEA-LETI (Grenoble, France), which associates 3 accelerometers and 3 magnetometers in a minimal volume (see Figure 3). This attitude sensor is able, through the processing algorithms associated, to reconstruct the orientation in space of the segment to which it is attached (Bonnet and Héliot, 2007). It is also possible to have access to accelerometer measurements, which often provide with reliable "signatures" of movements. A particular care was paid to an easy donning and doffing of these sensors on the subject. A wireless version of this sensor has been developed, which is suitable for motion capture.

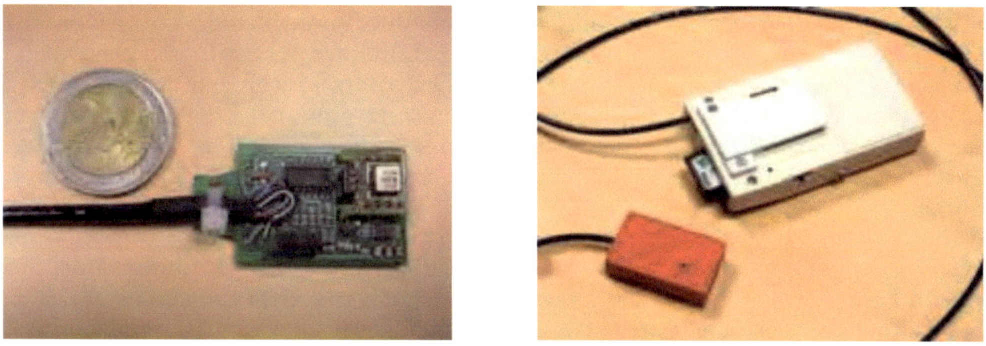

Fig. 3. CEA-LETI attitude sensor and its acquisition system. Left: Sensor size. Board is then embedded in a silicon-like material. Right: Final view of the sensor, with its datalogger.

3. Strategic level: intention detection

A first issue in our approach is to identify the intention of the patient, i.e. to detect as soon as possible the action (posture or movement) he/she is intending to perform. This can be done through motion observation, based on information from sensors placed on valid parts of the body. The operating scheme is thus the following: the patient uses his valid limbs to initiate or stop the movement, or switch from an action to another. Once the intended action recognized, the system triggers the correct command to apply (FES stimulation), so that the movement the patient intends to realize is achieved through both the valid and deficient parts of the body.

Of course, this scheme will work in a better way if the initial motion that the patient has to perform through is valid limbs is normally (i.e. in healthy subjects) occurring **before** the rest of the movement which will be artificially controlled on the deficient limbs. For this reason, an important issue is the understanding of the temporal organization of the whole movement, in order to place the sensors on the valid parts of the body which are normally involved in the initiation of the movement.

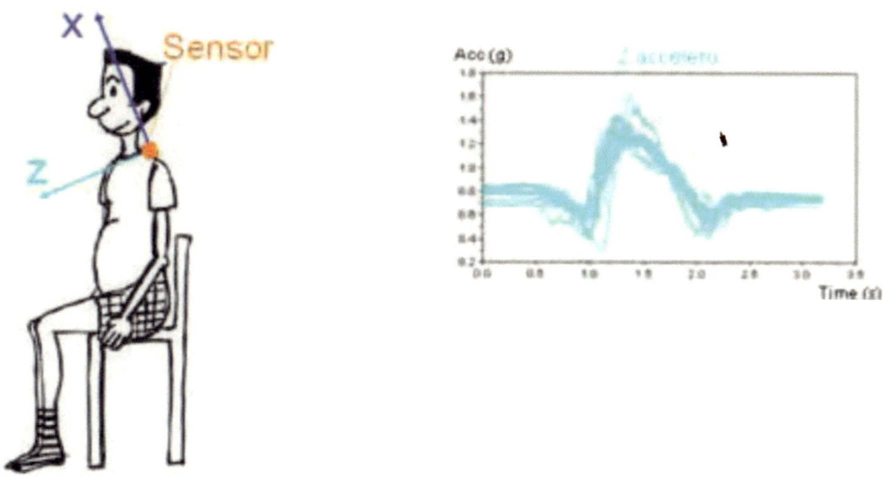

Fig. 4. Acceleration along Z axis during sit-to-stand transfer: 15 trials from one subject.

In this section, we will focus, without loss of generality, on one example: the **sit-to-stand transfer, for paraplegic patient's FES assisted rehabilitation**. Rising from a chair with the help of open-loop electrical stimulation of knee extensors is well accepted in paralyzed persons (Kuzelicki et al., 2000). However, electrically stimulated knee extensors only generate low joint moment during rising. Thus, the effort of upper extremities during standing-up is extensive. Excessive physical effort and large upper limb forces often lead to syndromes of shoulder overuse.

This movement is of great interest in a rehabilitation issue, since it is repeated many times in everyday activities and is usually a prerequisite to gait initiation (Kerr et al., 1997). In healthy subjects, the movement of the trunk precedes the action of the legs: sit-to-stand is impossible without arm support if trunk inertia is not used and associated with a proper postural preparation and action of the legs. **In a paraplegic patient, the coordination between the trunk and the legs, which is no more occurring, must be re-introduced**. Using a FES system, it is essential to optimize the sit-to-stand transfer, in terms of muscle fatigue. Indeed, minimizing the energy needed in rising up may improve the efficiency of the patient in his following activities. For this reason, classical techniques consisting in stimulating as strongly as possible the knee extensors throughout the rising process are inadequate with prolonged and functional standing. We therefore aim at proposing a solution where the global movement is "energetically" optimized, while the use of arm support is minimized.

Although the following will be illustrated through the sit-to-stand example, the proposed methodology can be applied for other types of transitions S from the framework described in Figure 2.

3.1 Movement characterization

In (Azevedo and Héliot, 2005), we demonstrated the pertinence of observing the trunk using a movement sensor system placed on the back of healthy subjects. Indeed, the trunk normally initiates the sit-to-stand transfer, and remains a healthy limb in paraplegic patients. We showed that trunk orientation and acceleration patterns present low intra and inter-variability as well as a high temporal reproducibility and could therefore be a nice characteristic "signature" of the sit-to-stand transfer (see Figure 4).

The next step is to develop a recognition algorithm able to robustly detect this sit-to-stand pattern; in the following section we propose and test two different algorithms for movement detection and recognition.

3.2 Proposed algorithms

3.2.1 Method 1 - monitoring a correlation coefficient

This first algorithm uses a correlation computation to compare the A_z acceleration (acceleration along the Z axis, see Figure 4) with a reference (the typical pattern characterizing the sit-to-stand transfer). This reference is built averaging the same accelerometric signal over several the trials from a given subject, truncated in a way that it only contains the initiation of the movement, stopped at the time when the legs actually start moving. Provided that the reference contains N samples, we compute at each instant k the correlation coefficient between the last N samples of the current A_z acceleration measurement and the reference:

$$C(k) = \frac{1}{N}\sum_{n=1}^{N}\frac{\left(A_z(k-N+n)-\overline{A}_z\right)\left(A_y(n)-\overline{A}_y\right)}{\sqrt{\sigma(A_z)?\sigma(A_y)?.}} \tag{1}$$

where A_z is the measured acceleration and A_y is the reference.

Once the movement begins, the correlation coefficient starts changing, and begins increasing after a while. When the A_z acceleration which we are testing reaches the instant corresponding to the point when the reference has been truncated, the correlation coefficient begins to decrease. Its maximum value should be very close from *1* if the acceleration pattern matches the reference. Thus, movement detection / recognition is achieved in an easy way: once the correlation coefficient reaches a value greater than $1 - \varepsilon$, ε being small, the movement is recognized as a sit-to-stand transition. The trigger for leg muscles activation should be set as soon as the correlation coefficient begins to decrease (see Figure 5).

3.2.2 Method 2 - sequential detection of abrupt changes

Abrupt changes theory has been widely explored by (Basseville and Nikiforov, 1993); we will introduce here only a simple application of this approach. Indeed, our detection issue belongs to the area of **detection of abrupt changes**, which itself relies on sequential Likelihood Ratio (SLR) estimates.

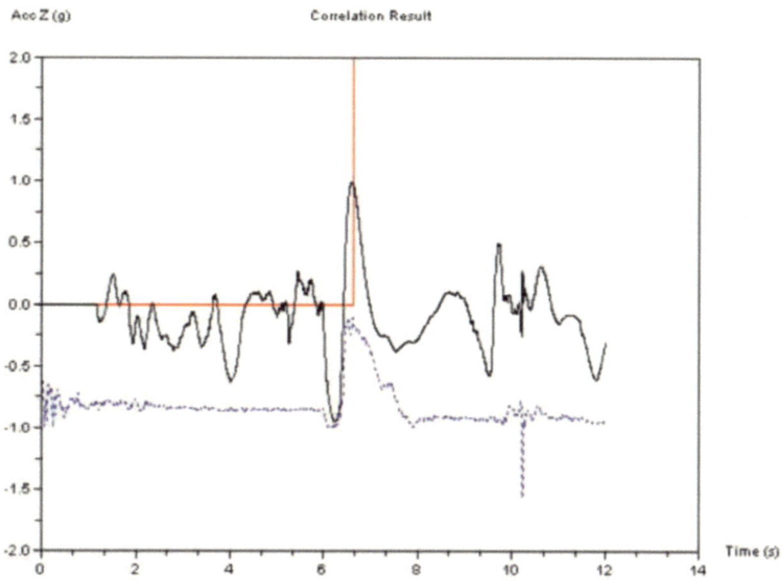

Fig. 5. Correlation computation over time (full line), from the accelerometric signal (dotted line). When the acceleration signal shows a pattern corresponding to the reference, the correlation coefficient increases and gets close to 1. The vertical line corresponds to the estimated time of leg movement onset, given by the maximum of correlation.

Given a **non-stationary** signal, one can ask **when** statistical changes occur. Computing a Likelihood Ratio (LR), we can test between two or more hypotheses and then check if some statistical characteristic of a signal belongs to one class or another. A sequential LR is then a way to look **online** for any changes in the signal properties.

We, here, apply this technique to detect a very simple change: transition from resting to moving. Assuming that the acceleration locally behaves as a signal with constant mean and variance σ^2, the computed LR allows to test between the two following hypotheses:

- *(H0)*: the acceleration is close to its "resting" value, μ_0
- *(H1)*: the acceleration is close to its "moving"' value, μ1

$$s_k = \ln \frac{P(H_1)}{P(H_0)} = \frac{(\mu_1 - \mu_0)}{\sigma?} \cdot \left(z(k) - \frac{\mu_0 + \mu_1}{2} \right) \tag{2}$$

Therefore, s_k is positive if *(H1)* is achieved, negative otherwise. Then the cumulative sum, SLR, is computed:

$$S_k = \sum_{n=1}^{k} s_n \tag{3}$$

Assuming that the signal starts at its resting value (hypothesis *(H0)*), SLR decreases until a change arises. Finally, let us set the following decision function, *g*:

$$\left\{ g_k = S_k - \min_{n=1}^{k} s_n \right\} > h \tag{4}$$

where h is an adequate threshold. As S_k first decreases, g_k stays around *0*; as soon as hypothesis *(H1)* appears to be the good one, S_k increases and *g* will become true. This threshold *h* reflects to what extent the signal has to be statistically close to □1: the higher this threshold is, the longer the signal will have to belong to *(H1)* before activating the detection event. This will make the algorithm more robust, but also introduce some delay in the detection. Finally, we are able with this method to robustly detect the movement initiation. Figure 6 shows an example.

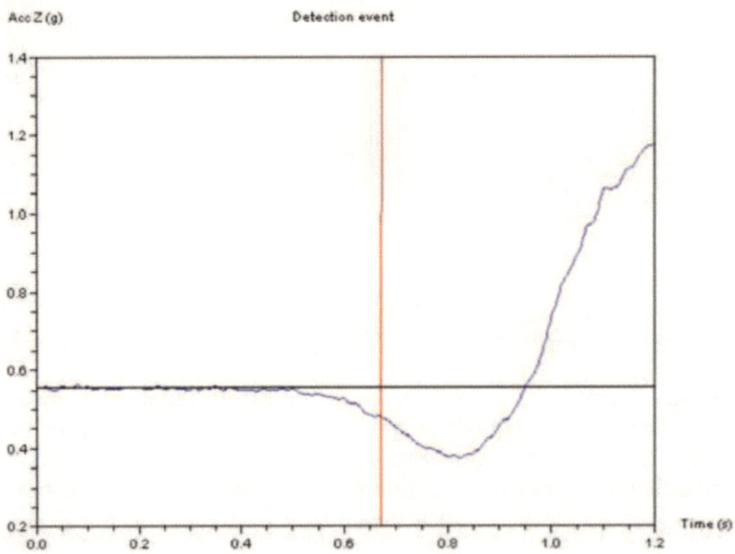

Fig. 6. Acceleration and its detected starting time.

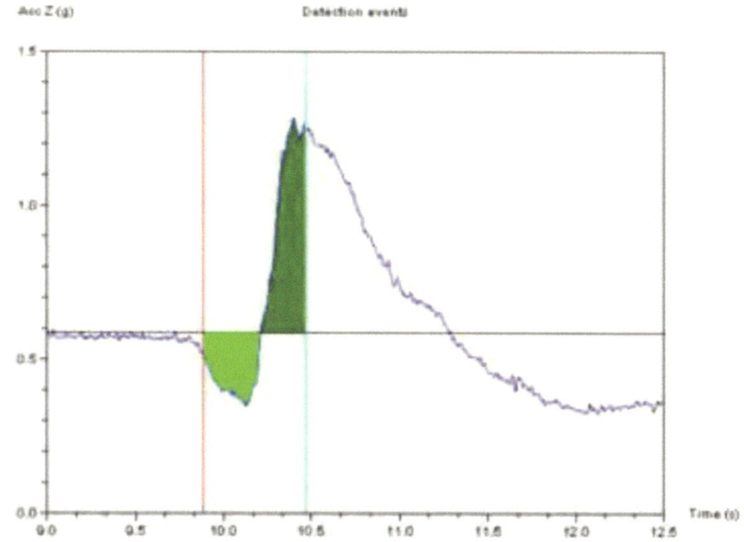

Fig. 7. Acceleration with its two detection events: starting time and integral ending value reached.

The next step is to compute the integral of the reference (the same reference as in section 3.2.1) between the two following boundaries, regarding to its baseline value:

- time when movement initiation is detected
- time when legs start moving (actually, end of reference, by definition)

This computation only has to be run once, and this can be done off-line. As we have one reference for each subject, we save one integral value per subject (called "ending value"), which will be useful. We finally apply the following processing to each trial:

- detection of movement initiation trough SLRs method. This is performed using the previously described method. Parameters for this detection **must be the same** than those used for the corresponding reference. Then, the acceleration integral is computed on line, regarding to its baseline value, between the detected onset of movement and current time.
- checking that, at the beginning of the movement, this integral goes below a given value, which means that the initial forward acceleration is significant. This will allow us to discriminate between a "true" and "false" sit-to-stand transition. These "false" movements can be for example the grasping of an object placed in front of the patient.
- the integral then increases, and finally reaches the corresponding reference ending value. In theory, if the measured acceleration has exactly the same dynamics as its reference, then this ending value is reached exactly as the time when legs start moving (Figure 7).

3.3 Results

Performance of the two proposed algorithms was evaluated, using sit-to-stand recordings from 10 valid subjects. Full details about these results can be found in (Héliot et al., 2005). Sensitivity (ability for the algorithm to recognize an effective sit-to-stand movement) and selectivity (ability for the algorithm to reject a "false" sit-to-stand movement, as grasping an object placed in front of the patient) were found identical for the two methods. Delays for recognition (elapsed time between the intended and actual detection time) are comparable, around 40 ms, which is very low regarding to the total duration of the movement (1.5 s).

	Correlation method	Abrupt changes method
Sensitivity	96.7 %	96.7 %
Selectivity	76.2 %	76.2 %
Delay for recognition (mean)	- 0.7 ms	1.47 ms
(standard deviation)	36.7 ms	39.3 ms

Table 1. Results summary for the two proposed algorithms.

3.4 Conclusion

In this section, we presented two methods for early motion identification, enabling to identify as soon as possible the action (posture or movement) he/she is intending to perform. Although presented through the specific sit-to-stand example, these methods remain applicable in a very large spectrum of actions.

Let us recall that it is particularly important to detect the transitions between activity modes as soon as possible after the patient has taken the decision to perform a new action. Normal postural control performance is largely based on the human capacity to anticipate. This anticipation could be relative to external events but also to internal disturbances. Indeed any movement is source of perturbation. To counteract these destabilizing effects, the initiation of a voluntary movement is preceded by dedicated muscular activities so-called Anticipated Postural Adjustments (APA) (Crenna and Frigo, 1991). In our sit-to-stand example, rising off a chair is normally preceded by the inhibition of the soleus muscle (ankle plantar-flexor) and the activation of the antagonist muscle, tibialis (ankle dorsi-flexor) without producing any movement, in preparation to the future change of support base when leaving the seat. Integrating these anticipatory corrections in artificial controllers of FES-systems appears to be a possible way of improving their performances.

4. Tactic level: movement monitoring

Once a movement has been detected, there is a need to monitor the ongoing action in order to provide with adapted commands (FES stimulation parameters), based on the information given by sensors placed on the patient. Again, the valid part of the body is of crucial importance, since it should be used to somehow "teleoperate" the deficient limbs.

Since coordination between limbs is critical during locomotion, we will focus on one example from that domain in the following: **gait monitoring in hemiplegic patients using multi-channel FET.** Today, in rehabilitation centres, pre-programmed stimulation patterns that are triggered by the therapist of the patient himself are used. One main problem is the fact that patients dramatically modify their gait all along the training session and some adaptability is therefore needed. Although some automatized triggering systems have been proposed, using heel switch detection through external sensors (Meadows et al. 1992) or implanted electrodes for nerve activity measurement (Burridge et al., 2005), the applied stimulation sequences are still pre-programmed.

When multi-channel FES is used for walking rehabilitation of hemiplegic individuals the **timing** of the stimulation needs to be set properly in order to optimize the use of preserved sensory-motor systems and lead to a symmetrical gait pattern. To this end, sensors are often used to get information concerning the ongoing movement. Of course there is a need for processing these input signals to provide with an adapted stimulation command.

4.1 CPG concept

This online timing adaptation issue can be seen as a trajectory generation problem, where the command has to be synchronized on sensory inputs. In the case of gait, the considered movement is cyclical. A classical way of generating cyclic motions for articulated systems is to synthesize a rhythm generator, called CPG (Central Pattern Generator) by reference to biological systems (Cohen et al., 1988). The CPG concept refers to a small neural network, probably located at the spinal level, able to generate rhythmic commands for the muscles. It can be divided into two parts: a rhythm generator, and a patterning mechanism. CPGs receive inputs from higher parts of the central nervous system, and also from peripheral afferents; thus, its functioning results from an interaction between central commands and local reflexes (see Figure 8). The CPG can be modelled either with a simulated neural network, for example using the Fitzhugh-Nagumo model (Matsuoka, 1985) or by using explicitly nonlinear differential equations. In both cases, the idea is to encode the desired behaviour in a stable limit cycle.

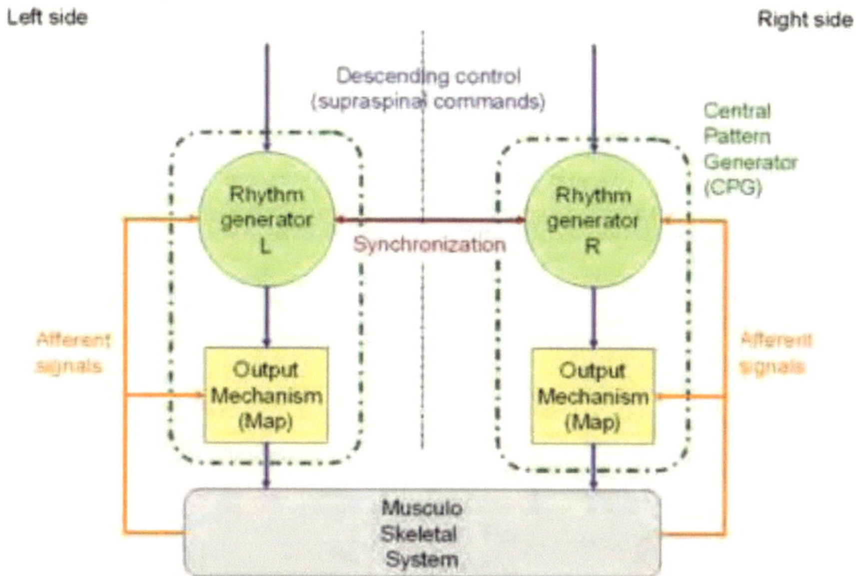

Fig. 8. CPG architecture for movement control in vertebrates.

In robotics, a CPG-based command structure has several advantages for the design of cyclic trajectories: the system is robust with respect to small perturbations, thanks to the intrinsic stability of the limit cycle; one can easily modulate the amplitude or the period of the trajectory; a multidimensional output can be generated for the same low computational price, which is helpful when dealing with robots with numerous Degrees Of Freedom (DOFs), having to exhibit multiple synchronized periodic motions, like walking machines.

For this kind of classical CPG-based approach, the literature is quite extensive (see for example (Williamson, 1998; Endo et al., 2004) as recent typical studies). However the need for adaptation of the system to environmental changes, external requirements or proprioceptive information through sensory signals is more rarely addressed. We can nevertheless refer the reader to a few recent papers in the field which give a good idea of the state of the art (Fukuoka et al., 2003; Dong et al., 2006; Simoni and DeWeerth, 2007). Actually, there is a lack of design tools in the framework of oscillators and synchronization.

A lot of analysis tools are available (Guckenheimer and Holmes, 1990; Pikovsky et al., 2001), but few design tools, as pointed out by (Bailey, 2004) and (Righetti et al. 2006). It appeared that the question of using **continuously** a set of sensor measurements as driving inputs to an artificial CPG aimed at controlling several links in a safe way is still an open question. In the following, we will focus on the input integration problem in the CPG framework: "How can we build a rhythm generator (oscillator) such as we can be sure it will synchronize with a given input?"

4.2 Oscillator design

Our working hypothesis is that we are dealing with a cyclical activity: this means that each signal (sensors, actuators …) can be described along a cycle. The phase ϕ can be introduced, as a coordinate along the limit cycle (Pikovsky et al., 2001), i.e a variable which grows uniformly in the direction of the motion and gains 2π during each rotation, thus obeying the equation:

$$\frac{d\varphi}{dt} = \omega_0 \tag{5}$$

where $\omega_0 = 2\pi / T_0$ is the frequency of the oscillations.

Our aim is to build an oscillator which will synchronize with a given cyclic sensory input. We present in this section a design methodology for such an oscillator. It can be synthesized in two steps:

- building a system as a phenomenological model, which simulates the sensor measurements
- building an observer of this system, in which are injected the real sensor measurements

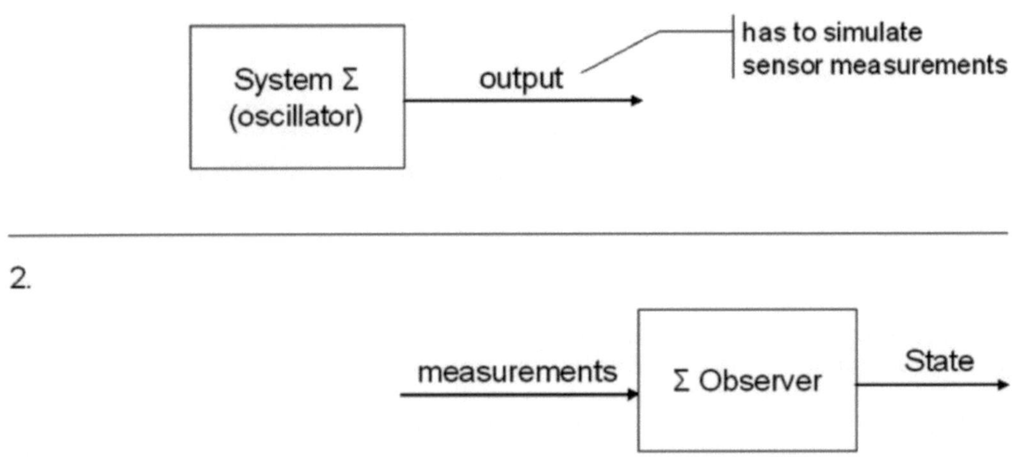

Fig. 9. A two-steps methodology for oscillator design.

To simulate a cyclical sensor measurement, one could choose a linear system as model, and provide it with a cyclical input u (for example, a sinusoidal input); in that case the linear system is shaping the input so as its output simulates the given measurement. A problem arises then: there is a need for providing with a cyclical input which has to be synchronous with the measurement. This problem has been explored previously (Righetti et al. 2006), but the proposed solutions adapt to the frequency changes too slowly for our targeted applications. For this reason, we chose a non-linear oscillator as a phenomenological model for our sensor measurements: it can **autonomously** (without input) generate a **cyclical** signal.

4.2.1 Non-linear oscillator model

The first step is to model the cyclical sensor signal with a nonlinear oscillator. In this section, we will focus on the modelling of one specific signal: **thigh inclination during human gait observation.**

a) Class of candidate oscillators

To some extent, and under the assumption of rigidity, a bipedal walking system can be modelled as a tree-structured n-link mechanical system free in space. Its dynamics can therefore be described through a Lagrange equation:

$$M(q)\ddot{q} + N(q,\dot{q}) + G(q) = -B(\dot{q}) + \Gamma + \Lambda^T C(q) \qquad (6)$$

where q is the set of joint coordinates, $q \in \Re^n f\ SE(3)$, M is a sdp. mass matrix, N gathers coriolis and centrifugal forces, B is the friction term, G the gravity vector, Γ the actuation input, and $\Lambda^T C(q)$ are the constraints of ground contacts, which are unilateral and time-varying. In the absence of constraints, friction and control, this equation becomes autonomous (i.e. with a right-hand side equal to zero), with mechanical energy as first integral, in which the continual exchange between kinetics energy and potential energy produces a periodic motion.

Let us now consider a single coordinate q_a, (the thigh inclination). Starting from the autonomous version of eq. (6), we can express its dynamics as:

$$H(.)\ddot{q}_a + F(q_a,.) = T(.) \qquad (7)$$

where T is a set of bounded perturbations depending on all the variables and their derivatives, $H(.)$ the equivalent of a mass term, F is analogous to a potential function. Therefore, the behaviour of q_a is the one of a periodic solution, issued from a nonlinear second-order equation, with a potential term and disturbances. This incitates to seek the nonlinear oscillator preferably within the class of modified and disturbed second-order mass-spring systems.

b) Need for a limit cycle

As seen previously, the natural behaviour of a mechanical robotic system without dissipative and other inputs is an oscillator with constant energy. Nevertheless, this does not correspond with the idea of an attractive limit cycle which underlies the oscillator-based approach. To justify this point of view, we have to refer to another class of mechanical systems: the passive walking machines. Indeed, let us consider the case of a planar compass, walking on a slope, with instantaneous and inelastic step transitions, as addressed in (Mcgeer et al. 1990) and several others (Goswami et al., 1998). It then can be shown that, for a given slope, such a system exhibits a limit walking cycle, with a rather large basin of attraction (see Figure 10). This behaviour can be compared to the concept of "natural gait" or "comfort gait" which is spontaneously reached and followed by a human in steady state walking, and which corresponds to a minimum of the metabolic energy consumption with respect to distance.

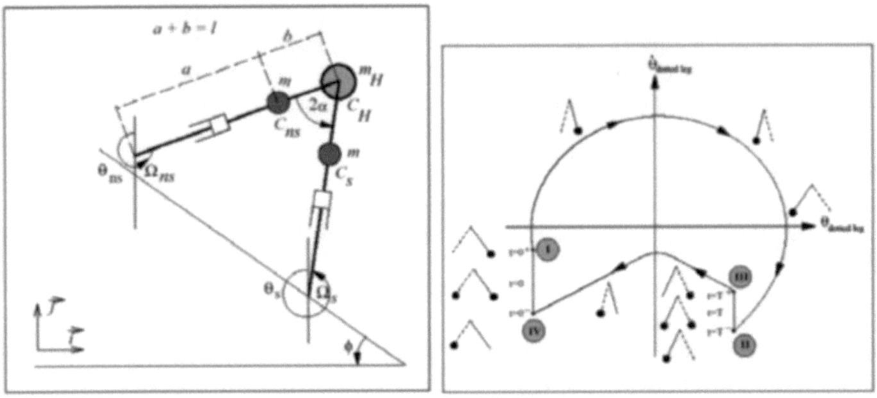

Fig.10. Mechanical model of a passive walking machine, and its stable limit cycle.

In conclusion, it appears that searching for an oscillator of second-order type and exhibiting a limit cycle is a natural way of modelling the periodic walking behaviour of a human link measured with an adequate sensor.

c) *Structure choice and parameters setting*

From the previous sections, we know that we have to choose a nonlinear oscillator which is derived from a second-order mass-spring system. Another requirement that will be explained in section 4.2.2, is that the oscillator has to belong to the Lur'e class. Two common oscillators fit these requirements: the van der Pol oscillator and the Rayleigh oscillator, which are very similar.

Let us start from the van der Pol equation in order to simulate our sensory input. However, depending on the sensor measurement, this equation has to be slightly modified to be able to correctly simulate it. For practical reasons due to our sensors (see section 2), we observe the thigh inclination with regards to vertical. During human gait, this inclination presents a dissymmetrical pattern, with an ascending phase shorter than the descending one. The van der Pol equation provides with symmetrical signals; thus, we have to introduce a new term in the equation:

$$\ddot{x} - \mu(1 - bx - x?)\dot{x} + \omega_0^2 x = 0 \tag{8}$$

Where *-bx* is the new introduced term. The idea is to modify the damping coefficient $\mu(1-bx-x?)$ so as it is different when $x<0$ or $x>0$. In that way, the output of the modified van der Pol oscillator won't be symmetrical anymore: for a given $|x|$ when $x<0$, $|\mu(1-bx-x?)|$ is higher than when $x>0$.

Once the structure of the nonlinear oscillator is chosen, we have to find the best parameters μ, b, and ω_0, so that the trajectory of the limit cycle of this oscillator will fit the sensor measurement. We write this identification problem as a least squares one: minimizing the error between the measurements and the output of the oscillator:

$$\begin{cases} \min\limits_{\mu,b,\omega_O,x_s^i} \sum\limits_{i=1}^{n} \left(x_s^i - x_m^i\right)^2 \\ \ddot{x}_s^i - \mu\left(1 - bx_s^i - x_s^i ?\right)\dot{x}_s^i + \omega_0^2 = 0 \end{cases} \tag{9}$$

where x_m^i are the discretized sensor measurements (for example, over one given cycle), and x_s^i are the simulated oscillator outputs, thus following the dynamics of eq. (8). One can notice that this problem is similar to an optimal control problem, which can be solved using a direct method (Betts, 1997). We include the discrete output of the oscillator in the parameters to optimize, and we add constraints on to follow the dynamical model of the oscillator. The discretization of this problem leads to a "nonlinear programming" problem which has been solved using a successive quadratic programming solver: FSQP (Lawrence et al., 1997). This method gave good results: we obtained a very good matching between measurement and oscillator output (Figure 11).

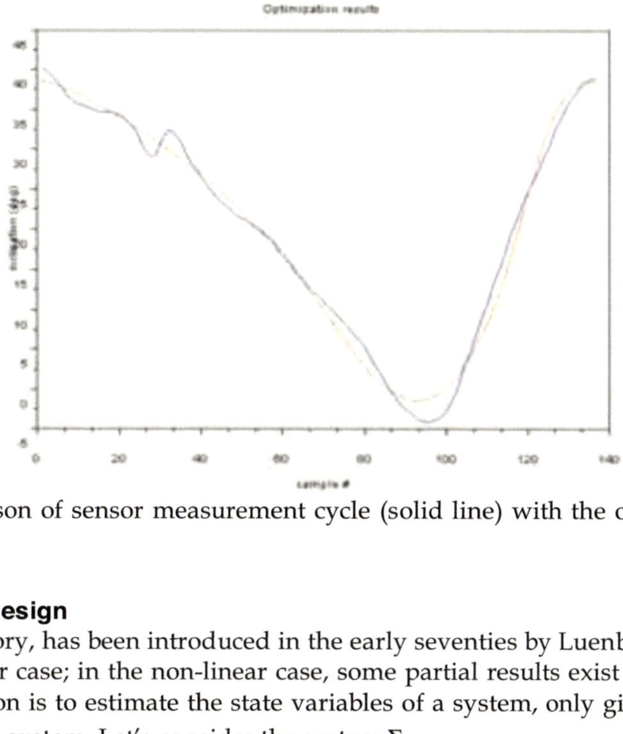

Fig. 11. Comparison of sensor measurement cycle (solid line) with the optimized oscillator output (dotted).

4.2.2 Observer design

The observer theory, has been introduced in the early seventies by Luenberger (Luenberger, 1971) in the linear case; in the non-linear case, some partial results exist (Isidori, 1995). The idea of observation is to estimate the state variables of a system, only given the inputs and the outputs of the system. Let's consider the system Σ:

$$\Sigma: \begin{cases} \dot{x} = f(x) + g(u) \\ y = h(x) \end{cases} \tag{10}$$

and build a copy of Σ with **output injection**:

$$\Sigma': \begin{cases} \dot{\hat{x}} = f(\hat{x}) + g(u) + K(\hat{y} - y) \\ \hat{y} = h(\hat{x}) \end{cases} \tag{11}$$

In the linear case, if the original system Σ is observable (see (Kailath, 1980) for a complete description of the observability conditions), and if gain K is correctly set, then the observer state will converge towards the original system state. When the output error $(\hat{y} - y)$ is cancelled, the observer state exactly matches Σ's state: the observer is synchronized with the observed system.

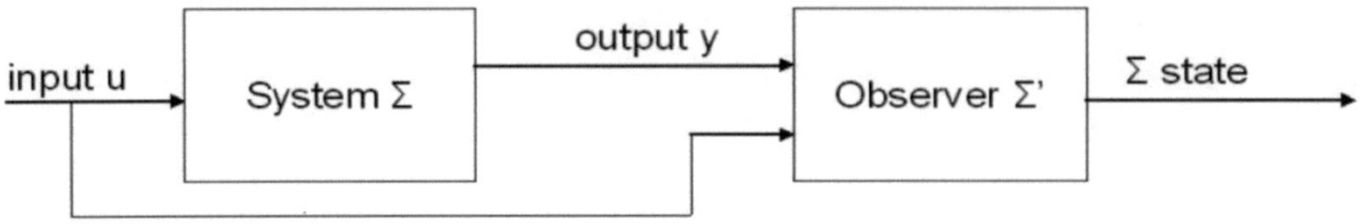

Fig.12. Observer principle.

In the non-linear case, there is no general result concerning the observer existence. However, it is sometimes possible to build a non-linear observer, when the error dynamics is feedback linearizable. To achieve this, the system has to belong to the ***Lur'e*** class (Lur'e and Postnikov, 1944), in which the non-linearity is a function of the output only:

$$\Sigma : \begin{cases} \dot{x} = A.x + f(y,t) + B.u \\ y = C.x \end{cases} \tag{12}$$

The observer is then given by:

$$\Sigma : \begin{cases} \dot{\hat{x}} = A.\hat{x} + f(y,t) + B.u + K(\hat{y} - y) \\ \hat{y} = C.\hat{x} \end{cases} \tag{13}$$

and the error dynamics can be linearized:

$$\begin{aligned} e &= \hat{x} - x \\ \dot{e} &= \dot{\hat{x}} - \dot{x} \\ &= A.\hat{x} + f(y,t) + B.u + K(\hat{y} - y) - A.x - f(x,t) - B.u \\ &= (A + KC)e \end{aligned} \tag{14}$$

We applied the observer theory to our specific case, and built an observer of the dynamical system described by the modified van der Pol equation (8), which can be written as:

$$\Sigma : \begin{cases} \dot{x}_1 = x_2 \\ \dot{x}_2 = \mu(1 - bx - x?)\dot{x} - \omega_0^2 x \\ y = x_1 \end{cases} \tag{15}$$

For practical reasons, mathematical details of the computation of the observer are not shown here, but can be found in (Nijmeijer and Mareels, 1997).

4.2.3 Phase estimation through isochrones

By injecting a measurement input in the computed observer, we get an estimation of the two state variables $\hat{x}_1$ and $\hat{x}_2$. Since this observer is also a (forced) oscillator, we can compute its phase based on its state variables. This can easily be done using isochrones.
We said earlier (in section 4.2) that the limit cycle of an oscillator can be parameterized using a phase variable ϕ. There is a natural way to define the phase variable not only on the limit cycle but in its neighbourhood as well. To this end, we define the so-called **isochrones** in the vicinity of the limit cycle. Observing the dynamical oscillatory system stroboscopically, with the time interval being exactly the period of the limit cycle T_0, we get a mapping:

$$x(t) \rightarrow x(t + T_0) \int \Phi(x) \tag{16}$$

This construction is illustrated by Figure 13. Let us choose a point X^* on the limit cycle and consider all the points in the vicinity that are attracted to X^* under the action of Φ. They form a hypersurface I called isochrone, crossing the limit cycle at X^*. An isochrone can be drawn at each point of the limit cycle, thus we can parameterize the hypersurface according to the phase as $I(\Phi)$. We now extend the definition of the phase to the vicinity of the limit cycle, demanding that the phase is constant on each isochrone. In this way, phase can be defined in the neighbourhood of the limit cycle.

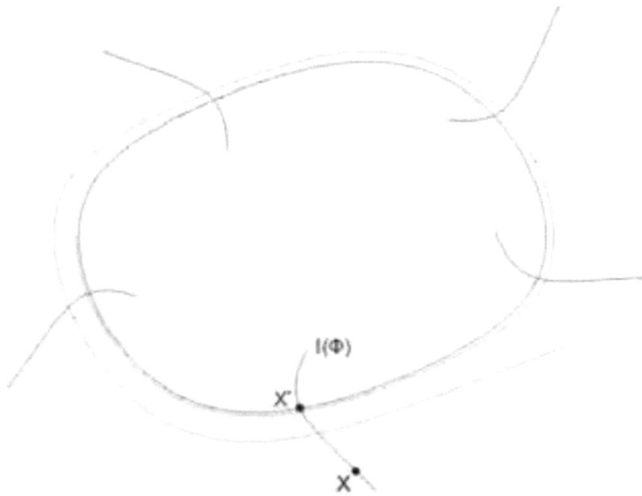

Fig. 13. Isochrones in the vicinity of the limit cycle.

Isochrones can be computed, using the free nonlinear oscillator equation (8), in two different ways. The first approach is to transform the oscillator equation in polar coordinates (R,θ), define the phase ϕ such as it grows uniformly, and compute the lines of constant phase on the (R,θ) plane. However, the resolution of this problem under an analytical form is possible only in a few simple cases. The second idea is to obtain them by simulation: first, let's assess the free oscillator period T_0. Then, for each point x_i on the phase plane which is in the vicinity of the limit cycle, simulate its trajectory under oscillator dynamics during a time $n.T_0$, with n being an integer large enough such that the distance from the point $x_i\,(n.T_0)$ to the limit cycle is small. In that case, the original point x_i has the same phase as $x_i\,(n.T_0)$, which is known, since it is on the limit cycle.

4.3 Summary: command generation

Finally, let's assume that the (cyclical) trajectory we want to generate is parameterized by its phase: we thus have a trajectory pattern $T(\phi)$ for $\phi = [0, 2\pi]$. The online computation scheme for command generation estimation is then the following (see Figure 14):

- inject the sensor measurement y_k in the adapted observer, to compute its state variables $\hat{x}_k$
- from the observer state variables $\hat{x}_k$, compute the phase ϕ of the oscillator through isochrones
- provide with the command desired trajectory $C = T(\phi)$

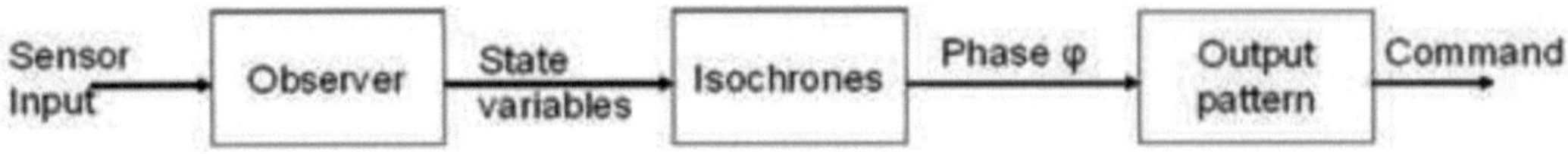

Fig. 14. Computation flow for command generation.

4.4 Results

The synchronization of the observer with the given input signal is **ensured**: thanks to observer theory, it can be assessed that the behaviour of the observer will match the behaviour of the observed system. In (Héliot and Espiau, 2007), we assessed the practical efficiency of the method, considering three important issues. First of all, we checked through a bifurcation analysis that the theoretical behaviour of the modified van der Pol oscillator was still the behaviour of an attractive limit cycle. We also evaluated the robustness of the approach with respect to errors in parameters; the estimation error was found to be linear w.r. to parameters. Finally, we validated the ability of the method to track changes in the input dynamics, thus allowing coping with transient walking stages and rapid rhythm changes; this issue is illustrated in Fig 15.

Robustness and accuracy can be improved using multidimensional sensory inputs, rather than a single sensor measurement. One can for example use thigh and shank inclinations, feet pressure as complementary inputs.

We ran an online experiment to test this method: by installing the sensor on the leg of a human, we observed the thigh angle and computed online a biped robot command, such that the robot "follows" the human gait, in a synchronous way. This was done by first generating with our oscillator-observer method a desired trajectory for each active DOF of the robot (in our case: ankle, knee and hip sagittal angles on both legs), and then following this trajectory with a PID controller. Such experiments were conducted on a biped robot, BIP (Azevedo and the Bip team, 2000). We thus fully validated the online trajectory generation based on sensor measurement. Thus, this method can be a useful design tool for sensory integration in CPG-type architectures.

4.5 Application

Providing bipedal locomotion by means of FES can be formulated as generating control inputs for the stimulator that acting via electrodes will result with adequate muscle contractions leading to functional movements. Muscle activations necessary to execute one reference step can be obtained by direct transposition of electro-myographic recordings or model-based transformation from the desired behaviour. Cloning able-bodied locomotion is not suitable because many neuro-muscular mechanisms are greatly modified due to the injury, and in a FES driven locomotion only one portion of the body is externally controlled. Reference trajectories should be adapted to each individual patient capability and should be adjusted to performance evolution along the training. The patterns we used are obtained with a modelling and simulation tool such as described in (Popovic et al., 1999). Muscles activities are optimized to perform the tracking of a reference walking trajectory with minimal level of activations with a prescribed level of co-contraction according to a model of the patient leg.

All the parameters of the model are identified for each individual subject. In this context our method resulted in perfect adaptation of stimulation patterns to walking rhythm changes within a range classically observed during walking. Observing valid leg in hemiplegic patients could lead to adaptation of the timing of the pre-programmed stimulation patterns in order to achieve a symmetric gait.

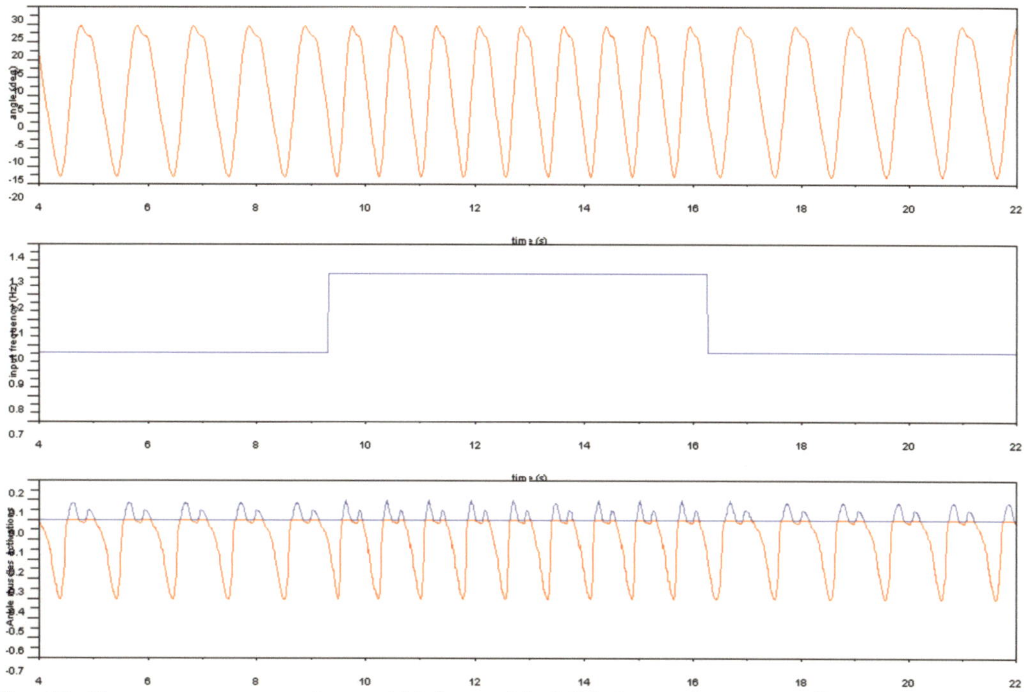

Fig. 15. Top: measurement input (thigh angle); Mid: input frequency; Bottom: computed ankle muscles activations for flexor/extensor muscles (the negative values in the muscle activation show the antagonistic muscle).

4.6 Conclusion

In this section, we presented a methodology for motion monitoring, enabling to provide with adapted commands corresponding to the ongoing action (in our example, FES stimulation amplitudes). This methodology in two steps (building a phenomenological model, and then an observer of this model; see Figure 9), is of course re-usable for monitoring any other action. In this framework, some important issues should be addressed, as transitions between different gait styles (flat ground, stairs, slope, …).

5. Full system design

5.1 An unified safe framework to merge strategic and tactic levels

The approach proposed in this chapter uses two levels of coordination. First, a strategic level, dealing with transitions from an action to another, thus expressing an ***event-driven*** behaviour. Secondly, a tactic level, which monitors the ongoing action and generates an adequate control, thus expressing a ***continuous*** behaviour. The final system has to encompass both aspects, thus falling into the *hybrid systems* class. Since the classical tools from automatic control theory are not directly applicable to hybrid systems, specific analysis tools have been developed in recent years (Brogliato and Heemels, 2003; Lygeros et al., 2003;

Morari et al., 2003). Other works propose a general formulation allowing to describe in a single framework all the systems expressing a continuous behaviour associated with discrete events (Johansson et al., 1999). This formulation is able to address various kinds of applications, from electronics (Brogliato and Heemels, 2003) to biology (De Jong et al., 2004)... However, the complexity of such applications often prevents from performing a formal analysis producing enough knowledge about the possible behaviour of the system, for anticipating its properties. In that case the most useful results come from simulation.
In addition, the application considered here, the rehabilitation, belongs to the class of *critical systems*. Indeed, system safety issues are critical because any dysfunction of the system can lead to dramatic injury. For example, the consequences of an inappropriate electrical stimulation on a paraplegic patient's leg, can possibly lead to bone breaking if he/she has fallen on the ground.

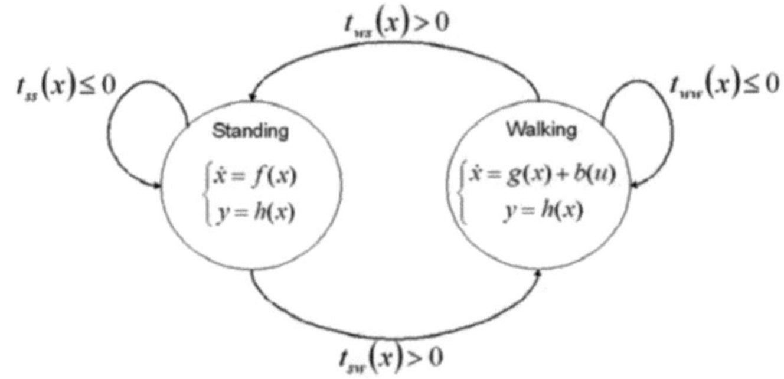

Fig. 16. Example of hybrid system. Two states are represented, with their associated transitions. From one state to another, evolution laws are structurally different, thus requiring a hybrid formulation.

As a consequence, there is a need for a system development approach that can handle both hybrid aspects as well as safety ones. It should be emphasized that safety involves many components: hardware (sensors, stimulator, computer, wiring), software (algorithms, programming, real-time implementation), human-machine interface (in order to prevent from wrong utilization). This requires that particular attention should be paid to the monitoring of possible dysfunctions, in order to anticipate the related actions to undertake. From a robotic point of view, this issue has already received much attention, mainly in the area of autonomous robots (Borrelly et al., 1998; Ingrand et al., 2001). Among the proposed approaches, the ORCCAD (Open Robot Control Computer Assisted Design) framework (Borrelly et al., 1998) presents interesting safety features; although it has been initially designed for classical robotics, it looks well suited for rehabilitation applications,

5.2 An ORCCAD-based Specification Approach

ORCCAD is a programming environment aimed at building complex robotics applications which are characterized by strong real-time issues and by high safety requirements. It is mainly organized around two key entities: a basic task, called *ROBOT-TASK*, which gathers elementary components called *MODULES*, and the *ROBOT-PROCEDURE*, which allows modular construction of complex applications. Thanks to the use of the synchronous language Esterel, ORCCAD offers tools of formal verification, simulation and visualization. It is also implementation-oriented, which means that it automatically produces real-time code to download. On the basis of ORCCAD concepts, we propose the following specification principles, which include two main hierarchical levels, i.e. from the bottom to the top:

An *ACTION*, kind of elementary task, is defined as the complete specification of:

- a control in continuous time, usually sensor-based, which has an invariant structure along the whole duration of the *ACTION*
- a set of events to be received and emitted at the beginning of the *ACTION*, during its execution, and at its end, and the associated processing.

The *ACTION* is made of communicating *COMPONENTS* which may have some genericity in their design: controller, observers, trajectory generators…

An *ACTIVITY* is used to logically and hierarchically compose *ACTIONS* into structures of increasing complexity. It is defined as:

- a main program, describing the logical and temporal arrangements of *ACTIONs* and other *ACTIVITIES*
- a set of triplets (event, processing, assertion) that specifies the processing to apply in order to handle each event and the related information to cast to an *APPLICATION* level.

Thus, the full specification of an application requires the description of both the continuous and discrete aspects, as well as their real-time features. The detailed specification of one of the applications presented earlier is beyond the scope of this chapter. However, as a short illustration of the instantiation of this architecture in the case of the sit-to-stand transition in a paraplegic patient, let us just give a correspondence between the generic entities defined above and their practical meaning The *APPLICATION* is for example the FES-assisted function: "going from a chair to another". It implies three *ACTIVITIES*: TO STAND UP; TO WALK; TO SIT DOWN. The "TO STAND UP" *ACTIVITY* involves itself three *ACTIONS* to be sequenced (figure 17). All details (used components, events, signals…) can be found in (Héliot et al., 2007).

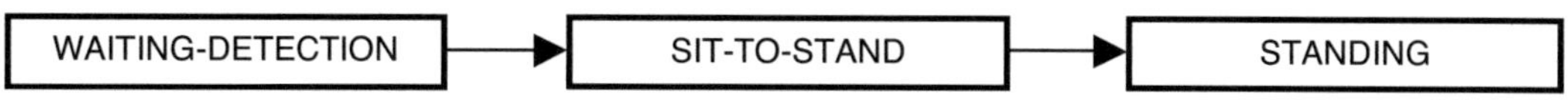

Fig. 17. One activity composed of three sequential actions can model the stand-up movement of a paraplegic patient.

6. Discussion

In the framework of FES-assisted rehabilitation and reeducation, we addressed in this chapter the problem of the interaction between artificial and natural systems co-existing within patient's body. Our approach consisted in placing micro-sensors on subject's healthy limbs (trunk, intact leg...) in order to observe voluntary actions at two stages: detecting patient's intention, and monitoring an ongoing action. We also formalized a unified framework to merge these strategic and tactic levels. We illustrated the approach by implementing solutions for two practical examples: detection of sit-to-stand transfer and gait monitoring, and validated the developed algorithms with online experiments performed on valid subjects.

Since the targeted application of these results is FES for disabled people, the next step is to adapt the developed techniques to patient characteristics. Detection of postural transitions and action monitoring are based on reference patterns which will have to be elicited by patients; thus, a phase of training will be needed in order to determine for each person the optimal valid limb motion according to lesion type and individual postural capabilities.

Another issue to keep in mind is that in hemiplegia and incomplete paraplegia, the paretic extremities are under influences of both artificial and biological controls. The patient can have a partial voluntary action on its deficient limbs with limited sensorial information. Coexistence of natural and artificial control loops is also true within the deficient limb itself. Indeed, even in complete paraplegia, spinal reflex loops often remain in somewhat modified form. Thus, contractures and spasticity can raise problems for FES applications.

The applications of the developed approach are not only restricted to FES. Prosthetic limb control could benefit from the presented algorithms. Not only deficiency affecting lower limbs could find interest, but also any type of disability which could be addressed through neuroprostheses and needing for sensory based control with phase monitoring and transition detection skills: respiratory control, suppression of seizures in epilepsy and tremor attenuation… Elderly activity monitoring and falls detection could also be a possible application.

The idea of using the real-time measurement of a human motion in the control device of another system can be also exploited in non-rehabilitation applications. Recalling that the considered sensors are embedded autonomous microsystems, they can for example be easily spread on a human for motion capture purposes in virtual reality. In robotics, we can imagine to teleoperate, in some sense, legged robots (or exoskeletons) from several sensor outputs, either in a master-slave mode if the addressed structure is anthropomorphic, or in a joystick-like approach in other cases.

7. References

Azevedo, C. and the Bip team. (2000). Control architecture and algorithms of the anthropomorphic biped bip2000. *Proc. Intl. Symposium on Mobile Climbing and Walking Robots (CLAWAR).*

Azevedo, C. and Héliot, R. (2005). Rehabilitation of Functional Posture and Walking: towards a coordination of healthy and Impaired Limbs. *Journal of Automatic Control.* Vol. 15 (Suppl), pp. 11-15.

Azevedo, C., Espiau, B., Amblard, B. and Assaiante, C. (2007) Bipedal Locomotion: Towards Unified Concepts in Robotics and Neuroscience. *Biological Cybernetics* Vol. 96, No. 2, pp. 209-228.

Barbeau, H., Ladouceur, M., Norman, K.E., Pepin, A., and Leroux, A. (1999). Walking after spinal cord injury: evaluation, treatment, and functional recovery. *Arch Phys Med Rehabil.* Vol. 80, No. 2, pp. 225-235.

M. Basseville and I. Nikiforov. (1993). *Detection of Abrupt Changes – Theory and Application.* Prentice-Hall.

Bayley, J.S., Cochran, T.P., Sledge, C.B. (1987) The weightbearing shoulder: The impingement syndrome in paraplegics. *J Bone Joint Surg.* Vol. 69, pp. 676-678.

Betts, J. (1997). Survey of numerical methods for trajectory optimization. *Journal of Guidance, Control, and Dynamics.*

Bonnet, S. and Heliot, R (2007). A magnetometer-based approach for studying human movements. *IEEE Trans. Biomedical Engineering,* to appear.

Borrelly, J.J., Coste-Manière, E., Espiau, B., Kapellos, K., Pissard-Gibollet, R., Simon, D. and Turro, N. (1998). The ORCCAD Architecture. *The International Journal of Robotics Research.* Vol. 17, No. 4, pp. 338-359.

Brogliato, B., and Heemels, W.P.M.H. (2003). The Complementarity Class of Hybrid Dynamical Systems. *European Journal of Control. Special issue on "fundamental issues in control"*, Vol. 9, No. 2-3, pp. 177-189.

Burridge, J., Haugland, M., Larsen, B., Svaneborg, N., Iversen, H., Brogger, P., Pickering, R., and Sinkjaer, T. (2005). Long-term follow-up of patients using the actigait implanted drop-foot stimulator. *10th IFES conference* Montreal, Canada.

Crenna, P. and Frigo, C. (1991). A motor programme for the initiation of forward-oriented movements in humans. *Journal Physiol.* pp. 635–653.

Cohen, A., Rossignol, S., and Grillner, S. (1988) *Neural control of rhythmic movements in vertebrates*. Wiley.

Cybulski, G.R. and Jaegger, R.J. (1986) Standing Performance of Persons with Paraplegia. *Arch. Phys. Med. Rehabil.* Vol. 67, pp. 103-108.

De Jong, H., Gouzé, J.L., Hernandez, C., Page, M., Sari, T. and Geiselmann, J. (2004). Qualitative simulation of genetic regulatory networks using piecewise-linear models. *Bulletin of Mathematical Biology*. Vol. 66, pp. 301-340.

Dong, H., Zhao, M., Zhang, J., and Zhang, N. (2006). Cpg-based adaptive dynamic control of a quadruped robot with sensory feedback. *Proc. 9th International Conference Climbing and Walking Robots*, pp. 77–81.

Endo, G., Morimoto, J., Nakanishi, J. and Cheng, G. (2004). An empirical exploration of a neural oscillator for biped locomotion control. *Proc. Intl. Conf. on Robotics and Automation (ICRA2004).*

Fukuoka, Y., Mimura, T. Yasuda, N. and Kimura, H. (2003). Integration of multi sensors for adaptive walking of a quadruped robot. *Proc.IEEE International Conference on Multisensor Fusion and Integration for Intelligent Systems*. pp. 21 - 26.

Goldstein, B., Young, J., Escobedo, E.M. (1997) Rotator cuff repairs in individuals with paraplegia. *Am J Phys Med & Rehab.* Vol. 76, pp. 316-322.

Goswami, A., Thuilot, B., and Espiau, B. (1998). A study of the passive gait of a compass-like biped robot: Symmetry and chaos. *The International Journal of Robotics Research*. Vol. 17, No. 12, pp. 1282–1301.

Guckenheimer, J. and Holmes, P. (1990) *Nonlinear Oscillations, Dynamical Systems and Bifurcations of Vector Fields*. Springer-Verlag.

Guiraud, D., Stieglitz, T., Koch, K.P., Divoux, J.L. and Rabischong, P. (2006) An implantable neuroprostheses for standing and walking in paraplegia: 5-year patient follow-up. *J. Neural Eng.* Vol. 3, pp. 268-275.

Héliot, R., Azevedo, C., Espiau, B. and David, D. (2005) Postural movement early detection and monitoring by observing one limb with micro-sensors. *3rd International Symposium on Adaptive Motion in Animals and Machines (AMAM),* Ilmenau, Germany, September 2005.

Heliot, R. and Espiau, B. (2007). Online generation of cyclic trajectories synchronized with sensor input. *Research Report No. 6101*. INRIA.

Heliot, R., Simon, D. and Espiau, B. (2007). ORRCAD specification of a FES assisted sit-to-stand transfer in a paraplegic patient. *Research Report*. INRIA.

Ingrand, F., Chatila, R., Alami, R. (2001). An Architecture for Dependable Autonomous Robots. *Proc. 1st IARP/IEEE-RAS Joint Workshop on Technical Challenges for Dependable Robots in Human Environments*. Seoul, Korea.

Isidori, A. (1995). *Nonlinear Control Systems*. Springer.

Johansson, K.H., Egerstedt, E., Lygeros, J. and Sastry, S. (1999). On the regularization of zenon hybrid automata. *Systems and Control Letters*. Vol. 38, pp. 141-150.

Kailath, T. (1980). *Linear Systems*. Prentice-Hall.

Kerr, K., White, J., Barr, D. and Mollan, R. (1997).Analysis of the sit-stand-sit movement cycle in normal subjects. *Clinical Biomechanics*. Vol. 12, No. 4, pp. 236-245.

Kuzelicki, J., Bajd, T., Kamnik, R., Obreza, P., and Benko, H. (2000). FES assisted sit-to-stand transfer in paraplegic person. *Proc. 22nd Annual International Conference of the IEEE Engineering in Medicine and Biology Society*. Vol. 3, pp. 2247 - 2250.

Lawrence, C., Zhou, J., and Tits, A. (1997). User's guide for cfsqp version 2.5 : A c code for solving (large scale) constrained nonlinear (minimax) optimization problems, generating iterates satisfying all inequality constraints. Electrical Engineering Dpt. and Institute for Systems Research, University of Maryland, Tech. Rep.

Luenberger, D. (1971). An introduction to observers. *IEEE trans. Automatic Control*, vol. 16, no. 6, pp. 596–602.

Luinge, H. and Veltink, P. (2004) Inclination measurement of human movement using a 3d accelerometer with autocalibration. *IEEE trans. neural sys. and rehabil. eng.* Vol. 12, pp. 112–121.

Lunenburger, L., Colombo, G., Riener, R. (2007). Biofeedback for robotic gait rehabilitation. *Journal of NeuroEngineering and Rehabilitation.*

Lur'e, A. I. and Postnikov, V. N. (1944). On the theory of stability of control systems. *Applied mathematics and mechanics*, vol. 8.

Lygeros, K.H., Johansson, J., Simic, J. Zhang, S.N. and Sastry, S.S. (2003). Dynamical properties of hybrid automata. *IEEE trans. Automatic Control*, Vol. 48, pp. 2-17.

Matsuoka, K. (1985). Sustained oscillations generated by mutually inhibiting neurons with adaptation. *Biological Cybernetics*. Vol. 52, No. 6, pp. 367–376.

Mauritz, K.H. (2002) Gait training in hemiplegia. *Eur. J. Neurol.* Vol. 1 (Suppl), pp. 23-29.

McGeer, T. (1990). Passive dynamic walking. *The International Journal of Robotics Research*, Vol. 9, No. 2, pp. 62–82.

Meadows, P., Campbell, J., Waters, R., Wederich, C., and Jordan, C. (1992). Multichannel electrical stimulation system for gait assist and exercise in the stroke and sci population. *Proceedings of the Annual International Conference of the IEEE Engineering in medicine and Biology Society*, 1992.

Morari, M., Baotic, M. and Borrelli, F. (2003). Hybrid systems modelling and control. *Eur. J. of Control. Special issue on "fundamental issues in control"*, Vol. 9, No. 2-3.

Nijmeijer, H., and Mareels, I. M. Y. (1997). An observer looks at synchronization. *IEEE Trans. on Circuits and Systems - Part I – Fundamental Theory and Applications*, Vol. 44, no. 10, pp. 882–890, 1997.

Pappas, I.P.I., Keller, T., and Mangold, S. (2002) A reliable, gyroscope based gait phase detection sensor embedded in a shoe insole. *Proceedings of IEEE Sensors 002, First IEEE International Conference on Sensors*. Vol. 2, pp 1085–1088.

Pikovsky, A., Rosenblumn, R. and Kurths, J. (2001). *Synchronization, a universal concept in nonlinear sciences*. Cambridge University press.

Popovic, D.B., Stein, R.B., Oguztreli, M.N., Lebiedowska, M., and Jonic. S. (1999) Optimal control of walking with functional electrical stimulation: A computer simulation study. *IEEE Trans Rehabil Eng.* Vol. 7, pp. 69–79.

Popovic, D.B. and Sinkjær, T. (2003) *Control of the movement for the physically disabled*. Aalborg University, ISBN: 87-90562-10-0, Aalborg, Denmark.

Righetti, L., Buchli, J. and Ijspeert, A. (2006). Dynamic hebbian learning in adaptive frequency oscillators. *Physica D*. Vol. 216, No. 2, pp. 269–28.

Simoni, M. F., and DeWeerth, S. (2007) Sensory feedback in a half-center oscillator model. *IEEE Transactions on Biomedical Engineering*. Vol. 54, pp. 193 – 204.

Williamson, M.M. (1998). Neural control of rhythmic arm movements. *Neural Networks*. Vol. 11, No. 7-8, pp. 1379–1394.

Zhang, D., and Zhu, K. (2007) Modeling biological motor control for human locomotion with functional electrical stimulation. *Biol. Cybern.* Vol. 96, pp 79-97.

11

Passive-type Intelligent Walker Controlled Based on Caster-like Dynamics

Yasuhisa Hirata, Asami Muraki & Kazuhiro Kosuge
Department of Bioengineering and Robotics, Tohoku University
Japan

1. Introduction

With the coming of aging societies, many elderly people have serious problems for their locomotion, because of the decline of the physical strength for walking. If they could not use their legs for walking, their physical strength would be weak gradually and they could not walk finally without assistance of other people or some assist system such as wheel chairs, etc. The walking using legs of themselves is very important for improving the quality of their lives, even if they use several kinds of tools for walking such as cane, walker, etc.

In this paper, we pay attention to the walker which support the human based on the physical interaction between the human and the walker. The simple walkers, which consist of support frame, wheels/casters and hand-brakes, are used commercially in many fields such as home, hospital, outside, and so on. On the other hand, to develop the intelligent walkers, many researchers have been proposed several kinds of walkers. Manuel et al. have proposed non-holonomic navigation system of a walking-aid robot referred to as "Care-O-bot II" [1]. Savaniti et al. have developed the motorized "Rollator" [2]. Dubowsky et al. have proposed "PAMM" system to provide a mobility assistance and monitoring for the health status of the user [3]. Fujie et al. have developed the power assisted walker for physical support during walking [4]. We have developed the motion control algorithm of intelligent walker with omni-directional mobile base in which the system is moved based on the intentional force/moment applied by user [5]. Kotani et al. have also proposed "HITOMI" system for permitting outdoor navigation of blind people [6].

The most of the conventional intelligent walkers utilize the servo motors and control them by using the information of sensors such as force/torque sensor, ultra sonic sensor, laser range finder, and so on, to realize the several kinds of functions. Although the active-type walkers using servo motors could realize many functions such as collision avoidance, path following, variable motion characteristics, and so on for supporting the user, the safety issues of this active-type system should also be considered. If we can not control the servo motors of the active-type walker appropriately, the system would move unintentionally and be a dangerous system for human being. In addition, the active-type system might be heavy and its structure might be complicated, because it consists of servo motors, reduction gears, sensors, controller, batteries, and so on. The battery problem is also very severe for its long time working, because the servo motors need much electricity to work. Therefore, the active-type systems still have many problems for their practical use.

To overcome these problems, we have introduced a concept of the passive robotics, in which the systems are developed without using the actuators for mobility. Most of the conventional passive-type walkers based on the passive robotics controlled its heading direction by using the servo motors attached to a steering wheel which can not generate the driving force of walkers [7], [8]. In these systems, the navigation function using sensors such as ultra sonic sensor, laser range finder, etc. could be realized by controlling the steering wheel. Since these kinds of system cannot move by themselves, and can only move when the user applies the force/moment to it, it is intrinsically safe system to support the user in walking similar to the simple walkers which consist of support frame and wheels/casters.

We have also proposed a passive type walker referred to as RT Walker in [9]. Different from the conventional passive-type walkers, RT Walker dose not have servo motors for steering wheel. In stead of it, the servo brakes are attached to the wheels of RT Walker as shown in Figure 1, which can change the brake torques of rear wheels proportionally with respect to the input current. By changing the brake torques of wheels appropriately, the motion of RT Walker could be controlled based on a condition of user and/or environmental information. The brake system is very important and essential functions for most of walkers to adjust their speed from the safety point of view. The controlling of the brakes is effective for developing the intelligent walkers without attaching the active device like servo motors.

Different from the conventional passive-type walkers, RT Walker could realize not only the navigation functions but also its variable motion characteristics by controlling the servo brakes of wheels without using the servo motors [9]. In this paper, we especially propose a motion control algorithm of RT Walker based on the caster-like dynamics, so that the maneuverability of the RT Walker could be improved. In the following part of this paper, first, we introduce the concept of passive robotics and the passive-type intelligent walker referred to as RT Walker developed based on the passive robotics concept. Next, we explain the fundamental motion control algorithm of RT Walker briefly and extend it to the motion control algorithm based on the caster-like dynamics for improving its maneuverability. Finally, we implement its motion control algorithm in RT Walker and illustrate its validity through the experiments.

2. Passive Robotics

For utilizing the intelligent systems practically in the real world environment, we have to consider two points mainly. One is the high performance of them and the other is the safety for users. Most of the conventional intelligent systems have servo motors and they are controlled based on the sensory information such as the force/torque sensor, ultrasonic sensor, laser range finder, etc. Therefore, the high performances for intelligent systems are realized based on the many functions such as power assist, collision avoidance, navigation, variable motion characteristics, and so on.

However, if we can not control the servo motors of the intelligent systems appropriately, they would move unintentionally and be a dangerous system for human being. Especially, in Japan, the legislation has to be formulated for using them in a living environment practically. On the other hand, Goswami et al. have proposed a concept of the passive robotics [10], in which the system moves passively based on the external force/moment without using the actuators, and have dealt with the passive wrist, whose components are springs, hydraulic cylinders, dampers, and so on. The passive wrist computes a particular motion in response to every applied force and changes the physical parameters of the components for realizing the desired motion.

A robot for direct physical interaction with a human operator within a shared workspace, referred to as COBOT, has been invented as an industrial application of the passive robotics especially for automobile industries [11]. A passive robot is intrinsically safe and its concept has been extended to many fields. PADyC, Passive Arm with Dynamic Constraints, has been proposed as an assistant tool for surgeons [12]. Other applications for surgical robots are seen in [13]. Applications to rehabilitation have been also considered by many researchers. One example is shown in [14]. Applications of the concept to haptic display have been proposed in [15], [16] etc.

In the fields of research on walker system, Wasson et al. [7] and Mac Namara et al. [8] have proposed passive-type intelligent walkers. In the most of them, the servo motor was attached to the steering wheel similar to Cobot system in order to control only the steering angle based on the information of an environment for navigating the user. RT Walker proposed in this paper also has a passive dynamics with respect to the force/moment applied to it. Different from the other passive-type walkers, RT Walker controls the servo brakes appropriately to realize the several functions without using any servo motors.

Many systems have been developed based on the concept of the passive robotics. These passive-type systems are intrinsically safe, since they do not move unintentionally. The passive robotics is a key concept when we consider real-world applications of the advanced robot technology.

3. RT Walker

The passive-type intelligent walker referred to as RT Walker developed based on the passive robotics concept is shown in Figure 1 (a). This prototype consists of a support frame, two passive casters, two wheels with powder brakes, laser range finders, tilt angle sensors, and controller. The part of the rear wheel with powder brake is shown in Figure 1 (b). The powder brakes can change the brake torques of rear wheels of RT Walker proportionally with respect to the input current as shown in Figure 1 (c) and they are transferred to the axes of wheels directly. RT Walker needs little electricity to work by using the servo brakes and is light weight, since its structure is relatively simple compared to the active-type walkers which utilize servo motors for controlling their motions.

By changing the brake torques of two rear wheels appropriately, the motion of RT Walker is controlled based on conditions of users. In addition, RT Walker could get environment information by using the laser range finder and the tilt angle sensors. Based on the information of the environment, RT Walker could realize a collision avoidance function, gravity compensation function, and so on.

In addition to the laser range finder for detecting the environment information, RT Walker has the other laser range finders for measuring the motion of the user, which is attached to the rear part of RT Walker. Based on the motion of the user, we could estimate the user state and change the several functions realized for the intelligent walkers [17].

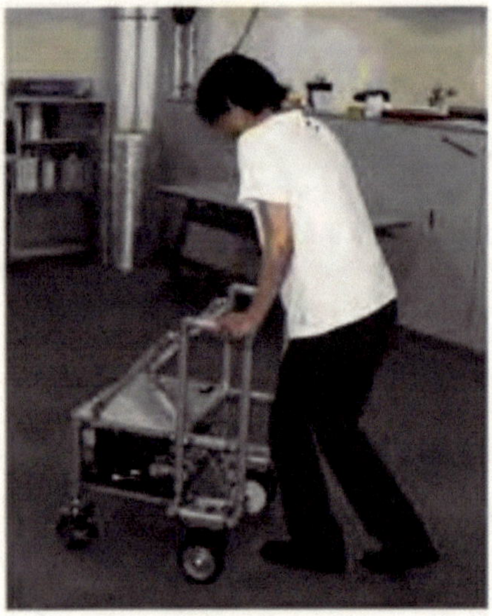

(a) RT Walker

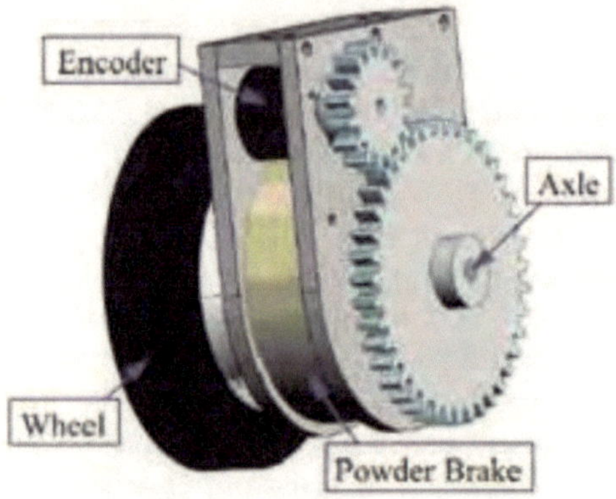

(b) Wheel with Servo Brake

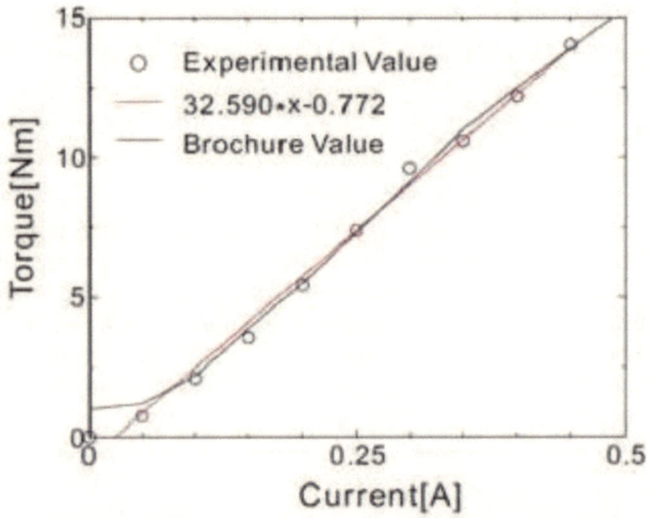

(c) Brake Torque Control based on Input Current

Fig. 1. Prototype of RT Walker.

4. Fundamental Motion Control Algorithm for RT Walker

First, we explain relationships among the brake torque, angular velocity, and applied torque of the wheel with servo brake for realizing the motion control of RT Walker. RT Walker can only move based on the external force/moment applied to it, because it does not have any actuators such as servo motors. To control the motion of RT Walker based on the external

force f_{ew} applied to the wheel with servo brake, we can derive the following relationships with respect to the angular velocity of the wheel with servo brakes ω_w.
for $\omega_w \neq 0$

$$t_{bw} = -k_b I_b \operatorname{sgn}(\omega_w) \tag{1}$$

for $\omega_w = 0$

$$t_{bw} = \begin{cases} -f_{ew} R_w & |f_{ew}| R_w \leq k_b I_b \\ -k_b I_b \operatorname{sgn}(f_{ew}) & |f_{ew}| R_w > k_b I_b \end{cases} \tag{2}$$

where t_{bw} is the brake torque generated by the servo brake of RT Walker, R_w is the radius of the wheel, I_b is the input current for the servo brakes, and k_b is the positive coefficient expressed the relationship between the brake torque and the input current. Different from the control of the servo motor, we can only control the motion of RT Walker under these relationships.
Next, we describe the fundamental motion control algorithm of RT Walker. Under the assumption that m_x and j_θ are the inertia coefficients, d_x and d_θ are the damping coefficients, and the velocity and the acceleration are defined as $\dot{x}$, $\dot{\theta}$ and $\ddot{x}$, $\ddot{\theta}$ respectively, the dynamics of RT Walker based on the force/moment f_h, n_h applied by the user and the brake force/moment f_h, n_h generated by the servo brakes is expressed as follows;

$$\begin{bmatrix} m_x & 0 \\ 0 & j_\theta \end{bmatrix} \begin{bmatrix} \ddot{x} \\ \ddot{\theta} \end{bmatrix} + \begin{bmatrix} d_x & 0 \\ 0 & d_\theta \end{bmatrix} \begin{bmatrix} \dot{x} \\ \dot{\theta} \end{bmatrix} = \begin{bmatrix} f_h \\ n_h \end{bmatrix} - \begin{bmatrix} f_b \\ n_b \end{bmatrix} \tag{3}$$

where x-axis is defined as the heading direction of RT Walker as shwon in Figure 2, and the moment and the rotational motion expressed in eq.(3) are defined around the middle point of the real wheel axis.
In this research, the brake force/moment f_h, n_h generated by the powder brakes is controlled for realizing an arbitrary motion of RT Walker, and we can derive the brake torques t_{br}, t_{bl} of each wheel of RT Walker as follows;

$$\begin{bmatrix} t_{br} \\ t_{bl} \end{bmatrix} = \begin{bmatrix} R_w/2 & R_w/T \\ R_w/2 & -R_w/T \end{bmatrix} \begin{bmatrix} f_b \\ n_b \end{bmatrix} \tag{4}$$

where T express the distance between each wheel with powder brake.
For realizing the variable motion characteristics of RT Walker, we derive the following equation with respect to the brake force/moment;

$$\begin{bmatrix} f_b \\ n_b \end{bmatrix} = \begin{bmatrix} m_{dx} - m_x & 0 \\ 0 & j_{d\theta} - j_\theta \end{bmatrix} \begin{bmatrix} \ddot{x} \\ \ddot{\theta} \end{bmatrix} + \begin{bmatrix} d_{dx} - d_x & 0 \\ 0 & d_{d\theta} - d_\theta \end{bmatrix} \begin{bmatrix} \dot{x} \\ \dot{\theta} \end{bmatrix} \tag{5}$$

where m_{dx}, $j_{d\theta}$ are the apparent inertia of RT Walker and d_{dx}, $d_{d\theta}$ are the apparent damping. When we derive the brake force/moment from eq.(5), and specified the brake torques of the servo brakes of RT Walker as shown in eq.(4), RT Walker could move as if it has the following apparent dynamics expressed by m_{dx}, $j_{d\theta}$, d_{dx} and $d_{d\theta}$.

$$\begin{bmatrix} m_{dx} & 0 \\ 0 & j_{d\theta} \end{bmatrix} \begin{bmatrix} \ddot{x} \\ \ddot{\theta} \end{bmatrix} + \begin{bmatrix} d_{dx} & 0 \\ 0 & d_{d\theta} \end{bmatrix} \begin{bmatrix} \dot{x} \\ \dot{\theta} \end{bmatrix} = \begin{bmatrix} f_h \\ n_h \end{bmatrix} \tag{6}$$

When we change the apparent dynamics of RT Walker using the brake system, we could realize many kinds of motion characteristics of RT Walker.

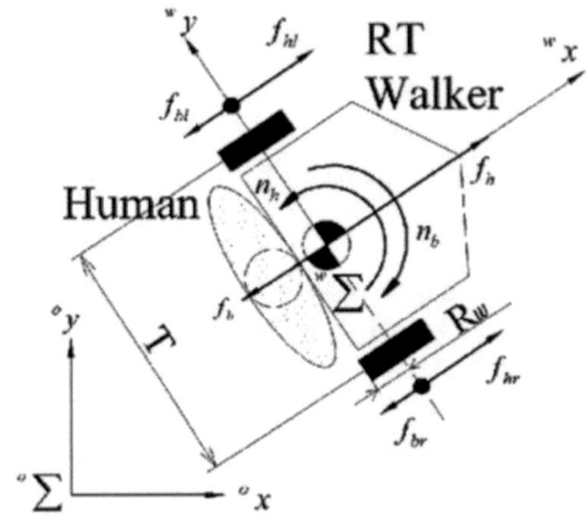

Fig. 2. Model of RT Walker.

5. Caster-like Motion

5.1 Human/Environment-adaptive Motion Control

In the conventional control algorithm of RT Walker proposed in [9], we realize the human-adaptive and the environment-adaptive motion control algorithms. In the human-adaptive motion control algorithm, the apparent dynamics of RT Walker could be specified to it by controlling the servo brakes appropriately, so that we could change its maneuverability, which is explained briefly in the previous section.

However, we have not considered that how RT Walker change its apparent dynamics based on the condition of users, though we have proposed the method for changing the parameters of RT Walker. In this paper, we introduce an example of a method that how we change the apparent dynamics of RT Walker based on its condition, which could be realized by using the caster-like dynamics.

In the environment-adaptive motion control algorithm proposed in [9], we realize the collision avoidance motion of RT Walker using the laser range finder. In this algorithm, to derive the brake torques of servo brakes for avoiding the obstacles, we utilize the method based on an artificial potential field proposed in [18], which is generally utilized by the research of the mobile robot system.

For intelligent walkers, this method is very effective to realize the collision avoidance motion. However, when we consider that intelligent walker utilize in the real world environment including doors, elevators, shelves, walls, and so on, we could not utilize it easily, unless we recognize the object in the real world environment. For example, if RT Walker could not recognize a door, an elevator, a shelf and so on, we could not close to them by using RT Walker implemented in the general collision avoidance methods, because these kinds of object are regarded as obstacles.

To overcome these problems, in this paper, we propose a motion control algorithm based on the caster-like dynamics. By considering the caster-like motion and extending its motion to the advanced motion characteristics of the caster, we could improve the maneuverability of RT Walker in the human-adaptive and the environment-adaptive motion control algorithms.

5.2 Caster-like Dynamics

The concept of the motion control of the robot based on the caster-like dynamics have been proposed in [19] for realizing the coordinative transportation of an object by using multiple mobile robots. In the algorithm proposed in [19], each mobile robot is controlled as if it has a caster-like dynamics as shown in Figure 3, and transports a single object together with other robots based on a intentional force/moment applied by a human. When the human applies the force/moment to the object, the wheel of each virtual caster rotates around the free rotational joint to the direction of the force applied by the human, so that the human could handle a single object together with multiple mobile robots. The caster-like dynamics is also robust against the inevitable positioning error of each robot, even if each robot has a slippage between the wheels of each mobile robot and the ground.

Intelligent walker realizes the physical interaction between the user and walker based on the force/moment applied by the user similar to the case of cooperative transportation of an object by a human and robots. In addition, the robustness with respect to the slippage between wheels of walker and the ground is required. In this paper, we extend the caster-like dynamics proposed in [19] and propose the control algorithm of RT Walker based on its caster-like dynamics for supporting the people who have walking difficulties.

In this section, we consider how the apparent dynamics of RT Walker are changed based on the condition of users or information of an environment. To realize the walker with good maneuverability, we propose Adaptive Caster Action in this paper, which is a control algorithm based on the caster-like dynamics. To realize the caster-like dynamics for RT Walker, first, we consider a motion of a real caster as shown in Figure 3.

The real caster consists of a wheel, a free rotational joint and a wheel support, which connects the wheel and the free rotational joint as shown in Figure 3. The motion of the caster is characterized by three kinds of motion. One is the translational motion of the wheel along the heading direction of its wheel, second one is the rotational motion of the wheel around a point where the wheel contacts with a ground, and third one is the rotational motion of the free rotational joint around its own.

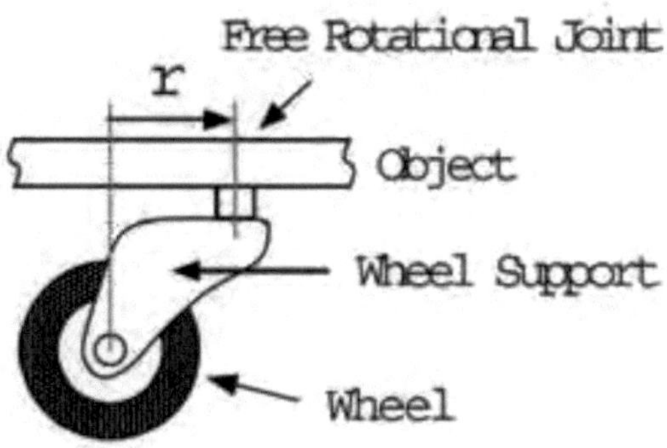

Fig. 3. Real Caster.

In this paper, we control the middle point of the axis of the rear wheels of RT Walker so as to have virtual caster wheel, and the virtual free joint is designed in the forward of RT

Walker along its heading direction as shown in Figure 4. To discuss the motion of the virtual caster, we define two coordinate systems as shown in Figure 4; a wheel coordinate system ${}^{w}\Sigma$ and a free rotational joint coordinate system ${}^{f}\Sigma$. ${}^{w}\Sigma$ is fixed on the virtual caster wheel, and ${}^{f}\Sigma$ is fixed on the virtual free rotational joint. The direction of x-axes of the wheel coordinate system and the free rotational joint coordinate system are defined as the heading direction of the virtual caster wheel as shown in Figure 4. The x-axis of the free rotational joint coordinate system is also defined as the heading direction of RT Walker.

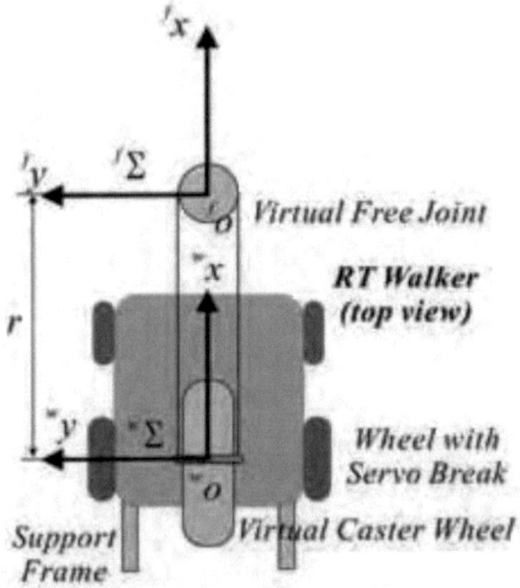

Fig. 4. Coordinate System of RT Walker.

To realize the caster-like dynamics based on two coordinate systems, first, we consider the translational motion of the virtual caster wheel around the free rotational joint based on the force applied to RT Walker along its heading direction as follows;

$$ {}^{f}f_{hx} = {}^{f}m_{x}\,{}^{f}\ddot{x} + {}^{f}d_{x}\,{}^{f}\dot{x} \tag{7} $$

where ${}^{f}m_{x}, {}^{f}d_{x}$ are positive inertia and damping coefficients and ${}^{f}\ddot{x}, {}^{f}\dot{x}$ are acceleration and velocity of virtual caster wheel with respect to the free rotational joint coordinate system. ${}^{f}f_{hx}$ is a force applied to x-axis of the free rotational joint coordinate system by the human.

Next, to mimic the rotational motion of the caster wheel around a point where the caster wheel contacts with a ground based on the force applied to the virtual free rotational joint perpendicular to the heading direction of RT Walker, we obtain the dynamics of the free rotational joint using the following equation;

$$ {}^{f}f_{hy} = {}^{f}m_{y}\,{}^{f}\ddot{y} + {}^{f}d_{y}\,{}^{f}\dot{y} \tag{8} $$

where ${}^{f}m_{y}, {}^{f}d_{y}$ are positive inertia and damping coefficients and ${}^{f}\ddot{y}, {}^{f}\dot{y}$ are acceleration and velocity of virtual free rotational joint. ${}^{f}f_{hy}$ is a force applied to y-axis of the free rotational joint coordinate system.

Actually, RT Walker is controlled around the middle of the axis of rear wheels of it, around which the virtual caster wheel is designed, based on the force/moment applied by the user. Therefore, we should derive the dynamics of the virtual caster with respect to the wheel coordinate system. When ${}^{w}f_x$, ${}^{w}n_\theta$, ${}^{w}\ddot{x}$, ${}^{w}\ddot{\theta}$, ${}^{w}\dot{x}$ and ${}^{w}\dot{\theta}$ are force/moment, accelerations, and velocities of the wheel coordinate system, the relations between the force, accelerations and velocities with respect to the free rotational joint coordinate system and the force/moment, accelerations and the velocities with respect to the wheel coordinate system are expressed as follows;

$$ {}^{w}f_h = {}^{f}f_{hx}, \quad {}^{w}n_h = {}^{f}f_{hy} r \tag{9}$$

$$ {}^{w}\ddot{x} = {}^{f}\ddot{x}, \quad {}^{w}\ddot{\theta} = \frac{{}^{f}\ddot{y}}{r} \tag{10}$$

$$ {}^{w}\dot{x} = {}^{f}\dot{x}, \quad {}^{w}\dot{\theta} = \frac{{}^{f}\dot{y}}{r} \tag{11}$$

where r is a offset of the virtual caster which is the distance between the virtual caste wheel and the free rotational joint as shown in Figure 4.

From eq.(9)-(11), the caster-like dynamics expressed in eq.(7) and (8) are modified as follows;

$$ \begin{bmatrix} {}^{w}m_x & 0 \\ 0 & {}^{w}j_\theta \end{bmatrix} \begin{bmatrix} {}^{w}\ddot{x} \\ {}^{w}\ddot{\theta} \end{bmatrix} + \begin{bmatrix} {}^{w}d_x & 0 \\ 0 & {}^{w}d_\theta \end{bmatrix} \begin{bmatrix} {}^{w}\dot{x} \\ {}^{w}\dot{\theta} \end{bmatrix} = \begin{bmatrix} {}^{w}f_h \\ {}^{w}n_h \end{bmatrix} \tag{12}$$

where

$$ {}^{w}m_x = {}^{f}m_x, \quad {}^{w}d_x = {}^{f}d_x \tag{13}$$

$$ {}^{w}j_\theta = r^2\, {}^{f}m_y, \quad {}^{w}d_\theta = r^2\, {}^{f}d_y \tag{14}$$

This equation is similar to eq.(6), so that we could realize the caster-like dynamics by controlling the brake torques of wheels using the method explained in the previous section. It should be noted that we do not consider the rotational motion of the free rotational joint of the real caster around its own for implementing the virtual caster, because it dose not effect to the motion of RT Walker actually.

5.3 Adaptive Caster Action

In this section, we consider the maneuverability of RT Walker and propose a control algorithm referred to as Adaptive Caster Action for utilizing it effectively. The apparent dynamics of RT Walker is determined by control parameters such as inertia and damping properties, or offset of virtual caster. Especially, the apparent dynamics is strongly affected by the caster offset r. Adaptive Caster Action adjusts the caster offset based on the condition of users or information of environments

5.3.1 Human-adaptive Control

When the offset is large, the angular acceleration and the velocity of the wheel coordinate system are small as shown in eq.(14) and Figure 5 (a). The larger offset will stabilize the straight line motion of RT Walker against disturbance force perpendicular to the motion direction, but it will make the motion direction change difficult. On the contrary, when the offset is small as shown in Figure 5 (b), the wheel coordinate system rotates to the direction of the intentional force easily, so that RT Walker could rotate to the intentional direction of user.

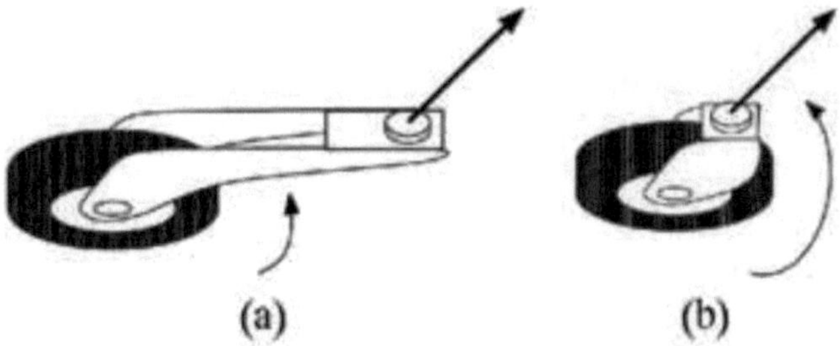

Fig. 5. Adaptive Caster Action.

Let us consider an example of Adaptive Caster Action based on the velocity of RT Walker along its heading direction. When a user moves in narrow space by using RT Walker, its velocity would be low and its easy rotation would be effective. In this case, the smaller caster offset is selected. On the other hand, when the user walks a long distance by using RT Walker, its velocity would be high and the straight line motion of RT Walker would be useful during the walking. In this case, the large caster offset is selected, so that the straight line motion is stabilized and the user could use RT Walker stably, even if the user applies the disturbance force to RT Walker by stumbling. To select the caster offset automatically based on these situations, we change the caster offset according to the velocity of the heading direction of RT Walker, which is expressed by the following equation as an example.

$$r = 0.6\sin({}^{W}\dot{x}) + 0.2 \quad ({}^{W}\dot{x} \geq 0) \tag{15}$$

$$r = -0.2 \quad ({}^{W}\dot{x} < 0) \tag{16}$$

5.3.2 Environment-adaptive Control

To apply the adaptive caster action to the environment-adaptive motion control, we modify eq.(7), (8) as follows;

$$^{f}f_{hx} - {}^{f}f_{vx} = {}^{f}m_{x}\,{}^{f}\ddot{x} + {}^{f}d_{x}\,{}^{f}\dot{x} \tag{17}$$

$$^{f}f_{hy} - {}^{f}f_{vy} = {}^{f}m_{y}\,{}^{f}\ddot{y} + {}^{f}d_{y}\,{}^{f}\dot{y} \tag{18}$$

where ${}^{f}f_{vx}$, ${}^{f}f_{vy}$ are the virtual forces generated based on the information of an environment. By deriving the virtual forces based on the distance between obstacles/steps and the system appropriately and generate the brakes torques by using its virtual force/moment, a user could avoid the collision with obstacles or prevent missing his/her steps in a difference in level [9]. We utilize the method referred to as artificial potential field proposed by Khatib in [18], which is utilized generally in the research on the collision avoidance of the mobile robot.

For measuring the distance between the system and the obstacles or between the system and steps to derive the artificial potential field in the environment, in this research, we utilize the laser range finder which is attached to RT Walker with an angle with respect to the horizontal plan as shown in Figure 6. By attaching the laser range finder with the angle with respect to the horizontal plan, RT Walker could detect the positions of both the obstacles and the steps based on the measured distance.

If the distance is constant d_H, which is derived in advance based on the attached angle and height of the laser range finder from the ground level, this constant measurement means that RT Walker is on the flat ground without obstacles and the steps. When the measured distance is smaller than the constant distance d_H, RT Walker detect the obstacles. In this case, the virtual force/moment is derived based on the measured length d_O, so that the obstacle avoidance motion of RT Walker could be realized. If the measured distance is larger than d_H, RT Walker could detect the steps. In this case, RT Walker generates the map information based on the boundary position of the difference in level, because the length d_S does not change after the detecting the edge of the steps different from the detection of the obstacles. By deriving the virtual force/moment based on the map, the user using RT Walker could avoid the missing his/her steps.

As shown in eq.(17), (18), the virtual force is applied to the free rotational joint of the virtual caster. When we utilize the Adaptive Caster Action, the position of the free joint is changed based on the velocity of RT Walker as shown in Figure 7. When the velocity of RT Walker is high, the larger offset is selected. In this case, RT Walker is influenced by the virtual forces and the avoiding motions with respect to the collision with obstacles and the falling down from the steps could be realized.

On the other hand, when the velocity of RT Walker is low, the smaller offset is selected. In this case, RT Walker would not be influenced by the virtual forces compared with the larger caster offset, so that RT Walker could close to a door, a elevator, a shelf and so on. Even if RT Walker collides with the obstacles with low speed, the dangerousness would also be reduced. It should be noted that the falling down from the step is dangerous situations compared with the collision with obstacles. If RT Walker detects the steps, the control parameters of Adaptive Caster Action should be changed to prevent the falling accident.

6. Experiments

In this research, we implemented Adaptive Caster Action in RT Walker and did several experiments to illustrate the validity of the proposed control algorithm. In this experiment, we move RT Walker to the wall by pushing based on the different kinds of force as shown in Figure 8, so that RT walker closes to the wall in the different kinds of velocity. Motion paths of RT Walker with high speed and low speed are shown in Figure 9 (a), and velocity, caster offset, brake force/moment based on the Adaptive Caster Action during experiments are shown in Figure 9 (b), (c), (d) and (e) respectively.

From these experiments, you can see that RT Walker generates the collision avoiding motion based on the larger caster offset, when its velocity is high. On the other hand, RT Walker can close to the wall, when its velocity is low based on the smaller caster offset. By using Adaptive Caster Action, we could change the apparent dynamics of RT Walker based on its velocity, so that we could use it with good maneuverability in the real world environment.

7. Conclusion

In this paper, we introduce the concept of the passive robotics and the passive-type intelligent walker referred to as RT Walker developed based on the passive robotics concept. For improving the maneuverability of the walker in an environment such as a home, an office, a hospital, etc., we proposed a motion control algorithm referred to as Adaptive Caster Action. The proposed control algorithm is experimentally applied to the developed RT Walker, and the validity of the proposed control algorithm was illustrated by the experimental results.

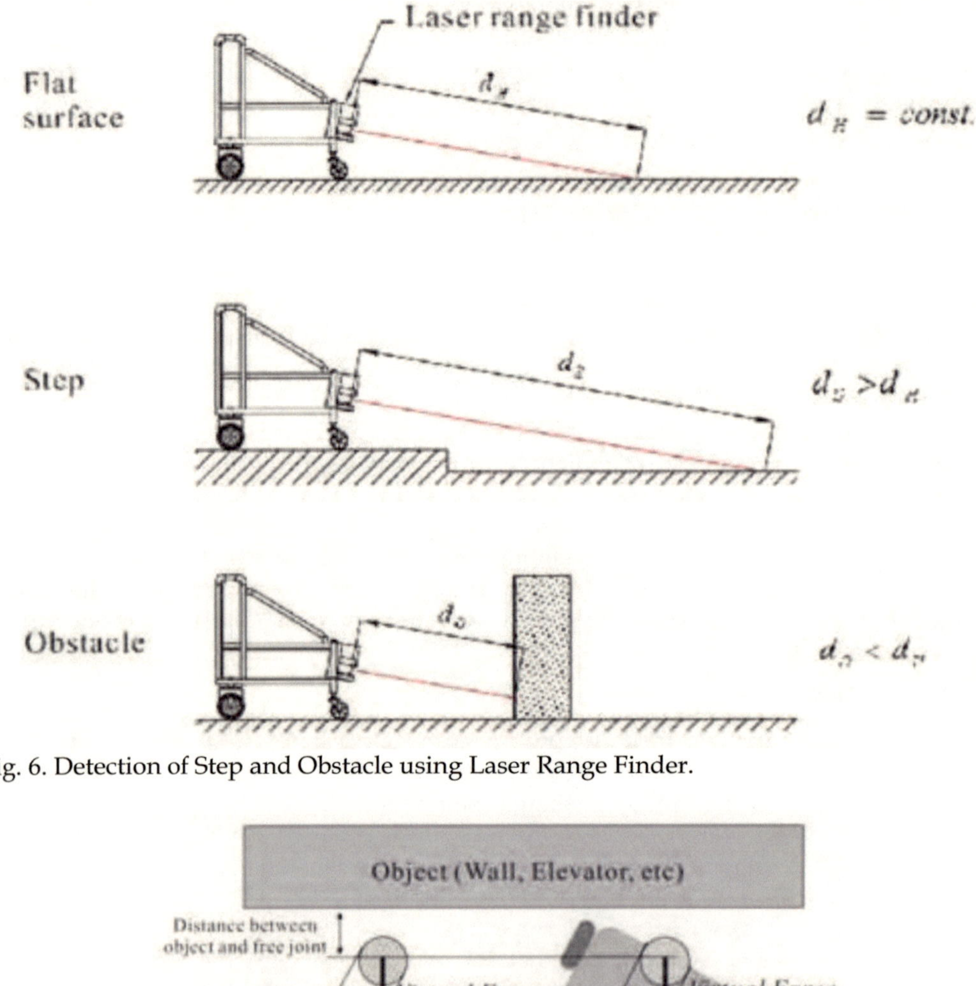

Fig. 6. Detection of Step and Obstacle using Laser Range Finder.

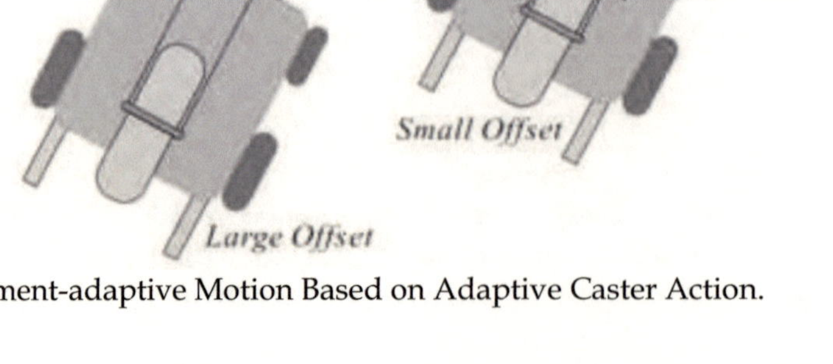

Fig. 7. Environment-adaptive Motion Based on Adaptive Caster Action.

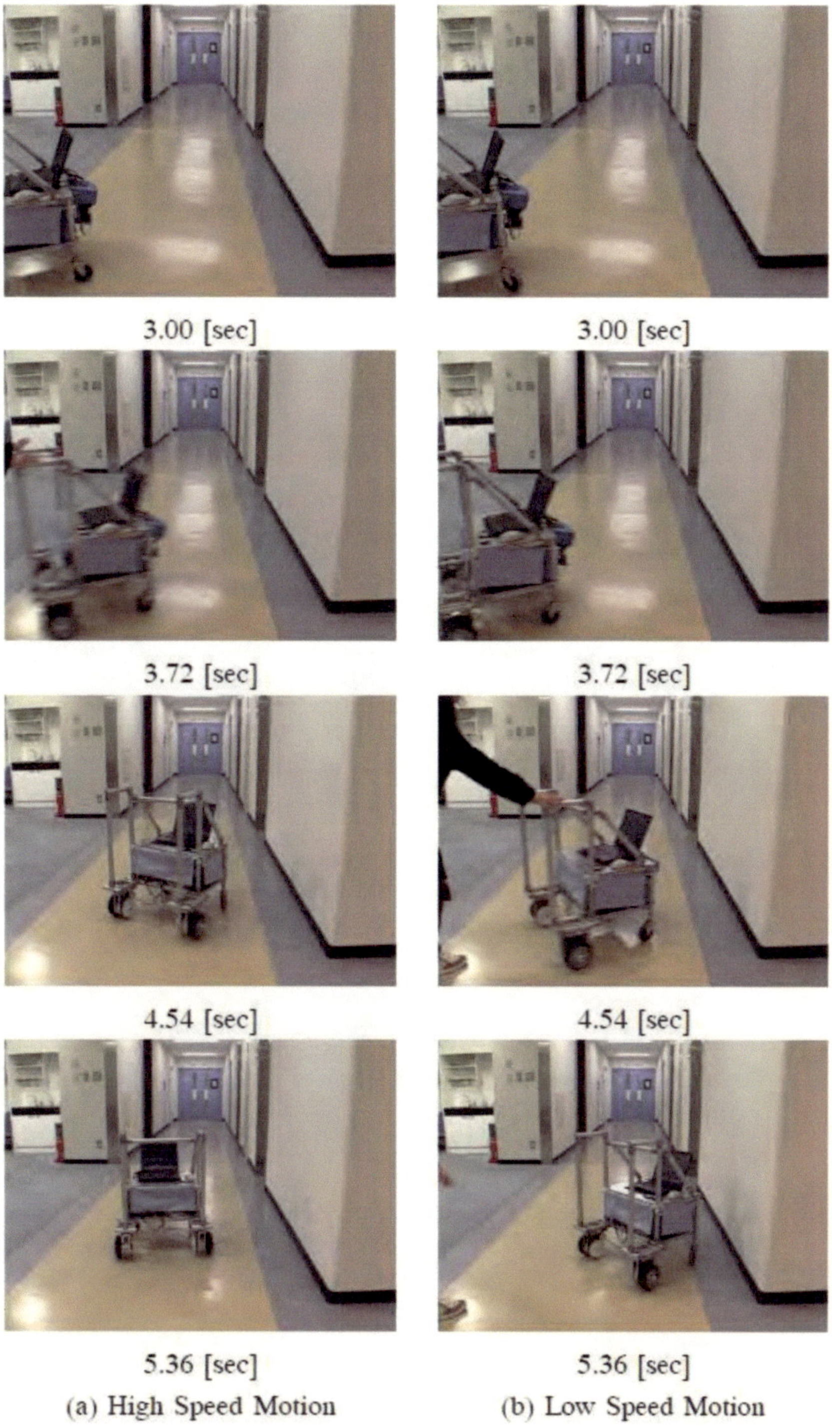

Fig. 8. Motion of RT Walker Based on Adaptive Caster Action.

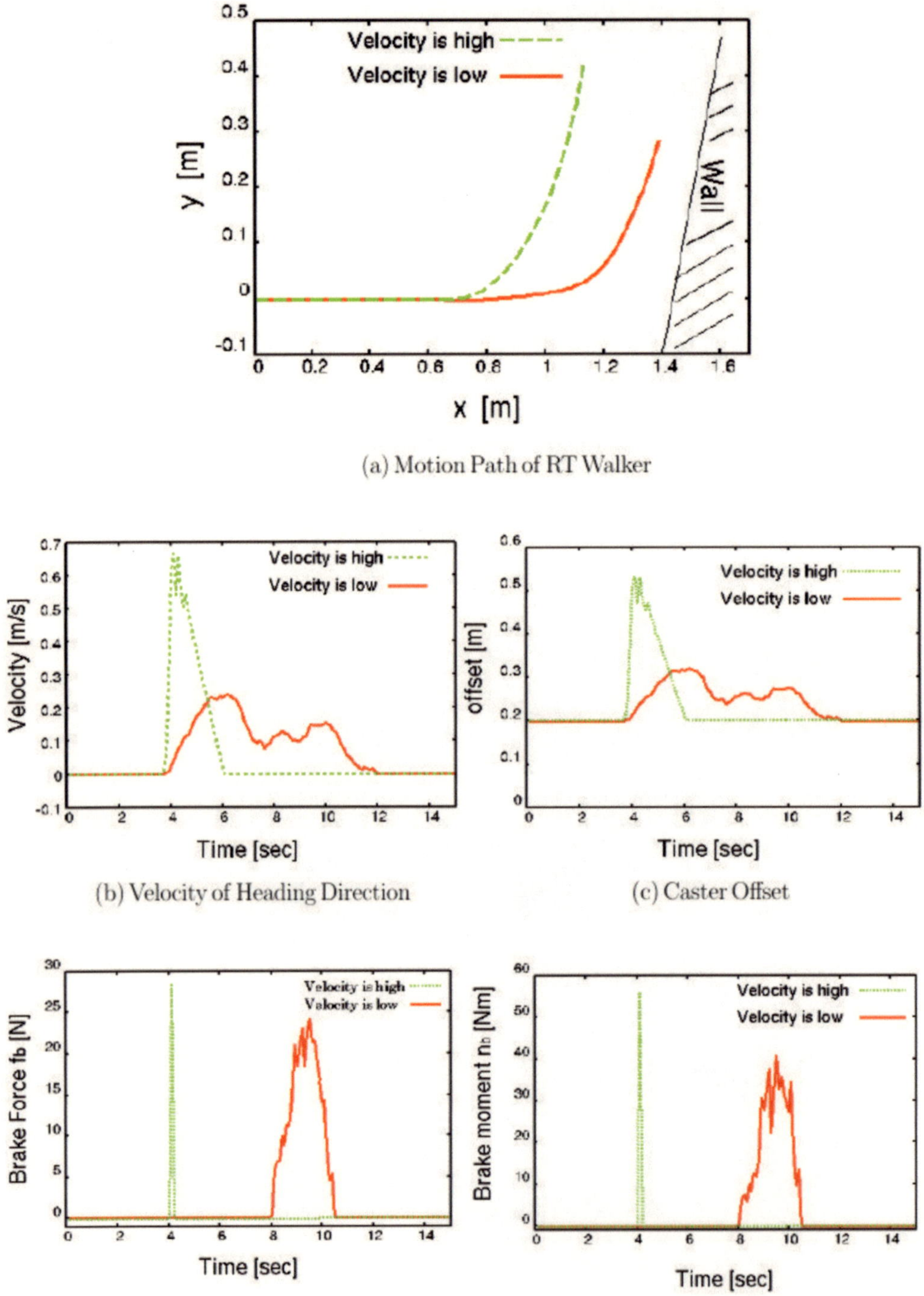

(a) Motion Path of RT Walker

(b) Velocity of Heading Direction

(c) Caster Offset

(d) Brake Force

(e) Brake Moment

Fig. 9. Experimental Results.

8. Reference

[1] J. Manuel, H. Wandosell, B. Graf, "Non-Holonomic Navigation System of a walking-Aid Robot", Proc. of IEEE International Workshop on Robot and Human Interactive Communication, pp.518-523, 2002.

[2] A. M. Sabatini, V. Genovese, E. Pacchierotti, "Mobility Aid for the Support to Walking and Object Transportation of People with Motor Impairments", Proc. of IEEE/RSJ International Conference on Intelligent Robots and Systems, pp.1349-1354, 2002.

[3] S. Dubowsky, F. Genot, S Godding, H. Kozono, A. Skwersky, H. Yu, L. S. Yu, "PAMM-A Robotic Aid to the Elderly for Mobility Assistance and Monioring: A "Helping-Hand" for the Elderly", Proc. of IEEE International Conference on Robotics and Automation, pp.570-576, 2000.

[4] M. Fujie, Y. Nemoto, S. Egawa, A. Sakai, S. Hattori, A.Koseki, T. Ishii, "Power Assisted Walking Support and Walk Rehabilitation", Proc. of 1st International Workshop on Humanoid and Human Friendly Robotics, 1998.

[5] Y. Hirata, T. Baba, K. Kosuge, "Motion Control of Omni-directional type Walking Support System "Walking Helper"", Proc. of IEEE Workshop on Robot and Human Interactive Communication, 2A5, 2003

[6] S. Kotani, H. Mori, N. Kyohiro, "Development of the robotic travel aid HITOMI", Proc. of IEEE Int. Conf. on Robotics and Automation, 1990

[7] G. Wasson, P. Sheth, M. Alwan, K. Granata, A. Ledoux, C. Huang, "User Intent in a Shared Control Framework for Pedestrian Mobility Aids", Proc. of the 2003 IEEE/RSJ Intl. Conf. on Intelligent Robots and Systems, 2003

[8] A. J. Rentschler, R. A. Cooper, B. Blaschm M. L. Boninger, "Intelligent walkers for the elderly : Performance and safety testing of VA-PAMAID robotic walker", Journal of Rehabilitation Research and Development, Vol. 40, No. 5, 2003

[9] Y. Hirata, A. Hara, K.Kosuge, "Passive-type Intelligent Walking Support System "RT Walker", Proceedings of the 2004 IEEE/RSJ International Conference on Intelligent Robots and Systems, (2004), pp.3871-3876, 2004.

[10] A. Goswami, M. A. Peshkin, J. Colgate, "Passive robotics: an exploration of mechanical computation (invited) ", Proc. of the IEEE Int. Conf. on Robotics and Automation, pp. 279-284, 1990.

[11] M. A. Peshkin, J. E. Colgate, W. Wannasuphoprasit, C. A. Moore, R. B. Gillespie, P.Akella, "Cobot Architecture", IEEE Transactions on Robotics and Automation, Vol. 17, No.4, 2001

[12] O.Schneider, T.Troccaz, O.Chavanon and D.Blin, "PADyC: a Synergistic Robot for Cardiac Puncturing", Proceedings of 2000 IEEE International Conference on Robotics and Auotmation, 2000.

[13] Jocelyne Troccaz, Peter Berkelman, Philippe Cinquin, Adriana Vilchis-Gonzales, "Surgical robot dependability: propositions and examples", 2nd IARP/IEEE-RAS Joint Workshop on Technical Challenge for Dependable Robots in Human Environments, 2002.

[14] J. Furusho, M. Sakaguchi and N. Takesue: Basic Study for Development of Muscular-Strength Estimation and Training System Using ER Brake ---Development of ER Brake and its Passive Velocity Control---, Journal of RSJ, Vol.20, No.1, pp.77-84 (2002), in Japanese.

[15] Michael A. Peshkin, J. Edward Colgate, Carl Moore, "Passive Robots and Haptic Displays based on Nonholonomic Elements", Proceedings of the 1996 IEEE International Conference on Robotics and Automation, pp.551-556, 1996
[16] Michael A. Peshkin, J. Edward Colgate, Carl Moore, "Passive Robots and Haptic Displays based on Nonholonomic Elements", Proceedings of the 1996 IEEE International Conference on Robotics and Automation, pp.551-556, 1996
[17] Y. Hirata, A. Muraki, K. Kosuge, "Motion Control of Intelligent Passive-type Walker for Fall-prevention Function based on Estimation of User State", Proceedings of the 2006 IEEE International Conference on Robotics and Automation,(2006),3498-3503
[18] Y. Hirata, K. Kosuge, "Distributed Robot Helpers Handling a Single Object in Cooperation with a Human", Proc. of IEEE International Conference on Robotics and Automation, pp.458-463, 2000.
[19] O. Khatib, "Real-Time Obstacle Avoidance for Manipulators and Mobile Robots", Int. Journal of Robotics Research, pp. 90--98, 1986.

12

Powered Human Gait Assistance

Kevin W. Hollander* and Thomas G. Sugar†
*Augspurger-Komm Engineering, Inc., Phoenix, Arizona
†Arizona State University, Mesa, Arizona
USA

1. Introduction

Wearable robots are computer-controlled, actuated devices that are worn by a person. The purpose of such a device is to enhance the strength or performance of the person that wears it, where performance can be speed or coordination or some other desired attribute. Potential uses of a wearable robot are in rehabilitation, training, strength augmentation or simply as an assistance device for normal daily living. The greatest potential impact that a wearable robot could have is in the rehabilitation or assistance of a weak or disabled person.

Within the growing elderly population, 20 to 50% are affected by abnormal gait, i.e. walking impairment (Rubenstein & Trueblood, 2004). Abnormal gait in the elderly does not have a specific cause; many age related factors can affect normal locomotion. Some examples include; 1) muscle weakness, 2) slow reaction times, and 3) impaired tactile sensation from the feet. The ability to balance is the first requirement for successful gait. Impaired sensory information, long processing times and weak actuation all lead eventually to an unstable balance control system.

Adaptation of powered actuated devices to assist elderly or weak individuals implies special design requirements (Hollander & Sugar, 2004). Use of the term `wearable' implies that such a robot be portable, lightweight and safe. In order for such a device to be accessible for home use, the additional implications are that the wearable robot be economical and easy to operate. In contrast, a factory floor robot is none of these things; therefore, simple adaptation of existing technology is not possible.

The goal of this work is to investigate these design requirements and to develop the methodologies necessary for their implementation to human gait assistance. This work will focus on the use of a novel spring based actuator, which is powerful, lightweight, energy efficient and above all safe to its wearer.

2. Background

The prevalence of powered assistance devices for the weak and elderly can be seen almost every day. Powered-seated scooters are increasingly popular and are available from a variety of commercial sources. Often these scooters require additional modifications to one's home and automobile to accommodate their use. The popularity of the seated scooter is testament to the need for powered assistance; however, the use of these devices are in direct conflict to the belief that long term health is maintained by the inclusion of "the types of activities that provide an adequate load-bearing stimulus" (ACSM, 1995). Powered assistance is required, but should come in a form that promotes and supports standing/walking activities. To maintain general health and wellbeing, load-bearing walking is essential.

However, the solution to developing a walking assistance robot is not trivial. It is well known that such a system would need the ability to produce large torques and be capable of high power. Such requirements raise the threshold for wearable robots to be successful in this application. Nevertheless, work in this area has already begun.

Projects in the area of assisted locomotion are the BLEEX (Berkely Lower Extremity Exoskeleton) robot (Kazerooni et al., 2006) and the HAL-3 (Hybrid Assistive Leg) robot (Kawamoto et al., 2003; Kawamoto & Sankai, 2002). Both devices are rigidly attached to the wearer and are directly driven, i.e. no compliant interface.

The BLEEX robot uses hybrid hydraulic actuators to drive the system, whereas the HAL-3 robot uses DC motors and gearboxes to provide power for movement to the user. In both projects, the same solution is used, providing both positive and negative forces to the user to achieve a desired movement pattern. For example in gait, sometimes the robot needs to push the user (positive) and sometimes for support the robot needs to resist the user (negative) and in either case the robot is putting power into the system.

In other work, a robotic powered knee, RoboKnee (Pratt et al., 2004), and an active ankle foot orthosis, AAFO (Blaya & Herr, 2004) have been developed to assist with an individual's gait. Each of these devices features the linear Series Elastic Actuator (Robinson et al., 1999) as the means of robotic control. The linear series elastic actuator features a helical spring in series with a ball screw mechanism, similar to the actuator developed by Sugar and Kumar (Sugar & Kumar, 1998) for grasping tasks. For the series elastic device, the inclusion of the spring aids greatly in force and impedance control task stability. However, even though the device uses a spring between the actuator and the environment (i.e. person), the compliance of this system is derived mostly from its controller. Based upon the geometry and length of the springs used, very little deflection or compliance would be possible in a passive situation and thus is still very nearly a directly driven system.

Common knowledge in the legged robot community is that inclusion of springs in robotics can effectively reduce both the power and energy requirements demanded of an actuator (Raibert, 1986; Hurst et al., 2004). This is because a spring can store and release energy efficiently during cyclic repetitive tasks and the power released from a spring is limited only by the natural frequency and stiffness of the system. In other literature, van den Bogert describes a theoretical, passive mechanism that reduces peak power for human gait by more than 70% (van den Bogert, 2003). The passive device uses a series of elastic cords and pulleys around multiple anatomical joints to accomplish reduced power requirements. As written, the specific implementation described would not likely be practical, but the point of including springs in the design of wearable robotic systems is beneficial.

In order to meet the demanding requirements stated above, a wearable robotic device must include lightweight, energy conservative, power reducing springs to be both portable and inherently safe.

3. Human Ankle Gait

A basic understanding of human ankle gait is required before a discussion of actuator strategies for ankle gait assistance can begin. Gait is the term used to describe the locomotion of legged animals. Gait is a reoccurring pattern of leg and foot movements, rotations, and torques. The discussion of gait is presented in terms of percentages of a gait cycle due to its repetitive nature. The basic description of gait analysis terms is illustrated in figure 1.

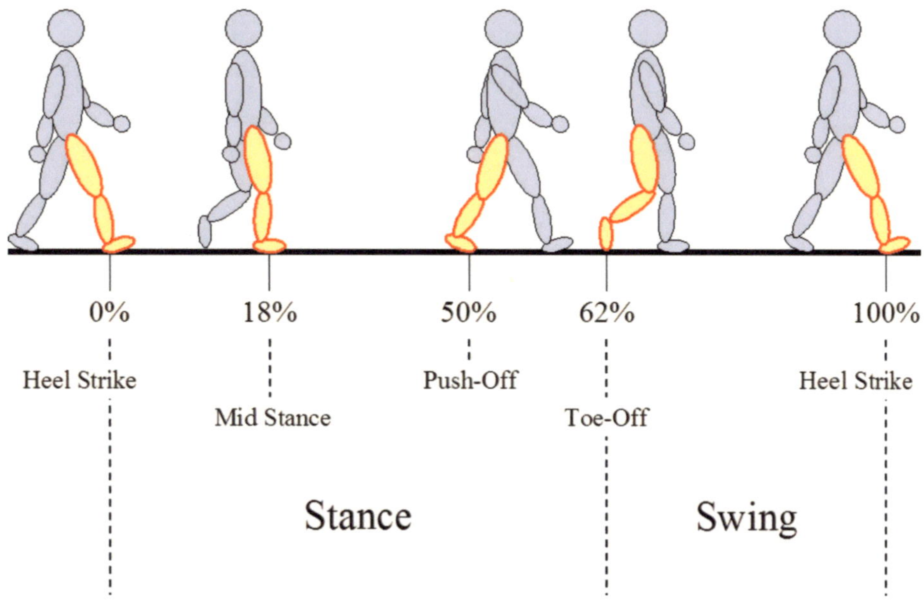

Fig. 1. Normal Gait Cycle.

As can be seen in the figure, a gait cycle is defined for a single leg and begins with the initial contact of the foot with the ground or `heel strike'. The conclusion of a cycle occurs as the same foot makes a second `heel strike'. The end of one gait cycle is of course the beginning of another.

Other key regions of the gait cycle are indicated in figure 1 as mid stance, push-off, and toe-off. In this case, the mid stance is shown with the leg perpendicular to the foot at the ankle. At this point in the gait cycle the body's weight is aligned over the primary supporting foot. The peak thrust of the push-off phase of gait is diagrammed at 50% of the gait cycle. Push-off is the propulsive phase of gait, giving the body its continued forward motion. The toe-off event begins at the completion of push-off, which is the beginning of leg swing. At toe-off, the hip is fully extended and the leg and foot are advanced to prepare for the next step or heel strike. To illustrate a typical pattern of gait, consider the kinematics and kinetics of a normal ankle (Whittle, 1996), figure 2; notice that the ankle moment (torque) data is normalized by body weight (kg).

In this figure, peak ankle moment occurs at roughly 45% of the gait cycle and at a value of -1.25 Nm/kg or for an 80 kg person, -100 Nm. The negative sign represents the physiological direction for which the moment occurs. In this case, peak moment is acting to move the foot in a toes-down direction. Interesting to note, the point at which the peak moment occurs, the ankle angle begins a rapid descent to its lowest overall value of -24° at 60% of the gait cycle. The region of gait approximately between 40% and 60% of the gait cycle is known as `push off' (highlighted on each plot).

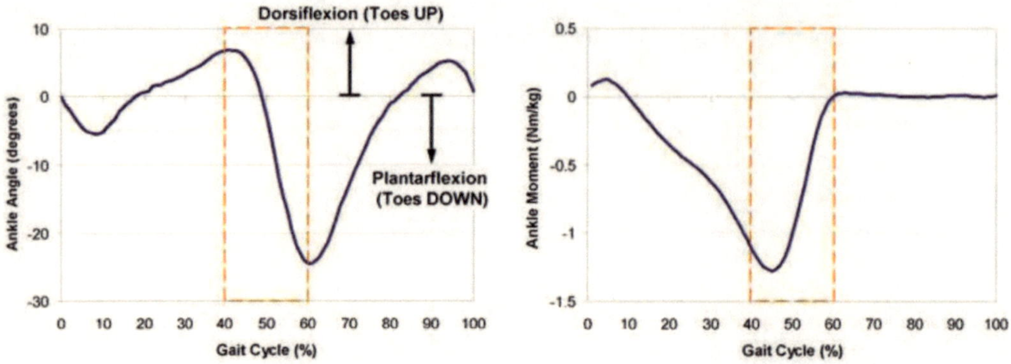

Fig. 2. Normal Ankle Gait: Kinematics and Kinetics.

This data provides information about the torques and angles required to achieve normal ankle gait. In terms of an actuator, these torques and angles can be converted into required forces and displacements. An actuator following this linear data will provide normal gait. Knowing the forces and positions necessary for gait is the first step. The next step is to determine the power requirements, which is used to size the motor for this task.
In order to determine the power of gait for the human ankle, it is necessary to assume a person's body weight and gait speed. This information, combined with the data for normal ankle gait, i.e. figure 2, are used to calculate ankle power for an ideal person who weighs 80 kg and walks at a frequency of 0.8 Hz, see figure 3.

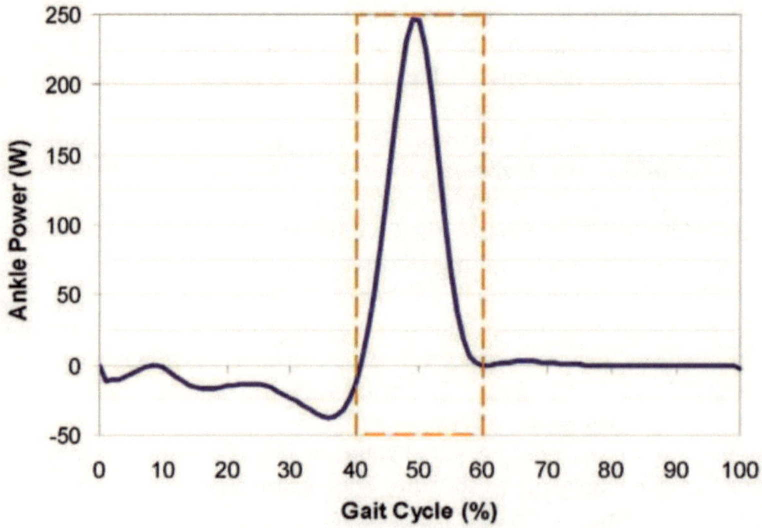

Fig. 3. Normal Ankle Gait Power, 80 kg person, 0.8 Hz gait frequency.

Notice that the ankle requires primarily positive power for the task of `push off' (i.e. 40%-60%). For most of the ankle's power needs the requirements are modest, but during the push off phase of gait it spikes to 250 W. Considering both the negative and positive portions of power, average power for this task is only 15 W. The power required during the swing phase of gait is minimal because little torque is needed to reposition the foot for the next heel strike. An integration of the power curve yields a total value of energy for each ankle to be 19.4 Joules/step.

Additionally, the primary source for this peak power or propulsion in normal gait is the gastrocnemius and soleus muscle groups. These muscle groups are located at on the backside of the lower leg and are often referred to as the calf muscles. Flexing these muscles produces a downward thrust of the foot or plantar flexion moment about the ankle. Experimental recordings of muscle activity are achieved via electromyography or EMG instrumentation. During a muscular contraction, positively charged calcium ions flow within the muscular tissue. The movement of these charged particles creates a change, or flux, in the magnetic field surrounding the muscles, and can be captured or measured by electromagnetically sensitive equipment, i.e. EMG electrodes.

Once captured, an EMG signal can be processed and observed. For the gastroncnemius muscle group, a rectified and processed EMG signal is shown for normal gait, see figure 4 (Hof et al., 2002).

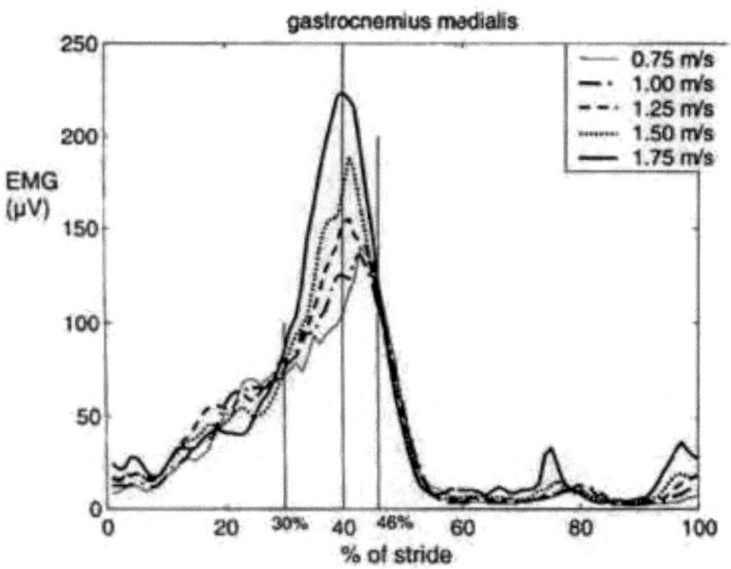

Fig. 4. Normal Ankle Gait EMG: Gastrocnemius Muscle Group (reprinted with permission from Hof et al., 2002).

Figure 4 shows several processed EMG signals, each for a different gait speed. Logically, the data shows higher amplitudes in muscular response for increases in gait speed. The raw signals for this data have been filtered for noise, rectified and enveloped as part of the processing. The result is the relatively clean looking signals displayed in the figure. EMG signal measurements are sensitive to many factors and thus its amplitude can be compared only under carefully considered situations.

For example, in the displayed data, the measurements were recorded sequentially during the same testing session. In this case, it is appropriate to compare the amplitudes of these signals. However, these same amplitudes have no real meaning for comparison to another subject or even the same subject on a different day. As such, the real usefulness of an EMG measure is in capturing the relative shape and timing of muscular activity and not its amplitude. From figure 4 it is apparent that peak amplitude of EMG activity of the gastrocnemius occurs just prior to the push-off phase of gait. In a later section, the significance of this shape and timing will be discussed.

4. Robotic Tendon Approach

The Robotic Tendon is the name given to our spring-based actuator (Hollander et al., 2006b). Use of the term Robotic Tendon implies an analogy to human physiology. The premise of the following development is that the human muscular system uses the advantages inherent in its elastic nature. Therefore, similar to a human muscle, the elastic nature of a spring is used to minimize both the work and peak power required to perform the task of ankle gait. A conceptual model of the Robotic Tendon can be seen in Figure 5. Conceptually, this model is same model described by Sugar and Kumar (Sugar & Kumar, 1998; Sugar, 2002) as well as the linear series elastic model described by Robinson (Robinson et al., 1999).

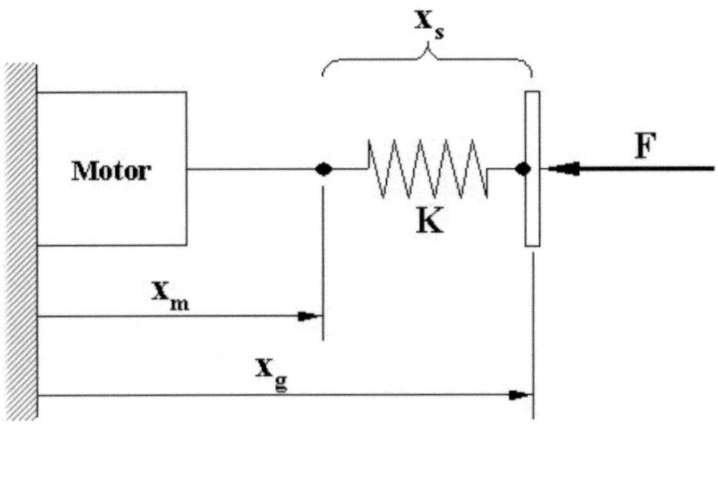

Fig. 5. Robotic Tendon Model: motor and spring in series.

From figure 5, a development of motor power requirements based upon stiffness K can be derived. The position of the environment, x_g, is given by converting the joint angles of gait to linear displacement using a simple lever arm. In the model, the position, the compression of the spring and the movement of the motor can achieve x_g. It is thus a combination of the position of the motor, x_m, and the position of the spring, x_s, see equation 1.

$$x_g = x_m + x_s \quad (1)$$

However, since a spring is a passive device its position is determined by the force, F, applied to it. The force, F, is calculated by converting the moment needed in gait using a simple lever arm. Consider the basic Hookean spring shown in equation 2.

$$F = K \cdot \Delta x_s \tag{2}$$

where, $\Delta x_s = d_o - x_s$.

The free un-deformed length of the spring is represented by d_o and is simply an offset value. Solving equation 2 for x_s, yields:

$$x_s = d_o - \frac{F}{K} \tag{3}$$

The length of the spring is based upon the environmental force and spring stiffness. Equation 3 can be substituted into the equation for environmental position, x_g, and solved for the required motor position, x_m. From this substitution equation 4 is determined,

$$x_m = x_g + \frac{F}{K} - d_o \tag{4}$$

and taking its derivative, yields the velocity required.

$$\dot{x}_m = \dot{x}_g + \frac{\dot{F}}{K} \tag{5}$$

Knowing the forces, F, required by the gait cycle and knowing the motor's required velocity, $\dot{x}_m$, the relationship for motor power, P_m, can be obtained. Power is simply force multiplied by velocity, thus multiplying F by equation 5 will yield a relationship for motor power.

$$P_m = \left| \underbrace{F \cdot \dot{x}_g}_{required\ gait\ power} + \underbrace{\frac{F \cdot \dot{F}}{K}}_{spring\ power} \right| \tag{6}$$

Human ankle gait power can be both negative and positive. When it is negative, a resistance motion is applied to the ankle, and when it is positive, a propelling motion is applied. A motor unit cannot typically provide negative power; therefore, it must provide power to both resist and propel human motion. For this reason, an absolute value in equation 6 is used. In addition, values for force, F, velocity, $\dot{x}_m$ and $\dot{F}$ can all be determined from human gait analysis data. Thus, stiffness, K, becomes the only design parameter.

Consider the case where spring stiffness, K, is nearly infinite (i.e. direct drive). In this example the spring power term drops to zero and the motor must provide the absolute value of normal gait power. In the opposite case, consider a spring with stiffness near zero. In this example, the power requirements tend toward infinity. If a straight line were assumed between these two cases, it would appear that a direct drive scenario is the best.

Fortunately, this simplistic relationship is not the case. On the contrary, if a spring is properly selected both energy and peak power for the motor required to perform human gait can be drastically reduced compared to the direct drive analogy.

4.1 Stiffness for Zero Motor Power at Peak Output

As a first approach to determining stiffness, consider the form of equation 6. In terms of a design, the only variable to pick is spring stiffness. The rest of the terms in this equation are dictated by ankle gait kinematics and kinetics. So, what is the best method for choosing stiffness?

One possibility is to try and minimize the motor's power demand during the most demanding portion of the gait cycle. If the peak motor requirement could be driven lower than 247 W described earlier, then a smaller and thus lighter motor could be chosen for the actuator. So as a first approach, equation 6 can be set equal to zero and solved for K.

$$K = \frac{\dot{F}}{\dot{x}_g} \tag{7}$$

Evaluating equation 7 for the example gait data, using a 0.12 m lever arm, yields a stiffness K_1 = 14,152 N/m. The peak power of gait occurs at 50% of the gait cycle. Using this calculated value of stiffness, power of the motor will equal zero during the peak power of gait. Initially, this may seem counter intuitive, but consider that a spring can store energy over time and yet release it very quickly (i.e. high power). In the case of the Robotic Tendon, at this stiffness, the spring is providing 100% of the power needed for gait at the instance of peak demand. Figure 6 shows the power profile that results from choosing this stiffness.

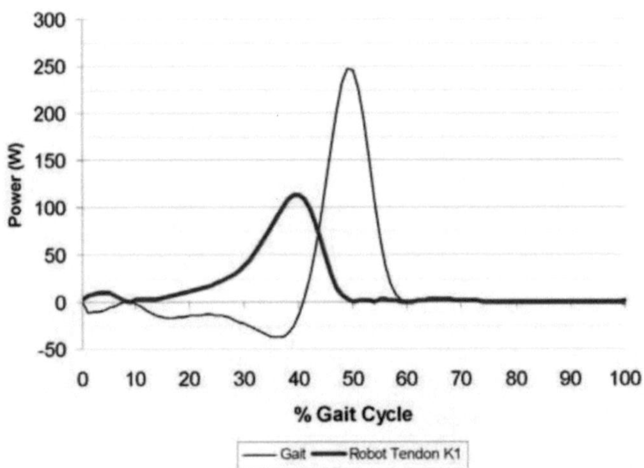

Fig. 6. Robotic Tendon Power with K_1 = 14,152 N/m: Zero motor power at peak gait power.

The figure shows a thick line for the Robotic Tendon power and a thin line for the power required for ankle gait. The resulting power curve for the Robotic Tendon differs significantly from the one developed for a lead screw only or direct drive actuator. In this case, the ankle gait curve and motor curve do not seem to match. The difference between these two curves is the addition of the spring power. The addition of spring power to the motor power will result in the appropriate ankle gait output.

Noteworthy in this graph is the much lower value of peak power for the motor compared to ankle gait. Even with the addition of efficiency of the lead screw, a motor sized below 150 W can easily perform this gait task. As an example, the Maxon RE40 DC motor is nominally rated for 150 W of continuous power and weighs only 0.48 kg. With a small 6 mm diameter lead screw design, the combined weight of the K_1 actuator is still less than 1 kg and would

consume only about 23 J per step. This provides a much better result than the lead screw only actuator, which would require a much larger motor and thus a heavier design.
Consider again the analogy of the Robotic Tendon to human muscle and its response to the task of ankle gait. Previously, figure 4 showed the timing and shape of the EMG response of gastrocnemius muscle during gait. EMG has often been correlated to muscular force. However, consider the shape and timing of the motor power curve for the Robotic Tendon compared to EMG signal of the gastrocnemius. Both of these actuators are performing a similar function and both use elasticity to minimize power and to conserve energy. For convenience, a scaled plot of both of these figures was constructed, see figure 7.

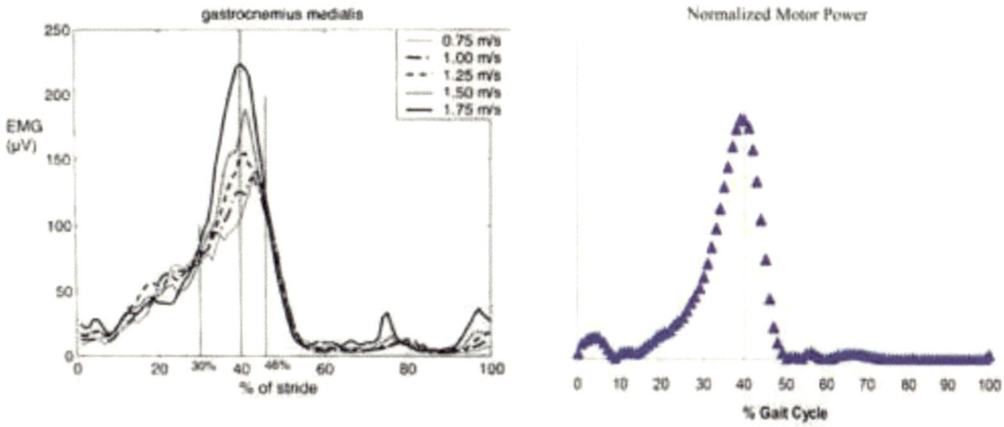

Fig. 7. Robotic Tendon Power and EMG Comparison: Triangles represent the calculated Robotic Tendon power data, scaled to fit the previously referenced EMG data plot of the gastrocnemius muscle group (reprinted with permission from Hof et al., 2002).

The magnitudes for these sets of plots have no meaning in the present comparison. Only the shape and timing need to be considered. It is remarkable to see the level of similarity between the two sets of plots. Although this is not a conclusive result, it is nonetheless a strong indication of relationships. If EMG is more closely related to power of the muscle than force, it is still not surprising to see that an EMG/force correlation would exist. Consider that power is defined as force multiplied by velocity and so EMG and power would each follow force closely. The significance of these similar graphs is that the models of a Robotic Tendon could provide a clean and simple explanation as to how the human uses his own muscle motors. This topic is a separate discussion to the present analysis, but still offers an interesting result to share.

4.2 Stiffness Optimization

Using the above method for selecting stiffness yields good results for the Robotic Tendon actuator. These results may even indicate that the human's gastrocnemius muscle group could be using a similar strategy. If this is the case, can a better result be obtained? To answer this question an exploration of the influence of stiffness, K, on peak motor power is required. Based upon equation 6, the relationship between stiffness, K, and 'peak' motor power is considered in equation 8.

$$\left(P_m\right)_{peak} = \max\left|F \cdot \dot{x}_g + \frac{F \cdot \dot{F}}{K}\right| \tag{8}$$

To run the optimization, a C++ program was written to calculate the maximum motor power during a gait cycle for a large range of spring stiffness values. The code was run for several iterations to further refine the optimization results. To explain these results, a plot of only peak motor power was produced for a successive range of spring stiffness's. This plot can be seen in figure 8.

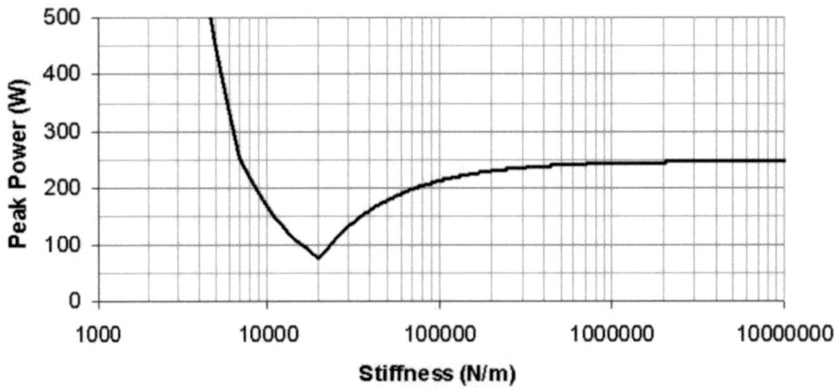

Fig. 8. Optimization of Stiffness, K, for an 80kg person.

Figure 8 reveals an interesting relationship. Extreme stiffness cases can be described by this graph and its corresponding equation. At a stiffness value near zero, infinite motor power would be required. The analogy is that the spring is absorbing all of the power that the motor can provide and is not providing any back to the environment. At the opposite extreme is infinite stiffness or direct drive (i.e. lead screw only design). It is seen that a high stiffness spring asymptotically approaches peak gait power near 250 W. However, rather than being a linear relationship between the two extremes, a minimum point or cusp occurs. The odd shape of this graph can be explained as follows. The driving profile for this plot is determined by a *–1/K* relationship with respect to power. The cusp is created as a function of the absolute value of this factor and hence a minimum is created. For the example problem, an optimal value of stiffness, K_2, is determined to be 20,278 N/m. Figure 9 shows the power profile that results from choosing this new stiffness.

The figure shows a thick line for the Robotic Tendon power and a thin line for the power required for ankle gait. The resulting power curve for the Robotic Tendon is very different from the one developed for a lead screw only actuator and is different still from the previous stiffness choice. The peak power for the motor using this stiffness is lower than was seen in the previous stiffness case. Including the effects of friction on this graph, a motor sized below 90 W can be used. As an example, the Maxon RE35 DC motor is nominally rated for 90 W of continuous power and weighs only 0.34 kg, that is 30% less weight than in the previous example. Again, considering the effects of friction, the K_2 actuator would still consume only about 23 J per step. Even though the power results have been improved between the K_1 and K_2 stiffness cases, the energy of either approach is the same.

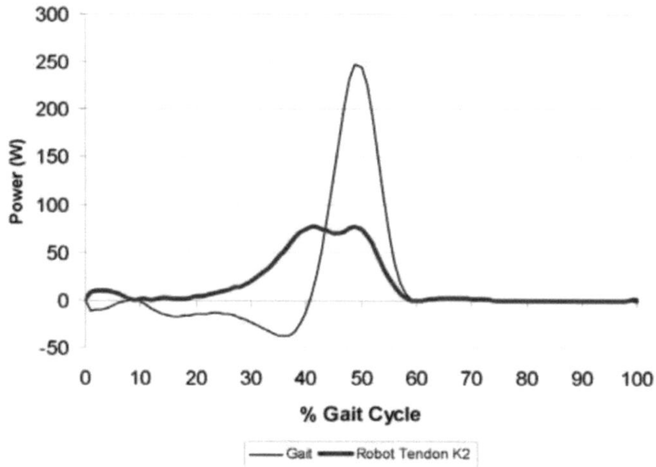

Fig. 9. Robotic Tendon Power with K2 = 20,278 N/m: Optimized stiffness.

4.3 Experimental Results

The Robotic Tendon actuator just described was used on a volunteer subject. As an additional means of safety during early testing, the ankle gait actuator was not allowed to drive the subject's ankle joint. Instead, the subject's foot was placed into a rigid and locked orthosis and the robot manipulated the position of its own separate ankle.

In this first prototype it was useful to separate the function of the robot from the function of the human ankle. This separation allows a clean comparison of results from the robot to the functional predicted expectations presented above. Had the robot been used to only assist in moving the subject's true joint, obtained results would not clearly separate the power supplied by the person from that of the robot.

For this experimental work, the subject tested was not the same size as our ideal subject.

Our ideal assumptions were developed for a typical young adult male, 80 kg. Our subject was slightly smaller and weighed just 65 kg. The significance of this difference is that the previously selected stiffness of K = 20,278 N/m would not be the optimal result for the tested subject. Nevertheless, using the same formulation as above, the response of the robot can still be predicted for this alternative set of conditions. In the following graphs, Figure 10, the predicted and measured positions of both the robot's end effector (lever) and the motor nut are presented.

The end effector position is the physical position of the forward end of the spring, i.e. the point at which the robot foot is attached. The motor nut position is the linear displacement of the nut along the lead screw; this is also coincident with the back end of the spring. Looking first at figure 10A, the thin line represents the end effector path through the gait cycle. The thick line in this plot represents the path of the motor nut. The difference between these lines is the deflection of the spring.

Comparing figure 10A with 10B reveals a very similar set of results. In general the measured data in figure 10B does not get the range of motion predicted, but still manages to get significant deflection of the spring. These results are quite remarkable in light of the fact that the only control variable for the robot was to maintain the thick lined path seen in figure

10B. The thin line in this plot was generated completely by the subject walking on the robot. This shows that the natural response of the human is to use the elastic compression spring similar to how his own elastic musculotendon complex would be used in gait. In a separate trial of data collection, the force and power profiles measured by the actuator were obtained. The results of these measurements are shown once again in comparison to predicted values, see figure 11.

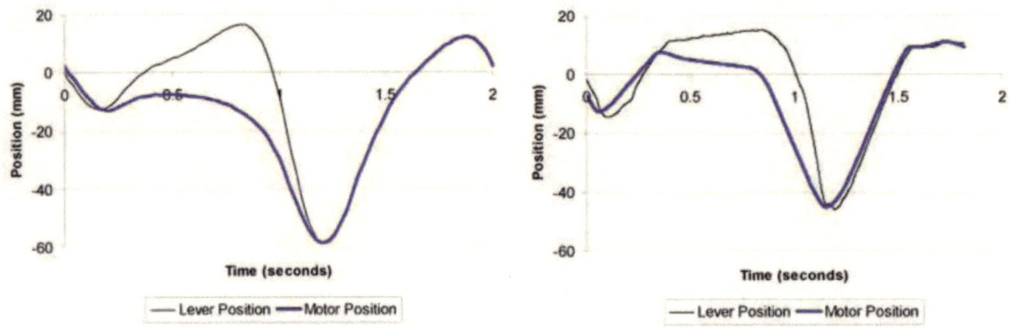

(A) (B)

Fig. 10. Robotic Tendon Experimental Results: Position, A) Predicted results of end effector (lever) and motor nut positions, B) Measured results of the same.

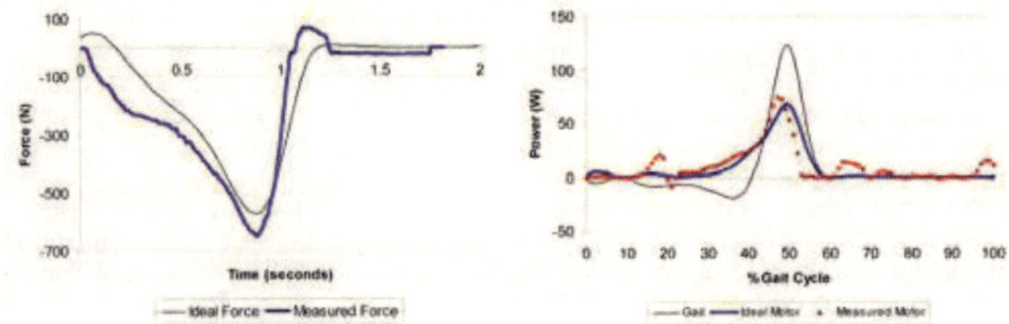

(A) (B)

Fig. 11. Robotic Tendon Experimental Results: A) Forces and B) Powers.

Again for both graphs the predicted and experimental results match very well. In figure 11A, the measured force is shown to slightly exceed predicted (ideal) and it descends to zero more rapidly from its peak. Figure 11B, shows a similar result for power as seen in force, a slightly higher peak is reached but drops to zero earlier in time. The result of power is shown with its ordinate axis as a percentage of a gait cycle, while forces were shown in seconds. During testing and comparisons, gait frequency was reduced to a just 0.5 Hz, for added safety.

In recent work, a 50% assistance ankle robot was constructed. Figure 12 shows this robot. The robot features a rear-mounted actuator that allows the user to easily don and doff the device. The Robotic Tendon actuator is tuned to provide 50% assistance to the wearer.

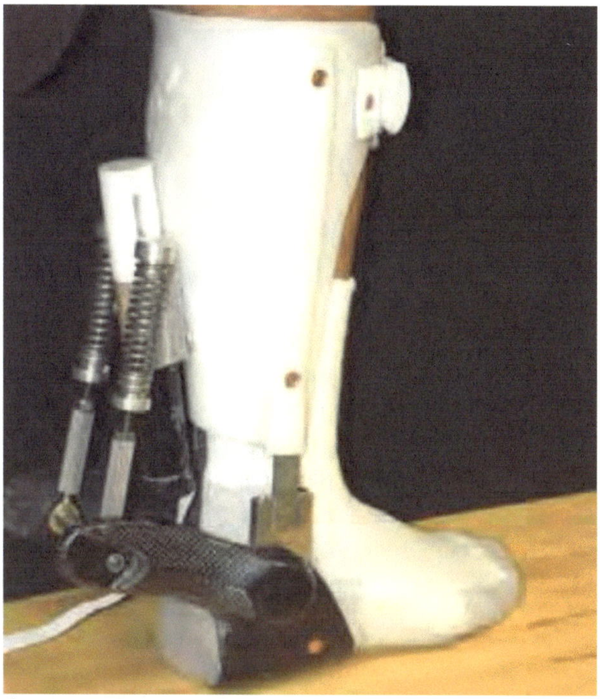

Fig. 12. Robotic Tendon prototype.

5. Application to Elderly Gait

Muscle weakness, slow reaction times, and impaired tactile or sensory information from the feet can affect a person's ability to balance and thus affect their ability to walk. For the complex tasks of balance and gait, significant deficiency in any of these factors pushes the limits of postural stability to `marginal' at best. The result of these factors is an increase in duration of double-limb support during gait, which leads to a decrease in walking speed.

This decrease in elderly gait is approximately 12-20% less than the speed of a typical young adult (Elble, 1997; Winter, 1991). It is interesting to note is that this decrease in speed is not due to a reduction in cadence (i.e. frequency of gait), but is attributed to a decrease in stride length, or reach. The term `cautious gait', coined by Nutt et al. (Nutt et al., 1993), describes this phenomenon as the response to a "real or perceived disequilibrium". Cautious gait is the result of apprehension to falling.

A wearable robot device can potentially aid in these difficulties. A wearable robot would provide strength where there is weakness, respond to stimuli quickly rather than slowly, and a wearable robot would sense problems early, rather than after it is too late. To assist elderly gait, a wearable robot based upon the idea of the Robotic Tendon actuator can be created.

The gait kinematics and kinetics for an elderly individual are different than for a younger able-bodied person. A shorter stride length, an increase in double stance time and ultimately a decrease in ankle power production are all hallmark characteristics of elderly gait (Winter, 1991; Devita & Hortobagyi, 2000). The gait kinematics and kinetics for an elderly individual (Devita & Hortobagyi, 2000) can be seen in Figure 13.

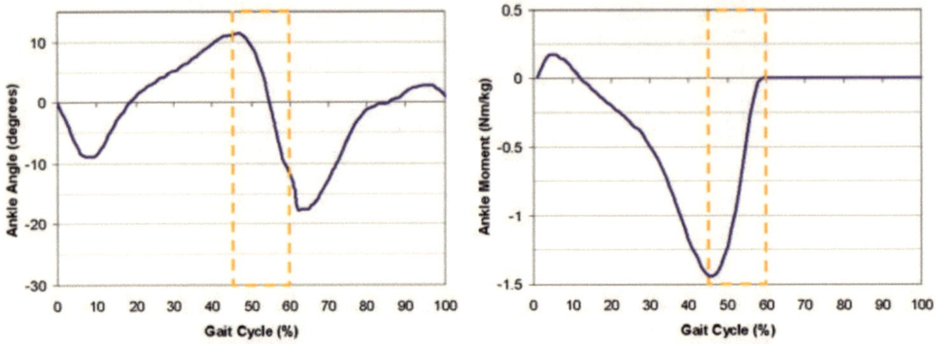

Fig. 13. Elderly Ankle Gait: Kinematics and Kinetics.

Different from the young able-bodied gait data, the elderly ankle gait kinematics has increased ankle dorsiflexion and reduced plantarflexion. Although the peak moments still occur roughly at 45% like young able-bodied gait, the peak moment is slightly greater. At a value of –1.44 Nm/kg the peak moment for an 80 kg person is -115 Nm. Also, the `push off' phase of elderly gait starts about 5% later than for young able-bodied gait and ranges from roughly 45% to 60% of the gait cycle (again highlighted on each plot).
In order to determine the power of elderly ankle gait, it is necessary to assume body weight and gait speed. Using the elderly ankle gait kinematics and kinectics presented in Figure 13, ankle gait power can be calculated for 80 kg individual that walks at a frequency of 0.8 Hz, see figure 14.

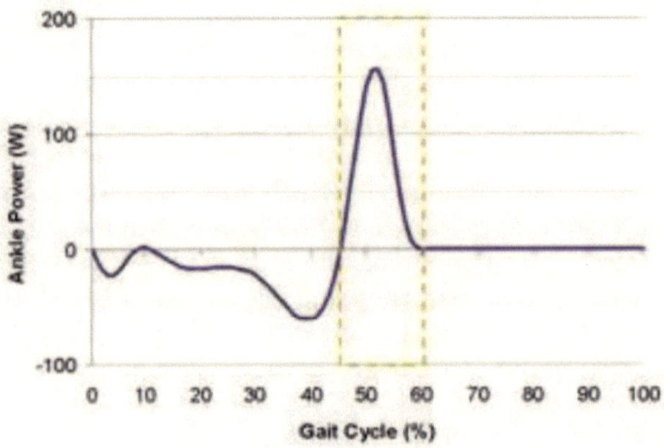

Fig. 14. Elderly Ankle Gait Power, 80 kg person, 0.8 Hz gait frequency.

Elderly ankle gait power has a lower positive peak power than does young able-bodied gait, 157 W compared to 250 W. Also, integration of the power curve yields a net energy of just 1.5 Joules/step. This is much less energy than is calculated for young able-bodied gait (19.5 Joules/step). A slightly greater amount negative peak power and 5% longer time allows an elderly ankle to store additional energy into its elastic structures. This combined with lower a positive peak power yields a very low combined or net positive energy added during each step.

Just like in the able-bodied Robotic Tendon actuator development, optimal spring stiffness can be chosen to reduce actuator motor peak power requirements for elderly gait and thus provide a very lightweight actuator design. A power optimization analysis for an 80 kg elderly individual, using a 0.12 m lever arm, yielded an ideal stiffness of K_3=29,929 N/m. The effect on the power input and output can be seen in Figure 15.

The figure shows a thick line for the Robotic Tendon power and a thin line for the power required for ankle gait. The peak power for the motor using this K_3 stiffness is less than 40 W. As an example, the Maxon RE30 DC motor is nominally rated for 60 W of continuous power and weighs only 0.238 kg. The RE30 motor weighs only half of the weight of the RE40 motor mentioned earlier. Motor energy calculated for this elderly gait assistance design is only about 12 Joules/step.

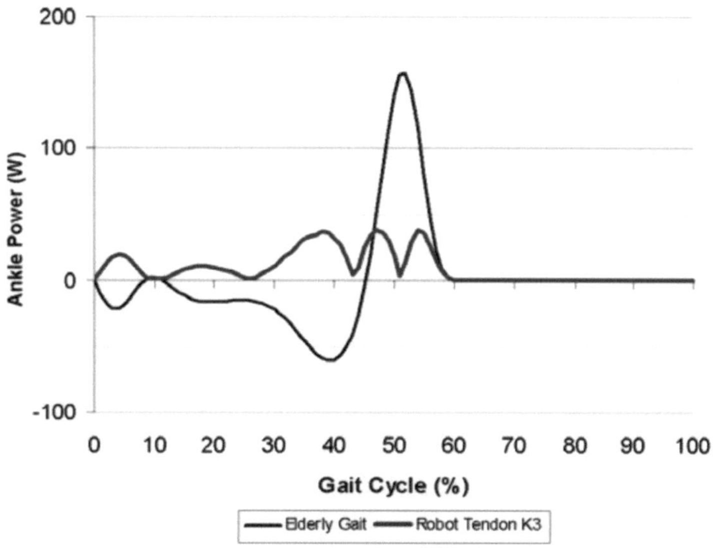

Fig. 15. Elderly Ankle Gait, Robotic Tendon Power with K3 = 29,929 N/m.

Providing correctly timed energy and power to an elderly individual's gait is the first step to assistance. It may be that powered gait assistance for the elderly must come in the form of the elderly gait pattern shown. However, if appropriate strength and timing is given to such a person, then maybe powered assistance can restore a young able-bodied gait profile to that elderly individual. Additional work in this area is still needed. The extent of influence such powered assistance has on elderly gait or even, pathological gait is simply not yet known.

6. Application to Hips and Knees

As seen in the previous development, the Robotic Tendon approach can be applied to alternative patterns of gait. In fact, the same method can be adapted to develop power-minimizing actuators for other joints, like the knees or hips. A Robotic Tendon actuator can be designed for any anatomical joint and provide a compliant, robust, powered assistance for a variety human movements. However, in order for a Robotic Tendon actuator to be designed to significantly minimize required motor power, special movement characteristics must exist.

As an example, the reason the Robotic Tendon approach successfully reduces motor power for the task of ankle gait is due to the nature of output movement of the ankle. Ankle gait patterns are asymmetrical in terms of power output. Relatively speaking, ankle power requirements are low and absorptive for the majority of the gait cycle and then during `push off' energy is released very quickly (high power).

In contrast, hip gait motion is much more symmetrical and as a result only minimal power savings are achieved by optimizing the spring stiffness. For the same 80 kg individual, walking at a 0.8 Hz rate the peak hip output power is 82 W. An optimization of the spring for hip gait assistance yields a stiffness value of 16,970 N/m. A Robotic Tendon actuator tuned for this stiffness would require a motor peak power value of just 60 W. In this example, the power savings is only on the order of 27%. Even considering only modest savings in peak power required, use of a spring-based actuator for powered hip assistance is still recommended. A spring is a compliant and an efficient form of energy storage, and thus will provide a good basis for most wearable robot designs.

Different from the hip and the ankle, knee power requirements for gait shows that the mean output is negative and the peak magnitude is around -80 W. With a majority of the output power requirements being negative, controlled damping (energy dissipation) can provide a good assistance solution. Examples of devices that control damping at the knee are the Rheo Knee (Ossur, Iceland) and the C-Leg (Otto Bock Healthcare, Germany) prosthetic knee devices.

A Robotic Tendon actuator can also provide controlled damping utilizing its spring. Mentioned previously, a using a spring is an efficient method of energy storage. However, since the motor is used to control the backside of the spring, this stored energy does not have to be completely returned to the environment. Imagine compressing a spring from one side and then allowing backside of the spring to slowly release that stored energy. Motorized control of a spring's total deflection is the fundamental nature of the Robotic Tendon approach.

Although the knee power profile is primarily negative, it still requires some positive power contribution. The Rheo Knee and C-Leg do not provide this additional required energy. A spring-based actuator can add, subtract or even store energy as needed and thus provide full powered walking assistance at the knees.

7. Control Methodology

Conceptually, the control approach used for the Robotic Tendon is an approach called `equilibrium control' (Hollander & Sugar, 2004). A linear actuator is used to drive the backside of the spring, effectively moving the un-deflected or equilibrium position of the spring. The basic premise of this approach is to position the spring into the right place, at the right time, so that the device operator (wearer) can take advantage of its elastic properties.

This method of control only dictates the position of the backside of the spring and does not force the wearer's ankle to follow any specific or predetermined pattern of motion. This is an important factor and is used to help insure the operator's safety while wearing the actuated device.

In our able-bodied testing, this control approach has worked remarkably well. The device wearer seems to naturally take advantage of the spring's aid and thus shares the walking workload. While walking on a treadmill and utilizing the device for several minutes, the device wearers' have commented that they do not really feel its aid. However, once the device is removed it takes several awkward steps to resume a natural, un-assisted pattern of gait. As seen previously in Section 4.3, data collected from the actuator device confirms that sharing of walking effort exists.

8. Conclusions

Adaptation of powered actuated devices to assist elderly or weak individuals implies special design requirements. These actuators must be powerful enough to perform the tasks required of them yet remain efficient, lightweight and safe to its wearer. A spring-based actuator can contribute to all of these things.

Springs are inherently powerful and lightweight. For the examples actuators developed above, the springs have `power to weight' ratios of approximately 300,000 W/kg. Springs are an efficient form of energy storage. For unstressed spring steel, its efficiency is reported to be 99.9% (Carlson, 1980). Springs are by nature compliant and back drivable, thus providing a natural measure of safety. Additionally, the other mechanical actuator elements, like a lead screw, can be designed to promote these design requirements as well (Hollander and Sugar, 2006a).

Methods that include the implementation of springs into wearable system designs are necessary to meet these special design requirements. The development presented here offers a robust approach to the design of actuators that fit a variety of powered assistance situations. The creation of lightweight and practical, powered assistance actuators is possible with today's technology. The era of robots serving a role in everyday life is close at hand and will likely be in the form of powered wearable assistance.

9. References

ACSM. (1995). ACSM position stand on osteoporosis and exercise, *Medicine And Science In Sports And Exercise*, Vol. 27, No. 4, i–vii

Blaya, J. & Herr, H. (2004). Adaptive control of a variable-impedance ankle-foot orthosis to assist drop-foot gait, *IEEE Transactions on Neural Systems and Rehabilitation Engineering*, Vol. 12, No. 1, 24–31

Carlson, H. (1980). *Springs troubleshooting and failure analysis*, 1st ed., Marcel Dekker, Inc., New York

DeVita, P. & Hortobagyi, T. (2000). Age causes a redistribution of joint torques and powers during gait, *Journal of Applied Physiology*, Vol. 88, 1804–1811

Elble, R. (1997). Changes in gait with normal aging, *Gait Disorders of Aging: Falls and Therapeutic Strategies* (Masdeu, Sudarsky, and Wolfson, eds.), Lippincott - Raven, Philadelphia, 93–105

Hof, A.; Elzinga, H.; Grimmius, W. & Halbertsma, J. (2002). Speed dependence of averaged EMG profiles in walking, *Gait and Posture*, Vol. 16, 78–86

Hollander, K. & Sugar, T. (2004). Concepts for compliant actuation in wearable robotic systems, *Proceedings of the US-Korea Conference* (UKC) CDROM, Research Triangle Park, North Carolina, August 2004

Hollander, K. & Sugar, T. (2006a). Design of lightweight lead screw actuators for wearable robotic applications, *ASME Journal of Mechanical Design*, Vol. 128, No. 3, 644-648

Hollander, K.; Ilg, R.; Sugar, T. & Herring, D. (2006b). An efficient robotic tendon for gait assistance, *ASME Journal of Biomechanical Engineering*, Vol. 128, No. 5, 788-791

Hurst, J.; Chestnutt, J. & Rizzi, A. (2004). An actuator with physically variable stiffness for highly dynamic legged locomotion, *IEEE International Conference on Robotics & Automation*(ICRA), New Orleans, LA, April 2004

Kawamoto, H. & Sankai, Y. (2002). Comfortable power assist control method for walking aid by HAL-3, *IEEE International Conference on Systems, Man and Cybernetics*, Vol. 4, pp. 6–11, Hammamet, Tunisia, October 2002

Kawamoto, H.; Kanbe, S. & Sankai, Y. (2003). Power assist method for HAL-3 estimating operator's intention based on motion information, *IEEE International Workshop on Robot and Human Interactive Communication*, pp. 67–72, Millbrae, CA, October 2003

Kazerooni, H.; Steger, R. & Huang, L. (2006). Hybrid control of the Berkeley lower extremity exoskeleton (BLEEX), *The International Journal of Robotics Research*, Vol. 25, 561-573

Nutt, J.; Marsden, C. & Thompson, P. (1993). Human walking and higher-level gait disorders, particularly in the elderly, *Neurology*, Vol. 43, 268–279

Pratt, J.; Krupp, B.; Morse, C. & Collins, S. (2004). The RoboKnee: An exoskeleton for enhancing strength and endurance during walking, *IEEE International Conference on Robotics and Automation* (ICRA), pp. 2430–2435, New Orleans, LA, April 2004

Raibert, M. (1986). *Legged Robots that Balance,* The MIT Press, Cambridge

Robinson, D.; Pratt, J.; Paluska, D. & Pratt, G. (1999). Series elastic actuator development for a biomimetric walking robot, *IEEE/ASME International Conference on Advanced Intelligent Mechatronics*, pp. 561–568, Atlanta, GA, September 1999

Rubenstein, L. & Trueblood, P. (2004). Gait and balance assessment in older persons, *Annals of Long-Term Care,* Vol. 12, No. 2, 39-45

Sugar, T. (2002). A novel selective compliant actuator, *Mechatronics*, Vol. 12, No. 9-10, 1157–1171

Sugar, T. & Kumar, V. (1998) Design and control of a compliant parallel manipulator for a mobile platform, *ASME Design Engineering Technical Conferences and Computers in Engineering Conference* (DETC), CDROM, Atlanta, GA, September 1998

Van Den Bogert, A. (2003). Exotendons for assistance of human locomotion, *BioMedical Engineering Online*, Vol. 2, 17

Whittle, M. (1996). *Gait analysis: an introduction*, 2nd ed., Butterworth-Heinemann, Oxford

Winter, D. (1991) *The biomechanics and motor control of human gait: normal, elderly and pathological*, 2nd ed., Waterloo Biomechanics, Waterloo

13

Task-oriented and Purposeful Robot-Assisted Therapy

Michelle J Johnson, PhD[1,2,3], Kimberly J Wisneski, MS[3], John Anderson[1,3], Dominic Nathan[2,3], Elaine Strachota[4], OTR, PhD, Judith Kosasih, MD[1,3], Jayne Johnston, OTR, RN[3], Roger O. Smith, OTR, PhD[5]

Medical College of Wisconsin[1], Marquette University[2], Clement Zablocki VA[3], Concordia University[4], University of Wisconsin, Milwaukee[5]
Milwaukee, Wisconsin, USA

1. Introduction

Robot-assisted therapy devices are available for rehabilitation of persons after stroke, which is the leading cause of disability among adults in the United States (AHA 2006, Volpe et al. 2002). Improving upper extremity function after stroke is critical for performance of one's life-role and the completion of unilateral and bilateral activities of daily living (ADLs). Carryover to real-life activities after rehabilitation training cannot be assumed (Sterr et al. 2000; Maclean et al. 2000; Ma and Trombly 2002; Trombly and Ma 2002; Prange et al. 2006). For example, the existence of learned non-use behavior indicates that motor gains after rehabilitation therapies may not transfer to long-term functioning on ADLs (Taub et al. 1994; Taub et al. 1999; Sterr et al. 2000). This behavior is present when persons with hemiparesis due to strokes demonstrate significant differences between residual movement capabilities and spontaneous use of the impaired arm in real world. There is a need to address barriers to the carryover of motor gains during training to stroke function in real life.

This chapter reviews examples of current upper arm robot-assisted therapy environments and present findings from case study experiments with a new task-oriented, robot therapy system focused on improving carryover of motor improvements to functional activities of daily living. We draw attention to influence of function on arm movements during robot training and explore how future environments can be more functional and engaging.

Robot-assisted therapy devices are now being used more frequently in the rehabilitation of persons with physical disabilities due to neurological trauma caused by stroke and spinal cord injury. These therapy robots provide semi- or fully-autonomous training and permit patients using them to engage in repeated and intense practice of goal-directed tasks (Volpe et al 2002; Prange et al 2006; Burgar et al. 2000; Loureiro et al. 2003; Patton et al. 2006; Krebs et al. 2003; MacClellan et al. 2005, Kahn et al. 2006). Typically, the automation of therapeutic exercises involves generating trajectories that guide reaching movements and the application of forces directly or indirectly to the impaired arm to assist, resist, and/or passively support it during the reaching exercise. For example, the MIT-MANUS (Krebs et al. 2003; MacClellan et al. 2005) therapy robot permits stroke survivors to practice two-dimensional (2-D) point-to-point (PTP) movements while systems like the Gentle/s (Loureiro et al. 2003) and MIME (Burgar et al. 2000) robots are capable of three dimensional (3-D) PTP training. Studies have shown that these early robotic therapy systems improve motor function as quantified by motor performance measures such as movement time and smoothness during reaching (Rohrer et al. 2002) and standard clinical measures of motor impairment such as the Upper Extremity Fugl-Meyer (UE-FM (Fugl-Meyer et al. 1975). Despite this, they have mixed impact on learned non-use and the ability to use the impaired arm in real tasks (Prange et al 2006). Given the promise of robot-assisted therapies, it is important to further investigate the mapping between practice and real-world ADL function and determine what mechanisms influence it.

Recent evidence from neuroscience literature suggests that enriched environments (Will et al 2004; Fisher and Sullivan 2001; Nudo et al. 2003), highly functional and task-oriented practice environment (Carr et al. 1985;Ada et al. 1995; Trombly et al. 1995; Aycock et al. 2004, Bayona et al. 2005; Wu et al. 2000; Woldag et al. 2003; Theilman et al. 2004), and highly motivating fun and game-based environments that increase task engagement (Bach-y-rita et al 2002, Wood et al. 2003) are important for motor re-learning, recovery after stroke and reduced learned non-use behavior. Task-oriented therapies facilitate the practice of a variety of simple and complex functional movements within a real context, with environment feedback to cue task success or failure. Occupational therapists Wu and colleagues have shown that the presence of real objects as the target of reach significantly influences the reaching kinematics of both neurologically normal and stroke impaired persons (Wu et al. 2000, 1998). In fact, reaching towards a real object is more likely to result in smoother movements, lower movement times, and higher peak velocities. These results were also verified by Wisneski and Johnson (Wisneski and Johnson 2006, 2007) for complex ADLs such as drinking and eating. Successful examples of novel task-oriented therapy are forced-use and Constrained-Induced Movement Therapy (CIMT) (Taub et al. 1994; Taub et al. 1999; Sterr et al. 2000; Liepert et al. 2002; Page et al. 2004; Aycock et al. 2004). The training is intense and repetitive, requiring the use of the impaired arm. Data indicate that CIMT therapies reduce learned non-use, increase ADL function, and often increase the size and change the location of the cortical area representative of a muscle function (Liepert et al. 2002). These forced-use therapies often induce changes in the motor areas especially in the motor cortex and the cerebellum.

A natural question is whether combining robot-assisted therapies with a task-oriented approach involving the practice of real ADLs would improve real world functional outcomes and whether current trajectory planning processes support functional retraining on complex ADLs such as drinking and eating. The trend in the field has been towards the development task-oriented, biofeedback mechanical systems with virtual environments that permit the practice of real ADL tasks and some form of biofeedback (Huang et al. 2006). Examples of such environments include Jiping He and colleagues's RUPERT upper arm exoskeleton (He et al. 2005) and Riener and colleagues's ARMIn upper arm exoskeleton (Nef et al. 2006) that embed robot assisted training into patient-centered, engaging, and focused on daily living activities with virtual functional objects.

Currently few clinical trials exist that test whether robot-assisted therapies can be more effective when combined with a highly task-oriented therapy paradigm that focuses on the practice of ADLs in virtual or real environments. One study did examine the effect of adding grasping to the planar manipulation environment of the MIT-MANUS (Fasoli et al 2005). No additive effect for the reach-to-grasp practice was found but this was most likely due to differences in the intensity of training administered to the two groups and the use of motor impairment measures (the UE-FM was used to judge motor gains) to evaluate between group differences. It is still not clear what gains were made in ADL functioning on real-world tasks or how robot-assisted practice may have influenced the CNS cortical changes.

The rehabilitation robotics lab at the Medical College of Wisconsin and Marquette University has developed the Activities of Daily Living Exercise Robot (ADLER) stroke training environment, which was inspired by the Gentle/s system set-up to accommodate reaching and grasping activities in the three-dimensions (Johnson et al. 2006). Here robot-assisted training is focused on improving carryover of motor gains to real life through ADL task practice and the trajectory models used to implement movement plans in 2-D and 3-D space. The chapter presents the design and several case studies to evaluate some of the main design concepts of the robot system. The ADLER was developed to train functional ADL-like tasks with and without physical objects. It capitalizes on the existing benefits of robot-assisted therapies while supporting more natural movements to position the wrist during ADL practice. Three case studies with a few able-bodied and stroke adults were conducted to evaluate the performance of the ADLER system. Case study 1 examined issues in repeatability and stability of kinematic measures such as movement time and smoothness. Case study 2 examined issues in modeling and trajectory planning of wrist movements for a real ADL task, the drink task. Case study 3 examined ADLER system's ability to reduce motor impairment and improve ADL function during the practice of point-to-point (PTP) movements that mimic real ADL tasks. Overall, these case studies show that the system has the potential to be effective in training of the upper arm after stroke with future work focused on the ability to improve both reaching and grasping abilities in the long-term.

2. Activities of Daily Living Exercise Robot (ADLER)

2.1 Hardware

ADLER is a robot therapy environment developed to permit training of real-life functional tasks involving reach, grasp, and object transportation in both 2-D and 3-D space (Fig. 1ab) (Johnson et al. 2006). The system is designed to support seated functional tasks such as grooming, drinking, eating, and desktop vocational tasks such as game playing tasks including tic-tac-toe. ADLER uses a HapticMaster robot (FCS Robotics) to assist an impaired arm along trajectories for real-life tasks and administer customized forces along programmed trajectories. The HapticMaster is an admittance-controlled, 6 degrees of freedom (DOFs) robot. Three active DOFs position the hand in space. The end-effector of the robot can pivot 1 full radian and has a vertical range of 0.40 m. The arm pivots about a post, with end-effector positions ranging between a radius of 0.28 m and 0.64 m. A three-axis force sensor located at the end-effector measures interaction forces (3 DOF) generated during the tasks. The three remaining DOFs orient the wrist passively through rotation of a three-axis gimbal. Fig. 1b illustrates the range of gimbal position in the ADLER environment with an approximation of the actual task space, which is often extended beyond the end-effector, depending on the orthosis used.

Several custom-designed orthoses have been designed for attaching an impaired limb to the gimbal at either the wrist or the forearm (close to the elbow) without impeding grasp. The configuration permits the subject to orient freely their hand as needed to grasp and use an object (Fig. 2ab). Orthoses have also been constructed to support lower-functioning stroke survivors that have no grasp capability, i.e. those that need to begin training in the reaching phase only (Fig. 2c).
A custom-made glove is designed to assist in functional grasping as needed (Nathan and Johnson 2007). The glove uses bend sensors (Flexpoint Sensor Systems) to detect finger joint angle changes between 0 and 90 degrees. Sensors measure the joint angles of the 2nd interphalangeal joint (PIP) of the index finger and the distal interphalangeal joint of the thumb during the tracking movements. At present only the index finger and thumb is incorporated since these are most often involved in ADLs to complete whole arm grasp, pinch and cyinder grips (Ada et al. 1995). The glove can be used with a functional electrical stimulation (FES) unit to assist in voluntary grasp and release or passive grasp and release. The current glove design is minimally evasive and does not interfere during task performance and to allow appropriate hand shaping before and during grasp with open-ended finger tips to allow haptic feedback and better grasping and shaping of the hand.
Patients using the ADLER system are asked to sit on a rail-mounted chair that can be easily pushed into position. The chair can be positioned on either side of the table. The table height is adjustable, and a custom-made harness is available to restrain motion of the trunk. To ensure subject safety during robot therapy, three safety systems are integrated into ADLER. First, power to the robot can be cut (halting any motion of the arm) and all systems shut down with the use of an emergency stop button held by an experimenter. The second safety system, controlled by the subject, is a foot pedal placed under the dominant foot that must be depressed during any operation of the robot. If at any time the subject lifts his or her foot off the pedal, the robot halts all motion. Finally, all orthoses attach to the gimbal magnetically with a pair of solenoids. Current through the two solenoids is automatically stopped if a force overload is detected and the orthoses detaches.

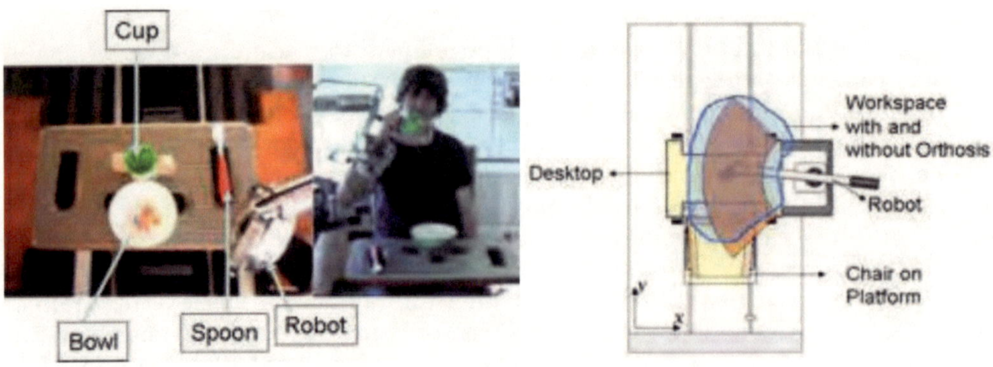

Fig. 1. The set-up for the ADLER stroke therapy system.

The system consists of an activity table and tray for selfcare-like tasks such as eating. The chair is on guide rails that permit it to be adjusted and mounted on either side of the table. The HapticMaster robot is the main system used and is customized wrist orthosis that permits the hands to be free for 3-D spatial functional movements such as drinking.

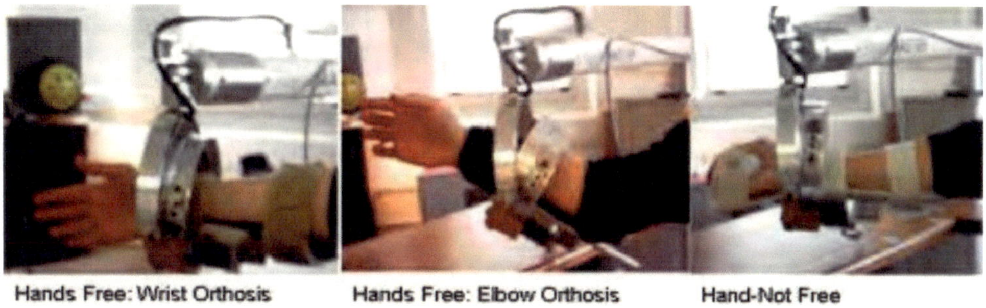

Fig. 2a-c. The ADLER Orthoses.

Three orthoses for ADLER; depending on the protocol used and tasks, these orthoses are interchangeable with the system.

2.2 Software

The ADLER system uses a custom-designed software called HERALD to implement various upper arm functional movements. The HERALD software, flow-charted in Fig. 3a, uses HapticAPI (FCS Robotics Manual 2003) to control the HapticMaster robot and Crystal Space v0.98 (Tyberghein et al. 2004), a freeware for creating graphical user interfaces (GUIs), to render the simulated environment. Crystal Space is an open-source engine that is platform and application programming interface (API) independent. In the ADLER system, we use this engine within a PC-based Windows XP environment. The safety signals from the foot pedal and emergency stop are also monitored by HERALD. The glove signals are also monitored so that the glove collection rate can be synchronized with the robot system.

In HERALD, the experimenter can define all the parameters for a task and the training modes. The experimenter is able to program arm movements on-the-fly using start, end, and multiple via points or upload the data from a file storing real or pre-defined trajectories. HERALD can also be used to set boundaries within the robotic workspace, for example, to prevent the gimbal from scraping against the table.

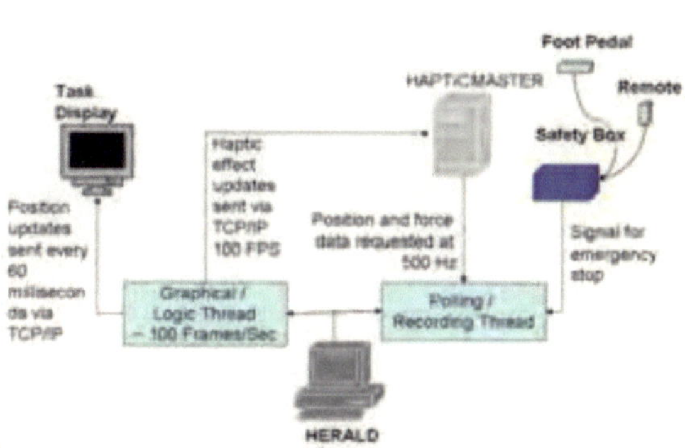

A.

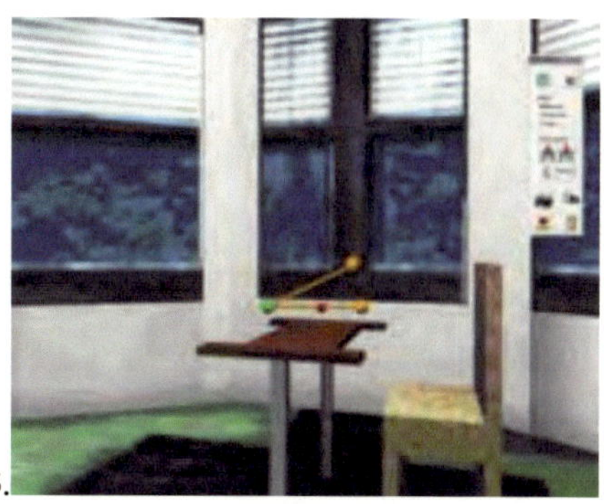

B.

Fig. 3. HERALD Control software.

a. Signal flow to and from HERALD. b. Graphical interface where spheres denote via-points with straight line trajectories. Colored dots indicate the gimbal position and the current target via-point.

HERALD's graphical interface displays a one-to-one mapping of the task environment, which consists of the platform, table, chair, and straight-line or curved connections to the key points in the trajectories (Fig. 3b). Typically, one of the experimenters operates the computer and monitors the therapy on-screen. Audio cues signal acquisition of key events that correspond to pre-programmed points in the real task, providing feedback to the user and experimenters. The system actively acquires the position and the orientation of the gimbal center as well as the forces on the end-effecter at up to 1250 Hz. Training session data are stored automatically.

2.3 Training Paradigms in ADLER

In order to accommodate a range of training protocols, ADLER is able to operate in three modes: normal, form, and function. Normal mode permits unconstrained subject motion anywhere within the robot workspace. In form mode the subject is constrained to move along a defined path between via-points. When a via-point is reached, the robot emits an audible cue and continues along a new path to the next point. The robot pulls the user with a spring force traveling at a minimum velocity set by the experimenters. In function mode the subject is constrained to a cylindrical space around the defined path between via-points, allowing more freedom than form mode. A spring force, again with a minimum velocity, pulls the user towards and along the axial path. When the user moves into a defined spherical volume around each via-point called a pull zone, a spring force pulls the user radially towards the via-point. Form and function modes are illustrated in Fig. 4. Assistance can be provided in form and function modes by increasing the spring constant, or removed entirely by setting the spring constant to zero. The robot can also resist user motion in any mode by setting a velocity-dependent damping coefficient.

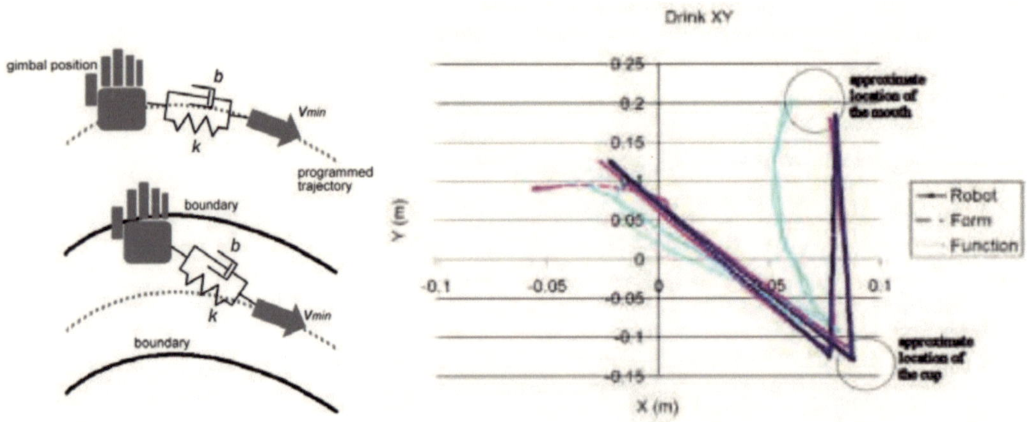

Fig. 4. Movement Modes.

Form (a) versus function (b) concept implemented in the ADLER training modes. The subject performed in function and form modes. The subject starts at location in upper left quadrant. The functional mode allowed for more natural trajectories.

Subjects using ADLER may be classified as high, medium, or low functioning. ADL training protocols have been developed for each. High functioning subjects train with tasks that involve grasping and manipulating objects. Medium and low-functioning subjects may begin by performing PTP tasks that mimic functional ADLs and then progress to performing reaching and grasping tasks with the FES Grasp glove integrated with ADLER. Table 1 displays some of the training tasks currently programmed in ADLER. Subjects are evaluated in the normal mode with the tasks from Table 1 or additional evaluation tasks as shown in Table 2.

2.3.1 Point-to-Point Reaching Robot Training

Two-dimensional reaching movements are guided by a flat-screen computer monitor on the activity table (Fig. 5a). Subjects move from one highlighted point to another, tracing predefined shapes and paths. While the entire monitor is contained within the robotic workspace, certain points can be excluded if the subject is not able to reach them. Three dimensional reaching movements are designed to be similar to those of functional activities. For instance, to mimic the actions of drinking from a cup, the subject may be asked to touch a point on the activity table, reach up to his/her mouth, touch the table again, and return his/her hand to rest. Subjects can practice these tasks repeatedly and at different levels of assistance or resistance.

2.3.2 Task-oriented Robot Training

Task-oriented robot training consists of functional, self-care tasks such as eating, drinking (Fig. 5 and Tables 1 and 2), combing hair, game-playing tasks such as tic-tac-toe (against the experiment or against the computer, and household manipulation tasks such as ringing a bell or opening doors and locks. Typically, game-playing tasks are only performed in normal mode, but robot impedance characteristics can be modified to react faster or slower in response to the forces on the end-effector. Task-oriented robot-assistance can be performed in any of the three modes.

	Task Name	**High-ADL**	**Low-ADL**
ADLs	Drink	Subject reaches, grasps and lifts a cup; drinks; returns cup.	Subject reaches, touches red dot; touches mouth; touches red dot.
	Comb	Subject reaches, grasps, and lifts a comb; lifts comb to side of head; combs up and down twice; returns comb.	Subject reaches, touches blue dot; touches side of head; touches blue dot.
PTP	Reaching	Subject reaches straight out, presses a buzzer	Subject reaches straight out to a colored dot
	Point-to-point	Subject traces a 2-D pattern with a pointer.	Subject follows a 2-D pattern without a pointer.
Other tasks	Doors	Subject performs a sequence of tasks that unlocks and opens nine different doors.	Subject reaches and touches nine sets of colored dots in specific sequences.
Fun	Tic-tac-toe	Subject plays tic-tac-toe in normal mode with custom-designed board and pieces	N/A
	Plinko	Subject plays drops a ping pong ball into plinko game in normal mode	N/A

Table 1. Examples of training tasks on ADLER.

ADLER supports several categories of task from selfcare tasks such as feeding and drinking, reaching tasks in 2D and 3D space and fun tasks.

Task Name	Description
Reach	Subject reaches outward to six points
Drink	Subject reaches, grasps and lifts a cup with one hand; drinks; returns cup.
Bilateral Drink	Subject reaches, grasps and lifts a cup with both hands; drinks; returns cup.
Point-to-Point	Subject traces circle and cross patterns
Jebsen-Taylor	Subject performs a Jebsen-Taylor evaluation task

Table 2. Evaluation tasks supported on ADLER.

ADLER supports several evaluation tasks that are performed without forces in the normal mode. From selfcare tasks such as feeding and drinking, reaching tasks in 2D and 3D space and fun tasks.

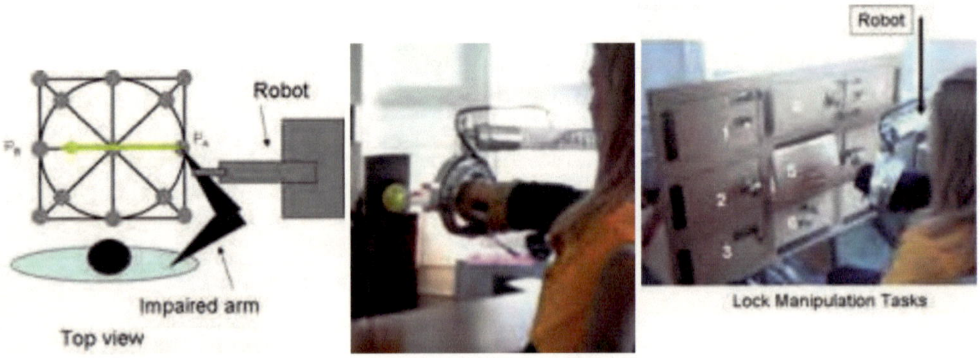

Fig. 5. ADLER Activities.

The ADL activity table set up in the ADLER environment; a. 2-D PTP reaching; b. patient practicing functional reaching; c. patient practicing manipulation.

2.4 Trajectory Planning for Functional and More Natural Wrist Movements

Typically, robot-mediated movements between via-points in reaching tasks are modeled on the minimum jerk theory of movement (Flash & Hogan, 1985; Flash & Hogan, 1987; Amirabdollahian et al. 2003; Loureiro et al. 2003). The minimum jerk algorithm defines straight-line movements and bell shaped velocity curves with zero starting and ending velocities. However, more complex models may be necessary to describe reaching during ADLs. The presence of a real object modifies the orientation of the wrist for the reach-to-grasp movement (Gentilucci et al. 1991, 1996, 2002; Gentilucci, 2005; Wu et al. 1998; Wu et al. 2000). Loureiro and colleagues, in their study of 3-D tracking in the Gentle/s robot-assisted therapy environment, proposed the use of 7th order polynomial curves with varying boundary conditions to better approximate reaching towards real objects (Loureiro et al. 2003; Amirabdollahian et al. 2003).

We had investigated the influence of objects on reaching movements and compared the results to a popular current trajectory model called the minimum-jerk model (Wisneski &

Johnson 2007). Wrist movements were significantly curved away from a predicted straight line and they were curved to accommodate task constraints such as the table, a cup handle, or an obstacle. Supporting real task trajectories means identifying trajectory planning models that better account for curvatures observed in real tasks. We have also developed a 5th order model based on curvature equations reported by Flash and Hogan with modified input conditions (Flash & Hogan, 1985; Flash & Hogan, 1987). The models are described in Fig. 6 and show the contrast in how accurately the models approximate the actual trajectories. Wisneski & Johnson demonstrated that the model with curvature consideration is adequate for functional task planning (providing the input conditions in Table 4 are well defined) however the basic minimum-jerk model without curvature is adequate for PTP movement and planar movements (Wisneski & Johnson 2007). Table 3 shows the relevant equations for these raw data along with the raw subject data. The minimum jerk model with curvature considerations combined with the model inputs for via points was a better fit than the basic model (Model A in Table 3). The model inputs lead to significant reduction of area between data curves; these area reductions were seen for all events as compared to the original minimum jerk paradigm (Model C - 5th order with initial conditions such as those seen in Table 4 for the drink task).

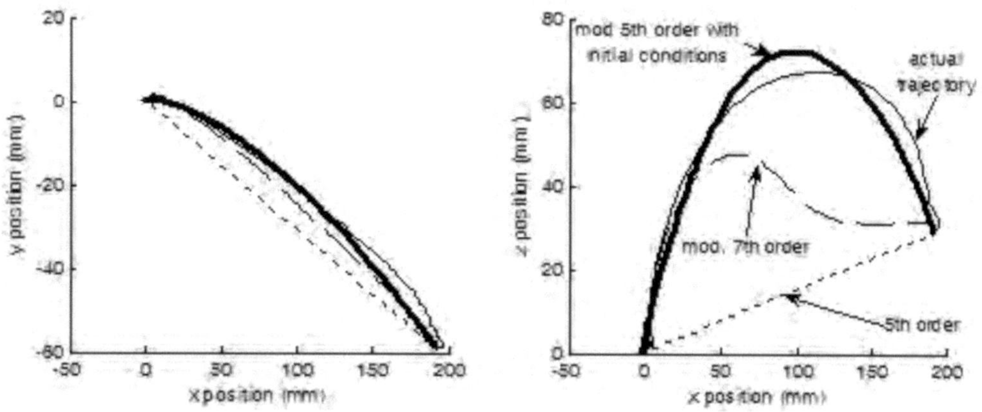

Fig. 6. Trajectory Planning Fits.

Three trajectory models supported by ADLER and an actual trajectory defined from motion analysis studies for a reach to a cup during drinking. Model C based on the 5th order trajectory with curvature and end-point considerations was the best fit for X-Y and X-Z planes.

3. Case Studies

3.1 Methods

Three case studies presented below examine how two healthy, right-handed normal-functioning adults and a low-functioning stroke survivor used and experienced ADLER and its various modes. All subjects gave informed consent for the study, which was approved by the Institutional Review Board of the Clement J. Zablocki VA Medical Center. Table 5 summarizes the able-bodied subjects in this case study.

Case study 1 examines issues in repeatability and stability of kinematic measures such as movement time and smoothness. Able-bodied subjects (age 59 - S1 and age 55-S2) experienced the ADLER robot three times at the beginning and end of one week. The tasks for this study were defined using the 5th order minimum jerk model (Model A, Tables 3). The subjects completed both reaching and grasping phases of a battery of ADLs. Only the drink task is shown and analyzed for kinematic parameters.

Model	Defining equations and boundary conditions	
A. 5th order minimum jerk	$x(t) = x_o + (x_o - x_f)(15\tau^4 - 6\tau^5 - 10\tau^3)$ $y(t) = y_o + (y_o - y_f)(15\tau^4 - 6\tau^5 - 10\tau^3)$ $z(t) = z_o + (z_o - z_f)(15\tau^4 - 6\tau^5 - 10\tau^3)$ Zero velocity, acceleration at initial and final points	The 5th order minimum jerk model for reaching is widely used in robotic therapy (Flash & Hogan, 1985; Flash & Hogan, 1987).
B. Modified 7th order minimum jerk	$p(\tau) = a + b\tau + d\tau^3 + f\tau^5 + h\tau^7$ where $a = \frac{1}{2}\sum p; b = v_{mid}; d = -3v_{mid} + \frac{35}{16}\Delta p$ $f = 3v_{mid} - \frac{21}{8}\Delta p; h = -v_{mid} + \frac{15}{16}\Delta p$ $\sum p = p_f + p_s; \Delta p = p_f - p_s$ Zero velocity, acceleration at initial and final points. Maximum velocity and zero acceleration at 50% reach.	This modified 7th order model was developed by Loureiro and colleagues as a better approximation of actual reach towards an object (Loureiro et al. 2003; Amirabdollahian et al. 2003).
C. 5th order curvature model	$x^-(\tau) = \frac{t_f^5}{720}(\pi_1(\tau_1^4(15\tau^4 - 30\tau^3) + \tau_1^3(80\tau^3 - 30\tau^4$ $- 60\tau^3\tau_1^2 + 30\tau^4\tau_1 - 6\tau^5) + c_1(15\tau^4 - 10\tau^3 - 6$ $x^+(\tau) = x^-(\tau) + \pi_1 \frac{t_f^5(\tau - \tau_1)^5}{120}$ where $c_1 = \frac{1}{t_f^5 \tau_1^2 (1-\tau_1)^5}((x_f - x_0)(300\tau_1^5 - 1200\tau_1^4 + 1600\tau_1^3)$ $+ \tau_1^2(-720x_f + 120x_1 + 600x_0) + (x_0 - x_1)(300\tau_1 - 2$ $\pi_1 = \frac{1}{t_f^5 \tau_1^5 (1-\tau_1)^5}((x_f - x_0)(120\tau_1^5 - 300\tau_1^4 + 200\tau_1^3) - 20(x_1 -$ Zero velocity, acceleration at initial and final points. Via point (x_1, y_1, z_1) defined at time $\tau_1 = 0.4$ (40% of reach).	This modified 5th order model is based on equations developed by Hogan and Flash to describe reaching. We have applied special inputs to the equations based on motion analysis studies to approximate functional reaching.

Table 3. Summary of Trajectory Planning Models Investigated.

Three trajectory models supported by ADLER and an actual trajectory defined from motion analysis studies. The critical time for via points and the Cartesian inputs are as X1, Y1, and Z1.

Model Input#	Purpose	Applicable Events	*t1*	X1	Y1	Z1
1	Table Constraint (TC)	'Reach' 'Rest'	.40 .40	N/A N/A	N/A N/A	42 mm 28 mm
2	TC+Cup Manipulation	'Reach' 'Rest'	.40 .40	39mm 39mm	N/A N/A	T.C. + 12 mm T.C. + 7mm
3	Movement out-of-the-plane (MOP)	'To Mouth' 'Return Object'	.40 .40	N/A N/A	N/A N/A	59mm 59mm
4	MOP + a cup-type object	'To Mouth' 'Return Object'	.23 .40	16mm 16mm	N/A N/A	10.5mm 10.5mm

Table 4. Settings of Model C for A Drink Task.

Summary of input and output points used to define Model B for a drinking task using a cup with one hand. This setting is also used with Case Study 2.

Case study 2 examines issues in modeling and trajectory planning of wrist movements for a real ADL task, the drink task. An able-bodied subject (age 22 – S3) experienced the ADLER robot with two different trajectory planning models in the same day and compared the results. The tasks for case study 2 were defined using either Model A or the curved model Model C with input as shown in Tables 4. These tasks were drink and feed (with spoon). They were repeated at least three times. First, the subject completed the reaching and grasping phases of the tasks without a trajectory model, i.e., the subject completed the task in normal mode with no assistance from the robot and the ADLER is only recording movement and forces. Next, the subject repeated the tasks with Models A and C and then answered questions about their experiences. Only the drink task is shown and analyzed for kinematic parameters.

Case study 3 examines ADLER system's ability to reduce motor impairment and improve ADL function during the practice of Low ADL movements (Table 1). The stroke survivor was 48 years old and sustained an ischemic stroke four years before with hemiparesis of the left side (Fig. 7).

Subjects	Gender	Trained with	Age	Mode	Robot Mode Assist/Resist	Motor Functional level	Trajectory Model Used
S1	Female	Left hand	59	Function	Assist	Able-Bodied	Model A (Table 3)
S2	Male	Left hand	55	Form	Assist	Able-Bodied	Model A (Table 3)
S3	Male	Left hand	22	Form	Assist	Able-Bodied	Model A Model C (Table 4)
S4	Male	Left Impaired hand	48	Form	Assist	Stroke(RCVA) UE-FT: Level2 UE-FM: 22	Model A (Table 3)

Table 5. Subjects for Case Studies 1-3.

Summary of able-bodied and stroke subjects ran on ADLER. The stroke survivor had a right CVA and motor functional level (UE-FM) of 22 of 66 and an ADL functional (UE-FT) of level 2 of 7.

The stroke subject participated in the reaching aspects of the functional tasks but was not able to participate in the grasping portion (the FES glove was not worn in this instant). The training was conducted in form mode using 2-D and 3-D PTP reaching tasks mimicking ADLs. These tasks were programmed using Model A. As the subject improved, the force assistance (gains on the spring forces) was gradually decreased. Training sessions were administered three times per week for six weeks, with each lasting for approximately one hour. Clinical and robotic evaluations sessions using tasks in Table 2 were completed in the first, third, and last weeks of training. Clinical evaluations included upper-extremity Fugl-Meyer (UE-FM) and functional test (UE-FT) evaluations administered by an occupational therapist (Fugl-Meyer et al. 1975; Wilson et al. 1994). A follow-up evaluation was conducted about one month after the final training period. The ADLER evaluations, completed in normal mode (without force assist), allow for quantification of kinematic improvement without the aid of robotic assistance.

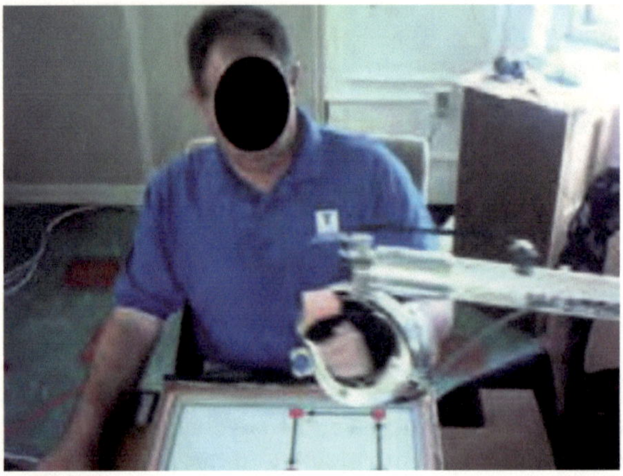

Fig. 7: Stroke Subject in ADLER.

Training takes place using ADLER to complete several low ADL tasks. The low functioning stroke is completing a 2-D PTP.

Force and position data recorded by HERALD were filtered (10 Hz Butterworth low pass) and analyzed using Matlab software (The MathWorks, Inc.). Several kinematic dependent variables were calculated for Case Studies 1 and 2. Total displacement (TD) is the total distance traveled during a given task. The total time required to complete a given task is the movement time (MT). Peak Velocity (PV) is the maximum velocity used in the task. Several measures of smoothness are calculated from the velocity profile, including the ratio of peak velocity (PV) to mean velocity. The movement smoothness (MS) is defined as the peak velocity divided by the average velocity (PV/MeanV) (Rohrer et al. 2002). Trajectories are charted on two position plots, where the initial starting position is normalized to point (0, 0, 0). The x-y plane is parallel to the activity table top, while the z axis points up. The responses to questions about Model A and C for case study 2 were analyzed and compared using t-test.

3.2 Results and Discussion of Cases

3.2.1 Case Study 1: Repeatability and Short-term Learning

Table 6 shows the results of the drink evaluation sessions. We expected that able-bodied subjects may have some short-term learning but that, in general, they would have minimum changes across the key kinematic variables. Subject 1 had consistent kinematics across all kinematic variables with low standard deviations. The fact that S2 had more variance than S1 may indicate that some subjects may require more time during training than others. In addition, we realized that a possible source of error is in the placement of artifacts during it repeatable task trial. It is important the artifacts are placed in the same location during these trials. On the other hand subject 2 only had consistent kinematics across total displacement and peak velocity. Figure 8 shows an example of the results for subject 1.

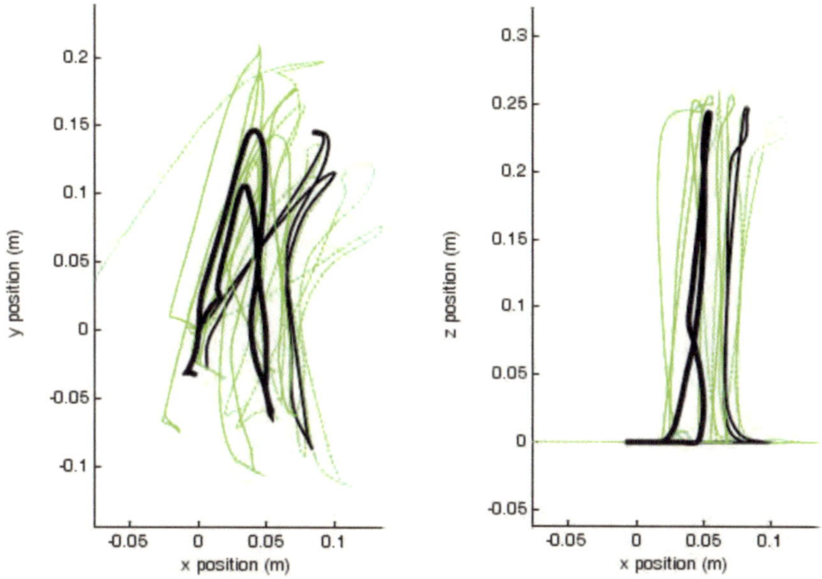

Fig. 8. XY and XZ plane data of the drink task for subject 1 for all trials for 1st and last evaluations.

The graphical data show all three trials and averages for days 1 and 4. Day 1 is solid lines (thick average line) and Day 4 is dash lines (thin line average). XY is the plane of the table and XZ in out of the plane of the table in the plane of the person's torso.

Subject	Initial				Final			
	MT (s)	TD (m)	PV (m/s)	MS	MT (s)	TD (m)	PV (m/s)	MS
S1	7.26	2.36	0.40	3.04	7.38	2.41	0.40	2.95
	±0.39	±0.13	±0.04	±0.23	±0.67	±0.13	±0.01	±0.23
S2	17.51	2.65	0.21	3.06	4.31	2.02	0.33	2.24
	±8.22	±0.65	±0.02	±0.38	±1.09	±0.12	±0.04	±0.18

Table 6. Able-bodied subjects' kinematics are shown. The evolution of Movement Time (MT), Peak Velocity (PV), Total Displacement (TD) and movement smoothness (MS) are shown across two evaluation sessions. S1 was more stable that S2

3.2.2 Case Study 2: Model Evaluation on ADLER

The results from the case study are presented in Figures 9 and 10. The area between curves was significantly reduced for all the drink events. The new model provides a more accurate prediction of the desired functional trajectory than the old paradigm of the minimum jerk model. These results show that this trajectory generation scheme provides more appropriate wrist center paths for implementing functional tasks in the ADLER environment. This improvement was noted by the subject as well.

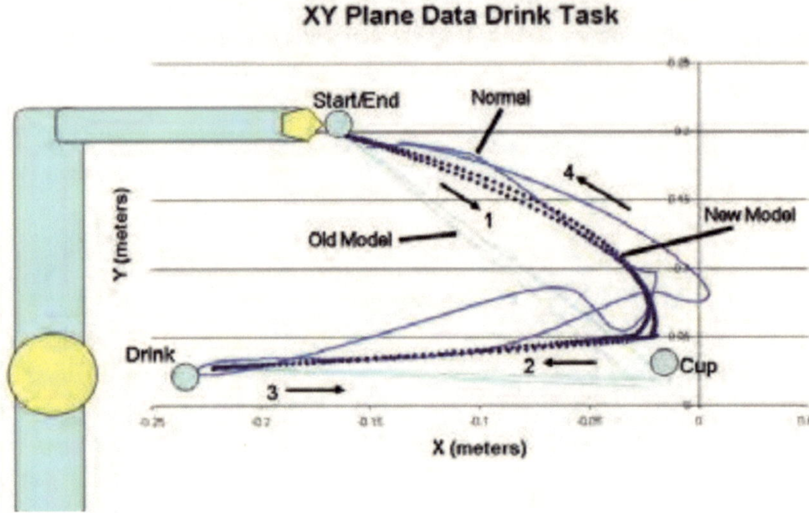

Fig. 9. XY plane data of (from top to bottom) the drink task on ADLER.

The data collected in normal mode is represented by a thick solid line, the data collected when using the old model is represented by a thin solid line (cyan), and the data collected when using the new model is represented by a dotted line. MT = 8.97 ±4.03 seconds, TD =2.23±0.33, PV= 0.29±4.03, and MS 3.70±0.73.

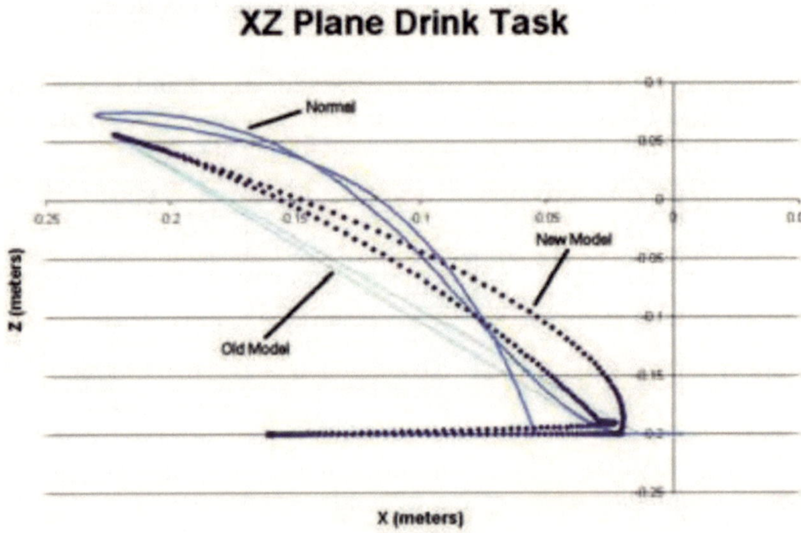

Fig. 10. XZ plane data of (from top to bottom) the drink task on ADLER.

The data collected in normal mode is represented by a thick solid line, the data collected when using the old model is represented by a thin solid line (cyan), and the data collected when using the new model is represented by a dotted line.

Table 7 shows the average responses to the questions presented to the subject after each trial. When using the new model and asked if the robot was moving the way he would have liked to move he answered with an average value of 7. This is a more positive response than for the old model, with which he answered 3. When using the new model and asked if he felt as though he had to work against the robot to complete the task he answered with an average value of 2. This is a more positive response than for the old model, with which he answered 5. His comments reveal that the old model did produce movements that did not feel natural.

Question	Response Range (1-10)	Average Response
Do you feel as though the robot is moving the way you would like to move?	10 = Yes, completely; 5 = About half the time; 1 = No, not at all	Model A: 3 +/-1 **Model C: 7 +/- 1 ***
Do you feel as though you need to fight against the robot to complete the task?	10 = Yes, all the time; 5 = About half the time; 1 = No, not at all	Model: 5 +/- 1 **Model: 2 +/- .5 ***

Table 7. Subject survey at the end of each trial.

The questions, possible responses, and average responses are listed. Representative comments were chosen for each model. If a result was statistically more successful by means of a t-Test it is marked with an asterisk and in bold.

The results from the questionnaire show that the differences seen between the new and old model can be felt by the subject and that using the new model provides for a more comfortable experience and more natural feeling movements. The obvious next step is to complete this analysis with stroke survivors to determine their response to the changes. Since stroke survivors are more likely to have decreased proprioception that affects their ability to sense their arm in space, we anticipate less sensitivity to changes in arm position in space. The question of whether training using these more accurate and natural movement paths will translate into the ability to dynamically position and orientate the impaired arm for various ADL artifacts (e.g., spoon, comb etc.) and the ability to use any performance improvements seen in less supervised environments.

3.2.3 Case Study 3: Training Evaluation on ADLER

Training improved the subject's ability to perform more functional reaching. The result of the 4 main evaluation sessions using the drink 3-D PTP patterns are illustrated in Fig. 11 and the biomechanical measures for kinematics and the clinical measures of ADL and motor function are shown in Table 8. The subject's UE-FT improved by two levels, while UE-FM scores did not change during training. However, this subject was low functioning and did not practice grasping objects, so improvement in UE-FM testing was not expected. A clinical evaluation 1 month (at about 6 weeks) after the end of training showed that the subject maintained a UE-FT score of level 4 and a UE-FM score of 24/66.

Table 8 summarizes the evolution of the key kinematic variables derived for S4. We expected that the kinematic variables of movement time and smoothness (Peak V/mean V) would consistently decrease as evaluation proceeded from pre to post to follow-up and approach normal values (Rohrer et al 2002; Krebs et al. 2002; Wu et al 2000). In general this expectation was met and can be seen from the data for S1 and S2 in Tables 7and S4 in Table 8.

We expected that the peak velocity and total displacement would consistently increase as evaluation proceeded from pre to post to follow-up and approach normal values. Table 8 clearly shows the gain in peak velocity over time. Overall total displacement was not consistent from pre- to post-training and follow-up because this measure as calculated evaluated the entire movement included those that were not useful to accomplish the task.
From Figure 11, it is clear that the subject's height off the table increased and the range of motion on the table also increased. This implies that although overall TD did not behave consistently, therefore, in the future, a better and more sensitive kinematic measure could be derived in terms of increases in height (z) and table top range of motion (x-y area). We anticipate that when we include the FES grasp glove, especially for low-functioning stroke survivors, we will add the inclusion of a curvature and orientation measure to detect changes in dynamic orientation of the hand during functional reaching to an ADL artifact such as the cup in the drink task.
The subject used the normal mode to complete the evaluation tasks and the training modes to complete the training tasks. The drink task is shown.

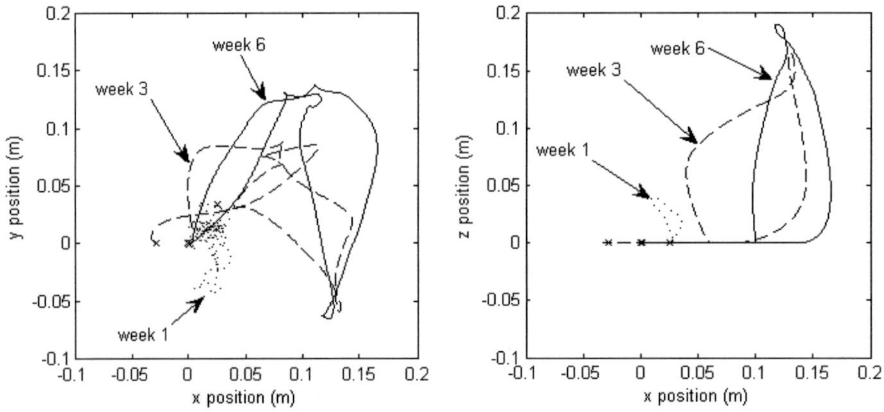

Fig. 11. Drinking Task Changes in XY and XZ planes.

The evolution of movement for the drink task are shown for the evaluation sessions from pre-training (Week 1) to follow-up (Week 6) for the drink task. The subject had increasingly more height in the Z direction as time passed and covered more table area in the X-Z area.

The key changes seen translated mainly into increased shoulder and elbow movement, which lead to change from level 2 to 4 on ADL function. This result is typical of systems that training only reaching performance (Loureiro et al. 2003; Krebs et al. 2002; Prange et al. 2006). Since grasp function did not improve and is required for ADL function on levels 5 through 7, we anticipate that training to assist opening and closing of the hand for grasping as well as reaching via the full integration of the FES game glove into the ADLER system will improve these results. In addition to gaining data from lower functioning stroke subjects, we are also evaluating the performance of higher-functioning stroke survivors with low to medium grasping capability on the ADLER system (with and without FES glove). We hope to see improvement in the UE-FM and UE-FT scores of these subjects due to more functional training. We also anticipate greater improvement following the full implementation of curved trajectory models (Model C especially). The first stroke subject was trained using PTP trajectories defined by the straight-line, 5th order minimum jerk model. We expect that the curved trajectories, which approximate better actual movements, will result in improved recovery.

Evaluation Session	Biomechanical and Clinical Measures					
	MT (s)	TD (m)	PV (m/s)	MS	UE-FM	UE-FT
Initial	15.78 ±5.65	2.51 ±0.46	0.26 ±0.01	3.90 ±0.68	23	Level 2
Week 1	12.75 ±4.01	2.05 ±0.23	0.23 ±0.10	4.32 ±1.32	27	Level 2
Week 3	8.14 ±1.42	1.88 ±0.37	0.28 ±0.031	2.93 ±0.20	23	Level 2
Week 6	6.38 ±0.13	2.08 ±0.13	0.27 ±0.03	2.97 ±0.54	23	Level 4
Follow-up	12.59 ±1.01	2.89 ±0.59	0.36 ±0.05	3.27 ±0.94	24	Level 4

Table 8. Evolution of the Kinematics of S3 (Stroke) on PTP drink task.

The table shows the changes in movement time (MT), total displacement (TD), smoothness (PV/MeanV), and clinical values for motor impairment (UE-FM with 66 as maximum) and ADL function (UE-FT: Level 7 maximum).

4. Conclusion

This chapter discussed the development of a task-oriented therapy robot focused on real ADL training and performance. The development of the software, HERALD, and the hardware platform and FES grasp glove has been discussed. We also presented training and trajectory planning models that have been implemented with the system along with defining the pros and cons of three possible models that can be used to accurately reflect natural movement of the wrist during ADL task. We presented three case studies that briefly examined how the system has repeatable performance and has the ability to train stroke survivors. A low functioning stroke survivor was successfully trained on the system using PTP ADL-like movement. The subject's kinematics, especially movement time and movement smoothness decreased reflecting motor impairment reduction and increased motor control. The ADL functioning was improved on tasks involving more shoulder and elbow function but not on task involving grasp. In the future, the FES glove will be fully integrated in the ADLER system to allow stroke clients on all levels of motor function and ADL ability to be trained in both reaching and grasping ADLs. As such we anticipate that a major impact will then be seen on both motor impairment and functional scales.

We also presented via case study 2 different trajectory models for planning and assisting movement of the wrist using ADLER. We demonstrated that models that included curvature and had customized inputs can improve a subject's movement kinematics for an ADL tasks such as drinking and can affect their perception of the ease or difficulty of the movement. In the case study performed on the ADLER system, the subject reported a "more natural" feel when operating with the new model rather than the old model. This shows that the model appears to meet the goal of providing a more natural prediction of functional wrist paths. Although these results are promising it is understood that much more work to be done and there is a need to examine movements from the perspective of the stroke survivor.

In the near future, we will be improving our models for trajectory planning of ADL movements as well as examining whether the ADLER system including the FES glove can improve both motor and ADL function.

5. References

(AHA) American Heart Association. Heart Disease and Stroke Statistics – 2005 Update. Dallas, TX: American Heart Association; 2005

Ada L., Canning C.G., Carr J.H., Kilbreath S.L., Shepherd R.B. "Task-specific training of reaching and manipulation." In Insights into Reach to Grasp movement. K.M.B. Bennett and U. Castiello (Editors). Elsevier Science B.V. 1994

Abend W, Bizzi E, Morasso P: Human arm trajectory formation. *Brain* 1982, Vol 105, pp. 331-348.

Amirabdollahian, F, (2003). An investigation of roboti-mediated therapies and therapy effects on the recovery of upper limb post stroke. *University of Reading, Department of Cybernetics, Dissertation Thesis*. September.

Amirabdollahian, F.; Loureiro, R. & Harwin, W., (2002). Minimum jerk trajectory control for rehabilitation and haptic applications. *Proceedings of IEEE Int Conf on Robotics Automation*, Washington DC, May, pp. 3380-3385.

Atkeson CG, Hollerbach JM: **Kinematic features of unrestrained vertical arm movements.** *Journal of Neuroscience* 1985, 5(9): 2318-2330.

Aycock DM. Blanton S. Clark PC. Wolf SL. What is constraint-induced therapy? *Rehabilitation Nursing*. 29(4):114-5, 121, 2004

Bach y Rita P, Wood S, Leder R, Paredes O, Bahr D, Bach-y-Rita EW, Murillo N. "Computer assisted motivating rehabilitation for institutional, home, and educational late stroke programs." *Top Stroke Rehabil*, Vol. 8, Issue 4, pp. 1–10, 2002

Barton, L. A. & Wolf, S. L., (1993). Learned nonuse in the hemiplegic upper extremity. In Gordon WA, Editor. *Advances in Stroke Rehabilitation*. Boston: Butterworth-Heinemann; pp. 79-87, 1993

Bayona, NA.;Bitensky, J.; Salter, K. & Teasell, R. (2005a). The role of task-specific training in rehabilitation therapies. *Topics in Stroke Rehabilitation,* Vol. 12, Issue 3, pp. 58-65, 2005a

Burgar, C.G.; Lum, P.S.; Shor, P.C. & Van der Loos, H.F.M., (2000) Development of robots for rehabilitation therapy:the Palo Alto VA/Stanford experience, *Journal of Rehabilitation R&D*, Vol. 36, Issue 6, November/December.

Carr J, Shepherd R. *A Motor Relearning Programme For Stroke*. 2nd edn. Heinemann Medical, Oxford; 1987

Calautti, C. & Baron, J., (2003). Functional neuroimaging studies of motor recovery after stroke in adults. A review. *Stroke*, Vol. 34, pp. 1553-66.

Fasoli, S.; Krebs, H.I.; Stein, J.; Frontera, W.R. & Hogan, N., (2003). Effects of robotic therapy on motor impairment and recovery in chronic stroke. *Archives of Phys Med Rehabil*, vol. 84, pp. 477-84.

Fasoli, S.;Krebs, H. I.; Hughes, R., Stein J. & Hogan N., (2005). Functionally-based rehabilitation: Benefits or Buzzwrod? *Proceedings of International Conference on Rehabilitation Robotics ICORR)*, Chicago, IL, June 28-July 1, pp. 223-226, 2005.

FCS Control Systems HapticAPI Programming Manual, Version 1.2, Schipol, The Netherlands: FCS Control Systems, 2003.

Fisher, B. E. and Sullivan, K. J., "Activity-Dependent factors affecting poststroke functional outcomes." *Top Stroke Rehabil*, Vol. 8, Issue 3, pp. 31-44, 2001

Flash, T. & Hogan, N., (1985). The coordination of arm movements: An experimentally confirmed mathematical model. *The Journal of Neuroscience*, Vol. 5, pp. 1688-1703.

Fugl-Meyer, A.R.; Jaasko L. & Leyman I:, (1975). The post-stroke hemiplegic patient. A method for evaluation of physical performance. *Scandinavian Journal of Rehabilitation Medicine*, Vol. 7, pp. 13-31.

Gentilucci, M.; Castiello, U.; Corradini ML., Scarpa M., Umilta C., & Rizzolatti G., (1991). Influence of different types of grasping on the transport component of prehension movements. *Neuropsychologia*. Vol. 29, Issue 5, 361-78.

Gentilucci, M., (2002). Object motor representation and reaching-grasping control." *Neuropsychologia*. Vol. 40, Issue 8, pp. 1139-53.

Gentilucci, M.; Daprati, E.; Gangitano, M.;Saetti, M.C. & Toni, I., (1996). On orientating the hand to reach and grasp an object. *Neuroreport*. Vol. 7, pp. 589-592.

Hogan, N. & Flash, T (1987). Moving gracefully: quantitative theories of motor coordination. *TINS*. Vol. 10, Issue 4, pp. 170-174.

Hogan, N. (1984) An organizing principle for a class of voluntary movements," *Journal of Neuroscience*, Vol. 4, pp. 2745-2754.

He Huang, H., Wolf, S.L. & He J. (2006) Recent developments in biofeedback for neuromotor rehabilitation. *Journal of NeuroEngineering and Rehabilitation*. Vol. **3**, Issue 11. doi:10.1186/1743-0003-3-11

He, J.; Koeneman, E.J.; Schultz, R.S.; Huang, H.; Wanberg, J.; Herring, D.E.; Sugar, T.; Herman, R.; & Koeneman, J.B., **(2005).** Design of a robotic upper extremity repetitive therapy device. *9th International Conference on Rehabilitation Robotics, 2005. (ICORR 2005)* Volume, Issue , 28 June-1 July 2005, pp. 95 - 98

Hunter, P.; Peckham, P. & Knutson, J.S., (2005). Functional electrical stimulation for neuromuscular applications. *Annu. Rev. Biomed. Eng.* Vol 7: pp. 327–60,

Johnson, M.J.; Wisneski, K.J.; Anderson. J.; Nathan, D., & Smith. R., (2006) Development of ADLER: The Activities of Daily Living Exercise Robot. *IEEE-EMBS Biomedical Robotics (BioRob 2006)*, February 2006, Pisa, Italy, pp. 881-886.

Kahn, L. E., Zygman, M. L., Rymer, W. Z. & Reinkensmeyer, D.J., (2006). Robot-assisted reaching exercise promotes arm movement recovery in chronic hemiparetic stroke: a randomized controlled pilot study. *Journal of NeuroEngineering and Rehabilitation* 2006, Vol. 3, Issue 12, doi:10.1186/1743-0003-3-12

Krebs, H.I.; Palazzolo, J.J.; Dipietro, L.; Ferraro, M.; Krol, J.; Rannekleiv, K.; Volpe, B.T. & Hogan, N., (2003). Rehabilitation robotics: Performance-based progressive robot-assisted therapy. *Autonomous Robots*, Vol. 15, pp. 7-20.

H.I. Krebs, B.T. Volpe, et al., "Robot-aided neurorehabilitation: from evidence-based to science-based rehabilitation," *Top Stroke Rehabil*, vol. 8, no. 4, pp. 54-70, 2002.

Latash, M. L. & Nicholas, J.J. (1996). Motor control research in rehabilitation medicine. *Disability & Rehabilitation*. Vol. 18, Issue 6, pp. 293-9.

Liepert, H.; Bauder, W., Miltner, H.R. ; Taub, E. & Weiller, C., (2002). Treatment-induced cortical reorganization after stroke in humans. *Stroke*, Vol. 31, pp. 1210-1216.

Loureiro, R.; Amirabdollahian, F.; Topping, M.; Driessen, B. & Harwin, W., (2003). Upper limb robot mediated stroke therapy-GENTLE/s approach. *Autonomous Robots* Vol. 15, Issue 1, pp. 35-51.

Ma, H. & Trombly, C. A. (2002). A synthesis of the effects of occupational therapy for persons with stroke, Part II: Restoration of roles, tasks, and activities. *Am J Occup Ther*, Vol. 56, No. 3, pp. 260-74

Maclean N, Pound P, Wolfe C, Rudd A: Qualitative analysis of stroke patients motivation for rehabilitation. British Medical Journal 2000, 321(7268):1051-1054.

MacClellan, L.R.; Bradham, D.D.; Whitall, J.; Volpe, B.; Wilson, P.; Ohlhoff, J.; Meister, C.; Hogan,N.; Krebs, H.I. & Bever Jr, C., (2006) Robotic upper-limb neurorehabilitation in chronic stroke patients. *Journal of Rehabilitation R&D*, Vol. 42, No. 6, November/December, pp. 717-722

Merians, A.S.; Jack, D.; Boian, R.; Tremaine, M.; Burdea,G.C.; Adamovich,S.V.; Recce, M. & Poizner H., (2002).Virtual Reality–Augmented Rehabilitation for Patients Following Stroke. *Physical Therapy*. Vol. 82, No. 9 . September 2002, pp. 898-915

Michaelsen, S.M.; Jacobs, S.; Roby-Brami, A. & Levin, M.F. (2004) Compensation for distal impairments of grasping in adults with hemiparesis." *Experimental Brain Research*, Vol. 157, Issue 2, pp. 162-73.

Nathan and Johnson - ICORR 2007

Nelles, G., W. Jentzen, et al. (2001) Arm training induced brain plasticity in stroke studied with serial positron emission tomography. *Neuroimage*, Vol. **13**, Issue 6 Pt 1, pp. 1146-54

Nef T, Mihelj M, Colombo G, Riener R. "ARMin - Robot for Rehabilitation of the Upper Extremities." *IEEE International Conference on Robotics and Automation*, pp. 3152—3157, Orlando, Florida, May 15-19, 2006

Page, S.J.; Sisto, S.; Levine, P.; & McGrath, R.E., (2004). Efficacy of modified constraint-induced movement therapy in chronic stroke: a single-blinded randomized controlled trial. *Arch Phys Med Rehabil* , Vol. 85, pp. 14-8.

Patton, J.L.; Kovic, M. & Mussa-Ivaldi, F.A. (2006). Custom-designed haptic training for restoring reaching ability to individuals with stroke. *Journal of Rehabilitation Research and Development*, In press, 2006.

Patton, J.L.; Stoykov, M.E.; Kovic, M. & Mussa-Ivaldi, F.A., (2006). Evaluation of robotic tr aining forces that either enhance or reduce er r or in chronic hemipar etic stroke survivor s. *Exp Brain Res*, Vol. 168, pp. 368-383.

Patton, J.L. & Mussa-Ivaldi, F.A. (2004) Robot-assisted adaptive training: custom force fields for teaching movement patterns. *IEEE Transactions on Biomedical Engineering*. Vol. 51, Issue 4, pp. 636-46.

Prange, G. B.; Jannink M. J. A; Groothuis-Oudshoorn, C. G. M.; Hermens, H. J. & IJzerman, M. J., (2006). Systematic review of the effect of robot-aided therapy on recovery of the hemiparetic arm after stroke. *Journal of Rehabilitation R&D*, Vol. 43, No. 2, March/April, pp. 171-184

Reinkensmeyer, D.J.; Takahashi, C.D.; Timoszyk, W.K.; Reinkensmeyer, A. N. & Kahn, L.E., (2001). Design of robot assistance for arm movement therapy following stroke. *Advanced Robotics*, Vol. 14, No. 7, pp. 625-637.

Roby-Brami, A.; Jacobs, S.; Bennis, N. & Levin, M.F., (2003) Hand orientation for grasping and arm joint rotation patterns in healthy subjects and hemiparetic stroke patients." *Brain Research*, Vol. 969, issues 1-2, pp. 217-29.

Rohrer, B.; Fasoli, S.; Krebs, H.I.; Hughes, R.; Volpe, B.; Frontera, W.R.; Stein, J. & Hogan, N., (2002). Movement smoothness changes during stroke recovery. *Journal of Neuroscience*, Vol. 22, Issue 18, pp. 8297-304.

Schaechter, J.D., (2004) .Motor rehabilitation and brain plasticity after hemiparetic stroke. *Progress in Neurobiology*. Vol. 73, Issue 1, pp. 61-72.

Simone, L.K. & Kamper, D.G., (2005) . Design considerations for a wearable monitor to measure finger posture. *Journal of NeuroEngineering and Rehabilitation*, Vol 2, Issue 5, doi:10.1186/1743-0003-2-5

Sterr, A.; Freivogel, S. & Schmalohr, D. (2000). Neurobehavioral aspects of recovery: Assessment of the learned nonuse phenomenon in hemiparetic adolescents. *Arch Phys Med Rehabil*. Vol. 83, No. 4, pp. 1726-31

Thielman G.T., Dean C.M., Gentile A.M. "Rehabilitation of reaching after stroke: task related training versus progressive resistive exercise.," *Arch Phys Med Rehabil*, Vol. 85, pp. 1613-1618. 2004.

Trombly, C. A. & Ma, H. (2002). A synthesis of the effects of occupational therapy for persons with stroke, Part I: Restoration of roles, tasks, and activities. *Am J Occup Ther*, Vol. 56, No. 3, pp. 250-59.

Trombly C. Occupational Therapy of Physical Dysfunction. Trombly C, editor. Baltimore (MD): Williams & Wilkins; 1995

Taub E, Uswatte G, Pidikiti R. Constraint-induced movement therapy: a new family of techniques with broad application to physical rehabilitation -- a clinical review. J Rehabil Res Dev. 36(3): 1-18, 1999

Taub, E.; Crago, J.E.; Burgio LD, et al., (1994). An operant approach to rehabilitation rehabilitation medicine: overcoming learned nonuse by shaping. Journal of Experiment Analysis of Behavior. Vol. 61, pp. 281-93.

Taub, E.; Lum, P. S.; Hardin, P.; Mark V. & Uswatte. G., (2005). AutoCITE, Automated delivery of CI therapy with reduced effort by therapists. *Stroke*, Vol. 36, pp. 1301.

Tyberghein J., E. Sunshine, (2004, Aug 13). "Crystal Space 0.98 manual," available: http://www.crystalspace3d.org/docs/online/manual-0.98/.

Wilson DJ, Baker LL, Craddock JA: Functional test for the hemipar etic upper extremity. *Am J Occup Ther* 1984, 38(3):159-164.

Wisneski, K.J. & Johnson, M.J. (2006) Insights into Modeling Functional Trajectories for Robot-Mediated Daily Living Exercise Environments." *IEEE-RAS Biomedical Robotics* (BioRob 2006), February 2006.

Wisneski K. Development of a Model for Functional Upper Extremity Trajectory Generation and Implementation on the Activities of Daily Living Exercise Robot (ADLER). Masters Thesis, *Marquette University, Department of Biomedical Engineering*, August 2006.

Wisneski, K.J. & Johnson, M.J. (2007). Quantifying kinematics of purposeful movements to real, imagined, or absent functional objects: Implications for modelling trajectories for robot-assisted ADL tasks. *Journal of NeuroEngineering and Rehabilitation*, Vol 4, Issue 7, doi:10.1186/1743-0003-4-7

Woldag, H.; Waldmann, G.; Heuschkel, G. & Hummelsheim, H., (2003). Is the repetitive training of complex hand and arm movements beneficial for motor recovery in stroke patients?. *Clinical Rehabilitation*. Vol. 17, Issue 7, pp. 723-30.

Wood, S. R., N. Murillo, et al., (2003). Motivating, game-based stroke rehabilitation: a brief report. *Top Stroke Rehabil*, Vol. 10, Issue 2, pp. 134-40.

Wu C., Trombly C.A,. Lin K, & Ticke-Degnen L. (1998). Effects of object affordances on reaching performance in persons with and without cerebrovascular accident. *Am J Occup Ther* 1998

Wu C., Trombly C.A., Lin K, et al., (2000). A kinematic study of contextual effects on reaching performance in persons with and without stroke: Influences of object availability. *Arch Phys Med Rehabil*, Vol. 81, Issue 1, pp. 95-101.

Volpe BT, Ferraro M, Lynch D, Christos P, Krol J, Trudell C, Krebs HI, Hogan N., (2002). Robotics and other devices in the treatment of patients recovering from stroke. *Current Neurology & Neuroscience Reports*, Vol. 5, Issue 6, pp. 465-70.

14

Applications of Robotics to Assessment and Physical Therapy of Upper Limbs of Stroke Patients

M.-S. Ju [1], C.-C. K. Lin [2], S.-M. Chen [3], I.-S. Hwang [4], P.-C. Kung[1], Z.-W. Wu[1]
[1] *Department of Mechanical Engineering,* [2] *Department of Neurology ,* [3] *Department of Physical Medicine & Rehabilitation* [4] *Department of Physical Therapy, National Cheng Kung University*
Taiwan, R.O.C.

1. Introduction

Cerebrovascular accident or stroke is one of the major causes of debilitation in the world. The major symptoms of stroke are loss of muscle power, spasticity and in-coordination of muscle activation. In the past, the assessment of above symptoms were quite subjective by using Medical Research Council scale, Brunnstrom's stage and modified Ashworth scale and the rehabilitation of these patients was a labor intensive work. In the past decade, a series of researches was conducted at National Cheng Kung University (**NCKU**) for applying robotic technology to biomechanical assessments of spasticity and the neuro-rehabilitation of stroke patients in chronic stage. In particular, applications of robotics to the assessments of functional recovery, the individualized rehabilitation program and modeling of the motor learning of normal subjects and stroke patients treated by a de novo robot developed in Taiwan will be presented. The advantages and impact of utilizing robots to assist physicians on treating stroke patients will be discussed.

1.1 Symptoms of stroke

Stroke is the primary cause of disability and the second leading cause of death in many countries, including Taiwan. Although the mortality rate of stroke has declined, the incidence and prevalence of stroke continue to rise. The goal of rehabilitation is to help stroke patients to achieve as much functional independence as possible and to maintain quality of life. Rehabilitation has an important role in reducing the burden of long-term stroke care on society. By definition, stroke is a non-traumatic brain injury, caused by occlusion or rupture of cerebral blood vessels, and manifests as sudden appearance of neurological deficits characterized by loss of motor control, altered sensation, cognition or language impairment and disequilibrium. Intracranial hemorrhage accounts for about 10-15% of all strokes, and the remaining 80-85% is caused by infarction.
Disability in stroke affects physical, cognitive and psychological functions in variable severity. No two strokes are identical and no two patients respond to treatments identically. Therefore, the therapeutic approach requires assessment of every individual patient and demands specialized professional knowledge, skills and creativity. Hemiplegia or hemiparesis caused

by a stroke in the middle cerebral artery distribution area is commonly seen within the rehabilitation setting. Initially, limb weakness and poor control of voluntary movement are noted and associated with reduced muscle tone. As voluntary movement improves, non-functional mass flexion and extension of the limbs becomes apparent, i.e., synergy patterns and mass contraction of multiple muscle groups. Later, synergistic movement patterns gradually disappear and, following the neurological motor recovery, more isolated joint movements gradually develop (Sawner & La Vigne, 1992). Spasticity is a velocity-dependent increase in resistance to muscle stretch that develops after an upper motor neuron lesion (Lance, 1981; Katz, 1992). Spasticity develops shortly after a completed stroke and usually persists if recovery is incomplete and it contributes to pain, motor impairment and disability. Jackson classified symptoms after a central nervous system lesion as positive or negative. Positive symptoms are spontaneous and exaggerated version of normal functions that reacts to specific external stimuli. They include spasticity, increased deep tendon reflexes and hyperactive flexion reflexes. In contrast, negative symptoms are deficits of normal behavior or performance and they include loss of dexterity, loss of strength, and restricted ability to move. Therapeutic interventions are performed under the assumption that a cause-and-effect relationship exists between these two groups of symptoms. And the major focus is to decrease the positive symptoms and improve the negative symptoms.

1.2 Biomechanical assessments of stroke

The motor deficits and functional capability of stroke patients are usually evaluated by qualitative and semi-quantitative scales, such as Brunnstrom's stage and Fugl-Meyer assessment. Spasticity, the abnormally increased muscle tone, is evaluated similarly by the modified Ashworth scale. Though quantitative assessment of motor functions in stroke patients is less developed due to its complexity, many biomechanical methods have been employed to quantify spasticity by measuring the muscle response to the passive stretch (Firoobakhsh, 1993, Otis, 1983, Rebersek, 1986). Three types of stretch methods are commonly utilized, i.e., pendular motion (Lin, 1991, Rack, 1983), sinusoidal excitation (Agrawal, 1977, Lehmann, 1989) and constant velocity stretch (Powers, 1989).

1.3 Therapeutic Exercise Training for Motor Recovery after Stroke

In consequence of lacking inhibition within the central nervous system, abnormal coordination of movement patterns combined with abnormal postural tone are two of the major plastic responses that impede restoration of motor functions for patients with post-stroke hemiparesis (Bobath 1990). On account of weakness-related neurological deficits, the patients would rely unconsciously on various compensatory attempts to move limb segments that result in atypical synergy patterns and enhanced hypertonus during the rehabilitation process (Lum et al., 2003). Therapeutic intervention therefore focuses on relearning normal movements through experience with active participation of the patients. Correct movement patterns can be facilitated with appropriate application of proprioceptive, cutaneous, or reflexive inputs in the beginning of the recovery phase. Reinforced successful sensorimotor experiences could expedite recovering from upper limb paralysis of stroke patients with manual stretch (Carey et al., 1990), tactile stimulation (Mark et al., 2005), or joint compression (Brouwer and Ambury, 1994). As the individual becomes more effective and independent in the motor task, this handling of external sensory inputs is gradually withdrawn, in replace of strengthening exercises against resistance (Ada et al., 2006) with designed patterns and training of goal-oriented and skilled movements (Bobath 1990).

A number of neurological treatment approaches have been proposed to facilitate motor recovery of stroke patients, including Bobath (Bobath 1990; Davies 1991), Brunnstrom (Sawner and Lavigne, 1992), Proprioceptive Neuromuscular Facilitation (PNF) (Dickstein et al., 1986), Motor Relearning Program (MRP) (Carr and Shepherd, 1989; Langhammer and Stanghelle, 2000), constraint-induced movement therapy (CIMT) (Blanton and Wolf , 1999; Taub and Uswatt 2006), task-related training (Dean and Shepherd, 1997; Jang et al., 2003) and bilateral training (Mudie and Matyas, 2000;Whitall et al., 2000; Tijs and Matyas, 2006). Forms of the rehabilitative practices claimed effective regain of motor control based on different conceptual assumptions that lead to a variety of technical emphases. For example, the Brunnstrom PNF and bilateral training approaches made use of resistance-induced associated movements or widespread mass synergies to strengthen unresponsive muscles (Whitall et al., 2000; Hwang et al., 2005). On the other hand, the Bobath approach which persisted to restore motor functions with functional activities according to neuro-developmental sequences and considered reflex-inhibiting patterns to counteract abnormal postural tone (Bobath 1990). According to the MRP, training in motor control of stroke patients contained two fundamental elements, i.e., anticipatory actions and ongoing practice (Carr and Shepherd, 1989). The patients practiced motor task of environment specific to enrich relearning (Davis et al., 2006). The CIMT approach addressed massed practice with the affected limb. The shaping technique was extensively employed in CIMT by using operant conditioning, so that successful performance was consistently rewarded to reverse of the "learn non-use" mechanism (Taub et al., 1999; Liepert et al., 2000). Although those different approaches showed some degree of improvements in multiple physiological domains and longitudinal outcomes after stroke, recent studies have not reached a consensus for any of prevailing prescription to optimize performance outcomes and neuromuscular adaptations (Pollock et al., 2003; Van Peppen et al., 2004).

1.4 Robot-aided Assessment and Rehabilitation

For the rehabilitation of stroke patients, many robotic systems have been developed (Noritsugu, 1997, Krebs, 1998, Ju, 2002, Cozens, 1999, Reinkensmeyer, 1999). One of the major difficulties in realizing robot-assisted rehabilitation is the controller design. Manual treatments usually involve complex maneuvers with resistive or assistive force imposed at specific points along a specific direction of the movement. Circular or more complex movements with predefined imposing force are difficult to implement by using either conventional position or force control alone. Three types of controllers have been employed, isotropic or impedance control that maintained a constant stiffness and damping at the end effector, hybrid position/force controller that controlled position in one direction and force in the orthogonal direction, and hardware method to constrain position in the direction orthogonal to the tangential velocity (Reinkensmeyer, 1999, Raibert, 1981, Suh, 1991, Lum, 2002, Burgar, 2000). In a robot-assisted rehabilitation program, the subject is part of the man-machine system and dynamic model of the subject is not as clear and invariant as the manipulator. To solve this problem fuzzy control was employed to develop a hybrid position/force control for a shoulder-elbow rehabilitation robot (Ju et al, 2005).
In recent years, the fast advancement in robotics has made the appearance of many sophisticated robots in industrial, home, entertainment and medical industries. Most of these robots are equipped with vision system, tactile sensors and hearing system and the control system even has some kind of artificial intelligence. It is believed that robotic technology may have a contribution to the assessment and neuro-rehabilitation of stroke

patients during the acute and the chronic stages. The long-term goals of these researches are three-folds. First, devices for biomechanical assessments of the syndromes of stroke are developed. Second, neuromuscular mechanism of the syndromes has to be explored. Third, based on the mechanism, a neuro-rehabilitation robot is developed to assist physicians and physical therapists to provide objective assessments and treatments of the stroke patients.

Organization of this chapter is summarized in the following. In section 2, two spasticity measuring systems for quantifying the degree of spasticity of stroke patients are presented. In section 3, a rehabilitation robot developed at NCKU and its applications to the assessments of motor functions and clinical treatment of patients is introduced. In section 4, a recent improvement of the above-mentioned robot for quantifying the abnormal synergistic forearm movement and model simulation of the subjects for monitoring the motor adaptation progress is presented. In the last section, the advantages and disadvantages of applying robotics on the assessments and treatment will be discussed followed by a description of the future aspects of neuro-rehabilitation robots.

2. Spasticity Measurement Systems

2-1 Single-axis manipulator for biomechanical assessment of spasticity

At NCKU, two devices were developed for the assessments of spasticity and tracking performance of stroke patients for time course study. Figure 1 shows the schematic and the control block diagram of a single-axis manipulator system for quantifying spasticity of stroke patients. The system was designed to perform passive stretch on spastic muscles of upper and lower limbs. The mechanism was capable of positioning and manipulation of elbow, knee or ankle joint. The DC servomotor could drive the manipulandum to perform constant velocity or ramp-and-hold, sinusoidal and arbitrary movements. A very sensitive torque sensor was utilized to measure the stretch reflex torque exerted on the manipulandum by the spastic muscles. The subjects were tested in the supine position. The hypothesis to be examined was that tonic stretch reflex of stroke patients was first decreased at the acute stage and latter increased at the chronic stage. Figure 2 shows the ramp-and-hold stretch of the elbow of a stroke patient. A simple method to eliminate the gravitational torque was developed. First, a baseline was measured when the manipulandum was driven at an average speed of 5 deg/s. Then, by subtracting the baseline from the reflex torques measured at 20, 40, 60 and 80 deg/s, we could eliminate the gravitational torque of the manipulandum and the forearm. Four stroke patients were recruited for a time course evaluation. The subjects were tested on the spasticity measurement system 72 hours, 1 week, 1 month, 3 months and 6 months from the onset of the last stroke. The protocol of the human tests was approved by the human study ethics committee of National Cheng Kung University Hospital. A biomechanical model for the spastic joint was written as:

$$\tau_r = I\ddot{\theta} + B\dot{\theta} + K\theta - \tau_g(\theta) \tag{1}$$

in which I was the inertia of forearm and manipulandum, B was the viscous damping coefficient of the robotic system, K was the stiffness constant, θ was the angular displacement of the manipulator, τ_g was the gravitational torque and τ_r was the stretch reflex torque. Figure 2 shows the stretch reflex torque of a typical stroke patient. Note that the area between the dotted baseline and the measured torque at various stretch speeds was proportional to the stretch speed. The averaged stretch reflex torque (ASRT) was found to be a suitable index for quantifying the degree of spasticity and the single-axis robot system provided an on-line examination of spasticity. Details of the development can be found in (Ju et al, 2000).

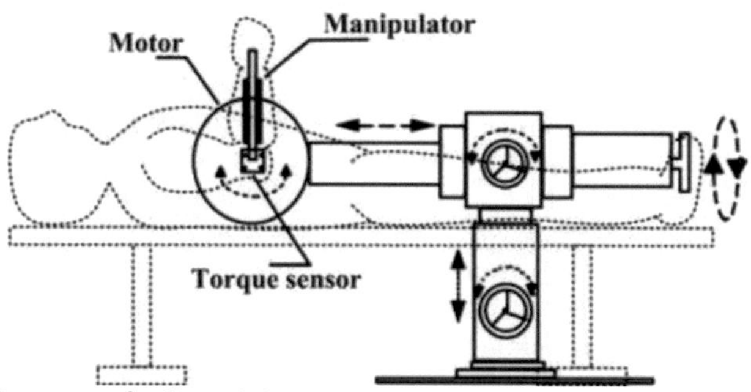

Fig. 1. Schematic diagram of a Spasticity.

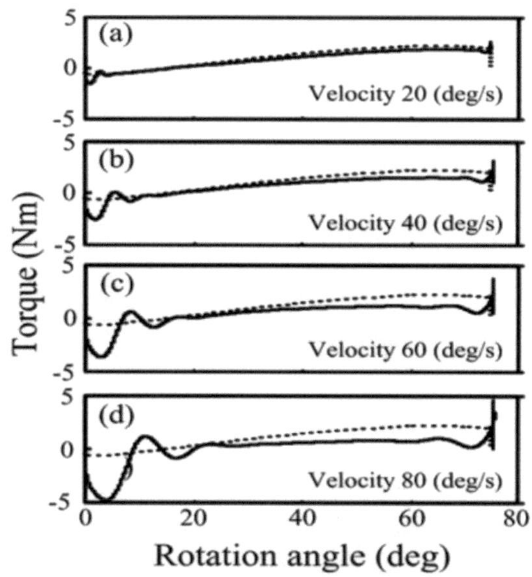

Fig. 2. Stretch reflex torques of a Stroke Patient Measurement System.

2-2 Pendulum test system for muscle tone

The other system that we developed was a pendulum test system for estimating the degree of spasticity of the elbow of the strokes. Figure 3 shows a picture of the pendulum system. In the past, the pendulum system was developed for the knee joint. The main difficulties of applying the conventional method to the elbow were the relatively small inertia of the forearm and the uncomfortable testing posture. The system was similar to a clock pendulum and a biomechanical model similar to Equation (1) was employed for off-line estimation of model parameters of the elbow. From the estimated parameters one could quantify the degree of spasticity. Eleven stable stroke patients and eleven normal subjects were recruited for the testing. Figure 4 shows the biomechanical model of the man-machine system. In this model, m_f was the mass of forearm, m_a was mass of the apparatus, K and C were stiffness and damping coefficients respectively. The subjects were asked to relax and the pendulum was released from an angle of 130° (full extension 0°). The angular trajectory of the pendulum was recorded and filtered with a fourth order Butterworth low pass filter (cutoff band 10Hz). The model was simulated with the same initial state as the experiment and the mean squared error between the model output and the experiment data was minimized by finding the optimal parameters K, C and θ_c. The sequential quadratic program method was utilized. Figure 5 shows that the damping ratio derived from the proposed model could differentiate spasticity from normotonus and it increased as spasticity increased. The system was also applied to a normal subject group and to a diabetic neuropathic patient group. The results from the normal group (n=192) showed that the biomechanical properties of the elbow joints (K and C) was similar in men and women when the body weight was adjusted and did not change with age until 70 years old. The results from the patients with diabetic neuropathy (n=53) indicated that the pendulum test could be used in this patient group to monitor the decreased muscle tone. Details of this development can be found in (Lin et al, 2003, 2005, 2006).

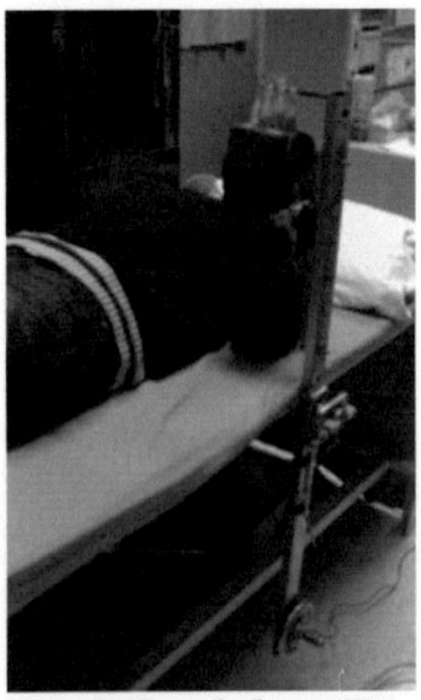

$$I\ddot{\theta} = -\tau_g - K(\theta - \theta_c) - C\dot{\theta}$$

$$I = I_a + I_f$$

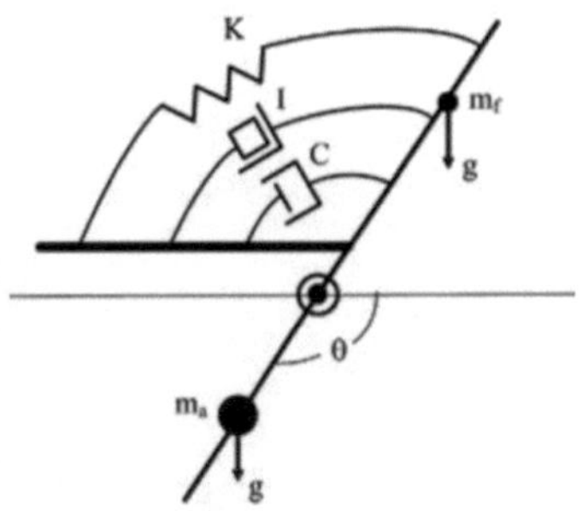

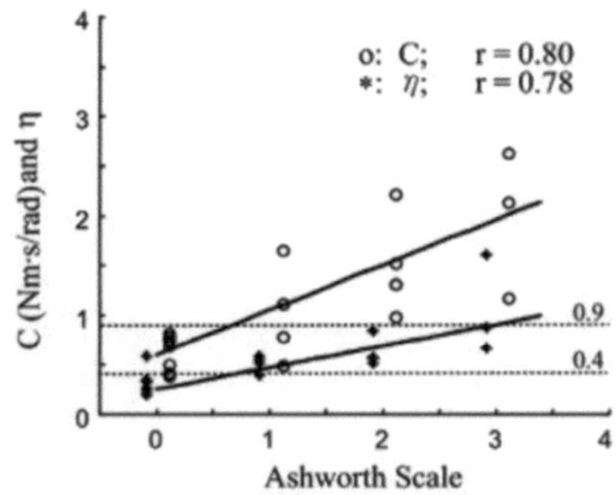

Fig. 3. Pendulum Fig. 4 Biomechanical Model Fig.5 Damping ratio vs Ashworth Scale.

3. Neuro-Rehabilitation Robot and Treatment Movements

3-1 Single axis robot for elbow

To investigate the influence of external constant torque on voluntary elbow movements of stroke and normal subjects, the spasticity measurement system was modified (Figure 6). A control system that could compensate gravitational torque and generate a constant-torque from the manipulandum was developed. Two groups of subjects were recruited, including six stroke patients and six normal subjects. Selection criterion of stroke patients were normotonic hemiparesis caused by one episode of stroke, clear consciousness and good cooperation and free from other central nervous system diseases. A voluntary tracking control test was designed for quantitative evaluation of the active tracking capability of the subjects. Target and actual elbow trajectories were displayed on a monitor. The target trajectory was a ramp-and-hold movement with a speed of 20°/sec. Both the intact and affected sides of the stroke patients were tested. The subjects were asked to extend the elbow joint from 55° to 110° under three, i.e., free, assistive and resistive, loading conditions. The intensity of the assistive/resistive torque was controlled to be 10% of the maximum isometric flexion/extension torque. Three tracking performance indices, namely, root mean squares (RMS) error, integration of squared jerks, integration of rectified electromyogram were compared. Figure 7 shows the comparison of the intact side with the affected side of a stroke patient. One may observe that the tracking performance of the affected side could be improved by either the resistive or assistive torque. Details of the developed techniques can be found in (Ju et al, 2002). The findings of this work paved the way for the development of a five-bar robot which could apply either assistive or resistive force to the wrist of a subject who was instructed to actively perform a therapeutic movement on the horizontal plane at the shoulder level.

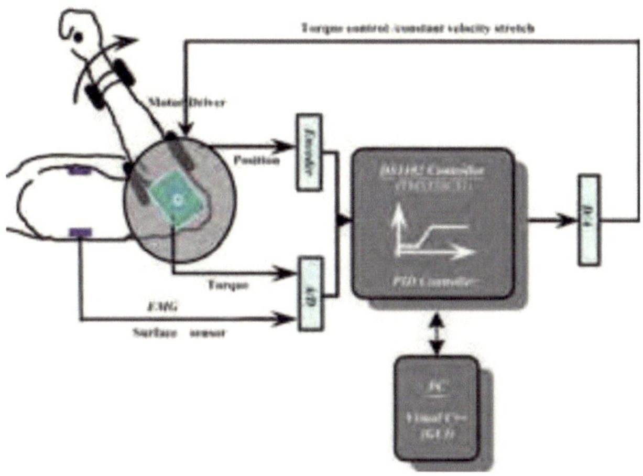

Fig. 6. Single-axis rehabilitation robot.

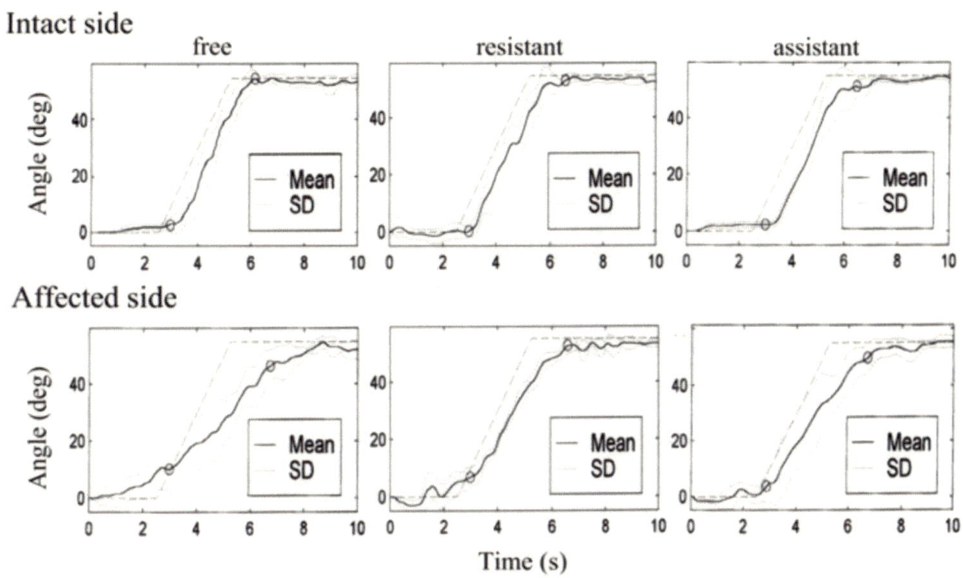

Fig. 7. Affected versus intact sides.

Various facilitation methods have been developed for the neuro-rehabilitation of paretic muscles. Up to now, the true mechanism of neuromuscular facilitation remains obscure. A possible explanation of the rehabilitation process was suggested (Reinkesmeyer, 2004). When the upper neurons are injured, the planner, controller and sensing elements of the neuromuscular system may loss their functions and the paths between the limbs and the sensing elements may be broken. The self repair of the human body is an adaptive process which can adjust the unused neurons in the planner, controller, sensing elements and limbs. To accelerate this adaptation process there are two approaches, one is to manipulate the paralyzed limbs and the other is to instruct the patient to move his/her paralyzed muscles and induce the desired movement. The facilitation processes of neuromuscular system include passively guiding the spastic limb movement, imposing resistance to strengthen muscle power and patterning of treatment movements.

3-2 Five-Axis Planar robot for shoulder and elbow

At NCKU a five-bar planar robot was developed for neuro-rehabilitation of shoulder and elbow joints of stroke subjects. Figure 8 shows a picture and the schematic diagram of the robot. The robot was able to guide patients' wrists to move along the planned linear or circular trajectories on the horizontal plan when the upper arm was abducted by 90°. A hybrid position/force controller incorporating fuzzy logic was implemented to control the movement in the desired direction and to maintain a constant force along the moving direction. Figure 9 shows the tangential and normal directions of movement and a block diagram of the hybrid controller. The circular trajectory, with a radius of 14cm, was chosen as the treatment movement. The movement involved coordination between shoulder and elbow joints and major muscle groups such as deltoid, pectoralis, biceps and triceps were all facilitated. A treatment protocol was developed and clinical tests on normal subjects and stroke patients have been performed at NCKU Hospital since 1999. Figure 10 shows the treatment protocol, in which graded resistive force ranged from 0N to 9N was applied by the robot on the wrist when the subject performed the horizontal circular movements.

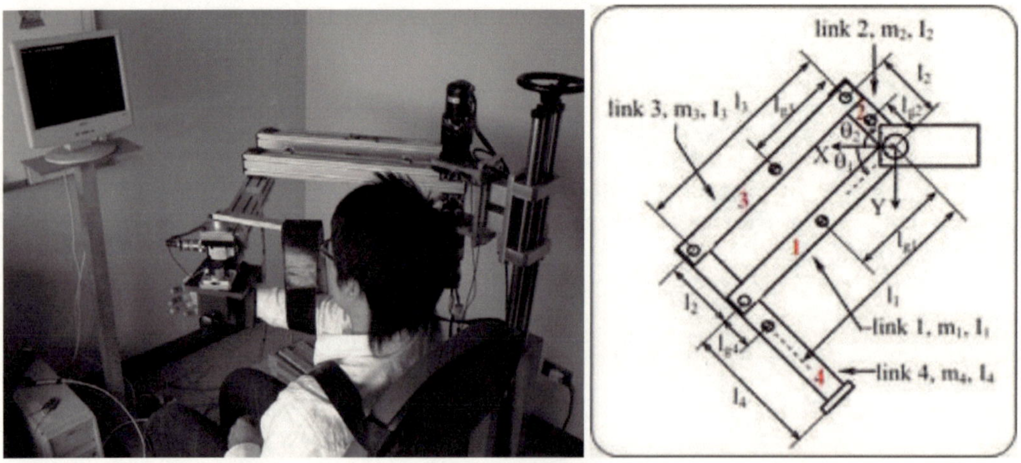

(a) (b)

Fig. 8. (a) Picture of the shoulder-elbow rehabilitation robot and (b) schematic diagram of the five-bar mechanism.

The average RMS tracking error of the movement from the normal group was utilized to score the performance. When the RMS tracking error was smaller than a threshold of the age-matched normal group, the resistance force was increased. An index called dynamic stiffness was employed to evaluate the goodness of motor coordination. The robot could apply a radial perturbing force at $\pm$ 45 degree from the far point (0 degree) of the circular trajectory. The subject would react to this unexpected perturbing force. By measuring the maximum perturbed displacement of the wrist and the perturbing force. A stiffness matrix could be calculated as:

$$K_e = \begin{bmatrix} K_{xx} & K_{xy} \\ K_{yx} & K_{yy} \end{bmatrix}, \quad K_{xx} \cong \frac{F_x}{\Delta x_e}, \quad K_{yy} \cong \frac{F_y}{\Delta y_e}, \quad K_{xy} \cong \frac{F_x}{\Delta y_e}, K_{yx} \cong \frac{F_y}{\Delta x_e} \tag{2}$$

Through the similarity transform the dynamic stiffness of the elbow and shoulder joints could be obtained,

$$K_j \equiv J^T K_e J = \begin{bmatrix} K_{ee} & K_{es} \\ K_{se} & K_{ss} \end{bmatrix} \tag{3}$$,

where K_{ee} and K_{ss} are the dynamic stiffness of the elbow and shoulder joints, respectively. Figure 11 shows the perturbed movement of a typical stroke patient and Figure 12 shows the time course variation of joint dynamic stiffness during the treatment period with the protocol depicted in Figure 10.

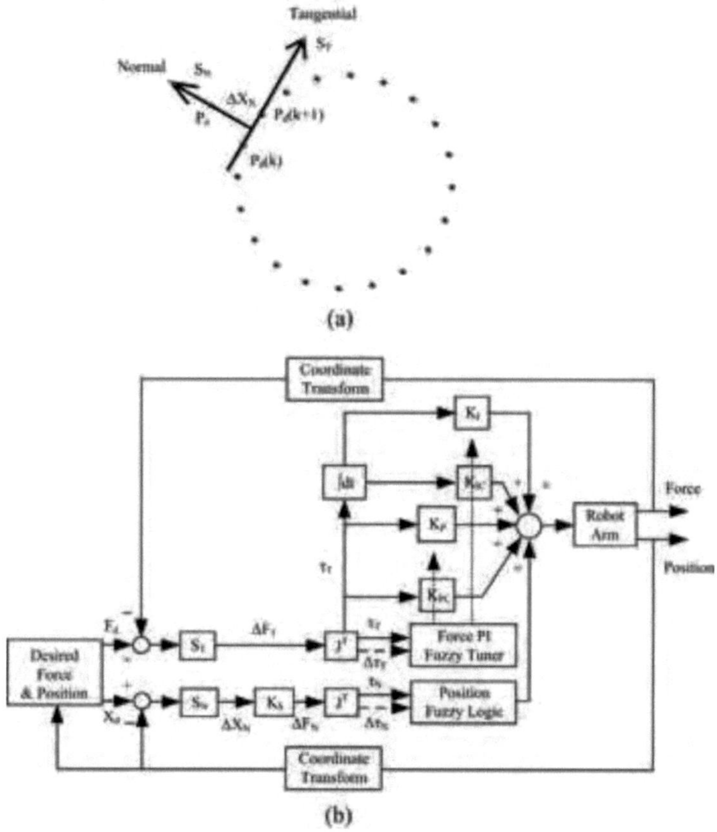

Fig.9 (a) Tangential and normal directions, (b) Control algorithm.

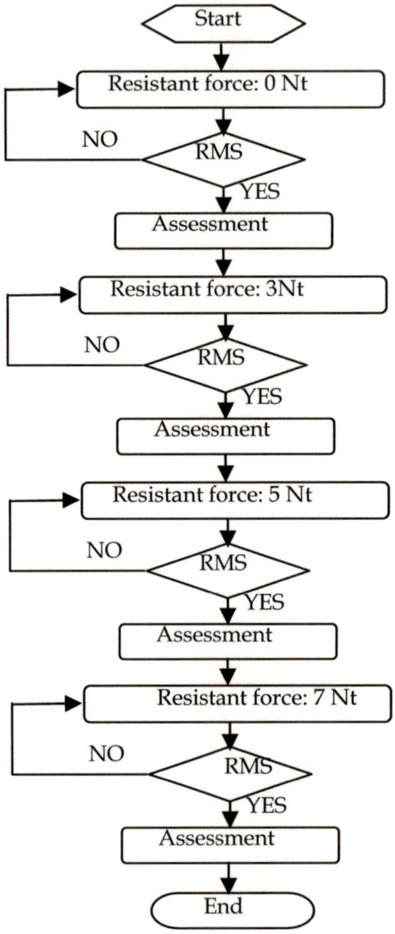

Fig.10 Clinical treatment protocol.

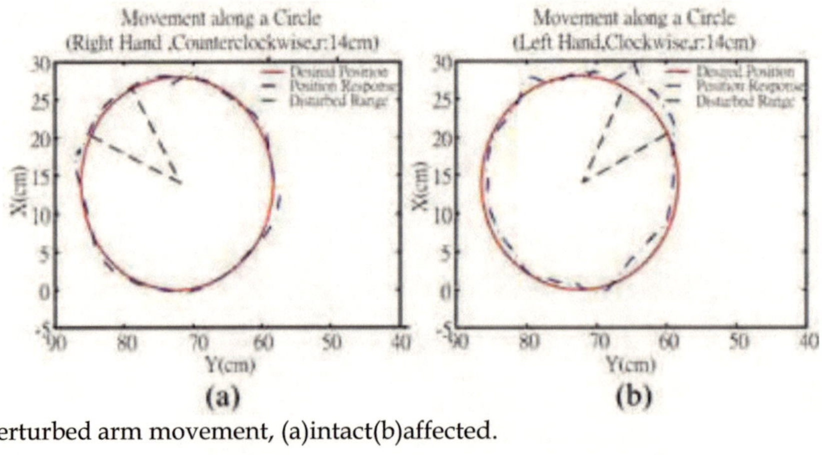

Fig. 11. Perturbed arm movement, (a)intact(b)affected.

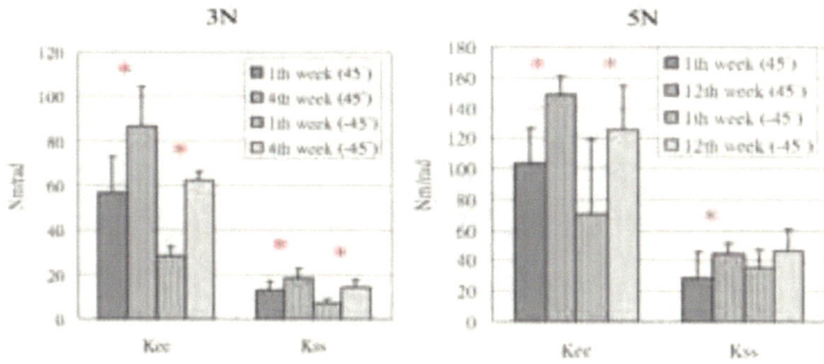

Fig. 12. Changes of dynamic stiffness.

3.3 Wrist Unit for assessing Forearm Synergistic Patterns

A new torque measurement system was developed to quantify the abnormal synergistic patterns of the strokes when they were performing upper limb movements on the horizontal plane. The same protocol for treatment was employed and the pronation/supination torque and the tracking trajectories were recorded. An index IADT (integration of absolute deviation torque) written as

$$IADT = \int_0^{2\pi} \left\| M_f \right| - \left| \overline{M}_f \right\| d\theta \tag{4}$$

was employed for quantifying the synergistic torque of the affected muscles. In Eqn. (4) Mf is the pronation/supination torque of forearm, over bar means the average, and θ is the angle that defines the position of wrist on the circular trajectory. We found that IADT could be utilized to quantify the degree of in-coordination of the affected joints. Two types of movements, namely, passive and active constrained movement were performed by the subjects. Figure 13 shows the comparison between four stroke patients and six normal subjects during the active constrained movements. The results showed that for three out of four stroke patients, IADT of affected side was higher than that of the intact side. Subject S3 had a motor capability very close to the normal level. We found that IADT could be used to quantify the degree of synergistic movement and the stroke patients manifested significant abnormal pronation/supination movements during the circular treatment exercise. Details of this research can be found in (Kung et al, 2005).

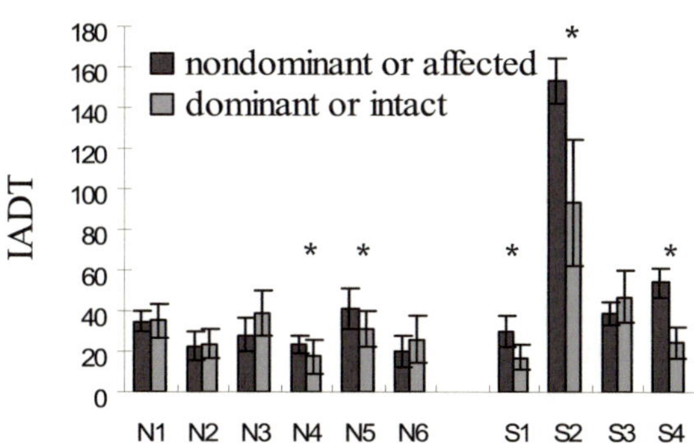

Fig. 13. IADT for normal group and stroke.

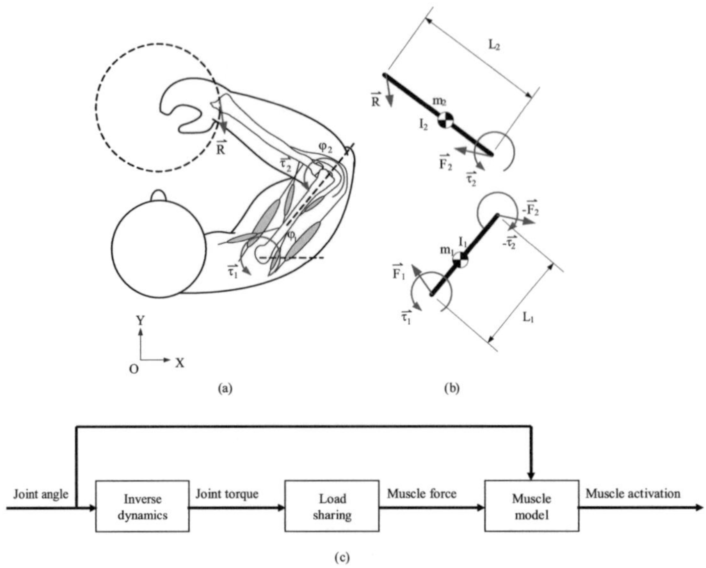

Fig. 14 Biomechanical model of subject.

4. Biocybernetic Models for Evaluating Motor Adaptation

4.1 Modeling of Subjects interacting with the Five-Axis Planar Robot

To explore the motor learning and adaptation of stroke patients during the time-course of robot-aided rehabilitation, a biomechanical model of the upper limb of a subject was developed (Figure 14). Simulations of the model could probe the interaction between the subject and the robot. The model consisted of the skeletal system and the Hill-type muscles. The inverse dynamics problem was solved by using the recursive Newton-Euler Equation to obtain the torque trajectories of shoulder and elbow. The static optimization problem was then solved to obtain the force distribution of the ten muscles. In the static optimization the objective function of sum of muscle stress squares which was an approach for minimum muscle fatigue was employed (Crowninshield et al, 1981). From the Hill-type muscle model and the angle trajectories of shoulder and elbow the neural excitation history of all muscles could be calculated.

4.2 Comparison of motor strategies between the normal and the stroke subjects

Seven subjects including a stroke and six normal subjects were recruited for a 6-week training program. All of them were new to the five-bar planar robot and they were asked to perform the transverse circular movement under a 10N resistive force. For the normal subjects, both speed and accuracy were improved progressively (Figures 15(a) and (b)). However, the performance of the stroke subject was not improved as steadily as that of the normal subjects (Figures 15(c) and (d)). Comparison between EMG signals and calculated activations showed that the normal subjects used minimum muscle fatigue strategy for the movements throughout the training program (Figures 16(a) and (b)). The stroke adopted a different strategy in the 2nd week and then returned to minimum muscle fatigue strategy in the later 4 weeks (Figures 16(c), (d), (e), and (f)). It might imply that the normal subjects could determine their motor strategies in the beginning for learning the movement and the training program might help the stroke subject to return to the "normal" strategy for the movement.

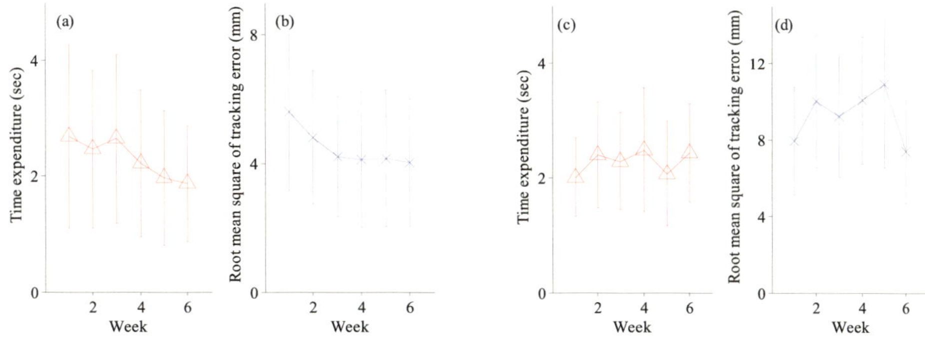

Fig. 15 Speed and accuracy of the subjects.

Normal, 1st~6th weeks Stroke, 2nd week Stroke, 3rd~6th weeks

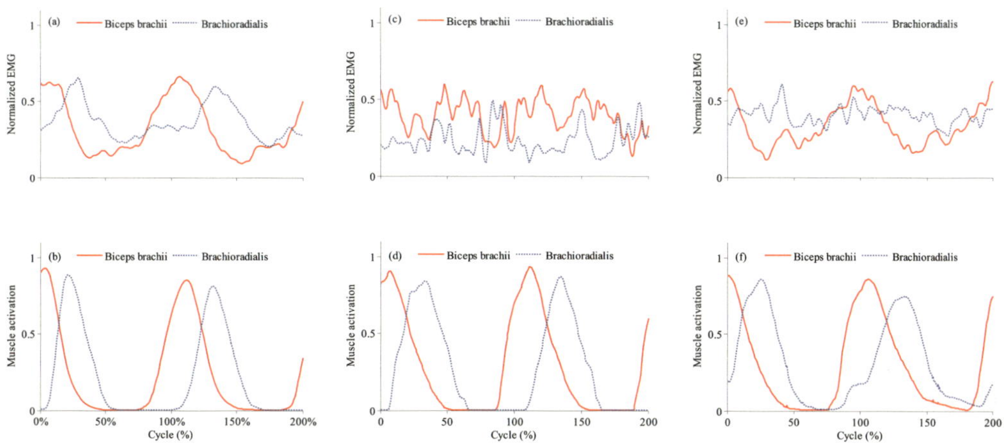

Fig. 16. Normalized EMG signals & calculated muscle activations.

5. Discussion

5-1 Advantages and Disadvantages of Robotics for Rehabilitation of Stroke Patients

One may find that robotics provides an integral solution to the treatments and objective assessments of some neurological diseases such as stroke. The robots can perform repeated treatment protocols without the need of continuous involvement of therapists. A robot can save therapists' arduous efforts by helping with heavy, challenging and repetitious movements. Physical strain and professional injury in therapists can be minimized. It is cost-effective to strengthen some basic elements, such as muscle strength, range of motion, and sensorimotor coordination, in preparation for higher skill-level movement patterns on a mass-practice basis. Robotic therapy techniques can mimic appropriate functional kinematics or apply novel patterns of force with precision, such as isokinetic contraction, that are potentially effective for muscle strengthening. More advanced robots can even provide tactile feedback that kinetically and kinematically corrects the impaired movements. Data collected during the robot training sessions can be quantified with ease to complement the subjective and qualitative observation of clinicians.

On the other hand, although biomedical robots have been used for surgery, life support and rehabilitation, the acceptance by patients and physicians are still low. There are several obstacles needing to be solved. Robotic training can just perform standard paradigm of limited combination of movement patterns in proximal joints. Currently, it cannot provide some sensory inputs, such as temperature, touch, stroking and psychological support. Robotic training is less flexible than hands-on therapy that most therapists consider essential to revitalize residual motor power of the arm and hand in neurologically impaired patients. The most central concern of patients about treatments is the beneficial effects on daily living activities, such as grooming, hygiene, dressing, undressing and toileting. The effects of robotic training might not be necessarily able to be translated into functional recovery. In the last, robotic therapy for shoulder and elbow joints can not be directly generalized to robotic therapy for the wrist and hand, which involves more degrees of freedom in joint space.

5-2 Future Aspects of Robotics in Rehabilitation Medicine

The challenge for the next step in robotic rehabilitation is to develop more creative, functional, interesting, task-oriented intervention with demonstrated effectiveness that maximize functioning and independence for stroke patients. The robotic system can be miniaturized for home and personal use and the interface can be more humanoid. Robotic therapy is convenient to combine several different prevailing techniques, such as functional electrical stimulation, biofeedback, and virtual reality, to optimize treatment effects for patients with different needs.

Studies of larger scale and more objective evaluating tools are necessary to firmly establish the efficacy of robotic rehabilitation. Recent development of function brain imaging methods such as the near infrared spectroscopy (NIR), functional magnetic resonance image (fMRI) and others have made possible the non-invasive functional imaging of cortex, especially the motor and sensory areas (Rolfe, 2000, Hu & Norris, 2004). We believe that direct observation of treatment effects on the specific areas of the cortex is essential for designing treatment protocols to provide more efficient rehabilitation of patients in the near future. However, there are several technical problems to be solved before the integration of rehabilitation robot with these imaging modalities. First, the strong magnetic field of MRI has a large disturbance on the sensors such as load cells, electromyography electrodes and electro-goniometer. Second, the metal structure and the actuators of the robots have high interference on the brain images and there is a need for developing rehabilitation devices that have less interference to fMRI.

6. Conclusions

In this paper a review on the biomechanical assessment of spasticity and the development of neuro-rehabilitation robots for stroke patients is presented. The robots provide precise physical therapy and objective evaluation of stroke patients. With the aid of emerging functional brain imaging tools and new robotic technologies, more effective treatments can be delivered in the future.

7. Acknowledgements

The research is supported by ROC National Science Council via contracts: NSC 89-2212-E-006-109, NSC 90-2212-E-006-078, NSC 91-2212-E-006-059, NSC 92-2320-B-006-074, NSC 93-2320-B-006-021, NSC 94-2320-B-006-004.

8. References

Ada, L., Dorsch, S. & Canning, C.G. (2006). Strengthening interventions increase strength and improve activity after stroke: a systematic review. *Aust J Physiother*, Vol. 52, No.4, pp. 241-248.

Agarwal, G.C. & Gottlieb, G.L. (1977). Oscillation of the human ankle joint in response to applied sinusoidal torque on the foot. *J Physiology*, Vol.268, No. 1, pp. 151-176.

Blanton, S. & Wolf, S.L. (1999). An application of upper-extremity constraint-induced movement therapy in a patient with subacute stroke. *Phys Therapy, Vol.* 79, No.9, pp. 847-53.

Bobath, B. (1990). *Adult hemiplegia. Evaluation and Treatment*, 3rd ed., Heinemann Medical, Oxford.

Brouwer, B.J. & Ambury, P. (1994). Upper extremity weight-bearing effect on corticospinal excitability following stroke. *Arch Phys Med Rehabil*, Vol. 75, pp. 861-866.

Burgar, C.G., Lum, PS, Shor, P, Van der Loos, HFM. (2000). Development of robots for rehabilitation therapy: The Palo Alto VA/Standord experience. *J. Rehab. Res. & Develop.*, Vol. 37, No. 6, pp. 663-673.

Carey, J.R. (1990). Manual stretch: effect on finger movement control and force control in stroke subjects with spastic extrinsic finger flexor muscles. *Arch Phys Med Rehabil.*, Vol. 71, No.11, pp. 888-894.

Carr, J.H. & Shepherd, R.B. (1989). A motor learning model for stroke rehabilitation. *Physiotherapy*, Vol. 89, pp. 372–80.

Cozens, J.A. (1999). Robotic assistance of an active upper limb exercise in neurological impaired patients. *IEEE Tran. Rehab. Eng.*, Vol. 7, pp. 254-256.

Crowninshield, RD, Brand RA. A physiologically based criterion of muscle force prediction in locomotion, J Biomech, Vol. 14, pp. 793-801, 1981.

Davies, P. (1991). *Right in the middle.* Heidelberg: Springer,.

Davis, J.Z. (2006). Task selection and enriched environments: a functional upper extremity training program for stroke survivors. *Top Stroke Rehabil.*, Vol. 13, No. 3, pp. 1-11.

Dean, C.M. & Shepherd, R.B. (1997). Task-related training improves performance of seated reaching tasks after stroke. *Stroke*, Vol. 28, No. 4, pp. 722–8.

Dickstein, R., Hocherman, S., Pillar, T., Shaham, R. (1986). Stroke rehabilitation. Three exercise therapy approaches. *Phys Ther.*, Vol. 66, No. 8, pp. 1233-1238.

Dobkin, B.H. (2004). Strategies for stroke rehabilitation. *Lancet Neurol.*, Vol. 3, No. 9, PP.528-536.

Firoozbakhsh, K.K. & Kunkel, C.F. (1993). Isokinetic Dynamometric technique for spasticity assessment. *Am J Phys Med Rehabil*, Vol. 72, pp. 379-385.

Hu, X. & Nossir, D.G. (2004) Advances in High-Field Magnetic Resonance Imaging. *Annual Review Biomedical Engineering*, Vol. 6, pp.157-184.

Hwang, I.S., Tung, L.C., Yang, J.F., Chen, Y.C., Yeh, C.Y., Wang, C.H. (2005). Electromyographic analyses of global synkinesis in the paretic upper limb after stroke. *Phys Ther*, Vol. 85, No.8, pp. 755-765.

Jang, S.H., Kim, Y.H., Cho, S.H., Lee, J.H., Park, J.W., Kwon, Y.H. (2003). Cortical reorganization induced by task-oriented training in chronic hemiplegic stroke patients. *Neuroreport* , Vol. 20, No. 14(1), pp. 137-141.

Ju, M.S., Chen, J.J., Lee, H.M., Lin, T.S., Lin, C.C.K., Huang, Y.Z. (2000). Time-course analysis of stretch reflexes in hemiparetic subjects using an on-line spasticity measurement system. *J Electromyography & Kinesiolology*, Vol. 10, pp.1-14,.

Ju, M.S., Lin, C.C.K., Chen, J.R., Cheng, H.S., Lin, C.W. (2002). Performance of elbow tracking under constant torque disturbance in normotonic stroke patients and normal subjects. *Clinical Biomech*, Vol. 17, pp. 640-649.

Ju, M.S., Lin, C.C.K., Lin, D.H., Hwang, I.S., Chen, S.M. (2005). A rehabilitation robot with force-position hybrid fuzzy controller: hybrid fuzzy control of rehabilitation robot. *IEEE Trans Neural Sys & Rehabil Eng*, Vol. 13, No.3, pp.349-358.

Katz, R.T., Rovai, G.P., Rymer, W.Z.(1992). Objective quantification of spastic hypertonia, correlation with clinical findings. *Arch Phys Med Rehabil*, Vol. 73, pp. 339-347.

Krebs, H.I., Hogan, N., Aisen, M.L., Volpe, B.T. (1998). Robot-aided neurorehabilitation. *IEEE Trans. Rehab. Eng.*, Vol. 6, pp. 75-87.

Kung, P.C., Ju, M.S., Lin, C.C.K., Chen, S.M. (2005). Clinical Assessment of Forearm Pronation/Supination Torque in Stroke Patients. *J Med. and Biol. Eng.*, Vol. 25, No. 1, pp. 39-43.

Lance, J.W. (1981). Disordered muscle tone and movement. *Clin Exp Neurol*, Vol. 18, pp. 27-35.

Langhammer, B., Stanghelle, J.K. (2000). Bobath or motor relearning programme? A comparison of two different approaches of physiotherapy in stroke rehabilitation: a randomized controlled study. *Clin Rehabil*, Vol. 14, No. 4, pp. 361-369.

Lehmann, J.F., Price, R., DeLateur, B.J., Hinderer, S., Traunor, C. (1989). Spasticity: quantative measurement as a basis for assessing effectiveness of therapeutic intervention. *Arch Phys med Rehabil*, Vol. 70, pp. 6-15.

Liepert, J., Bauder, H., Wolfgang, H.R., Miltner, W.H., Taub, E., Weiller, C. (2000). Treatment-induced cortical reorganization after stroke in humans. *Stroke*, Vol. 31, No.6, pp. 1210-6.

Lin, C.C., Ju, M.S., Lin, C.W. (2003). The pendulum test for evaluating spasticity of the elbow joint. *Arch Phys Med Rehabil*, Vol. 84, pp. 69-74.

Lin, C.C.K., Ju, M.S., Huang, H.W. (2005). Gender and age effects on elbow joint stiffness of normal subjects. *Arch Phys Med & Rehab*, Vol. 86, pp. 82-85.

Lin, C.C.K., Ju, M.S., Huang, H.W. (2006). Hypotonia in diabetic polyneuropathy evaluated by quantitative pendulum test, *Arch Phys Med & Rehab.* (accepted).

Lin, D.C. & Rymer, W.Z. (1991). A quantitative analysis of pendular motion of the lower leg in spastic human subjects. *IEEE Trans Biomed Eng*, Vol. 38, No. 9, pp. 906-918.

Luke, C., Dodd, K.J., Brock, K. (2004). Outcomes of the Bobath concept on upper limb recovery following stroke. *Clin Rehabil*; Vol. 18, No. 8, pp. 888-98.

Lum, P.S., Burga, C.G., Shor, P.C., Majmundar, M., Van der Loos, H.F.M. (2002). Robot-assisted movement training compared with conventional therapy techniques for the rehabilitation of upper-limb motor function after stroke. *Arch. Phys. Med. & Rehab.*, Vol. 83, No. 7, pp. 952-959.

Lum, P.S., Burgar, C.G., Shor, P.C. (2003). Evidence for strength imbalances as a significant contributor to abnormal synergies in hemiparetic subjects. *Muscle Nerve*, Vol. 27, No. 2, pp. 211-221.

Mark, V.W., Oberheu, A.M., Henderson, C., Woods, A.J. (2005). Ballism after stroke responds to standard physical therapeutic interventions. *Arch Phys Med Rehabil*, Vol. 86, No. 6, pp. 1226-1233.

Mudie, M.H. & Matyas, T.A. (2000). Can simultaneous bilateral movement involve the undamaged hemisphere in reconstruction of neural networks damaged by stroke?. *Disabil Rehabil*, Vol. 22, No. 1/2, pp. 23-37.

Noritsugu, T., Tanaka, T. (1997). Application of rubber artificial muscle manipulator as a rehabilitation robot. *IEEE/ASME Trans. Mechatronics*, Vol. 2, pp. 259-267.

Otis, J.C., Root, L., Pamilla, J.R., Krol, M.A. (1983). Biomechanical measurement of spastic plantarflexors. *Develop Med Child Neurol*, Vol. 25, pp. 60-66.

Pollock, A., Baer, G., Pomeroy, V., Langhorne, P. (2003). Physiotherapy treatment approaches for the recovery of postural control and lower limb function following stroke. *Cochrane Database Syst Rev*, Vol.2, CD001920.

Powers, R.K., Campbell, D.L., Rymer, W.Z. (1989). Stretch reflex dynamics in spastic elbow flexion muscles. *Ann Neurol*, Vol. 25, pp. 32-33.

Rack, P.M.H., Ross, H.F., Thilmann, A.F., Walters, D.K. (1983). Reflex responses at the human ankle: the importance of tendon compliance. *J Physiol*, Vol. 344, pp. 503-524.

Raibert, M.H. & Craig, J.J. (1981). Hybrid position/force control of manipulators, *Trans. ASME J. Dyn. Syst., Meas. Contr.*, Vol. 102, pp. 126-133.

Rebersek, S., Stefanovska, A., Vodovnik, L. (1986). Some properties of spastic ankle joint muscles in hemiplegia. *Med and Biol Eng and Comput*, Vol. 24, pp. 19-26.

Reinkensmeyer, D., Takahashi, C., Timoszyk, W. (1999). Evaluation of an assistive controller for reaching following brain injury. *Proc. 1st Joint BMES/EMBS Conf.*, p. 631.

Reinkensmeyer, D.J., Emken, J.L., Cramer, S.C. (2004). Robotics, Motor Learning, and Neurologic Recovery. *Ann Rev Biomed Eng*, Vol. 6, pp.497-526.

Rolfe, P. (2002). In Vivo Near-Infrared Spectroscopy. *Ann Rev Biomed Eng*, Vol. 2, pp. 715-754.

Sawner, K.A. & Lavigne, J.M. (1992). Brunnstrom's Movement Therapy in Hemiplegia: *A Neurophysiological Approach*. Lippincott Williams & Wilkins; 2nd ed.

Suh, H., Hong, J.H., Oh, S.R., Kim, K.B. (1991). Fuzzy rule based position/force control of industrial manipulators. *IEEE/RSJ Int. Workshop on Intelligent Robots Systems*, Vol. 3, pp. 1617–1622.

Taub, E. & Uswatt, G. (2006). Constraint-Induced Movement therapy: answers and questions after two decades of research. *NeuroRehabilitation*, Vol. 21, No. 2, pp. 93-95.

Taub, E., Uswatte, G., Pidikiti, R. (1999). Constraint-Induced Movement Therapy: a new family of techniques with broad application to physical rehabilitation--a clinical review. *J Rehabil Res Dev*, Vol. 36, No. 3, pp.237-251.

Tijs, E., Matyas, T.A. (2006). Bilateral training does not facilitate performance of copying tasks in poststroke hemiplegia. *Neurorehabil Neural Repair*, Vol. 20, No. 4, pp. 473-483.

Van Peppen, R.P., Kwakkel, G., Wood-Dauphinee, S., Hendriks, H.J., Van der Wees, P.J., Dekker, J. (2004). The impact of physical therapy on functional outcomes after stroke: what's the evidence?. *Clin Rehabil*, Vol. 18, No. 8, pp. 833-862.

Whitall, J., McCombe, W.S., Silver, K.H., Macko, R.F. (2000). Repetitive bilateral arm training with rhythmic auditory cueing improves motor function in chronic hemiparetic stroke. *Stroke*, Vol. 31, No. 10, pp. 2390-2395.

15

Applications of a Fluidic Artificial Hand in the Field of Rehabilitation

Artem Kargov[1], Oleg Ivlev[2], Christian Pylatiuk[1], Tamim Asfour[3], Stefan Schulz[1], Axel Gräser[2], Rüdiger Dillmann[3] and Georg Bretthauer[1]
[1]*Institute for Applied Computer Science, Forschungszentrum Karlsruhe, Germany*
[2]*Institute of Automation, University of Bremen, Germany*
[3]*Institute of Computer Science and Engineering, University of Karlsruhe, Germany*

1. Introduction

Since the early middle of last century, use of artificial robotic hands in the field of rehabilitation has been associated with prosthetic devices used for the therapy of upper limb deficiency. Artificial manipulators of the last century were used in general for industrial applications or for service tasks of telemanipulation.

In the last three decades, service robotics developed very rapidly. In recent years, robotic systems which are able to complete service tasks in direct cooperation with humans became popular [Yuta at al., (2006)].

Modern robotic rehabilitation devices are intelligent systems used for movement assistance, physical support and indoor navigation, physical rehabilitation, vocational rehabilitation, and interactive entertainment [Bien, Stefanov (2004)].

Dextrous manipulation has become the subject of research for many scientists around the world and artificial hands are used in a wide area of applications [Venkataraman, Iberall (1990)].

Investigations of hand construction, artificial design, and manipulation abilities resulted in the development of different hand prototypes for service robotics, prosthetics, and rehabilitation [Muzumdar (2004); DeLaurentis et al., (2000); Pons et al., (1998); Pons et al., (2000); Lee et al., (2000); Light, Chappell, (2000); Weir *ff* et al., (2001); Kyberd et al., (2003); Walker (2003); Boblan et al., (1999); Plettenburg (2002); Hirzinger et al., (2004); Jacobsen et al. (1986); Townsend (2000)].

In view of the dexterity of natural hands, it may be assumed that there are problems in the development of dextrous artificial hands, including controllability, hand geometry, hand functionality, development and placement of sensors; sensory fusion, and the need for better actuators [Subramanian T. Venkataraman, Thea Iberall (1990)].

As regards the different criteria related to artificial manipulators, which were discussed in research literature, we share the opinion that acceptance of robotic devices by the user plays a very important role in the development of manipulator constructions. Safety and simplicity of usage are no less important aspects of device architectures. Universality of components, their modularity and changeability should be taken into account and can allow for reducing the energy consumption and production costs of whole systems.

This chapter will highlight applications of an artificial robotic hand actuated by flexible fluidic actuators developed at the Forschungszentrum Karlsruhe (Karlsruhe Research Centre, Germany) [Kargov et al., 2006].
Flexible fluidic actuators were developed as an alternative to other actuation principles of today, such as electromotors, shape memory alloys, or McKibben muscles.
Up to date, fluidic actuators have impeded the design of artificial actuation systems due to their relatively high weight and low power. Modern fluidic actuators have already been identified as being particularly suitable for macrorobotics, compared to other actuator technologies and considering several criteria, including stress improvements, bandwidth, intrinsic compliance, packaging, good power to weight ratio, and high dynamics [Hollerbach et al., 1992].

2. Fluidic artificial hand

2.1 System components and mechatronic design

Since 1999, a multifunctional artificial hand has been developed at the Karlsruhe Research Centre that meets modern technical standards. This development was based on the invention of new flexible fluidic actuators [Schulz at al, 1999]. The construction of first actuators was easy. They were built of thin plastic films in a very compact manner as a two-layered body with two separated chambers which contained a small pipe for fluid supply. The elastic chambers were expanded when the pressure was applied to the actuator. This expansion behaviour was taken into account by a new concept of an artificial finger joint, which was presented in 2000. The functional principle of such artificial joints consists in converting the energy of chamber inflation into a rotational movement between two thin plates that are connected to each other (Fig. 1a,b). Different prototypes of fluid actuators based on this principle have been built by the Institute of Applied Computer Science up to date [Schulz at al, 1999].

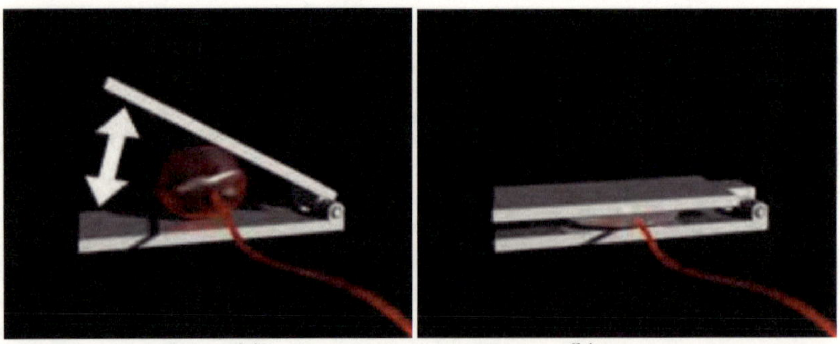

(a) (b)

Fig. 1a,b. Functional principle of flexible fluidic actuators.

The current model of an artificial finger joint consists of a flexible fluidic actuator made of a reinforced flexible bellow. Both fronts of the actuator are attached to solid fittings mounted on the joint, which transmit the pulling force of axial expansion to the joint (Fig. 2.). A special tissue covers the bellow and reduces the radial expansion of the actuator under pressure.
Two major advantages of these actuators are their low weight and inherent compliance. Each actuator weighs only 2.6 grams and is built of lightweight materials. In comparison

with fluid cylinders, flexible fluidic actuators can transmit energy in the same manner, but have a higher power-to-weight ratio at the same pressure and volume. Small dimensions of actuators of 12 mm in diameter and 12 mm in length allow for an integration directly in the artificial finger joint. A torque of up to 0.8 Nm can be achieved for such joint at 6 bar pressure.

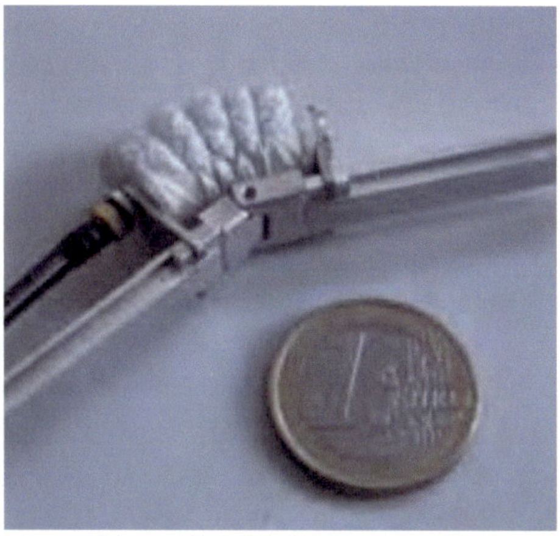

Fig. 2. Flexible fluidic actuator with artificial joint.

The development of artificial joints led to the design of a multi-articulated artificial hand (Fig. 3.). Biometric data of a natural hand were used to design the prototype of this robot hand. Made of lightweight aluminium with high tensile strength properties, the basic construction consists of the 5-fingered durable and stable mechanical framework with a natural appearance. The artificial metacarpus with the fingers is made up of artificial bones and joints. The number of joints can be varied for other prototypes and optimised for special applications without almost any losses of the anthropomorphic appearance of the hand, its dexterity, functioning, and high dynamics.

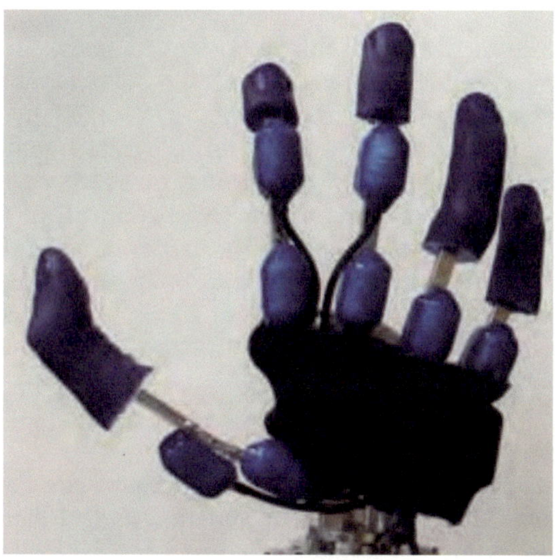

Fig. 3. Current prototype of a fluid hand

All joints and actuators in the hand are constructed identically. This makes the hand construction modular, actuators can be interchanged with each other, and the number of degrees of freedom can be changed. Consequently, redesigning of the end manipulator and the whole reconstruction of the system are not necessary.
Current prototypes of a fluid hand have 8 active actuated joints and 3 passive joints which are not actuated. The index and middle fingers have four active joints. The ring and small fingers have one actuated joint and one passive joint each. The thumb is actuated by two joints. The base joint of the thumb is placed perpendicular to the middle joint to achieve an opposite movement.
Other important components of the fluid hand are electronic valves and the control unit (Fig. 4.), which are integrated in the artificial metacarpus. Valves and electronics are custom-made, as suitable commercially available devices are lacking.

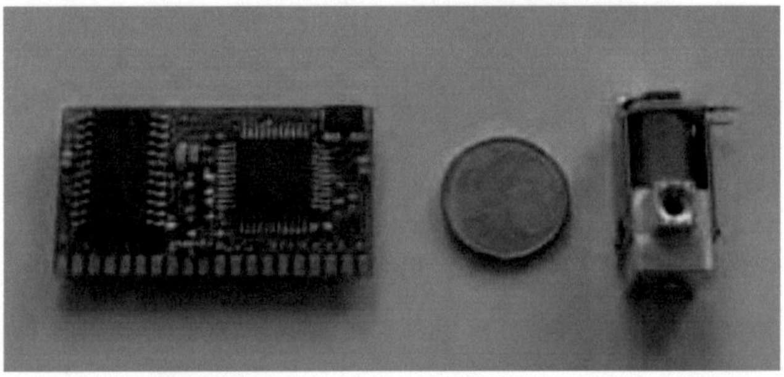

Fig. 4. Electric valve and control unit.

Valves are operated according to the mono-stable principle. They supply the fluid for fluidic actuators and keep the fluid pipeline closed, if no current is applied. In this way, the position of fingers can be saved during grasping. Small dimensions of valves of 23x11x13 mm allow for their integration in the hand. Low power consumption of the valves of 1 Watt saves energy and a flow rate of 14 l/min (by air) ensures a high dynamics of hand movements.
The electronic unit is built by SMD technology, except for some few discrete components, and arranged on a four-layered circuit board. With the dimensions of 51 mm / 40 mm / 9 mm, it consists of a programmable microcontroller PIC16F877 by Microchip (Microchip Technology Inc., USA), drivers for the valves, an integrated analogue-digital converter which can digitize 8 signals collected by positioning, pressure, and tactile sensors as well as mini connectors which allow for the direct connection of all periphery units to the electronics. Sensors can be integrated optionally in the hand and use analogue/digital ports to communicate with the control unit. Additionally, the electronics offers I2C, CAN, and SPI interfaces to interact with external robotic devices, such as the robot arm and an RS232 interface for programming the control unit and diagnosing the whole control system from a PC.

2.2 Control architecture and functioning

Communication and data transfer between the controller and external devices take place via serial CAN, SPI, I2C or RS232 interfaces. In general, control signals, such as the joint number, angles for positioning the joints or a number of programmed grip types are transmitted from the external control system to the fluid hand in this way.

A fluid hand works as follows: the controller collects external control signals and operates four mono-stable valves via the respective driver modules. Microvalves provide the corresponding flexible fluidic actuators with external air pressure. The actuators are inflated under pressure, forces of expansion are generated, and the flexion movement of hand digits is achieved. The extension movement is performed by a spring element.

2.3 Performance and functionality

Due to the use of fluidic actuators and the possibility of controlling each joint separately, a large operating range of hand motion is achieved. Every digit of the hand with an active base joint can be flexed by up to 90°. All actuators can be flexed independently of each other.

The possibility of moving each finger joint or joint group separately during grasping is a very important advantage of artificial hands with an anthropomorphic appearance and functionality. Using this benefit, artificial manipulators can perform in general all basic grasping patterns of human hands.

Different tasks of daily life, such as grasping and manipulating differently sized household objects, can be performed using a large number of combinations of movable joints. A cylindrical power grasp, precision grasp, tripod grasp, hook grasp, and spherical grasp can be performed. (Fig. 5.). The important functions of the index finger, such as pressing a key or operating a switch, can be implemented as well.

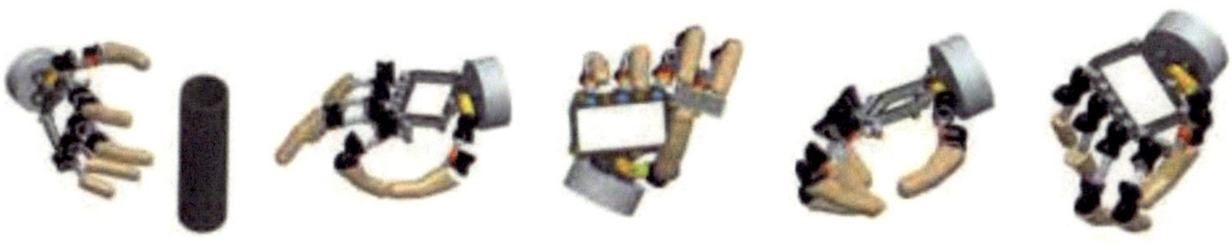

a b c d e

Fig. 5. Grip types which can be performed by the fluid hand. a - cylindrical power grasp, b - precision grasp, c - tripod grasp, d - hook grasp, and e - spherical grasp.

A multiple number of degrees of freedom (DOF) and compliance of the fluidic actuators and elastic finger pads give rise to a fluid hand with the specific feature of adaptive grasping. Artificial fingers conform to the shape of an object when grasping it. Additionally, the self-adapting properties of the hand provide for a correct distribution of contact force when grasping and manipulating objects, which is similar to that of natural hands.

2.4 Technical characteristics

The technical characteristics of the hand are presented in Table I. Small-sized and low-weight components were used for the mechanical construction of the hand, resulting in a low total weight of 350 g. The weight of the skeletal framework is 245 g, including 8 fluidic actuators and the elastic finger pads.

Prehension forces are distributed over a large contact area during grasping and stable holding with low grip forces is possible. Hence, a cylindrical object simulating the handle of a suitcase can be held with a maximum of 110 N in a hook grasp.

Using the custom-made valves, the hand can be closed within two seconds.

The fluid hand has different interfaces and can be integrated in different systems for service robotics and rehabilitation, which use different control interfaces.

The fluid hand requires an external power supply of 7.5V up to 12 V and air pressure supply of 6 bar.

3. Applications of a fluidic artificial hand

3.1 Humanoid robot for the household environment

3.1.1 System overview

The humanoid robot ARMAR-III [Asfour et al., 2006] has been developed within the German Humanoid Project (SFB 588: Collaborative Research Center on Humanoid Robots). The goal of this project is the development of humanoid robots which safely coexist with humans, interactively communicate with humans, and usefully manipulate objects in built-for-human environments. In particular, it is focussed on the integration of motor, perception, and cognition components, such as multimodal human-humanoid interaction and human-humanoid co-operation in order to be able to demonstrate robot tasks in a kitchen environment. Designing the robot is aimed at obtaining a humanoid that closely mimics the sensory and sensory-motor capabilities of the human being. The robot should be able to deal with a household environment and the wide variety of objects and activities encountered in it. Therefore, the robot must be designed in a comprehensive manner, such that a wide range of tasks (and not only a particular task) can be performed.

The humanoid robot ARMAR-III (Fig. 6) has 43 mechanical degrees of freedom (DoF): the head has a total number of 7 DoFs, the waist has 3 DoFs, each arm has 7 DoFs, each hand has 8 DoFs. The mobile platform has 3 DoFs. In addition, the hands consist of 16 DoFs. From the kinematics control point of view, the robot consists of seven sub-systems: head, left arm, right arm, left hand, right hand, torso, and a mobile platform. The upper body has been designed to be modular and light-weight while retaining a size and proportion similar to those of an average person. For locomotion, a mobile platform is used, which allows for holonomic movability in the application area. The head has seven DoFs and is equipped with two eyes.

The eyes have a common tilt and can sway independently. The visual system is mounted on a four-DoF neck mechanism. Each eye is equipped with two digital colour cameras (wide and narrow angle) to allow for simple visual-motor behaviours, such as tracking and saccadic motions towards salient regions as well as for more complex visual tasks, such as hand-eye co-ordination.

The head features human-like characteristics in motion and response, that is, the neck and the eyes have a human-like speed and range of motion. Furthermore, the head is equipped with a microphone array, consisting of six microphones (two in the ears, two in the front, and two in back of the head). This is necessary for 3D acoustic localisation.

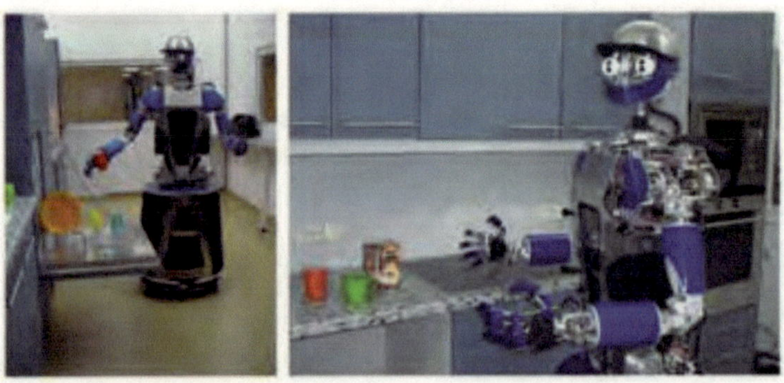

Fig. 6. The humanoid robot ARMAR-III in the demonstration environment (kitchen). The robot consists of seven sub-systems: head, left arm, right arm, left hand, right hand, torso, and a mobile platform.

The main goal of our research is to build humanoid robots which support people in their daily life. The main component of such a robot for handling objects is its manipulation system. The design of the arms is based on the observation of the motion range of a human arm. From the mechanical point of view, the human arm can be modelled by a first-order approximation as a mechanical manipulator with seven DoFs.
The sections of the arm are linked by one-DoF rotational joints, each specifying a selective motion. Consequently, the arms have been designed in an anthropomorphic way: three DoFs in the shoulder, two DoFs in the elbow, and two DoFs in the wrist. Each arm is equipped with a five-fingered hand with eight DoFs ([Schulz et al., 2004]). The goal of performing tasks in human-centred environments results in a number of requirements on the sensor system, especially on that of the manipulation system. To achieve different control modalities, different sensors are integrated in the arm. Each joint is equipped with motor encoders, axis sensors, and joint torque sensors to allow for position, velocity, and torque control. Due to space restrictions and mechanical limitations, the sensor configuration differs. For example, a sensor fitting into the elbow will most likely be too large for the wrist. In the current version of the arms, motor revolution speed, position of axis, and axis torque are monitored in each joint. In the wrists 6D force/torque sensors (ATI Industrial Automation, www.ati-ia.com) are used for position and force control. Four planar skin pads (see [Kerpa et al., 2003]) are mounted to the front and back side of each shoulder, thus also serving as a protective cover for the shoulder joints. Similarly, cylindrical skin pads are mounted to the upper and lower arms, respectively.

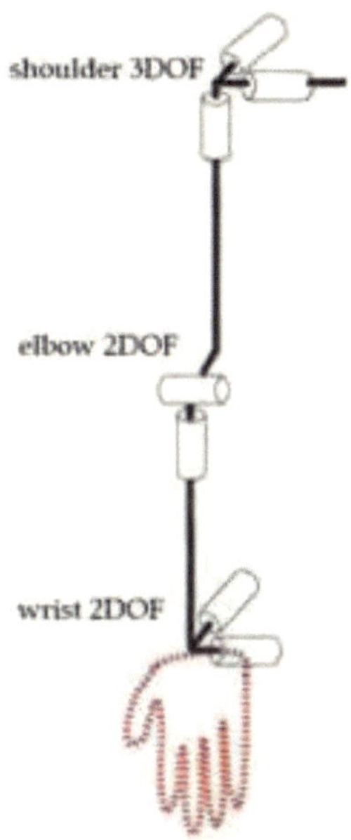

Fig. 7. Kinematics of the arm with 7 DOFs.

3.1.2 Control architecture

The control architecture comprises the following three levels: task planning level, synchronisation and coordination level, and sensor-actor level [Asfour et al., 2005]. A given task is decomposed into several sub-tasks. These represent sequences of actions the sub-systems of the humanoid robot must carry out to accomplish the task goal. The co-ordinated execution of a task requires the scheduling of the sub-tasks and their synchronisation with logical conditions, external and internal events.

Fig. 8 shows the block diagram of the control architecture with three levels, global and active models, and a multi-modal user interface [Asfour et al., 2005]:

- The task planning level specifies the sub-tasks for the multiple sub-systems of the robot. This level represents the highest level with functions of task representation and is responsible for the scheduling of tasks and management of resources and skills. It generates the sub-tasks for the different sub-systems of the robot autonomously or interactively by a human operator. The sub-tasks generated for the lower level contain the information necessary for the task execution, e.g. parameters of objects to be manipulated in the task or the 3D information about the environment. According to the task description, the sub-system's controllers are selected here and activated to achieve the given task goal.

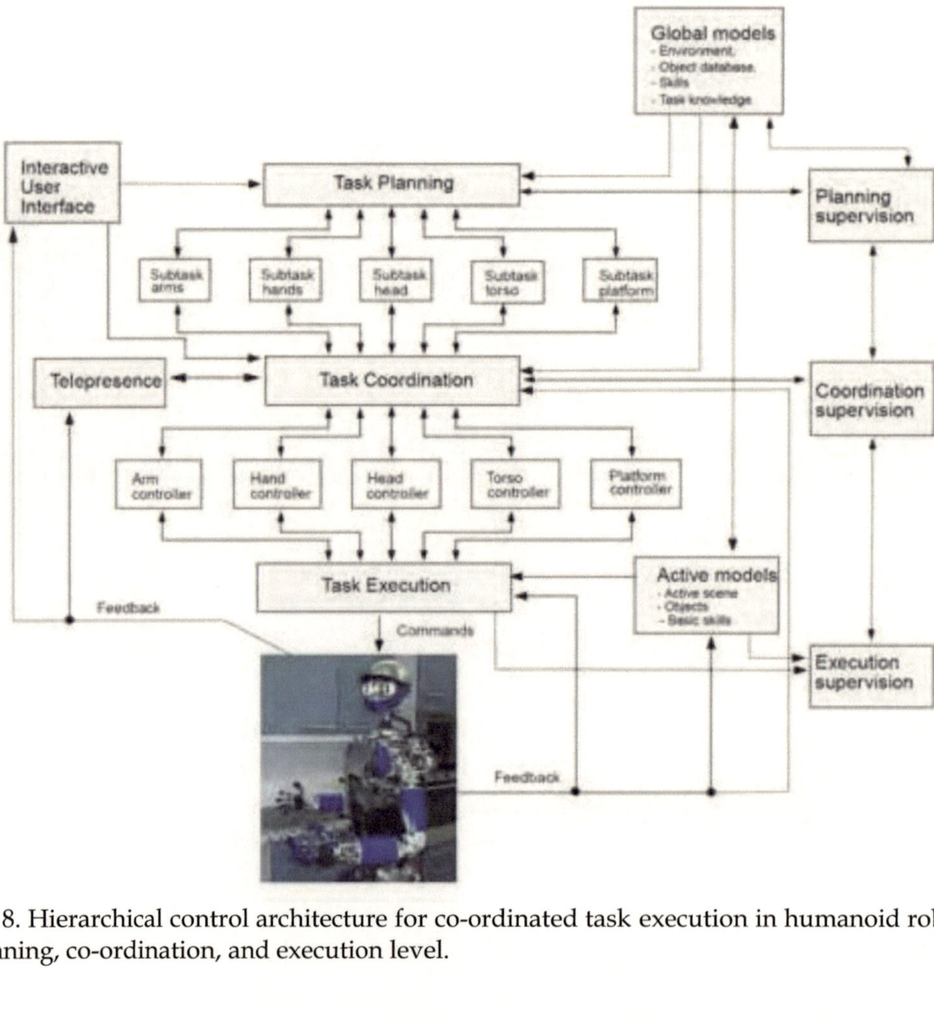

Fig. 8. Hierarchical control architecture for co-ordinated task execution in humanoid robots: planning, co-ordination, and execution level.

The task co-ordination level activates sequential/parallel actions for the execution level in order to achieve the given task goal. The sub-tasks are provided by the task planning level. As on the planning level, the execution of the sub-tasks in an appropriate schedule can be modified/reorganised by a tele-operator or user via an interactive user interface.

- The task execution level is characterised by control theory to execute specified sensor-motor control commands. This level uses task-specific local models of the environment and objects. Hereinafter, these models shall be referred to as *active models*.
- The active models (*short-term memory*) play a central role in this architecture. They are first initialised by the global models (*long-term memory*) and can be updated mainly by the perception system. The novel idea of the active models, as they are suggested here, is their independent actualisation and reorganisation. An active model consists of the internal knowledge representation, interfaces, inputs and outputs for information extraction, and optionally active parts for actualisation/reorganisation (update strategies, correlation with other active models or global models, learning procedure, logical reasoning, etc.).
- Internal system events and execution errors are detected among local sensor data. These events/errors are used as feedback to the task co-ordination level in order to take appropriate measures. For example, a new alternative execution plan can be generated to react to internal events of the robot sub-systems or to environmental stimuli.

In addition to graphical user interfaces (GUIs), the user interface provides the possibility for an interaction using natural language. Telepresence techniques enable the operator to supervise and tele-operate the robot and, thus, to solve exceptions which can arise for various reasons.

3.1.3 Integrated grasp planning and visual object localisation

As a first step towards a complete humanoid grasping system, an integrated approach to grasp planning has been developed [Morales et al., 2006]. The central idea of this system is the existence of a database with the models of all the objects present in the robot workspace. Based on this central fact, two necessary modules are developed: a visual system able to locate and recognise the objects and an offline grasp analyser that provides the most feasible grasp configurations for each object. The results provided by these modules are stored and used by the control system of the humanoid to decide and execute the grasp of a particular object. Fig. 9 gives an overview of the grasp planning system.

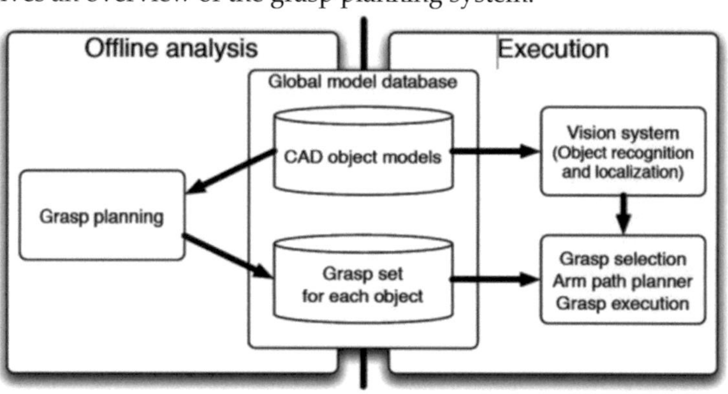

Fig. 9. An overview of the grasp planning system.

The grasp planning system consists of three components (see [Morales et al., 2006]):

- The **global model database**. It is the core of our approach. It does not only contain the CAD models of all the objects, but also stores a set of feasible grasps for each object. Moreover, this database is the interface between the different modules of the system.
- The offline **grasp analyser** that uses the model of the objects and of the hand to compute in a simulation environment a set of stable grasps. The results produced by this analysis are stored in the grasps database to be used by the other modules.
- A **online visual procedure to identify objects in stereo images** by matching the features of a pair of images with the 3D pre-built models of such objects. After recognising the target object, it determines its location and pose. This information is necessary to reach the object (see [Azad et al., 2006].

Once an object has been localised in the work scene, a grasp for that object is selected from the set of pre-computed stable grasps. This is instanced to a particular arm/hand configuration that takes into account the particular pose and reachability conditions of the object. This results in an approaching position and orientation. A path planner reaches that specified grasp location and orientation. Finally, the grasp is executed. These modules are not described in this paper, since they are still under development.

3.1.4 Outlook

The robot represents a highly integrated system suitable not only for research on manipulation, sensor-motor co-ordination, and human-robot interaction, but also for real applications in human-centred environments that make higher requirements on perception and action abilities of the robot. These are different scientific and technical problems, such as navigation, humanoid manipulation and grasping with a 5-finger hand, object recognition and localisation, task co-ordination as well as multi-modal interaction. The term multi-modality includes the communication modalities intuitive for the user, such as speech, gesture, and haptics (physical contact between the human and the robot), which will be used to command or instruct the robot system directly. Concerning the co-operation between the user and the robot - for example in the joint manipulation of objects - it is important for the robot to recognise the human's intention, to remember the acts that have already been carried out together, and to apply this knowledge correctly in the individual case. Great effort is spent on safety, as this is a very important aspect of the man-machine co-operation.

An outstanding property of the system is its ability to learn. As a result, the system can be led to new, formerly unknown problems, for example to new terms and new objects. Even new motions will be learned with the aid of the human and they can be corrected in an interactive way by the user.

3.2 Rehabilitation wheelchair system / Rehabilitation robot FRIEND-II equipped with the FZK hand: dexterous and safe manipulation

3.2.1. System description

The rehabilitation robotics system FRIEND developed by the Institute of Automation of the University of Bremen (IAT) can be used by disabled people, for instance, with upper limb impairments, to act more autonomously in daily life as well as in the working environment. For the detailed description of this robotics system, its main components, and envisaged functionalities see another chapter in this book about FRIEND I+II.

Service robots in general and rehabilitation robots in particular have to act in the real world and not in a specially installed working cell, i.e. an artificial world, as common industrial robots. To act safely and effectively in a real unstructured environment, this kind of robots requires dexterous manipulators with at least 7 joints (degrees of freedom or DoF) like a human arm. The effects of the limited motion repertoire of "Manus"-ARM, the 6-joint kinematic structure of which corresponds to that of an ordinary industrial robot, were demonstrated during the experiments with FRIEND-I [Martens et al., 2001]. The next generation of this rehabilitation robotics system, FRIEND-II (Fig. 10), therefore is equipped with a dexterous lightweight robot arm with 7 joints [Ivlev et al., 2005]. This electrically driven robot arm was developed by *amtec robotics*, Berlin (www.amtec-robotics.com) with the functional specification given by the IAT. To implement humanlike kinematics, the arm is composed of a series of turn and pan joints with perpendicular axes. The combination of a turn-pan-turn-joint is kinematically equivalent to a spherical joint like the human shoulder or the wrist joint. The middle (4th) pan joint corresponds to the elbow (Fig. 11). At the wrist, a multi-axis force/torque sensor of the type Gamma by ATI-Industrial Automation (NC, USA) is integrated. To increase the grasping capabilities, the arm may be equipped optionally with a 5-finger artificial fluid hand instead of a conventional two-finger gripper. In this way, the range of objects which can be grasped is extended and manipulation safety is improved thanks to the hand compliancy. Although it operates very closely to the user, this "soft" hand is safe and cannot harm a human or objects in the workspace. FRIEND-II also is equipped with a stereo pan-tilt-zoom camera system and a "smart tray" which is able to detect objects. The rack shown in Fig. 10, on which the cameras are mounted, was chosen to determine the optimal location of the cameras and will later be exchanged for a more ergonomic rack. The multi-processor control PC is mounted at the rear of the wheelchair.

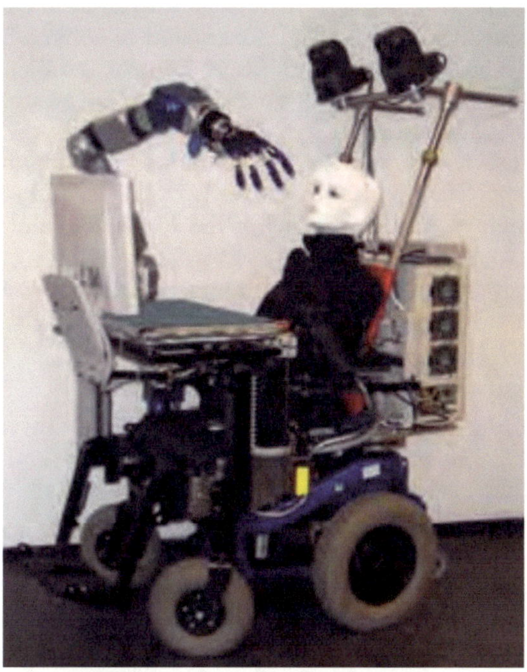

Fig. 10. Rehabilitation Robot FRIEND-II with fluidic Hand.

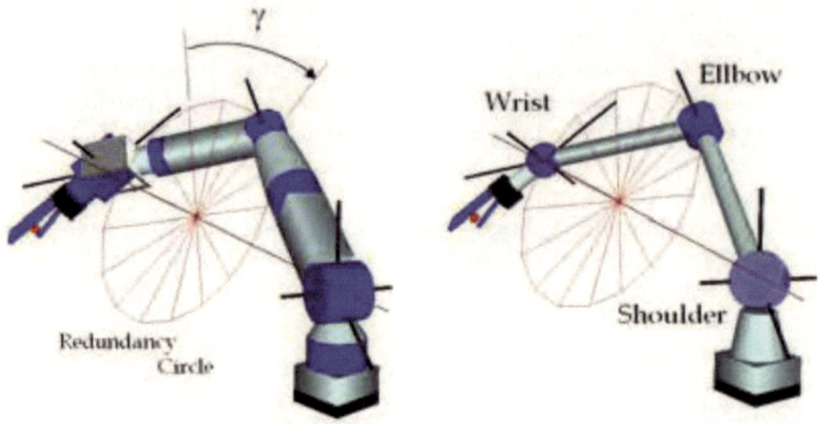

Fig. 11. Kinematic structure of a 7-joint manipulator and its self-motion manifold.

3.2.2. Grasping cases and dexterous arm control

Similar to a human arm, a dexterous manipulator with humanlike 7-joint kinematics allows for changes of the Cartesian elbow position in space without influencing the hand location. This feature is called *self-motion* and characterises in general the manipulative manifold of dexterous robots. In a 7-joint robot arm a manipulative manifold is a circle – the so-called redundancy circle, with the centre on the line connecting the intersection points of the shoulder and wrist joints (Fig. 11). The elbow position on the redundancy circle usually is determined by the redundancy angle γ. By varying γ, the arm configuration is changed without changing the hand location. This feature is utilised by the configuration control of dexterous 7-joint manipulators [Seraji, 1989]. Compared to conventional 6-joint kinematics, however, kinematic dexterity causes significant control problems, because dexterous kinematic structures with more than 6 DoFs are described by an underdetermined systems of non-linear algebraic equations.

For the successful and practically useable control of dexterous manipulators, a new control concept, called Kinematic Configuration Control (*KCC*), has been developed [Ivlev et al., 2000]. The concept combines the advantages of the kinematic control paradigm, enabling exact regulation of tool motion and typically used by conventional robots with 6 DoFs, with the possibility of precisely controllable changes of the robot configuration.

The standard algorithm of kinematic control is based on the following vector equation:

$$_{(s)}g = f(_{(n)}q), \tag{1}$$

which describes the relationship between the *n*-dimensional joint variables vector $_{(n)}q$ and the *s*-dimensional vector $_{(s)}g$ representing the location of the end effector (hand) in the workspace. The non-linear vector function f consists of s scalar functions specifying the kinematic structure of the robot as an open kinematic chain.

For non-redundant robots with $n=s$, the equation system (1) can be solved in a closed form: $_{(s)}q = f^{-1}(_{(s)}g)$. For each end effector location $_{(s)}g$ within the robot workspace $W \in \Re^s$, this solution yields a finite number of possible configurations. In the case of redundant kinematics n>s, the equation system (1) is underdetermined and can be solved in a so-called functionally closed form, when the inverse functions $f^{-1}(_{(s)}g, _{(r)}q)$ contain $r = n - s$ joint

variables as parameters. In order to fully specify the equation system (1), r additional conditions (scalar equations) are needed.
In the case of 7 DoF kinematics n=7. The dimension s of the vector $_{(s)}g$ depends on the manipulation and/or grasping task. If the manipulation task follows a fully defined trajectory in the 3D Cartesian working space $W \in \Re^3$, the three Cartesian coordinates as well as the hand orientation angles are specified unambiguously and the vector is $_{(6)}g = [X, Y, Z, Yaw, Pitch, Roll]$ with s=6. The same condition results when grasping objects of parallelepiped shape, as for example a book (Fig. 12a). The hand location here may also be considered as having been determined completely, because the object may be gripped in the middle for equilibrium reasons. In this case, s=6 as well. Therefore, just one additional condition to resolve the redundancy will be needed for such kind of manipulation and grasping tasks.
However, such a fully defined specification of the hand location is encountered rather rarely in service and rehabilitation robotics. Figures 12b and 12c show two other typical grasping cases. If a cylinder (e.g. a glass or a bottle) must be grasped, the orientation angle *Yaw* cannot be defined precisely: in general, it may have an arbitrary value between 0° and ±180°. In this case, $_{(5)}g = [X, Y, Z, Pitch, Roll]$ with s = 5 and for redundancy, two additional conditions are required. When grasping a ball-shaped object, such as an apple or an egg, all three orientation angles are free, $_{(3)}g$ = [X, Y, Z], s = 3 and three additional conditions already will be needed to resolve the redundancy.

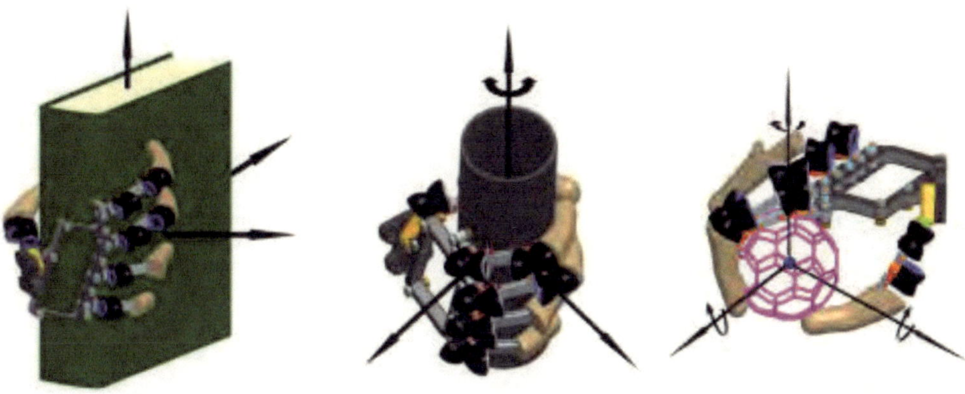

a b c

Fig. 12. a - completely defined hand location when grasping a book (s=6), b - Partly defined hand orientation when grasping a glass (s=5), c - Undefined hand orientation when grasping a ball (s=3).

The main idea of resolving redundancy in *KCC* in contrast to other concepts of closed solutions for 7-joint kinematics [Dahm 1997, Asfour 1999] is to control the robot arm relative to the actual robot pose (spatial posture) instead of the actual configuration, as it is typical of other control methods. The difference between a robot configuration and a robot pose is defined as follows: a pose is the placement of robot links and joints in the 3D Cartesian working space, while a configuration is a set of joint angles - i.e. a point in the 7D configuration space for a robot arm with 7 joints.
To control the robot arm relative to the current pose, the kinematic chain with a number of additional virtual (imaginary) links [Ivlev et al.,1997, Ivlev et al., 1999] is applied, such that

the constrained kinematic structure becomes non-redundant – this means that the number of degrees of freedom becomes equal to the working space dimension. For the case of $_{(6)}g$ = [*X, Y, Z, Yaw, Pitch, Roll*], just one imaginary link will be needed. In the case of 7-joint kinematics, it connects the robot elbow with the Cartesian point, where the elbow was placed by the previous control cycle (Fig. 13). For this kinematic structure, the kinematic equations can be solved analytically – like for conventional robots with 6 joints, and the desired hand position can be achieved with high accuracy.

The optimised KCC algorithm described in [Ivlev et al., 2000] allows to calculate exactly the elbow position E_{min} on the redundancy circle with the minimal distance to the previous elbow position E' – say, with minimal length of the imaginary link. The implemented routine contains only 21 multiplications, 11 additions as well as 1 square root and, hence, is very fast: the calculation requires only 40 µs on a PC with a 1 GHz Intel processor [Ivlev et al., 2004]. Within a typical robot control cycle of 16 ms, enough time remains to simulate the variation of the elbow position on the redundant circle and to generate other valid robot configurations. After this, the best robot pose considering the current spatial situation can be selected.

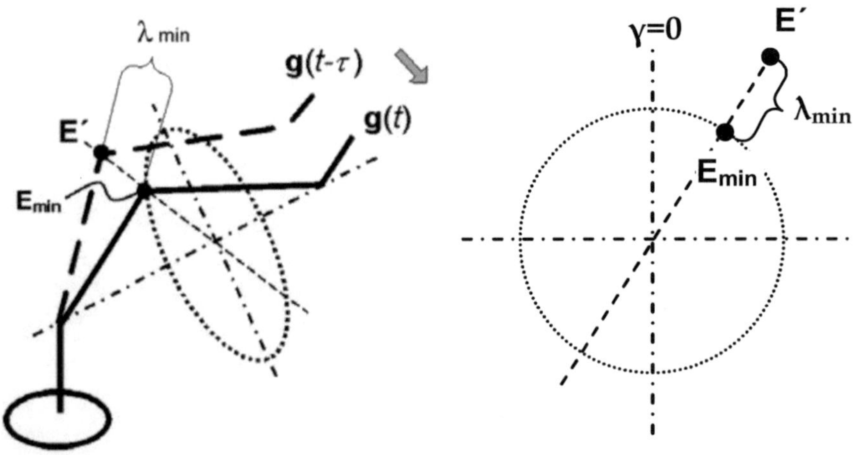

Fig. 13. Method of redundancy resolving in KCC.

In the grasping cases with s=5 and s=3, the new kinematic structures with two and four imaginary links, respectively, have to be assembled and the new inverse functions generated. In these functions, one or three parameters (lengths of imaginary links), respectively, must be chosen according to the current spatial situation. Alternatively, the inverse functions for the case s=6 (i.e. the fast optimised KCC algorithm) can be used. In this case, one (*Yaw*) or all three hand orientation angles *Yaw, Pitch,* and *Roll* (Fig. 12b and Fig. 12c) have to be varied in the hand location vector $_{(6)}g$ = [*X, Y, Z, Yaw, Pitch, Roll*] in addition to variations of the elbow position on the redundancy circle.

To simulate these variations and to choose a suitable hand orientation as well as an elbow position, the working environment, including the grasping object as well as the relevant obstacles, has to be mapped. To select a collision-free hand location and arm pose during the simulation process, the distances between obstacles and robot arm, including hand, have to be calculated permanently. In FRIEND, this problem has been solved by the so-called Mapped Virtual Reality (MVR) which models the spatial situation in an extremely simplified form and, at the same time, reflects the main spatial correlations [Feuser et al.,

2005]. The objects from the real world – obstacles, objects to be grasped as well as robot arm and hand - are mapped into this virtual reality as simple shapes covering the real objects. Only three simple 3D bodies are used in the MVR: cuboid, cylinder, and sphere. By combining these basic bodies, nearly any complex structure can be assembled. For object-oriented design, a base-class body is introduced, which provides the attributes all 3D bodies have. These are the position and the rotation. For the three simple 3D bodies, three classes are introduced, which all inherit from the base-class body: Cuboid, Cylinder, and Sphere. These classes add attributes which are needed for the description of the corresponding 3D body. For the cuboid, these are height, depth, and width, for the cylinder, height and radius, and for the sphere, only the radius.

For modelling robot links, a class CLink is used, which holds information about the transformation with respect to the previous link. This transformation is described by conventional DH parameters. To model the body structure of a link, a list is used, which holds objects of the three simple 3D bodies introduced before. Generally, a virtual robot consists of a certain number of links, where the number of links specifies the robot DoF. Therefore, the virtual robot is modelled by a list of CLink objects, where the order in the list describes the order of the links and their transformations, i.e. the kinematics of the virtual robot. The list and all needed methods are combined in the class CRobotModel.

The virtual obstacles are also modelled by the three simple 3D bodies and their class representatives and are stored in a list. The needed functionality is combined in the class CRobotWorld which inherits from CRobotModel. The result is a class which offers methods and attributes for modelling a robot and its environment.

The information in the class CRobotWorld can be used to calculate distances between the virtual robot and virtual obstacles. For this task, the GJK algorithm [Gilbert et al., 1988] is used. It provides information about the minimal distance between two convex polyhedrons and the minimal distance vector. The GJK algorithm only works with points (vertices) that describe the polyhedrons. For this purpose, a class Distance is introduced, which encapsulates the GJK algorithm and provides for a conversion of the classes describing the simple 3D bodies in a set of points. A cuboid can be described simply by eight vertices points, a cylinder has to be approximated by a set of points. To describe a sphere, it is not needed to approximate its surface by a polyhedron: its centre point and radius are sufficient. After computation by the GJK algorithm, the distance up to the sphere surface can be calculated by subtraction of the radius.

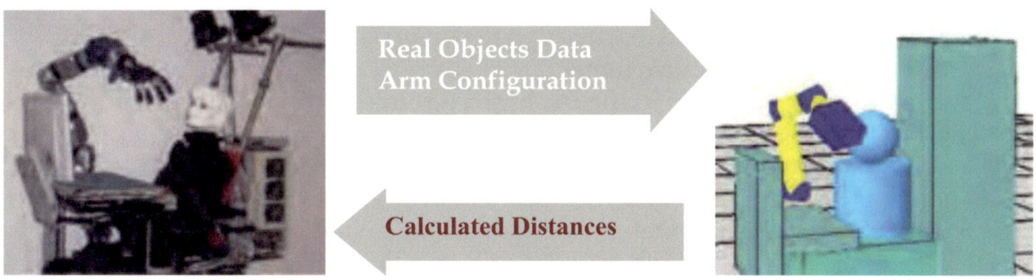

Fig. 14. Concept of Mapped Virtual reality (MVR).

The minimal distance to an obstacle can be obtained by calculating the distance between the obstacle and all body elements of each link of the robot and then choosing the smallest distance.

The classes CRobotModel and CRobotWorld both to render the virtual scene via OpenGL, but the main task of the MVR is to approximate a robot and its environment exactly enough to calculate the distances to obstacles. Therefore, very detailed graphical representation is not desired and not necessary.

In contrast to common VR, the task of which is to reflect the real world as exactly as possible and usually without influencing a situation in the real world, MVR interacts with the real world (Fig. 14). The robot configuration is transferred from the real robot and permanently updated. So, the virtual world reflects the real macro-situation and the distance can be calculated now without any difficulty instead of being measured. The task of external sensors (e.g. cameras) can be reduced to the detection of new objects which have to be mapped into the MVR instead of observing all obstacles in the workspace and measuring distances. Such task distribution increases the safety of manipulation by reduction of technical complexity.

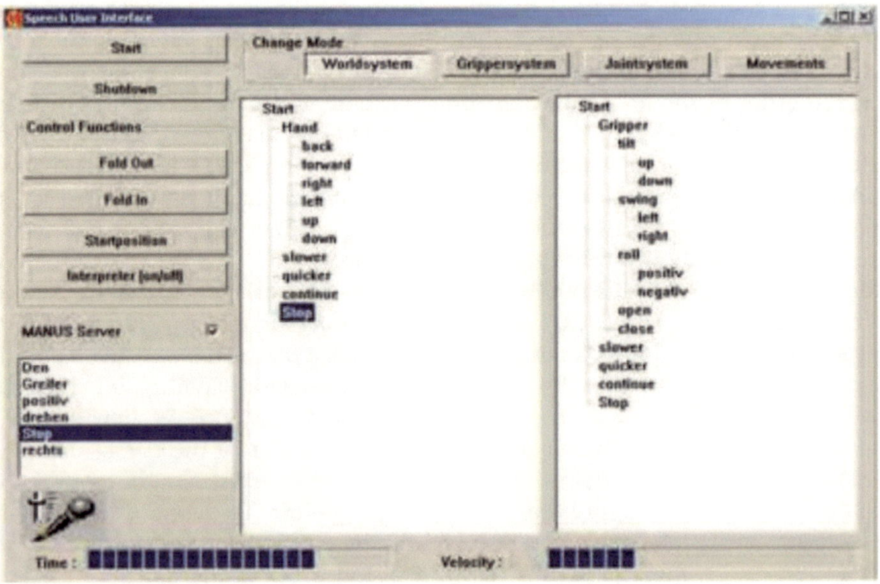

Fig. 15. Man-machine-interface with a speech command tree for the control of hand movements.

3.2.3. User–controlled hand movements

Many specific interfaces adapted to specific handicaps exist to control devices, e.g. devices which are controlled by the chin, tongue, eye position, etc. Speech recognition also is among these devices. An important requirement for the selection of the user interface is the general control philosophy "shared autonomy" which will be used in FRIEND-II [Volosyak et al., 2005]. Shared autonomy means that the robot acts autonomously at any possible time. But to restrict the complexity of the automation system and to enhance the overall robustness, a fall-back level is introduced. If the system detects a situation which cannot be resolved within the system's autonomy, it asks the user actively for support. This means that the system then relies on the mental capabilities of the user. The user can also actively take control of the robot and suspend the automation system. Speech recognition fulfils the requirement of a user interface for shared control. This is the reason why FRIEND-II is

equipped with a speech control interface shown in Fig. 15, which was also used in FRIEND-I [Martens et al., 2001].
The speech processing system translates naturally spoken words into commands. It consists of the two modules of speech recogniser and command interpreter. The speech recogniser consists of the speech recognition software ViaVoice Gold™ by IBM® , which translates naturally spoken commands entered via a microphone into specific words using pre-determined grammar. The recognised words are transmitted to the command interpreter which translates the words or text sequences received into system commands.
For safety reasons, the set of commands is organised in a hierarchical command tree. To suppress the misinterpretation of commands, such as interpreted noise or misspelled words, a path in the tree must be completed to cause a system action. This minimises the possibility of erroneous interpretations. If the system is in the user command mode and the command interpreter does not receive a permissible command within a fixed period of time, the system automatically returns to a safe state. The entire tree and the current state of the command are represented graphically on the flat screen, because the user can easily recognise the state of the system, if it is presented in the form of pictograms (Fig. 15).
Speech input allows for the control of the robot on different levels of complexity. Low-level commands which control directly a single robot joint or the robot tool (like "gripper up") are as possible as high-level commands like "pour in a drink". If the system is not able to recognise objects in the environment or if inconsistent data are retrieved from object recognition, the system may ask the user for support. In this case, the user may control e.g. the pan-tilt heads of the cameras.

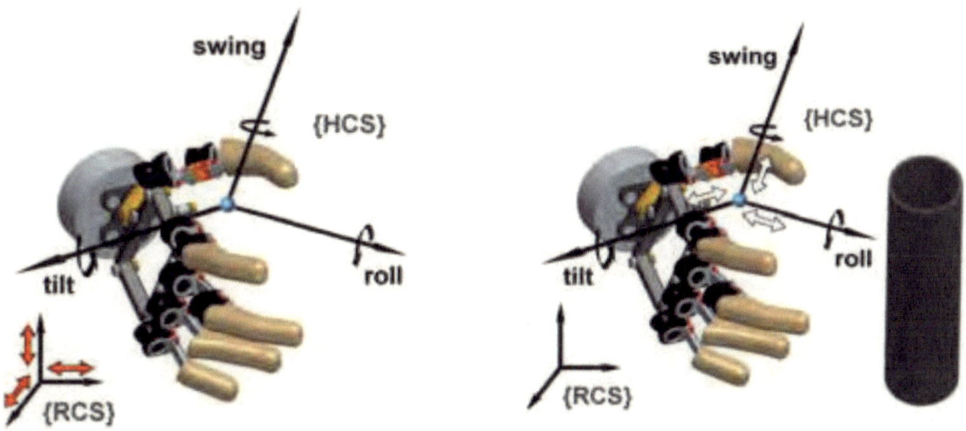

Fig. 16. Different reference coordinate systems during user-controlled hand movements: "mixed" motion directions (left), hand-fixed approaching movements (right).

By means of simple speech commands, the robot may be operated as usual by tele-operation of robot arms with respect to different coordinate systems: a reference coordinate system fixed to the robot arm base (RCS) as well as a coordinate system fixed at the hand (HCS). As shown in [Ivlev et al., 2004], the accuracy and stability of the end effector movements in the tele-operation mode increase due to the use of KCC compared to the so-called resolved-rate control which is used by default for the dexterous manipulator. The individual control of all joints is an alternative control variant and very useful, if complete arm reconfiguration

through the manipulation is required. Such a situation may occur for example during manipulation in a cluster environment, while avoiding obstacles. The pre-condition is that the hand orientation can be changed freely. This means, for example, no filled glass has been grasped before.
In the manual control of some rehabilitation robots, for example "Manus"-ARM (www.exactdynamics.nl), translational Cartesian movement defaults occur relative to the RCS, the rotary ones occur for the HCS. These "mixed" motion directions are shown in Fig. 16, left. If the approaching movement of the hand to an object is commanded, however, the HCS system is significantly more comfortable for the user than the RCS coordinate system, as was found out in the first experiments with FRIEND. Figure 16 (right) shows the directions of the approaching motion to the object.
With the help of the speech control interface, the complete control sequences can be carried out. For example, if the user wants to pick up an object placed on the tray, a possible command sequence might be *Hand right – Hand left - Hand down – Stop - Hand open - Hand forward – Stop - Hand close*. With the last command, the power hook grip can be activated to grasp, for example, cylindrical objects, such as a bottle or a glass (Fig. 12b). To activate other kinds of grips of the dexterous fluidic hand, for example a "precision grip" or a "spherical grip", special commands can be programmed. Due to the general compliancy of the fluidic hand, however, the majority of relevant objects, such as a book or a ball (Fig. 12a and Fig. 12c), handled by FRIEND can be grasped safely with the power hook grip.
The elbow position on the redundancy circle can be commanded in the same way. Possible commands for this action may be "Elbow left"–"Elbow right" or "Elbow up"–"Elbow down" depending on the current position of the elbow. The first command set corresponds to the situation when the elbow is located close to the upper point of the redundancy circle (i.e. the position with redundancy angle $\gamma \approx 0°$, s. Fig. 17), where the "down" direction is not unique. In all other elbow placements, the second two commands are more convenient from the user's point of view and can be used for controlling the elbow without loss of safety. Since the user observes the actions of the robot arm continuously, he or she can interrupt its actions in erroneous situations at any moment. As the user is supported by MVR which observes the current spatial situation and anyway stops the arm movement when a collision with the user or the environment may occur, safety of the manipulation processes increases significantly and can be classified as dependable.
The extended manipulatory facility of the dexterous robotic system FRIEND-II in comparison with conventional 6-joint kinematics is illustrated in Fig. 17. In the spatial situation shown, it is possible to grasp the glass without colliding with the bottle only by a skillful use of all 7 joints.

3.2.4. Outlook

FRIEND II is intended to increase the usability of service robots designed for paralysed people with quadriplegia or similar disabilities (paralysis down from the neck due to spinal cord injuries above vertebra C6 and movement of arms, hands, and fingers is impossible). FRIEND II helps to be independent of nursing staff for several uninterrupted hours in professional and private life. To achieve this goal, a range of new technical solutions is introduced. Keywords for the new technology are: manipulative as well as sensory redundancy, shared autonomy, smart devices, and ambient intelligence [Volosyak et al., 2005]. Figure 18 presents the concept of an "intelligent kitchen". A large number of different action sequences like "pour in and serve a drink", "take, prepare, and serve a frozen meal", "support eating", "open a drawer", "fetch and handle a book", "fetch and handle some tool" are necessary to fulfill the user's demands, to overcome the complaints about the existing systems, and to give the user a minimum of independence of the nursing staff for several uninterrupted hours. As additional requirements, FRIEND II will have a human-like robustness and flexibility for the autonomous control of unforeseen variations in the environment. Use of the dexterous 7-joint arm with human-like kinematic configuration control and a compliant fluidic 5-finger hand will help at least to solve the problems of manipulative robustness, flexibility in handling objects, and safety.

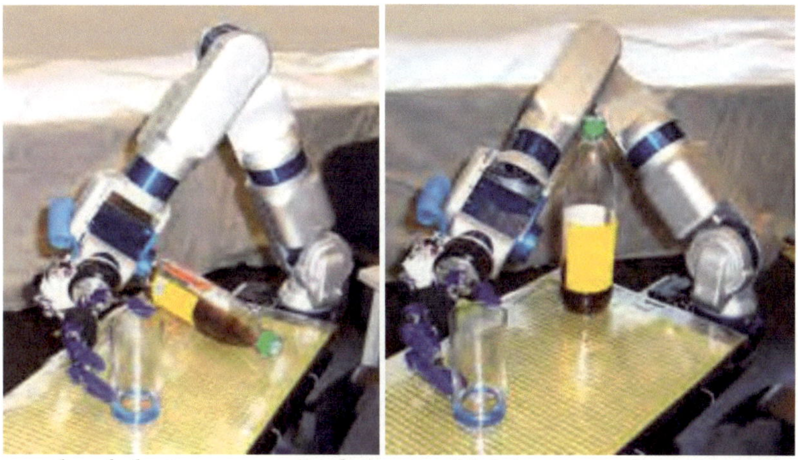

Fig. 17. Example of dexterous manipulation: a 6-joint arm can't grasp a glass without collision with a bottle (left); by controllable movement of elbow it will be possible (right).

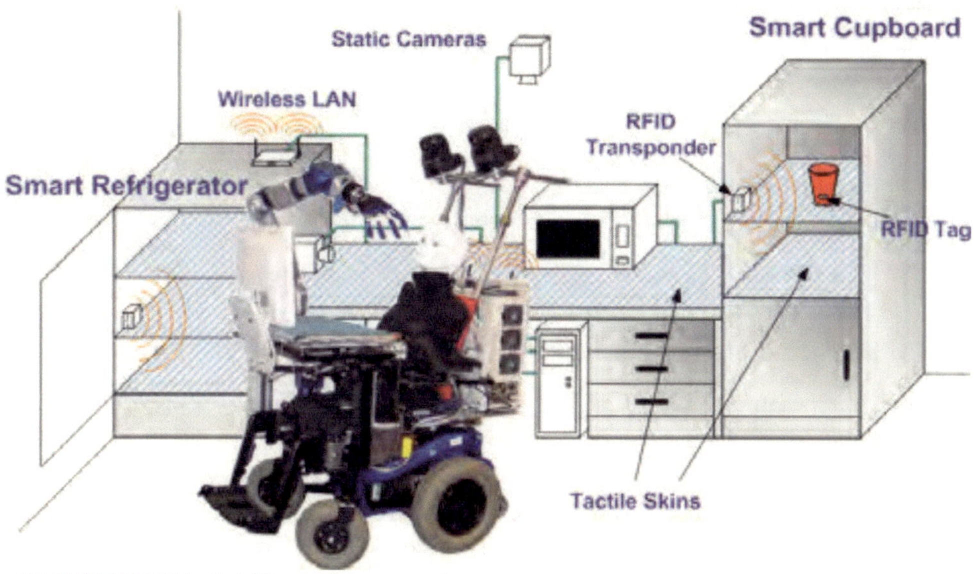

Fig. 18. FRIEND II in intelligent home environment.

3.3 Upper limb prosthesis

The loss of an upper limb implies a significant restriction of function and the individual has to cope with the stigma of being perceived as incomplete. Currently, upper limb-deficient individuals can either be fitted with a hook-type terminal device that provides good functionality and grasping force feedback, but poor cosmetics that are not accepted by most potential users in Europe. Therefore, most persons are fitted with a purely cosmetic hand or with an electrically driven hand that provides at least some cosmetic, but limited functionality. Since externally driven prostheses have been introduced to the market in the early 1970s an increasing number of patients have been fitted with these hands. However; approximately one third of all limb-deficient persons do not use their prosthesis at all [Atkins 1996]. In the last two decades, some of the achievements in the development of new materials and technologies were integrated in the design of artificial robot hands, resulting in higher dexterity. Artificial hands that are used in prosthetics have only very little in common with robot hands, which will be demonstrated in this chapter.
The following constraints should be considered when designing a prosthetic hand. They are based on the experience of different projects dealing with prosthetic hand design [Keller 1947, Peizer 1969, Weir 2003, Kyberd 2004, Pylatiuk 2007).

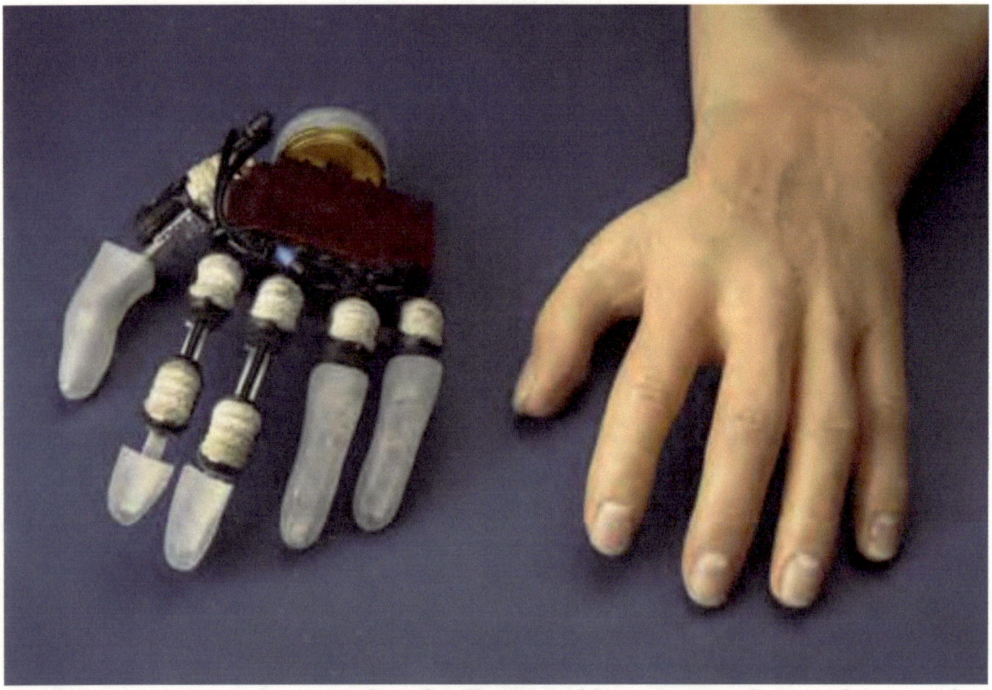

Fig. 19. A cosmetic glove made of silicone rubber covers the mechanics of the multifunctional prosthesis [Schulz 2005]. The thumb can be moved in a plane transverse to the index and middle finger.

- *Weight:* The mass of a prosthetic hand has to be below 500 grams. Otherwise, most users would not accept the technical aid. Every gram is perceived as an external load that must be carried, so the lighter a prosthetic hand is, the better accepted it will be. Although a lightweight design of robot grippers is also wanted in order to reduce the moments in the joints of the robot arm needed to move the terminal device, most commercial robot hands have a mass that considerably exceeds 500 g.

- *Compact design:* In prosthetic hands a very compact design is needed to allow for the fitting of a maximum number of upper limb-deficient persons. If not all requisite components were within the artificial hand, the large number of individuals with a transradial amputation could not be fitted. By contrast, many robot hands use the space at the forelimb to actuate the hand.
- *Appearance*: As most users of prosthetic hands, especially female users, do not want to attract attention to themselves, the design of a prosthetic hand should mimic a natural hand as closely as possible (Fig. 19). This includes different colours used to match the cosmetic glove to that of the user's skin. The design of robot hands usually is very technical. Additionally, the position of the thumb has a large impact on the appearance of the hand. In most commercial prostheses, the thumb's plane of motion is in direct opposition to the index and middle finger instead of a more natural transverse plane of motion.
- *Sound:* Any sound that originates from a prosthesis may annoy the user and should therefore be avoided. The noise level of commercial prosthetic hands is less than 45 dB at 1 m distance, which is almost imperceptible in surroundings with background noise, like an office.
- *Price*: The resources in most national health care systems are increasingly limited and in clinical practice, health insurance judges the therapeutic effects against the costs of a compensatory aid individually for every patient. In terms of economic efficiency, a prosthetic hand has to be a simple, but functional device, whereas robot hands typically are much more complex and, as a consequence, the expenses may be up to 20 times those of a prosthetic hand.
- *Power consumption*: The energy to process control signals and move the fingers of a prosthetic hand is typically supplied by rechargeable batteries of limited capacity. Therefore, efficient use of the battery energy is required and can be achieved by turning the controller to a stand-by mode when not used as well as by using actuators that do not require energy as soon as an object is grasped.
- *Sensors*: Robot hands need information from sensors about the flexion angle of each joint of the hand and about the occurring grasping forces, whereas commercial prosthetic hands do not have sensors, as the hand position is controlled visually by the user.
- *Grasping patterns:* The human hand is capable of grasping an object reliably with a vast number of different prehension patterns due to its versatility and ability to conform to the shape of an object. Commercial prosthetic hands only have one degree of freedom and, hence, can grasp only with a cylindrical power grasp or with the tip of the thumb, index, and middle finger. Multifunctional hands as described in detail in [Schulz 2005] offer additional prehension patterns (Fig. 20).
- *Grasping force:* A minimum pinch force of 67 N was proposed to enable the users to perform all activities with their artificial hands. If the fingers of a prosthetic hand have more than 1 DOF and, thus, can conform to the shape of an object, the requisite grasping force is significantly lower [Kargov 2004].

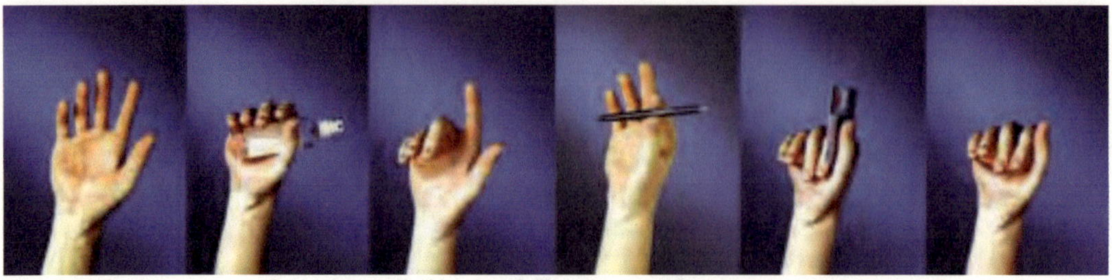

Fig. 20. From a neutral position (left), the following prehension patterns can be performed: cylindrical power grasp, index position, tip grasp, lateral grasp, and hook grasp.

- *Grasping speed:* Since their introduction in the 1970s, commercial prostheses have closed the fingers within one second, which can be taken as a benchmark. Just recently, prosthetic hands were introduced, which allow for much more speedy grasping.
- *Sensory feedback:* The lack of sensory information in electrically driven prosthetic hands is one of the main reasons for prosthesis rejection. The user has to estimate the force exerted by the prosthesis while grasping and the posture of the fingers has to be controlled visually.
- *Control:* Prosthetic upper limbs are typically controlled by switches, pressure sensors or myoelectric surface electrodes that are operated by the residual limb in the socket. The control of several independent DOFs has been a challenge, but with the introduction of microprocessors and new methods of biosignal analysis, future control systems will be easier for the patient to be learned and operation of the prosthetic aid will be more intuitive [Reischl 2004, Englehart 2003].
- *Reliability: Both* prosthetic and robotic hand users usually favour a reliable, but simple technical aid to a more sophisticated, independent device that malfunctions regularly. Especially users with a bilateral upper limb loss depend on their prosthetic hands.

Just recently, new prosthetic hands with increased functionality were presented [Schulz 2005, www.touchbionics.com]. For example the multifunctional prosthesis from the Forschungszentrum Karlsruhe, Germany allows for different prehension patterns and also includes sensory feedback [Schulz 2005, Pylatiuk 2006]. It is based on the same actuators described in 2.1 (Fig. 2), but it is driven by a micro hydraulic system (Fig. 4, 21), that is housed within the metacarpus of the hand.

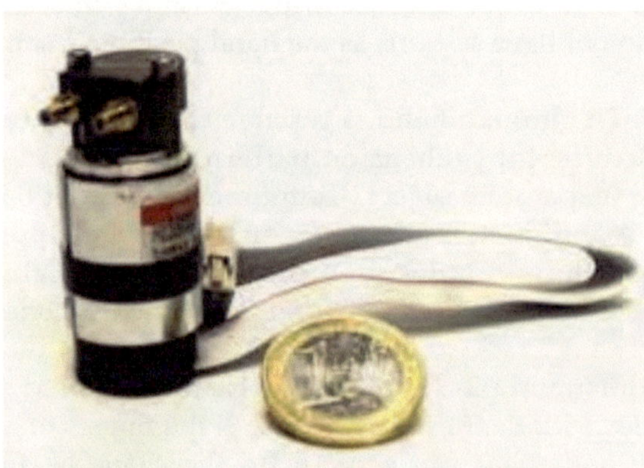

Fig. 21. A custom-made hydraulic pump.

4. References

Bien Z. Zenn; Stefanov Dimitar (Eds.) (2004). *Advances in Rehabilitation Robotics. Human friendly Technologies on Movement Assistance and Restoration for People with Disabilities.* Springer-Verlag Berlin, Heidelberg, New York, Hong Kong, London, Milan, Paris, Tokyo, 2004.

Venkataraman Subramanian T.; Iberall Thea (Eds.) (1990). *Dextrous Robot Hands.* Springer-Verlag New York, Berlin, Heidelberg, London, Paris, Tokyo, Hong Kong, 1990.

Muzumdar Ashok (Ed.) (2004). *Powered Upper Limb Prostheses. Control, Implementation and Clinical Application.* Springer-Verlag Berlin, Heidelberg, New York, 2004.

Shin'ichi Yuta; Hajime Asama; Sebastian Thrun; Erwin Prassler; Takashi Tsubouchi (Eds.) (2006) *Field and Service Robotics. Recent Advances in Research and Applications.* Springer-Verlag Berlin, Heidelberg, New York, 2006.

DeLaurentis KJ, Mavroidis C (2000). Development of a shape memory alloy actuated hand. In: Actuator `2000, S. 281-284, Bremen, Germany, 2000.

Pons JL, Rodriguez H, Ceres R, Van Moorleghem W, Reynaerts D (1998). Study of SMA Actuation to develop a Modular, User-adaptable Hand Prosthesis. 6th Int. Conference on New Actuators, 490-493, Bremen, Germany, 1998.

Pons JL, Rodriguez H, Duarte A, Luyckx, Reynaerts D, Ceres R, Van Brussel H (2000) High torque ultra-sonic motors for hand prosthetics: current status and trends. 7th Int. Conference on New Actuators, 285-288, Bremen, Germany, 2000.

Lee YK, Shimoyama I (2000). A micro rubber artificial muscle driven by a micro compressor for artificial limbs, Actuator 2000, 7th Int. Conf. on New Actuators, Bremen, Germany S. 272-275, 2000.

C.M. Light, P.H. Chappell, (2000). Development of a Lightweight and Adaptable Multiple-axis Hand Prosthesis, Med. Eng. & Phys., 10, 679-84, 2000.

Weir R.F. *ff*, Grahn E.C., Duff S.J., (2001). A New Externally-Powered, Myoelectrically Controlled Prosthesis for Persons with Partial Hand Amputations at the Metacarpals, J. Prosth. & Orth., 12(2), 26-31, 2001.

Kyberd P.J., Pons J.L. (2003). A Comparison of the Oxford and Manus Intelligent Hand Prosthesis. Proceedings of the IEEE (ICRA), Taipei, Taiwan, September 14 - 19, 2003.

Walker Rich (Shadow Robot Company) (2003). Design of a dextrous hand for advanced CLAWAR applications, In: Proceedings of the 6th International Conference on Climbing and Walking Robots (CLAWAR2003), Catania, Italy, 17.-19. Sept. 2003.

Boblan, I. Bannasch R., Schwenk H., Prietzel F., Miertsch L., Schulz A. (2004). A human-like robot hand and arm with fluidic muscles: Biologically inspired construction and functionality Embodied Artificial Intelligence Lecture Notes In Artificial Intelligence 3139: pp. 160-179, 2004.

Lee Y.K., Shimoyama I. (1999). A Skeletal Framework Artificial Hand Actuated by Pneumatic Artificial Muscles, Proceedings of the 1999 IEEE Int. Conf. On Robotics & Automation, Detroit, Michigan, May 1999.

Plettenburg DH (2002). A sizzling hand prosthesis. On the design and development of a pneumatically powered hand prosthesis for children. PhD-thesis, Delft University of Technology, The Netherlands, ISBN 90-370-0196-3, 2002.

Hirzinger G., Sporer N., Schedl M., Butterfaß J., Grebenstein M. (2004). Torque-controlled lightweight arms and articulated hands: do we reach technological limits, The International Journal of Robotics Research, vol. 23, No. 4-5, April-May 2004, pp. 331-340.

Jacobsen S., Iversen E., Knutti D., Johnson R., and Bigger K. (1986). Design of the Utah/MIT Dextrous Hand. In Proceedings of the 1986 IEEE International Conference on Robotics and Automation, pp. 96-102, 1986.

Townsend WT (2000). The BarrettHand grasper - programmably flexible part handling and assembly-Industrial Robot - An International Journal, 27(3), pp. 181-8, 2000.

Kargov A., Pylatiuk C., Schulz S (2006). Study of fluidic actuators in prosthetic hands. Proceedings of the 10th international conference on new actuators "Actuator 2006", Bremen, Germany, 14-16 June 2006. pp. 312-315.

Hollerbach J., Hunter I., Ballantyne J. (1992). A comparative analysis of actuator technologies for robotics, In: O. Khatib, J. Craig, Losano-Perez (Eds.), The robotics review 2, MIT Press, Cambridge, MA, USA, pp. 299-342, 1992.

Schulz S., Pylatiuk C., Bretthauer G. (1999). A New Class of Flexible Fluidic Actuators and their Applications in Medical Engineering. At 47 (8), Seite 390-395, 1999.

Martens C., Ruchel N., Lang O., Ivlev O., Graeser A. (2001). A FRIEND for Assisting Handicapped People, IEEE Robotics & Automation Magazine, Vol. 7, No.1, March 2001, pp. 57-65.

Ivlev O. Martens C., Graeser A. (2005). Rehabilitation Robots FRIEND-I and FRIEND-II with the dexterous lightweight manipulator. Technology and Disability (Special Issue), Vol. 17, 2, 2005, pp. 111-123.

Seraji H. (1989). Configuration Control of Manipulators: Theory and Implementation, IEEE Trans. on Robotics and Automation, Vol. 5, No.4, 1989, S. 472-490.

Ivlev O., Graeser A. (2000). The Optimized Kinematic Configuration Control Algorithm for Redundant Robots. Proc. 16th IMACS World Congress on Scientific Computation, Applied Mathematics and Simulation, Lausanne, Switzerland, August 21-25, 2000.

Dahm P., Joublin F. (1997). Closed form solution for the inverse kinematics of a redundant robot arm. Technical Report 8, Institut für Neuroinformatik, Ruhr-Universität Bochum, 1997.

Asfour T., Berns K., Albiez J., Dillmann R. (1999). Programming of Manipulation Tasks of the Humanoid Robot ARMAR. The 9th International Conference on Advanced Robotics (ICAR'99), Tokyo, Japan, October 25-27, 1999, pp. 107-112.

Ivlev O, Graeser A. (1997). An Analytical Method for the Inverse Kinematics of Redundant Robots. Proc. 3d ECPD International Conference on Advanced Robots, Intelligent Automation and Active Systems, Bremen, 1997, pp. 416-421.

Ivlev O., Graeser A. (1999). Explicit Symbolic Solution of the Inverse Kinematics for Redundant Robotic Systems, at-Automatisierungstechnik, 47, 11, 1999, pp. 523-531 (*in German*).

Ivlev O., Rixen K., Graeser A. (2004). Kinematic Configuration Control of Redundant Robots with 7 Joints, Robotik 2004, VDI-Report Nr. 1841, pp. 543-550 (*in German*).

Feuser J., Ivlev O., Graeser A. (2005). Mapped Virtual Reality for a Safe Manipulation in Rehabilitation Robotics", Assistive Technology: From Virtuality to Reality (AAATE 2005); IOS Press, Amsterdam, 2005, pp. 666-671.

Martens C., Ivlev O., Graeser A. (2001). Interactive Controlled Robotic System FRIEND to Assist Disabled People. 7th International Conference On Rehabilitation Robotics (ICORR 2001); Evry Cedex, France, April 25-27, 2001, pp. 148-54.

Volosyak I., Ivlev O., Graeser A. (2005). Rehabilitation Robot FRIEND II - The General Concept and Current Implementation", Proc. of the IEEE 9th Int. Conf. On Rehabilitation Robotics (ICORR 2005); Chicago, Illinois, pp. 540-544.

Gilbert E. G., Johnson D. W., Keerthi S. S. (1988). A Fast Procedure for Computing the Distance between Complex Objects in Three Dimensional Space. IEEE Journal of Robotics and Automation, Vol. 4, No. 2, April 1988, pp. 192-203.

Atkins DJ, Heard DCY, Donovan WH (1996). Epidemiologic overview of individuals with upper-limb loss and their reported research priorities. J Prosthet Orthot 8(1):2–11, 1996.

Englehart K, Hudgins B (2003). A robust, real-time control scheme for multifunction myoelectric control., IEEE Transactions on Biomedical Engineering, 50(7):848- 854, 2003.

Kargov A, Pylatiuk C, Martin J, et al. (2004). A comparison of the grip force distribution in natural hands and in prosthetic hands. Disabil Rehabil 26(12):705–711, 2004.

Keller A, Tyalor C, Zahm V (1947). Studies to Determine the Functional Requirements for Hand and Arm Prosthesis. Dept. of Engineering, UCLA, July 1947.

Kyberd PJ (2004). Research and the future in myoelectric prosthetics. In: Ashok Muzumdar (ed) Powered upper limb prostheses: control, implementation and clinical application. Springer, Berlin Heidelberg New York, pp 175–190, ISBN 3540404066, 2004.

Asfour, T., Regenstein, K., Azad, P., Schröder, J., Bierbaum, A., Vahrenkamp, N. and Dillmann, R. ARMAR-III (2006). An Integrated Humanoid Platform for Sensory-Motor Control. In IEEE-RAS International Conference on Humanoid Robots (Humanoids 2006), Genoa, Italy, December 2006.

Azad, P., Asfour, T. and Dillmann, R. (2006). Combining Appearance-based and Model-based Methods for Real-Time Object Recognition and 6D Localization. In Proc. International Conference on Intelligent Robots and Systems (IROS 06), Beijing, China, October 2006.

Asfour, T.; Ly, D.N.; Regenstein, K.; Dillmann, R. (2005). Coordinated Task Execution for Humanoid Robots. In Experimental Robotics IX, STAR, Springer Tracts in Advanced Robotics, Vol. 21, pp. 259-267, 2005.

Morales, M., Asfour, T., Azad, P., Knoop, S. and Dillmann, R. (2006). Integrated Grasp Planning and Visual Object Localization for a Humanoid Robot with Five-Fingered Hands. In Proc. International Conference on Intelligent Robots and Systems (IROS 06), Beijing, China, October 2006.

Schulz, S. , Pylatiuk, Ch., Kargov, A., Oberle, R. and Bretthauer, G. (2004). Progress in the development of anthropomorphic fluidic hands for a humanoid robot, In IEEE/RAS International Conference on Humanoid Robots, Los Angeles, Nov 2004.

Kerpa, O., Weiss, K. and Wörn, H. (2003). Development of a flexible tactile sensor for a humanid robot," in IEEE/RSJ International. Conference on Intelligent Robots and Systems, Las Vegas, Nevada, Oct. 2003, pp. 1-6.

16

Upper-Limb Exoskeletons for Physically Weak Persons

Kazuo Kiguchi[*1] & Toshio Fukuda[*2]
**1: Saga University*
Japan
**2: Nagoya University*
Japan

1. Introduction

Robotics technology is expected to play an important role not only in industries, but also in welfare and medicine. A power-assist exoskeleton, which is directly attached to the human body and assist the motion in accordance with the user's motion intension, is one of the most effective assist robots for the physically weak persons. A study of power-assist exoskeletons has been carried out for a long time (Mosher & Wendel, 1960). The power-assist exoskeletons, which are sometimes called as power suits, man amplifiers, man magnifiers, or power-assist systems, have been studied for the purpose of military, industry, or medial use (Cloud, 1965; Mosher, 1967; Vukobratovic, 1975; Kazerooni & Mahoney, 1991). Recently, many studies on power-assist robots have been carried out to help the motion of physically weak persons such as disabled, injured, and/or elderly persons in daily activities or rehabilitation (Nagai *et al.*, 1998, Kiguchi *et al.*, 2001-2007; Rosen *et al.*, 2001; Tsagarkis & Caldwell, 2003; Sasaki *et al.*, 2004).
EMG-based control (i.e., control based on the skin surface electromyogram (EMG) signals of the user) is often used for control of the robotic systems (Farry *et al.*, 1996; Suryanarayanan, 1996; Fukuda *et al.*, 2003) since EMG signals of user's muscles directly reflect the user's motion intension. When certain motion is performed, the EMG signals of the related muscles show the unique pattern. Therefore, upper-limb motion of the user could be predicted by monitoring EMG signals of certain muscles of the user since the amount of EMG signal is proportional to the activity level of the muscle. Consequently, the EMG-based control is good at automatically activating the power-assist exoskeletons in accordance with user's motion intention. However, the EMG-based control is not easy to be realized for multi-DOF power-assist exoskeletons because 1: obtaining the same EMG signals for the same motion is difficult even with the same person, 2: activity level of each muscle and the way of using each muscle for a certain motion is different between persons, 3: real time motion prediction is not easy since many muscles are involved in a joint motion, 4: one muscle is not only concerned with one motion but also another kinds of motion, 5: role of each muscle for a certain motion varies in accordance with joint angles (Dominici *et al.*, 2005), and 6: the activity level of some muscles such as bi-articular muscles are affected by

the motion of the other joint. The most of the above mentioned problems can be cleared by applying neuro-fuzzy control (i.e., the combination of adaptive neuro control and flexible fuzzy control).
The design and control method of upper-limb exoskeletons are explained in this chapter. Four-DOF upper-limb power-assist exoskeletons are introduced as examples of effective exoskeletons.

2. Exoskeletons for Upper-Limb Assist

Assist of upper-limb motion is important in daily activities. Therefore, many kinds of upper-limb exoskeletons have been proposed up to the present (Kiguchi *et al.*, 2001-2007) in order to improve the quality of life of physically weak persons. In exoskeletons, it is not easy to locate actuators and links in appropriate positions since the user's body is usually placed in the center of the system. Furthermore, the actuators and links of the exoskeletons must be located not to prevent the user motion, although the position of the rotational center of the exoskeleton's joints must be the same as that of the user's joint. In the case of the elbow joint, the joint is modeled as a uniaxial hinge joint (London, 1981) although it consists of three bones (humerus, ulna, and radius). Therefore, it is not difficult to locate the axis of the rotational center of the exoskeleton's elbow joint to be the same as that of the user's elbow joint. In the case of the shoulder joint, however, it is not easy to locate the position of the rotational center of the exoskeleton's shoulder joint to be the same as that of the user's shoulder joint since the joint is modeled as a spherical joint (Kiguchi *et al.*, 2003a, 2003b, 2004, 2006a).
A 4DOF power-assist exoskeleton (Kiguchi *et al.*, 2006c), which assists shoulder vertical and horizontal flexion/extension motion, elbow flexion/extension motion, and forearm pronation/supination motion, is depicted in Fig. 1 (a) as an example of the upper-limb power-assist exoskeleton robot. It mainly consists of a shoulder motion assist mechanism, an elbow motion assist mechanism, a forearm motion assist mechanism, four DC motors, the shoulder mechanism of the moving center of rotation, and a wrist force sensor, and is installed on a mobile wheel chair. In this system, the mobile wheel chair itself is able to generate 2DOF motion.
Another 4DOF power-assist exoskeleton (Kiguchi *et al.*, 2006b), which assists shoulder 3DOF motion (vertical and horizontal flexion/extension, and internal/external rotation motion) and elbow flexion/extension motion, is shown in Fig. 1 (b) as another example of the upper-limb power assist exoskeleton. It mainly consists of four main links, an upper-arm holder, a wrist holder, four DC motors, the shoulder mechanism of the moving center of rotation, the mechanism for shoulder inner/outer rotation motion assist, an elbow joint, a wrist force sensor, and driving wires. The shoulder vertical/horizontal motion is assisted by controlling the tension of driving wires connected to the upper-arm holder, and the shoulder rotational motion is assisted by the DC motor in the upper-arm holder in this robotic system. The mechanism for shoulder inner/outer rotation motion assist consists of a stator, a bearing holder, and a rotor. The rotor consists of a half cylinder, sliders, and a rack gear. The DC motor makes shoulder internal/external rotation motion by moving the rotor with respect to the stator. The DC motor and the mechanism for shoulder inner/outer rotation motion assist are installed in the arm holder. The details of the mechanism are shown in Fig. 2.

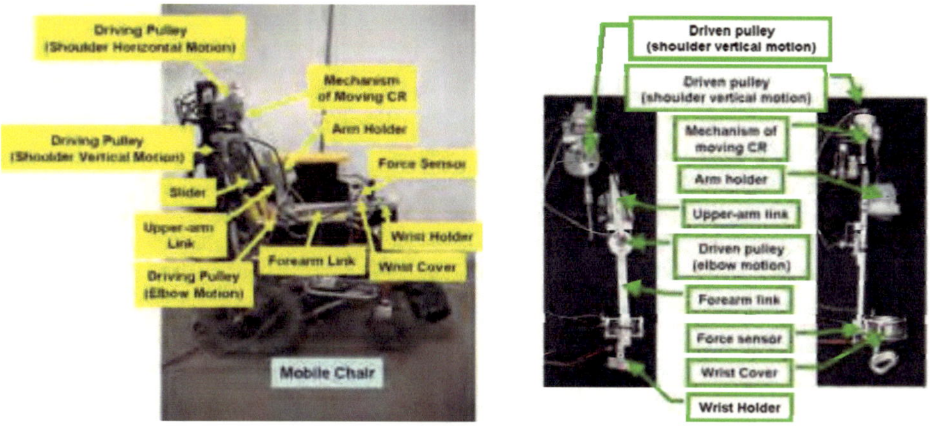

(a) Exoskeleton 1

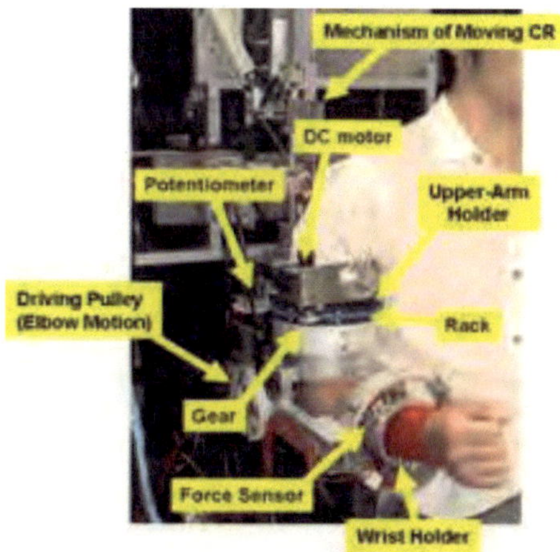

(b) Exoskeleton 2

Fig. 1 Examples of 4DOF upper-limb power-assist exoskeletons.

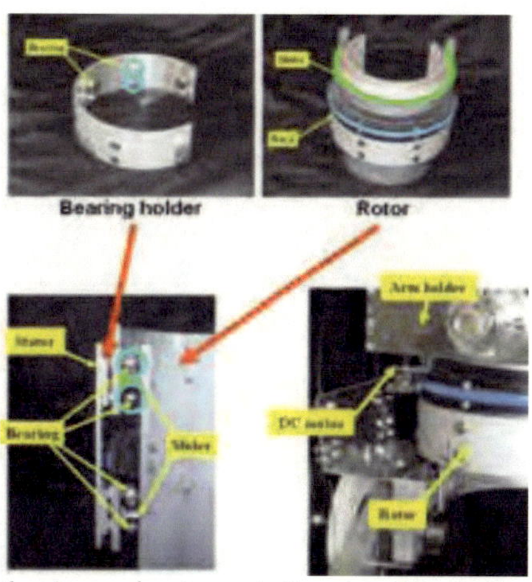

Fig. 2 Mechanism for shoulder inner/outer rotation motion assist.

The mechanism of the moving center of rotation of the shoulder joint (CR mechanism) used in the exoskeleton shown in Fig. 1 (a) is depicted in Fig. 3. The CR mechanism consists of a slider (made of ball-spline mechanism) and two links (link1 and link2, as shown in Fig. 3). The slider is installed between link1 and link2 of the exoskeleton and the upper-arm holder is installed on it.

The shoulder joint of the exoskeleton (i.e., joint between the link1 and the link2) is supposed to be located just behind the armpit of the user. This CR mechanism makes the CR of the exoskeleton shoulder joint move behind (farther position from the arm holder) in accordance with to the shoulder flexion angle in the case of flexion motion, and move inward (closer position of arm holder) in accordance with the shoulder abduction angle in the case of abduction motion. The link work mechanism is applied to realize this mechanism. In the case of shoulder flexion/extension motion, the link2 is vertically rotated with respect to the joint between the link1 and link2. As the link2 rotates vertically, the additional link (the link for the slider) is rotated with respect to joint2 (universal joint). The other end of the link for the slider is attached on the slider on the link2. Since the radius of the link2 and the link for the slider is different, the slider moves along the link2 according to the shoulder flexion angle.

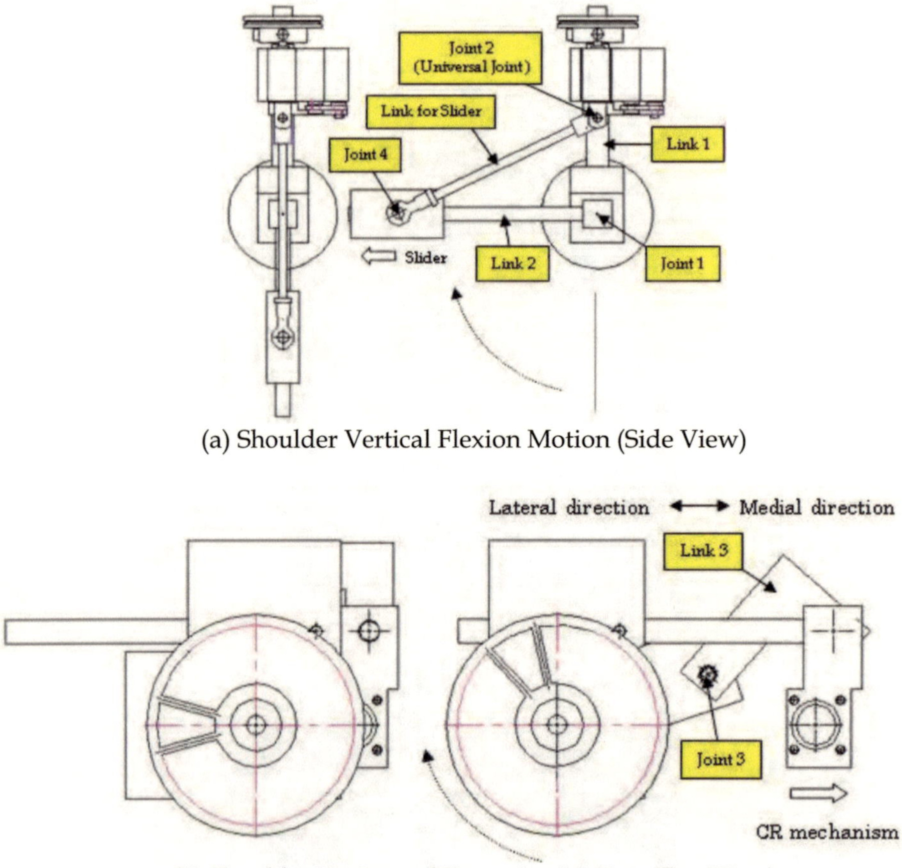

(a) Shoulder Vertical Flexion Motion (Side View)

(b) Shoulder Horizontal Extension Motion (Top View)

Fig. 3 Motion of Centre of Rotation (CR) Mechanism.

In the case of shoulder abduction/adduction motion, the link1 is rotated about its axis according to the abduction/adduction angle. As the link1 rotates, joint3 is rotated with respect to the axis of the link1. The rotation of the joint3 causes the movement of the position of the joint2 along the lateral-medial direction as shown in Fig. 3 (b). As the position of the joint moves along the lateral-medial direction, the slider moves along the link2 since the link for the slider is connected to the joint2.
Usually, the movable range of human shoulder is 180° in flexion, 60° in extension, 180° in abduction, 75° in adduction, 100-110° in internal rotation, and 80-90° in external rotation. The limitation of the movable range of forearm pronation-supination motion is 50-80 degrees in pronation and 80-90 degrees in supination, and that of elbow flexion-extension motion is 145 degrees in flexion and -5 degrees in extension. Considering the minimally required motion in everyday life and the safety of the user, the shoulder motion of the 4DOF exoskeleton shown in Fig. 1 (a) is limited to 0° in extension and adduction, 90° in flexion, and 90° in abduction. The limitation of its forearm motion is decided to be 50° in pronation and 80° in supination, and that of elbow motion is decided to be 120° in flexion and 0° in extension. In the case of 4DOF exoskeleton shown in Fig. 1 (b), the elbow joint motion of the exoskeleton system is limited between 0° and 120°, and the limitation of the shoulder joint motion of the exoskeleton system are decided to be 0° in extension and adduction, 90° in flexion, 90° in abduction, 90° in internal rotation, and 50° in external rotation.
Those exoskeletons are controlled to assist the upper-limb motion of the user in accordance with the user's motion intention by monitoring the EMG signals of certain muscles involved in the upper-limb motion. In order to assist all upper-limb motion except the wrist dorso-palmar flexion and radio-ulnar deviation motion, at least 5DOF motion must be provided assuming that the location of the rotational center of the shoulder joint of the exoskeleton is the same as that of the user. As a matter of fact, more DOF is required to assist all upper-limb motion since human shoulder complex, which consists of the scapula, clavicle, and humerus and moves conjointly, itself provides 7 DOF for the upper-limb motion (Zatsiorsky, 1998). Therefore, some kind of adjustment mechanism is usually required to compensate for the ill-effect caused by the difference of the shoulder rotational center between the exoskeleton and the user (Kiguchi *et al.*, 2003a, 2003b, 2004, 2006a).
As far as the hardware of the exoskeletons is concerned, both mechanisms shown in Fig. 1 can be easily combined to make a 5DOF power assist exoskeleton that assists shoulder 3DOF motion (vertical and horizontal flexion/extension, and internal/external rotation motion), elbow flexion/extension motion, and forearm pronation/supination motion. As far as the controller (EMG-based controller) of the exoskeleton concerned, however, it is not easy to control the combined 5DOF motion based on the EMG signals because certain muscles are involved in several motions in the 5DOF. The details are discussed in the next section.

3. Electromyogram (EMG)

Electromyogram (EMG) signal (0.01-10mV, 10-2,000Hz) is one of the most important biological signals to understand human motion intention it is generated when the muscles contract. Features must be extracted from the raw EMG data since it is difficult to use the raw EMG data for input information of the controller. There are many kinds of feature extraction methods, e.g., Mean Absolute Value, Mean Absolute Value Slope, Zero

Crossings, Slope Sign Changes, Waveform Length, or Root Mean Square (Hudgins, 1993). Root Mean Square (RMS), one of the best feature extraction methods, is applied in this study because of its simplicity and effectiveness.

$$RMS = \sqrt{\frac{1}{N}\sum_{i=1}^{N} v_i^2} \tag{1}$$

where, v_i is the voltage value at the ith sampling and N is the number of sample in a segment. The number of sample is set to be 100 and the sampling time is 500μsec in this study. Applying the RMS, the feature of the EMG signal can be effectively extracted in real-time as shown in Fig. 4.

Fig. 4. Feature extraction of EMG signal.

The magnitude of the RMS of the EMG signal is proportional to the activity level of the muscle. When the magnitude of the RMS of the EMG signals is not so large, the exoskeleton is controlled based on the wrist force sensor of the exoskeleton to avoid the misoperation (Kiguchi *et al.*, 2001-2002 & 2004-2007). When the user activates the muscles, the force sensor signals are ignored and the EMG-based control is applied. By applying sensor fusion with the EMG signals and the wrist force sensor signals, error motion caused by little EMG levels and the external force affecting to the user arm can be avoided.
Human elbow is mainly actuated by two antagonist muscles: biceps and triceps, although it consists of more muscles. The origin of the long head of biceps is connected to supraglenoid tubercle of the scapula, and that of the short head of biceps is connected to coracoid process of the scapula. The other side of biceps is connected to tuberosity of the radius and the bicipital aponeurosis. In the case of triceps, the origin of the long head is connected to infraglenoid tubercle of the scapula, that of the lateral head is connected to posterior surface and lateral border of the humerus and the lateral intermuscular septum, and that of the medial head is connected to posterior surface and medial border of the humerus and the medial intermuscular septum. The other side of triceps is connected to posterior part of the olecranon process of the ulna and the deep fascia of the dorsal forearm. Consequently, biceps and a part triceps are bi-articular muscles. For example, biceps is used to generate elbow flexion motion, shoulder vertical flexion motion, and also forearm supination motion especially when the elbow joint is in the flexed position. Therefore, when those motions are generated simultaneously, the EMG-based control of power-assist exoskeleton is not very easy to be realized.

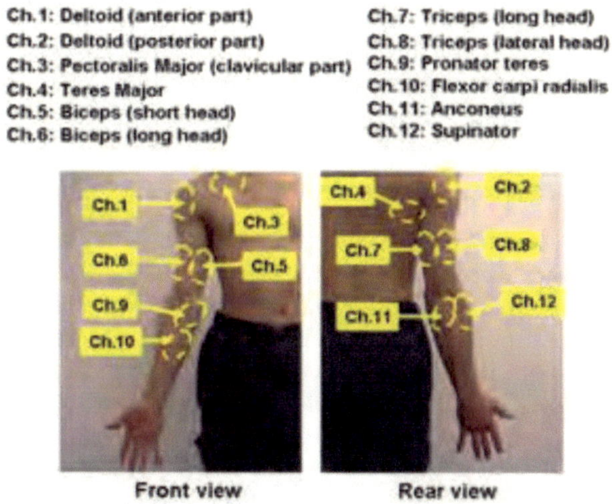

(a) Electrodes for the exoskeleton 1

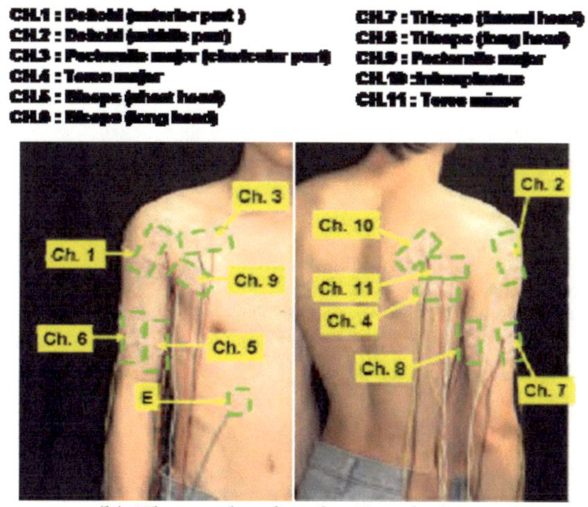

(b) Electrodes for the exoskeleton 2

Fig. 5 Location of each electrode.

In order to assist the 4DOF motion (shoulder vertical flexion/extension, shoulder horizontal flexion/extension, elbow flexion/extension, and forearm supination/pronation) of the exoskeleton1 shown in Fig. 1 (a), the EMG signals measured at 12 points (Deltoid - anterior part, Deltoid - posterior part, Pectoralis Major - clavicular part, Teres Major, Biceps - short head, Bicesp - long head, Triceps - long head, Triceps - lateral head, Pronator Teres, Flexor Carpi Radialis, Anconeus, and Supinator) of the related muscles are measured with the electrodes (NE-101A: Nihon Koden Co.) through the amplifier (MEG-6108: Nihon Koden Co.) and analyzed in the controller of the exoskeleton. The location of each electrode is depicted in Fig. 5 (a).

In order to assist the 4DOF motion (shoulder vertical flexion/extension, shoulder horizontal flexion/extension, shoulder internal/external rotation, and elbow flexion/extension) of the exoskeleton2 shown in Fig. 1 (b), the EMG signals measured at 11 points (Deltoid - anterior part, Deltoid - medial part, Pectoralis major - clavicular part, Teres major, Biceps - short head, Bicesp - long head, Triceps - long head, Triceps - lateral head, Pectoralis major, Infraspinatus, and Teres minor) of the related muscles are measured with the electrodes through the amplifier and analyzed in the controller of the exoskeleton. The location of each electrode is depicted in Fig. 5 (b).

4. Control of Upper-Limb Exoskeletons

In order to control the upper-limb exoskeleton in accordance with the user's motion intention, EMG-based control is mainly applied. In order to cope with the problems of the EMG-based control caused from human anatomy, multiple neuro-fuzzy controllers are applied. When the magnitude of the muscle activity levels of the user is little, however, the exoskeleton is controlled based on the wrist force sensor to avoid the misoperation (Kiguchi *et al.*, 2001-2002 & 2004-2007). When the user activates the muscles, the force sensor signals are ignored and the EMG-based control is applied. The basic architecture of the whole control system for the exoskeletons shown in Fig. 1 (a) is shown in Fig. 6. The controller basically consists of three stages (first stage: input signal selection stage, second stage: posture region selection stage, and third stage: neuro-fuzzy control stage). In the first stage of the controller, the EMG based control or the wrist sensor based control is applied in accordance with the muscle activity levels of the user. In the second stage of the controller, a proper neuro-fuzzy controller is selected according to the shoulder and the elbow angle region. In the third stage of the controller, the desired torque command for each joint is calculated with the selected neuro-fuzzy controllers to realize the effective motion assist for the user.

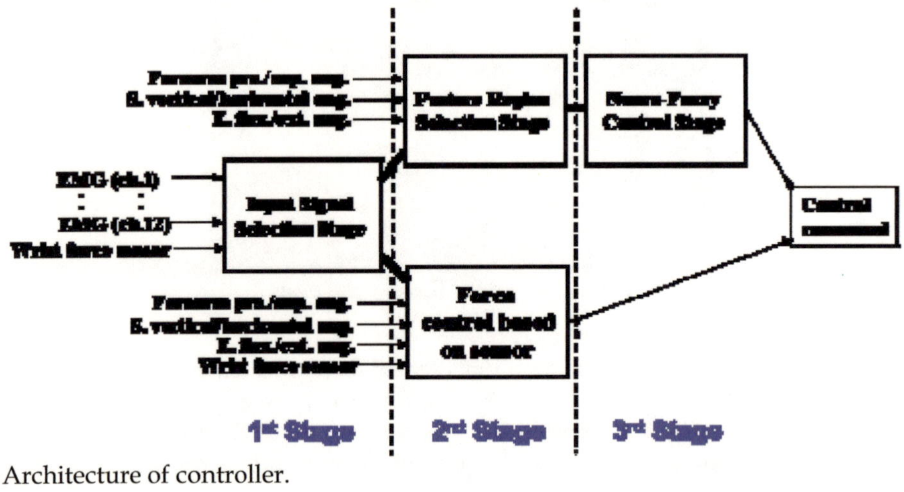

Fig. 6 Architecture of controller.

In the first stage of the controller, proper input information for the controller is selected according to the user's muscle activity levels. The EMG-based control or the wrist sensor based control is selected in this stage in accordance with the muscle activity levels of the user. If the activity level of every muscle is little, the wrist sensor based control is selected in this stage. When the user activates the muscles, the EMG-based control is selected. These control methods are gradually switched according to the situation by applying the fuzzy switching. The membership function (PB: Positive Big) of each muscle is used to switch the controller input information.

The EMG-based control rules are sometimes different when the arm posture is changed since role of each muscle is changed according to the arm posture because of anatomical reason. In order to cope with this problem, multiple neuro-fuzzy controllers are designed and applied under certain arm posture region in the second stage (Kiguchi, 2002, 2003a, 2004). A properly designed neuro-fuzzy controller is prepared for each elbow and shoulder angle region. Based on the joint angle, the movable range of elbow angle, shoulder vertical angle, and shoulder horizontal angle regions is divided into three regions (FA: flexed angle, IA: intermediate angle, and EA: extended angle), respectively. By applying the membership functions, the appropriate controllers are moderately selected in accordance with the upper-limb posture of the user.

In the third stage, selected neuro-fuzzy controllers generate the required torque command for each joint. The architecture of the neuro-fuzzy controller for the exoskeleton shown in Fig. 1 (a) is depicted in Fig. 7. Here, Σ means the summation of the inputs and Π means the multiplication of the inputs. Two kinds of nonlinear functions (f_G and f_S) are applied to express the membership function of the neuro-fuzzy controller.

$$f_s(u_s) = \frac{1}{1+e^{-u_s}} \tag{2}$$

$$u_s(x) = w_0 + w_i x \tag{3}$$

$$f_G(u_G) = e^{-u_G^2} \tag{4}$$

$$u_G(x) = \frac{w_0 + x}{w_i} \tag{5}$$

where w_0 is a threshold value and w_i is a weight.

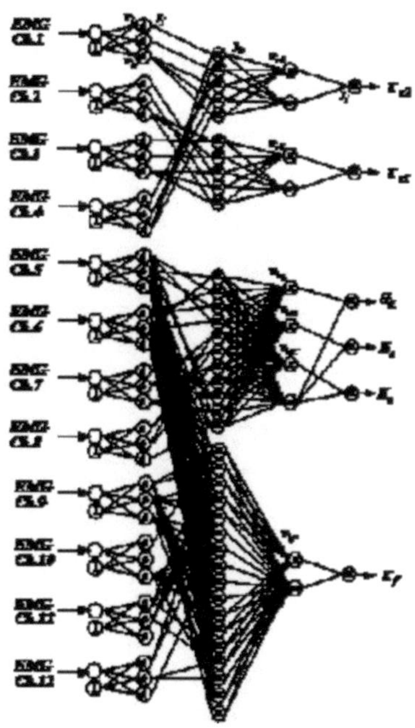

Fig. 7 Neuro-fuzzy controller.

The structure of the neuro-fuzzy controller is basically the same as the conventional simplified fuzzy controller since it can be easily designed based on our anatomical knowledge and the results of previously performed experiment. The neuro-fuzzy controller consists of five layers (input layer, fuzzifier layer, rule layer, defuzzifier layer, and output layer). In the fuzzifier layer, the degree of fitness of each input signal (each RMS) for each fuzzy set (ZO: ZERO, PS: Positive Small, and PB: Positive Big) is calculated. In the rule layer, the degree of fitness of each rule is calculated. The output from the neuro-fuzzy controller (i.e., the desired torque for shoulder and forearm motion, and the desired impedance and angle change of elbow motion) is calculated in the defuzzifier layer.

The amount of weights of consequence part of the control rules, which are concerned with elbow flexion motion, in the neuro-fuzzy controllers are defined as functions of the activity levels of the related muscles used for the shoulder vertical motion and forearm supination motion. So that the activity levels of the related muscles used for the other motion modify the related control rules effectively (Kiguchi, 2007).

When the user of the exoskeleton is changed, the controller is adjusted for the user's condition using the error back-propagation learning algorithm (Rumelhart, 1986). The evaluation function is written as:

$$E = \frac{1}{2}((\theta_d - \theta)^2 + \alpha \sum (RMS_d - RMS)^2) \tag{6}$$

where θ_d is the desired joint angle indicated by the user using the motion indicator, θ is the measured shoulder and elbow angle, α is a coefficient which changes the degree of consideration of the muscle activity minimization, RMS_d is the desired muscle activity level of certain muscle, and RMS is the measured muscle activity level of certain muscle. The desired joint angles are indicated by the user's hand motion (the other side of the assisted upper-limb) using the motion indicator shown in Fig. 8. The weights in all of antecedent part and some of consequence part of neuro-fuzzy controllers are modified to minimize the amount of the evaluation function. After the controller adjustment, appropriate power-assist can be carried out with the desired assist level.

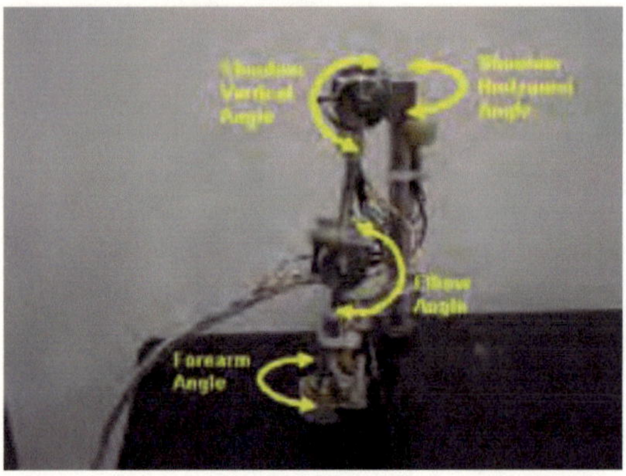

Fig. 8 Motion indicator.

5. Upper-Limb Motion Assist

Upper-limb motion assist experiment has been carried out with and without assist of the 4DOF active exoskeleton1 (Fig. 1 (a)) to evaluate its effectiveness. Two kinds of motion are carried out by healthy young male subjects in the experiment. If the motion is properly assisted by the proposed exoskeleton, the magnitude of the muscle activity level is supposed to be reduced for the same motion when the motion is assisted by the exoskeleton.

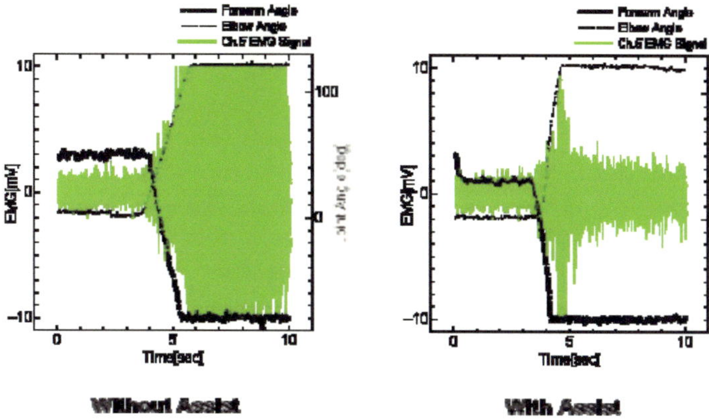

(a) Biceps (short head) - ch.5

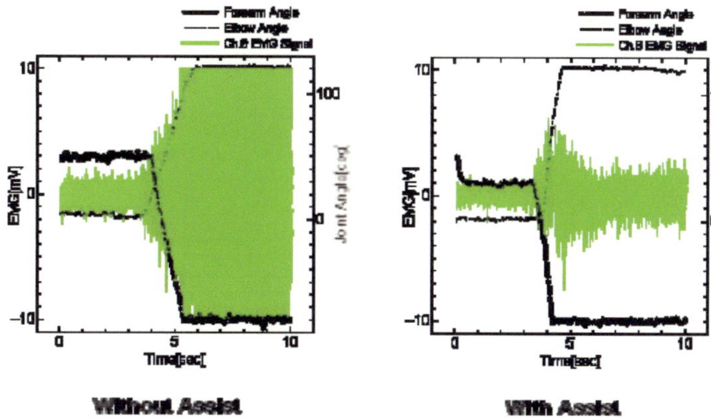

(b) Biceps (long head) - ch.6

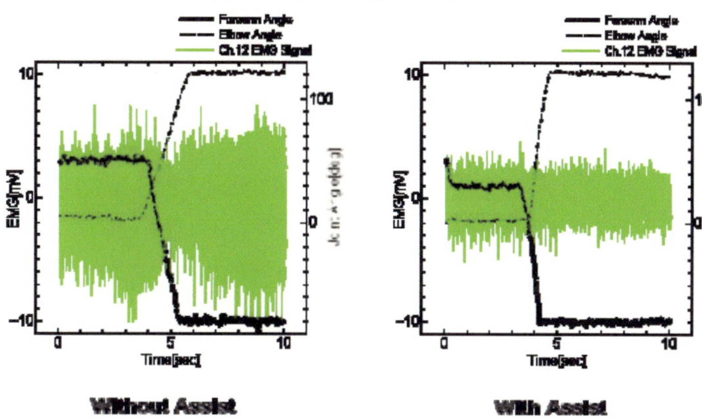

(c) Supinator - ch.12

Fig. 9. Experimental results of motion 1.

For the first motion (motion 1) in the experiment, cooperative motion of elbow flexion motion and forearm supination motion is performed with and without assist of the exoskeleton1. The results are shown in Fig. 9. Here, only the results of biceps (ch.5 & ch.6) and supinator (ch.12) are shown as representative results, since these are the most active muscles for this motion.

One can see that the activity level of each muscle is reduced for the same motion when the motion is assisted by the exoskeleton.

For the second motion (motion 2) in the experiment, cooperative motion of shoulder vertical motion, shoulder horizontal motion, elbow motion, and forearm motion is performed with and without assist of the exoskeleton1. The results are shown in Fig. 10. Here, only the results of deltoid anterior part (ch.1), teres major (ch.4), biceps short head (ch.5), triceps long head (ch.7) and pronator teres (ch.9) are shown as representative results.

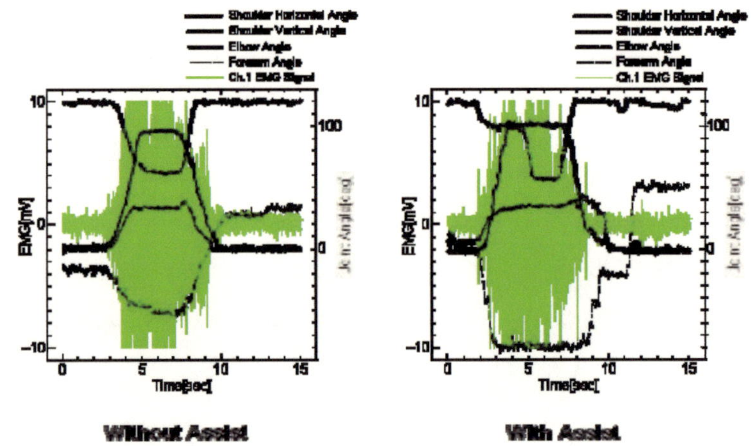

(a) Deltoid (anterior part) - ch.1

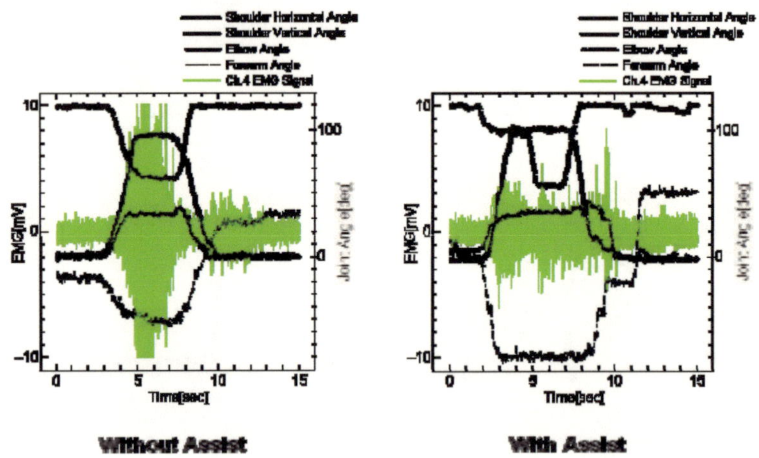

(b) Teres major - ch.4

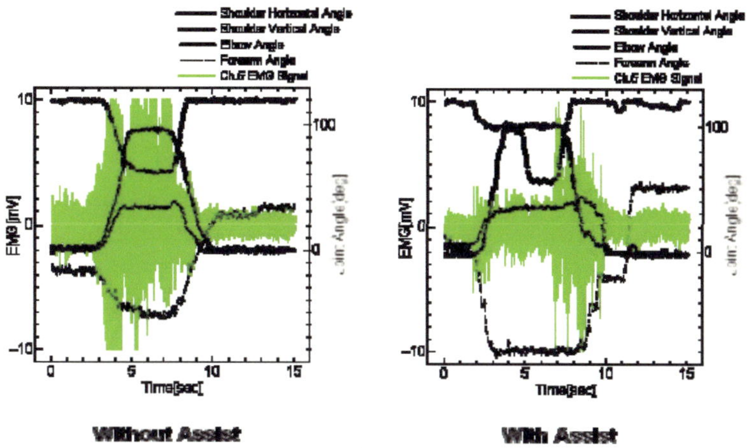

(c) Biceps (short head) - ch.5

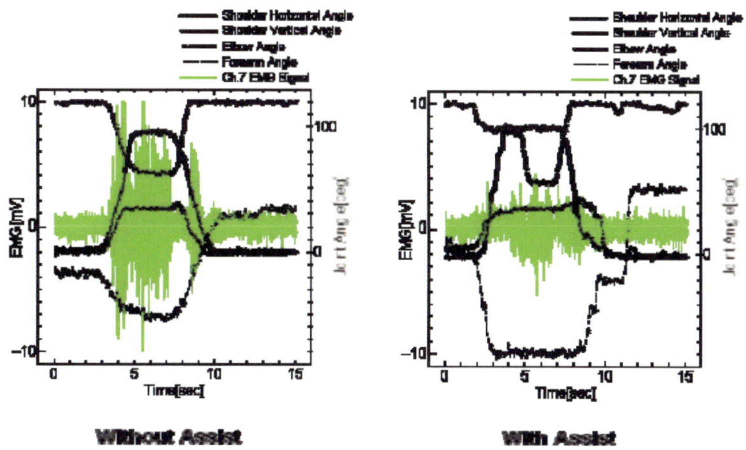

(d) Triceps (long head) - ch.7

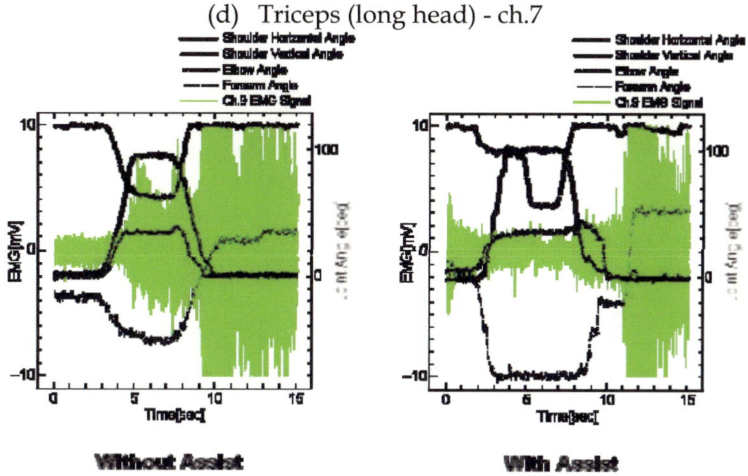

(e) Pronator teres - ch.9

Fig. 10. Experimental results of motion 2.

These experimental results also show that the activity level of each muscle is reduced for the same motion when the motion is assisted by the exoskeleton. Consequently, the effectiveness of the 4DOF upper-limb power-assist exoskeleton is verified by the experiment.

6. Conclusion

The design and control method of 4DOF upper-limb power-assist exoskeletons are explained in this chapter. Two kinds of 4DOF upper-limb power-assist exoskeletons are introduced as examples of the effective exoskeletons. The EMG-based control method is explained in order to activate the exoskeletons according the user's motion intention. The effectiveness of the power-assist exoskeleton is verified by the experiment.

As far as upper-limb motion assist for physically weak persons is concerned, not all users need full (7DOF) upper-limb motion assist since symptom of each user is different. Consequently, only the required motion assist for each user should be provided by the power-assist exoskeleton.

7. References

Cloud W. (1965). Man Amplifiers: Machines That Let You Carry a Ton, *Popular Science*, Vol.187, No.5, pp.70-73&204.

Dominici F.; Popa T.; Ginanneschi F. & Mazzocchio R. (2005). Cortico-Motoneuronal Output to Intrinsic Hand Muscles is Differentially Influenced by Static Changes in Shoulder Positions, *Experimental Brain Research*, Vol.164, pp.500-504.

Farry K.A.; Walker I.D. & Baraniuk R.G. (1996) Myoelectric Teleoperation of a Complex Robotic Hand, *IEEE Trans. on Robotics and Automation*, Vol.12, No.5, pp.775-788, ISSN 1042-296X.

Flash T. & Hogan N. (1985). The Coordination of Arm Movements: An Experimental Confirmed Mathematical Model, *Journal of Neuroscience*, Vol.5, pp.1688-1703.

Fukuda O.; Tsuji T.; Kaneko M. & Otsuka A. (2003). A Human-Assisting Manipulator Teleoperated by EMG Signals and Arm Motions, *IEEE Trans. on Robotics and Automation*, Vol. 19, No. 2, pp.210-222, ISSN 1042-296X.

Guizzo E. & Goldstein H. (2005) The Rise of the Body Bots, *IEEE Spectrum*, Vol.42, No.10, pp.42-48, ISSN 0018-9235.

Hudgins B.; Parker P. & Scott R.N. (1993) A New Strategy for Multifunction Myoelectric Control, *IEEE Trans. on Biomedical Engineering*, Vol.40, No.1, pp.82-94, ISSN 0018-9294.

Kazerooni H. & Mahoney S.L. (1991). Dynamics and Control of Robotic Systems Worn by Humans, *Trans. of the ASME, Journal of Dynamic Systems, Measurement, and Control*, Vol.113, No.3, pp.379-387.

Kiguchi K.; Kariya S.; Watanabe K.; Izumi K. & Fukuda T. (2001). An Exoskeletal Robot for Human Elbow Motion Support – Sensor Fusion, Adaptation, and Control, *IEEE Trans. on Systems, Man, and Cybernetics, Part B*, Vol.31, No.3, pp.353-361, ISSN 1083-4419.

Kiguchi K.; Kariya S.; Watanabe K. & Fukuda T. (2002). Application of Multiple Neuro-fuzzy Controllers of an Exoskeletal Robot for Human Elbow Motion Support, *Trans. on Control, Automation and Systems Engineers*, Vol.4, No.1, pp.49-55.

Kiguchi K.; Iwami K.; Yasuda M.; Watanabe K. & Fukuda T. (2003a). An Exoskeletal Robot for Human Shoulder Joint Motion Assist, *IEEE/ASME Trans. on Mechatronics*, Vol.8, No.1, pp.125-135.

Kiguchi K.; Iwami K.; Watanabe K. & Fukuda T. (2003b). An Assist Level Adjustment Method of an Active Shoulder Orthosis, *International Journal of Human-friendly Welfare Robotic Systems*, Vol. 4, No. 2, pp.8-12.

Kiguchi K.; Tanaka T. & Fukuda T. (2004). Neuro-Fuzzy Control of a Robotic Exoskeleton with EMG Signals, *IEEE Trans. on Fuzzy Systems*, Vol.12, No.4, pp.481-490, ISSN 1063-6706.

Kiguchi K.; Esaki R. & Fukuda T. (2005). Development of a Wearable Exoskeleton for Daily Forearm Motion Assist, *Advanced Robotics*, Vol.19, No.7, pp.751-771.

Kiguchi K.; Rahman M.H. & Sasaki M. (2006a). Neuro-Fuzzy based Motion Control of a Robotic Exoskeleton: Considering End-effector Force Vectors, *Proc. of 2006 IEEE International Conf. on Robotics and Automation*, pp.3146-3151, Orlando, May 2006.

Kiguchi K.; Yamaguchi T. & Sasaki M. (2006b). Development of a 4DOF Exoskeleton Robot for Upper-limb Motion Assist, *Proc. of 2006 ASME/JSME Joint Conf. on Micromechatronics for Information and Precision Equipment*, S10_03, June 2006.

Kiguchi K.; Miyamoto K. & Imada Y. (2006c). Intelligent Control of a 4DOF Upper-Limb Motion Assist Robot, *Proc. of Joint 3rd International Conf. on Soft Computing and Intelligent Systems and 7th International Symposium on advanced Intelligent Systems*, pp.907-912, Tokyo, September 2006.

Kiguchi K. (2007). Active Exoskeletons for Upper-Limb Motion Assist, *International Journal of Humanoid Robotics*. (to be published)

London J.T. (1981). Kinematics of the Elbow, *Journal of Bone and Joint Surgery*, Vol.63-A, No.4, pp.529-535.

Mosher R.S. & Wendel B. (1960). Force-Reflecting Electrohydraulic Servomanipulator, *Electro-Technology*, pp.138-141.

Mosher R.S (1967). Handyman to Hardiman, *Society of Automotive Engineers publication* MS670088.

Nagai K.; Nakanishi I.; Hanafusa H.; Kawamura S.; Makikawa M. & Tejima N. (1998). Development of an 8 DOF Robotic Orthosis for Assisting Human Upper Limb Motion, *Proc. of 1998 IEEE International Conference on Robotics and Automation*, pp.4386-4391, Belgium, 1998.

Rumelhart D.E.; Hinton G.E. & Williams R.J. (1986). Learning Internal Representations by Error Propagation, *Parallel Distributed Processing*, MIT Press, pp.45-76.

Rosen J.; Brand M.; Fuchs M.B. & Arcan M. (2001). A Myosignal-Based Powered Exoskeleton System, *IEEE Trans. on Systems, Man, and Cybernetics, Part A*, Vol.31, No.3, pp.210-222, ISSN 1083-4427.

Sasaki D.; Noritsugu T. & Takaiwa M. (2004). Development of Active Support Splint Driven by Pneumatic Soft Actuator (ASSIST), *Journal of Robotics and Mechatronics*, Vol.16, No.5, pp.497-503, ISSN 0915-3942.

Suryanarayanan S. (1996). *An Intelligent System for Surface EMG-Based Position Tracking of Human Arm Movements for the Control of Manipulators*, Ph.D. Dissertation, University of Akron.

Tsagarkis N.G. & Caldwell D.G. (2003). Development and Control of a 'Soft-Actuated' Exoskeleton for Use in Physiotherapy and Training, *Autonomous Robots*, Vol.15, No.3, pp.21–33, ISSN 0929-5593.
Vukobratovic M. (1975). *Legged Locomotion Robots and Anthropomorphic Mechanisms*, Mihailo Pupin Institute, Belgrade.
Zatsiorsky V.M. (1998). *Kinematics of Human Motion*, Human Kinematics.

17

Cyberthosis™ : Rehabilitation Robotics With Controlled Electrical Muscle Stimulation

Patrick Métrailler, Roland Brodard, Yves Stauffer, Reymond Clavel & Rolf Frischknecht
Fondation Suisse pour les Cyberthèses, Monthey, Switzerland
Laboratoire de Systèmes Robotiques, EPFL, Lausanne, Switzerland
Unité de Neuroréhabilitation, CHUV, Lausanne, Switzerland

1. Introduction

Each year, following an accident or illness, over 200 new cases of paraplegia occur in Switzerland, and 1000 in France. This makes 7'000, respectively 40'000 para-tetraplegic patients in these countries. Since the Second World War, methods available for the treatment of medullar trauma at the moment of lesion, and for re-education, have evolved considerably. Nowadays, these methods allow in around 80% of medullar injuries, limitation of the damage to a partial lesion of the spinal cord. Unfortunately, only 10% of these patients ever recover autonomous walking [Zäch G.A., 2000].
Today paraplegics often benefit from walking re-education programmes on treadmills. Two, occasionally three physiotherapists are required to mobilise the patient's legs and pelvis. Unfortunately this work is extremely hard on the staff, and the movements are difficult to reproduce and obviously non-quantifiable. These manual treatments are slowly being replaced by robotic rehabilitation [Reinkensmeyer et al., 2004], much more capable of providing the repetitive and precise exercises demanded by modern methods. However, in cases where residual voluntary capacity is absent, or where there is muscular atrophy, the movements made are purely passive. The Cyberthosis Project presented below, allows active re-education, and preliminary testing has confirmed its great efficacy.

2. Cyberthosis Project

An orthosis is a device intended to correct or improve a deficient function or compensate for incapacity of a part of the body - trunk, member or segment of a member. A hybrid orthosis has the addition of one or several motors and sensors. The latter serves as a mechanical interface with the patient and allow the measurement of a limb's position, as well as the force generated by the subject. Its motors assist or resist the movement according to the therapy being applied. A new dimension has appeared with cyberthosis, this being a hybrid orthosis assisted by controlled neuromuscular electrostimulation.
Initiated by the Fondation Suisse pour les Cyberthèses (FSC), the Cyberthosis Project aims to combine closed-loop electrical muscle stimulation with motorised orthoses. This innovative concept not only allows automation of the treatment, but also an active participation of the patient's muscles. From this concept new devices have been developed in a general re-

education process where recovery of walking did not feature as the only aim. It also integrated the benefits of electro-stimulated physical activity within an improvement to the quality of life for sufferers from medullar trauma and hemiplegics [Takahashi & Reinkensmeyer, 2003] through the reduction of complications due to immobilisation of the lower limbs.
The benefits of such treatment are obvious for the patient, but also for physiotherapists by releasing them from difficult and repetitive mobilisations.
The philosophy of Cyberthosis is founded on treatment in three stages. A dedicated re-education device corresponds to each phase; they are described in part 3, 4 and 5 of this chapter.

2.1 Medullar lesion

Medullar lesion is the result of an injury to the spinal cord. Its origin is usually traumatic, but it can also originate from an illness or an anomaly in the development such as discal hernia, tumour and spina bifida for example. The term paraplegic covers patients with paralysis of the lower limbs (dorsal, lumber or sacral lesions) as well as quadriplegics with paralysis of the four limbs (cervical lesions). Most patients with para- or quadriplegia have to get about in wheelchairs, but this is only the most visible consequence [Maury, 1981], [Grundy et al., 2002]. Several deficiencies, often hidden, result from the paralysis. At motor system level, these complications can be cardiovascular (adaptation to effort), muscular (atrophy), articular (limited movements), osseous (osteoporosis) and sensory. The resulting physical condition in these patients is insufficient for the recuperation of walking. The active muscular participation of the patient [Fitzwater, 2002] as well as their verticalisation [Postans et al., 2003], (basic principles of the Cyberthosis concept), permits the reduction of these secondary effects and in certain cases of incomplete lesions, to regain voluntary mobility.

2.2 CLEMS™ [1]

CLEMS™ (Closed Loop Electrical Muscle Stimulation) is one of the basic principles of the Cyberthosis concept.
The benefits of the addition of functional electrical stimulation (FES) to mobilisation have been shown for the last 10 years [Frischknecht & Chantraine, 1989], [Belanger et al., 2000], [Rushton, 2003]. FES is used to stimulate the recuperation of a certain voluntary activity, especially in cases of incomplete paraplegia, as well as to reduce muscular atrophy and spasticity. To maximise the chances of recuperation, controlled electro-induced contractions are essential. They allow the respect of coherence between movement and the proprioceptive impulses generated by the muscular-tendinous system (Golgi apparatus and neuromuscular spindles). Information about amplitude and position supplied to the nervous system during a movement resembles as closely as possible to that produced by muscular contractions observed during a voluntary movement.
Classical FES, as it is open loop, is capable of following the activation sequences of muscles concerned in a movement. However, it is unable to adapt its intensity during the execution of the movement. A closed-loop control of the FES is therefore necessary to accomplish complex and repetitive movements such as the leg-press, pedalling, or walking in a similar manner to that produced naturally. Thus, CLEMS technology allows the closest possible reproduction of the kinematics and dynamics of natural movements. This can have considerable impact on the plasticity of the nervous system at both spinal and cerebral levels.

---

[1] Cyberthosis™, CLEMS™, StimMaker™, MotionMaker™, WalkTrainer™ and WalkMaker™ are commercial trade marks belonging to the Swiss Foundation for Cyberthosis

2.3 The Cyberthosis devices

The aim of research conducted for the Cyberthosis project is the re-education of paraplegic and hemiplegic patients; ideally as soon as possible after stabilisation of the acute phase so as to avoid muscular atrophy, but also during the chronic phase. For this, a process in three stages has been evolved.

MotionMaker™ is the first element in the process of rehabilitation [Schmitt et al., 2004a]; it is described in part 3 of this chapter. The patient's limbs can be mobilised passively or work actively in an electro-stimulated manner and/or voluntarily against resistance loads created by the motors. The aim of MotionMaker is to treat patients as quickly as possible, so as to limit the effects of an absence of movement. This means maintaining, or increasing muscular volume and capacity for patients in the chronic phase, to reinstate mobility of the joints, to train cardiac capacity and prevent neurological osteoporosis.

Once the subject has successfully completed training on MotionMaker, and attained sufficient physical condition, re-education of the motor patterns for over-ground walking can begin using the mobile device WalkTrainer™. This device is presented in part 4 of this chapter. Equipped with orthoses for the legs and pelvis, body weight support, and with CLEMS, this system allows near perfect mimicking of walking movements with the aim of stimulating nervous system plasticity.

WalkMaker™ is the third cyberthosis. This is a walking assistance device using CLEMS type electrostimulation. It offers people who have not regained sufficient walking autonomy with WalkTrainer, a functional orthotic gait [Goldfarb et al., 2003].

3. MotionMaker™

It consists of a couch and two orthoses enabling a controlled movement of the hip, knee, and ankle joints. The feet move in arcs parallel to the sagittal plane.

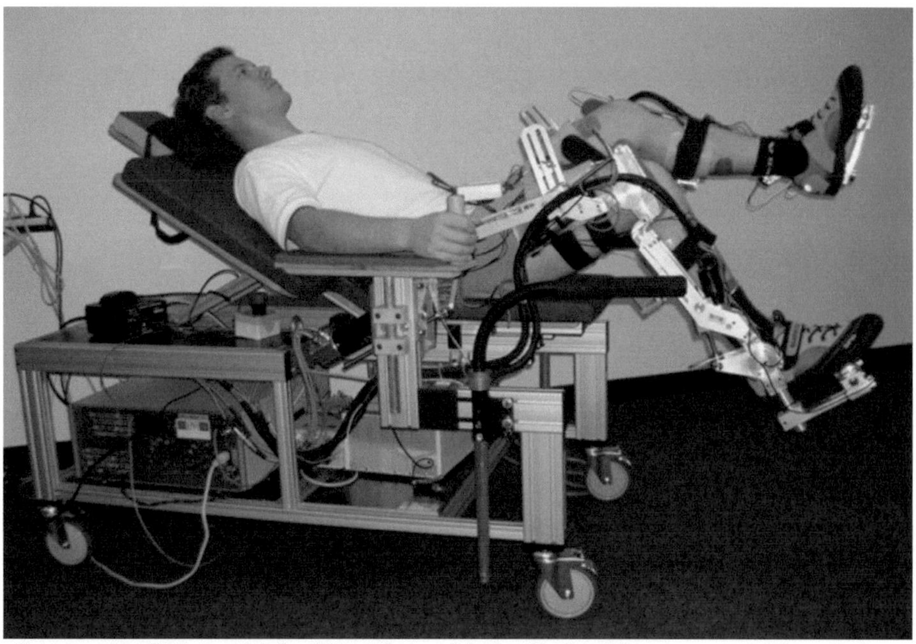

Fig. 1. Prototype of MotionMaker™ with an able-bodied subject.

MotionMaker is marketed by SWORTEC SA, a company dedicated to production and commercialization of the methods developed by the FSC.

3.1. An innovative concept

What is new about MotionMaker is essentially the coupling between the motorised orthoses, and the electrostimulation with closed-loop control. Each joint is motorised and equipped with sensors of position and articular moment. The sensors provide the control unit with the necessary information for the real-time adjustment of the electrical stimulation (CLEMS), during the execution of the movement. This adjustment takes into account the forces developed by the effect of electrostimulation, as well as the voluntary efforts made by the patients themselves. The aim of this control is to attain the level of force prescribed by the practitioner at the beginning of the exercise. According to the patient's muscular participation, the motors either assist or resist the movement. This allows active training throughout the articular range even in cases of great physical deficiency.

3.2. Technical description

The articulations of the orthosis are based on the principle of the variable length connecting rod and crank as shown in Fig. 2.

This type of orthotic joint allows the non-linear physiological curve of moment to be followed, according to the articular angle, and thus optimisation of the actuators' size. Calculation of the articular moments is made through the force sensors measuring axial amplitude in the actuator screw.

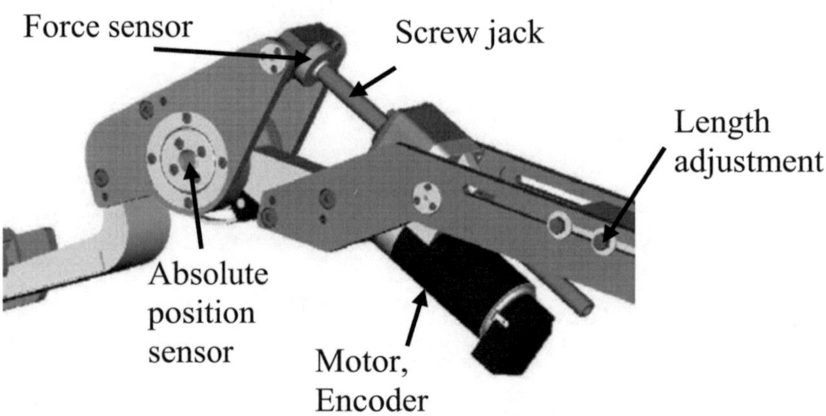

Fig. 2. Details of a MotionMaker joint.

Geometrical alignment between the robot and the patient's legs is ensured by adjustment to the length of the orthosis segments.

A dedicated electrostimulator has been developed to attain the performance required by the CLEMS control. The StimMaker™ has 20 channels of stimulation and allows modification of the electrostimulation parameters on 20 muscles with a reaction time of 0.5ms per channel.

Two systems are monitored on MotionMaker: the orthosis and the leg. Both being rigidly linked, their respective control loops must be uncoupled so that each system has its own physical

quantity to adjust. The choice is based on verification of the robot's position, and on the force of the legs. The CLEMS algorithm calculates the articular moments corresponding to the force prescribed at the level of the foot, or gets them from the initial instruction for a purely articular movement. The CLEMS algorithm uses these moments to define which muscles are to be stimulated, and then adjusts the amplitude of stimulation current supplied to these muscles throughout the movement. The stimulation technique is carried out by surface electrodes.
The comparison between the prescribed moments and those measured on the orthosis allows the adjustment of the electrostimulation but also the detection of disruptive elements such as spasms and clonus. In fact, electrostimulation and mobilisation can encourage involuntary reflex contractions that in certain patients can be considerable. To ensure the safety of the patient during an exercise, the system behaves in a carefully programmed manner following detection of a spasm. MotionMaker reacts to interrupt this spasm by reducing stimulation current, and lessening the osteo-tendinous constraints engendered by a compliant adjustment of the orthosis.

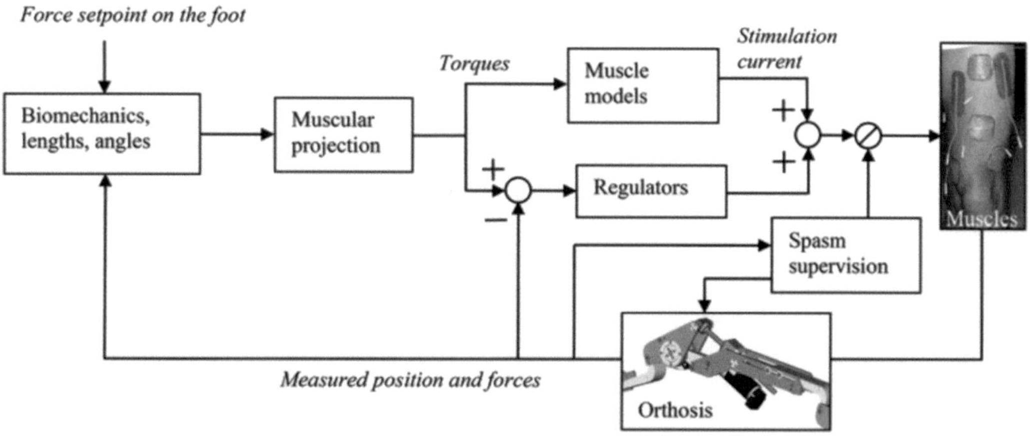

Fig. 3. Diagram of the CLEMS electrostimulation control unit.

3.3 Pilot clinical study

After having evaluated CLEMS with paraplegic patients using a simple knee orthosis [Schmitt et al., 2004b], the algorithm was tested using MotionMaker on able-bodied subjects [Metrailler et al., 2006a] with a leg-press type movement of extension-flexion. The results being satisfactory, a pilot clinical study was carried out [Metrailler et al., 2006b].
5 paraplegic patients (with lesions over 4 years old) - 4 with incomplete lesions and 1 with a complete lesion - conducted training sessions of 60 minutes on MotionMaker, 2 to 3 times a week over 2 months. The movements were leg-press type with alternate stimulation of the extensor muscles (Gluteus Maximus, Quadriceps and Gastrocnemius) and the flexors (Hamstrings and Tibialis Anterior). The principal aims of these tests were:

1. To confirm the inoffensiveness of the device.
2. To evaluate the possibility of carrying out controlled movements with paraplegic patients,
3. To confirm the possibility of increasing voluntary force and electro-induced force of subjects with incomplete medullar lesions,
4. To study the effect of movements with CLEMS on spasticity.

3.4 Results

All subjects were able to complete the whole training, there was no drop out. None of the participants felt unsafe at any time during the training sessions and they all appreciated the safety features of the MotionMaker™.

Fig. 4 shows the position of the patient during leg-press exercises. The patient is lying in dorsal decubitus position and pushes or pulls on his feet on a horizontal movement. Torque is measured on each joint and the resulting forces on the feet are obtained through biomechanical calculus.

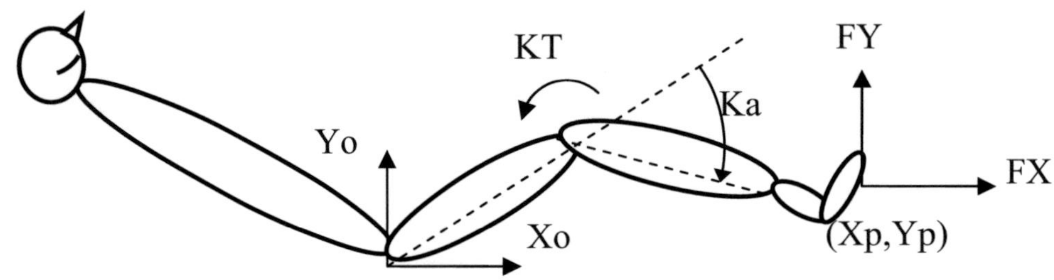

Fig. 4. Position of the foot (Xp, Yp), angle of the knee (Ka) and torque at the knee (KT).

The result of controlling the electro-induced force during extension and flexion of a leg-press exercise with a completely paraplegic patient is presented in the following diagrams. Fig. 5 (a) shows the X position of the foot (Xp), the horizontal force setpoint (FXs) and measured (FXm), the vertical force measures (FYm). The vertical setpoint force stays constant at 0N, the vertical (Yp) position remaining constant. Fig. 5 (b) shows the effects of theses forces on the foot at knee level. There one finds the torques setpoint (KTs) and measured (KTm), the angle (Ka) and the stimulation current of the quadriceps (KSc). It should be noted that the great differences between setpoint and measured values are due to saturation of the stimulation current at 70mA for safety reasons.

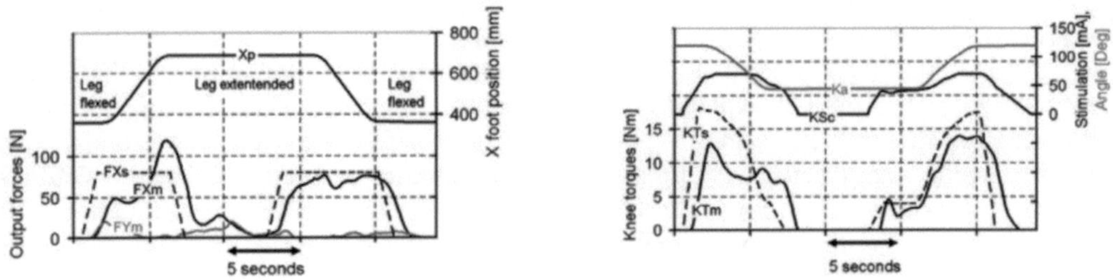

a) b)

Fig. 5. a) Extension and flexion, with the position of the foot (Xp), the command force (FXs) the measured forces (FXm) horizontal and (FYm) vertical. b) Torques setpoint (KTs) and corresponding measurements at the knee (KTm), angle of the knee (Ka) and stimulation current of the quadriceps (KSc).

Through these measurements, it has been demonstrated that the force resulting from several muscular contractions can be controlled in amplitude and in direction and that the CLEMS algorithm is judicious.

During mobilisation exercises with CLEMS stimulation and voluntary force, the subjects with incomplete lesions experienced greater awareness in their limbs than when doing purely voluntary exercises. This increase in sensation seems to be due to better stimulation of the proprioceptive receptors with CLEMS stimulation. Thus, they could develop greater voluntary force with electric stimulation. The improvement in perception of their limbs enabled them also to increase their purely voluntary force in the course of the exercises.

After the two months of training, all the subjects with incomplete lesions (P1, P2, P4 and P5) had more than doubled their voluntary force, without electrostimulation, on at least one leg. Fig. 6 shows the evolution of their average voluntary force by series of exercise, in % between the first and last sessions. This increase in performance can be explained by an improvement of muscular function, by improved function of the spinal motor system linked to the neuronal plasticity, to a central motor control improved by the reactivation of dormant motor patterns or by a combination of these three elements.

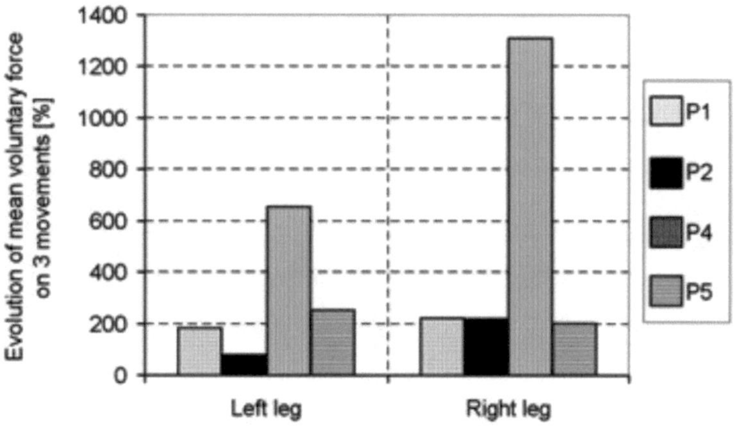

Fig. 6. Evolution, in % between the first and the last session, of the mean force developed voluntarily by the 4 incomplete paraplegic subjects, for the left and right legs, without electrical stimulation.

Fig. 7 shows the evolution of their average electro-induced force, in % between the first and last session. This increase in performance can be explained by an improvement of muscular function and by the increased stimulation current allowed by the patient's accommodation to electrical stimulation and the diminution of occurrence of spasms along the training program.

The activation of muscles in exercises of neurological re-education brings patients not only the recovery/conservation of good physical condition, but also the proprioceptive information essential for recovering the ability to activate of their own muscles. The example of patient P4 in our pilot study is particularly revealing. Fig. 8 shows the mean output power developed according to the type of exercise and the number of training sessions. The grey curve corresponds to the results of exercises with electrostimulation but without voluntary contribution, and the black curve shows the results of exercises with voluntary contribution but without electrostimulation.

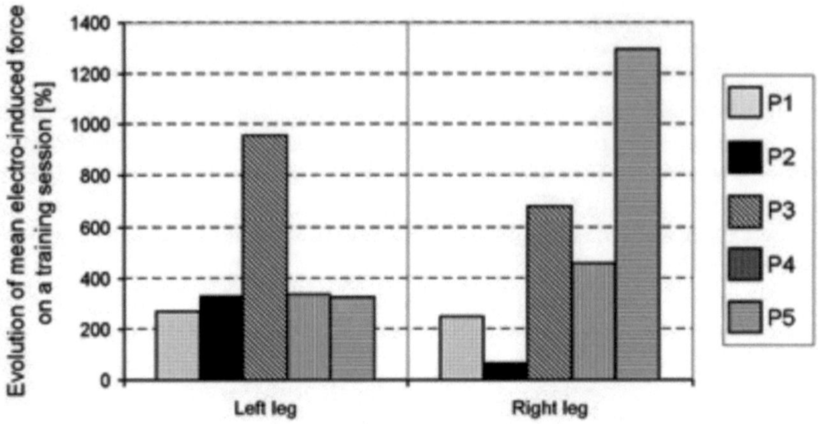

Fig. 7. Evolution, in % between the first and the last session, of the mean electro-induced force developed without voluntary participation, for the left and right legs.

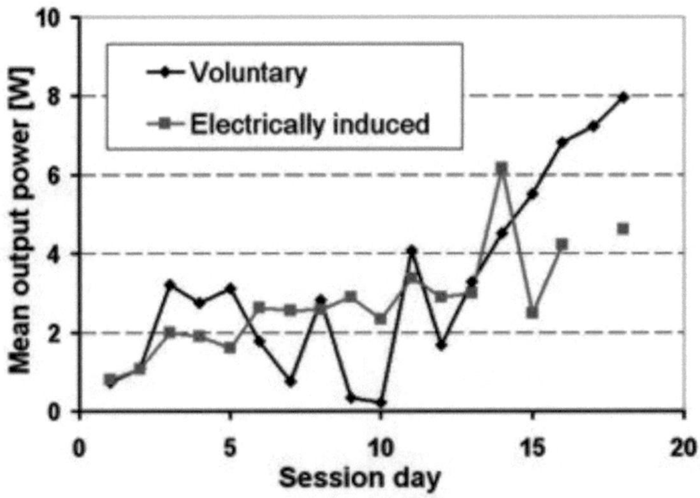

Fig. 8. Evolution of voluntary and electro-induced power for subject P4 in the clinical trial.

The evolution of voluntary force from session 10 shows a sudden and significant improvement in P4's voluntary power. This progress, being not related to the electrically induced evolution, tends to demonstrate the recovery of P4's motor pattern. This hypothesis was consolidated by the comments made by P4 concerning his capacity to use the muscles affected by his injury.

The mobilisation of the legs with electrostimulation has also had beneficial effects on the reduction of rigidity in the limbs due to hypertonia. Three of the five subjects were known to have considerable spasticity. Fig. 9 shows the evolution of mean spasticity measurements before and after each exercise session. The physiotherapists carried out manual mobilisations and graduated the resistance to movement according to the modified Ashworth Scale [Bohannon & Smith, 1987]. The reduction of spasticity lasted 2 to 3 hours after the session. This reduction was significant, hypertonia returning to levels close to those of able-bodied subjects, and it was felt to be most pleasant by the subjects concerned.

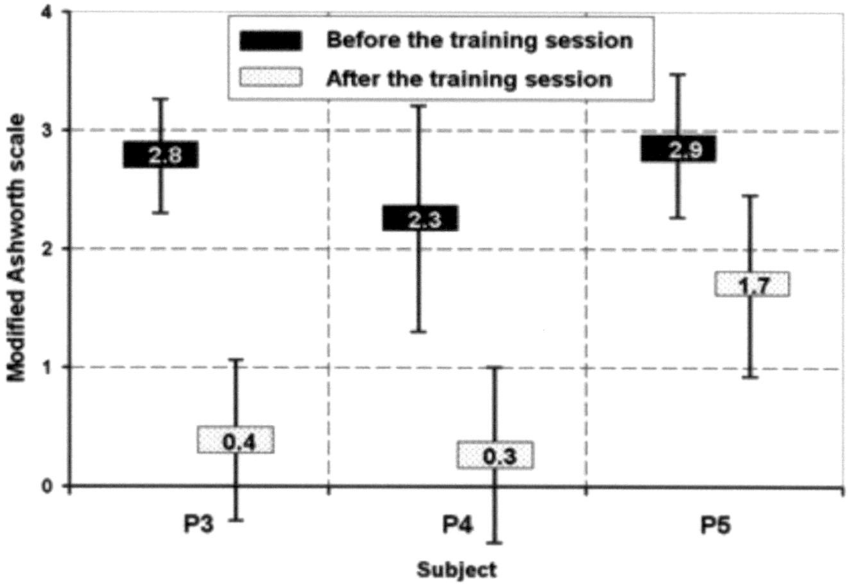

Fig. 9. Mean and standard deviation measures of spasticity before and after an exercise session.

4. WalkTrainer™

4.1. Concept

The technological developments and the promising results obtained from the clinical tests of MotionMaker, have led to the development of the second phase of the Cyberthosis project: WalkTrainer™.

The basic principle, namely closed-loop electrical muscle stimulation in conjunction with robotic assistance, is common to both these projects. The re-education of the walking motor patterns demands perfect emulation of the natural gait, which is why WalkTrainer offers training for over-ground walking. In fact, the kinematics and dynamics of the walking movement being different on a treadmill (modification of stride length [Dingwell et al., 2001] and of Electromyogram EMG [Arsenault et al., 2001]), the proprioceptive information differs. Motor patterns trained like this find themselves disrupted for over-ground walking. Locomotion with the subject moving in his environment, will not only stimulate the re-learning of over-ground walking functional motor patterns in the best possible way, but also its motivation, which constitutes an indispensable factor to the efficacy of re-education. Pelvic movement is essential to guarantee natural gait, which is why a pelvic orthosis was designed.

4.2. Components

WalkTrainer is composed of five mechatronic sub-assemblies that interact with the subject in two ways:

- Mechanically: the walking frame, the leg orthosis, the pelvic orthosis and the active suspension.
- Electrically: the CLEMS.

The main function of the walking frame is to follow the patient while moving. It serves as a mobile support for all the other components. Equipped with two differentially mounted wheels, it can operate in the plane and thus perfectly accomplish its task of following. Future versions will also have batteries on board to allow more freedom during training.

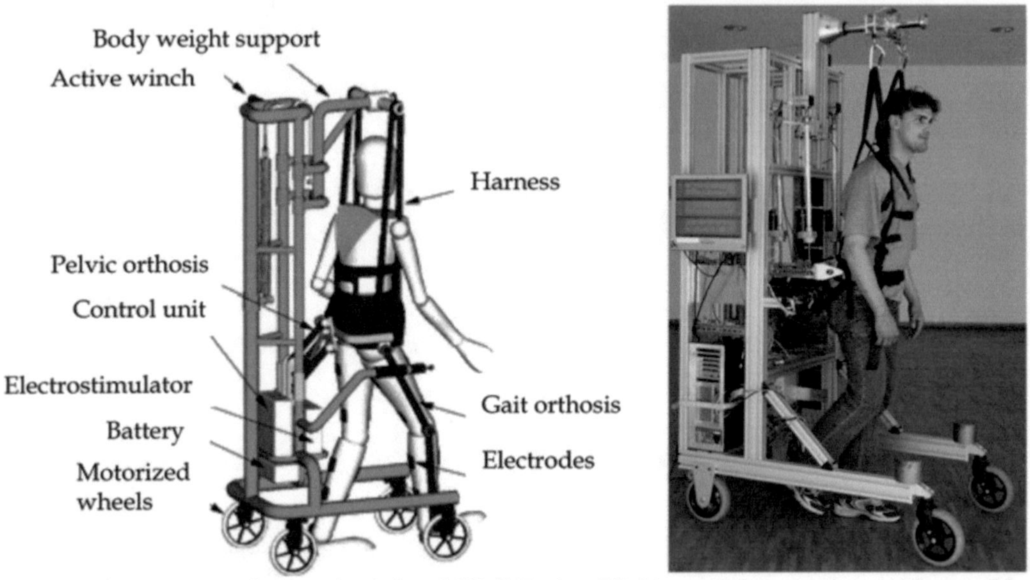

Fig. 10. a) Diagram of the principle of WalkTrainer™, b) partial execution with an able-bodied subject, without the leg orthosis.

The muscular condition of paraplegics, sometimes severe atrophy of the leg muscles, together with poor control of the postural muscles, must be taken into account. A harness allows controlled unloading of the legs, while supporting the patient's trunk. This suspension is termed 'active' as a motor combined with force and position sensors enable compensation of irregularities and force oscillations, due mainly to the preloaded spring and the different inertias at play.
The chosen kinematics for the pelvic orthosis is that of a parallel robot with six degrees of freedom. It is therefore possible for us to accompany the subject according to the three rotations and the three translations of space. The aim is to initiate the movements through the patient's pelvis and to guide it in a similar way to the work of a physiotherapist. The force sensors allow precise monitoring of the forces exerted on the subject. The work done by the pelvic orthosis is thus perfectly quantifiable, and can equally well be used in a diagnostic context.
The leg orthosis fulfils two functions of major importance. Firstly, positional measurement of the limbs of the subject is supplied in real time by the latter through the attached position sensors. The force the subject exerts on the orthosis is also measured by the force sensors. These two types of information are indispensable for the adjustment of the closed-loop muscular stimulation. Secondly, equipped with motors, the leg orthosis allows the patient's movements to be assisted.
The real-time muscular stimulator StimMaker, as described in 3.2 is also used with WalkTrainer. In this application the main muscles responsible for walking are targeted, i.e.:

Gluteus Maximus, Vastus Medialis, Vastus Lateralis, Rectus Femoris, Hamstrings, Tibialis Anterior and Gastrocnemius.

4.3. Global coordination

All the components described under section 4.2 must be coordinated to allow an interactive gait with the active participation of the subject, but without the latter being rushed by the machine.

Different strategies of co-ordination are envisaged. That currently employed consists of a master/slave relationship between the different components. The master component serves as a guiding element to the others. A logical choice for this function is the leg orthosis. In fact this latter is the keystone of CLEMS, thus of active re-education. Moreover, it includes all the necessary sensors for the measurement of the subject's activity (force and position). The master/slave relationship could therefore resemble that shown in Fig. 11.

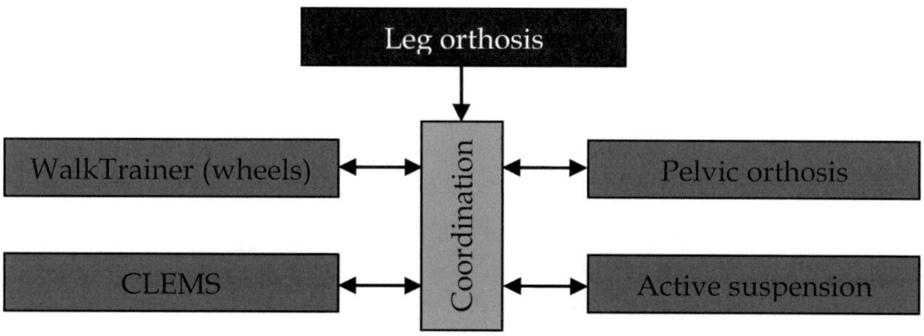

Fig. 11. Strategy of coordination between WalkTrainer's different components.

At the time of writing the leg orthosis was not available. However, an initial installation of the coordination strategy was set up. Instead of the leg orthosis, a footswitch placed under the subject's right leg served as the proprioceptive sensor to establish the position of the leg. Knowing the latter, it was possible to coordinate the movement of the pelvic orthosis with the subject's gait. The contact on the right heel was used to obtain two fundamental pieces of information: the frequency of steps and the phase difference between the legs and the pelvic orthosis. Knowledge of these two values then allows a trajectory of the pelvic orthosis guaranteeing synchronisation to be generated, under the condition that it does not rush the subject. This means that the synchronisation operates on a whole cycle and not instantaneously, which would induce acceleration that would be extremely unpleasant for the user.

The pelvic orthosis, Fig. 13, is able to guide the subject according to the six spatial degrees of freedom. These movements can be obtained with millimetric precision. However, to impose such movements in an inflexible way could generate great force on the subject, so to be considered negative, even counterproductive. It could thus be interesting to make the structure compliant in a controlled manner. One must however control these deviations exactly, and for this reason an algorithm allowing each degree of freedom in the orthosis to be made compliant independently and in a controlled manner, was installed.

This unit can be used to control interaction between the orthosis and the subjects so as not to rush them. Moreover, such an algorithm can be made progressive. It also allows the subject's progress to be evaluated. In fact, it is possible to adapt the compliance to the subject's evolution. If subjects follow good trajectories with a compliant controller, this means that they are capable of generating these trajectories themselves.

The basic principle of this algorithm is the calculation of return forces in the operational space (OP), then their projection into the articular space (ART). In this paragraph, we assume this process takes place around a fixed point, but the same reasoning remains valid for any trajectory.

The OP error of the pelvic orthosis is calculated, then converted into OP force (in the case of a spring : Force = k•error). This force is projected into the ART space by means of the Jacobian matrix of kinematical structure [Sciavicco & Siciliano, 2001]. Finally the ART forces are applied to the pelvic orthosis, as illustrated in Fig. 12. It then remains to measure the ART so as to calculate a new OP error and so on.

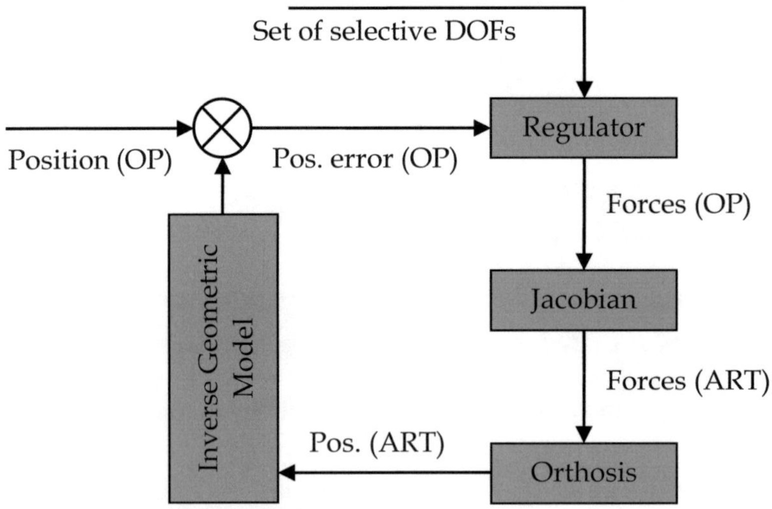

Fig. 12. Principle of selective compliance.

Initially static tests were carried out. A transverse force, Fig. 13, was applied to the orthosis and displacement in the operational space was measured.

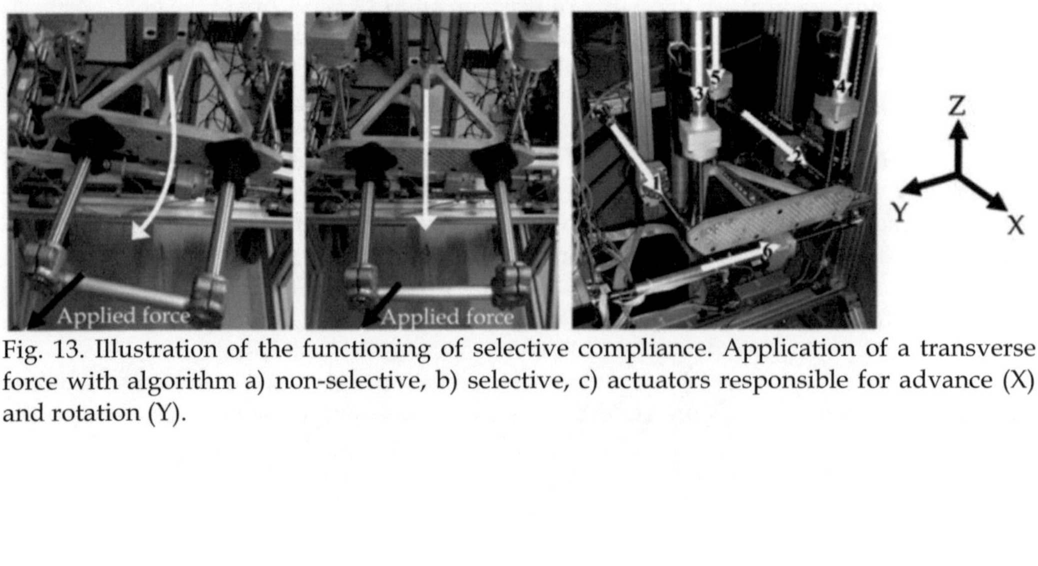

Fig. 13. Illustration of the functioning of selective compliance. Application of a transverse force with algorithm a) non-selective, b) selective, c) actuators responsible for advance (X) and rotation (Y).

In one case, Fig. 13(a), the advance axis (X) was made compliant in a non-selective manner by reducing the rigidity of the motors responsible for this translation. In the other case, Fig. 13(b), the advance axis (X) was made compliant in a selective manner. It can be clearly seen that with non-selective compliance, the translation (X) is added to by rotation around the vertical axis (Y). This originates from coupling of the translation (X) and the rotation (Y). The selective regulator however, guarantees a pure translation.

4.4. WalkTrainer and analysis of pelvic movement

WalkTrainer can also be used as a device for measuring pelvic movement for research or therapeutic purpose. To do this the addition of three sensors is necessary:

- An easyTrack200 6 axes sensor, which allows the real-time acquisition of the six degrees of freedom of the pelvis.
- A footswitch, which is placed under the subject's right heel. This signal is used to identify heel strike and lift and to compute the temporal measures in a repetitive gait cycle.
- Two potentiometric sensors, which link the subject to WalkTrainer, and actuate its servomechanism according to the subject's speed/position.

The easyTrack200 sensor is marketed by Atracsys SA. It enables, through an active tracer and linear cameras, the measurement of the 6 degrees of freedom of an object in space. A flexible pelvic belt, specially developed by an orthopaedist, is worn by the subject to carry the active tracer and also the mounting for the potentiometers, Fig. 14.

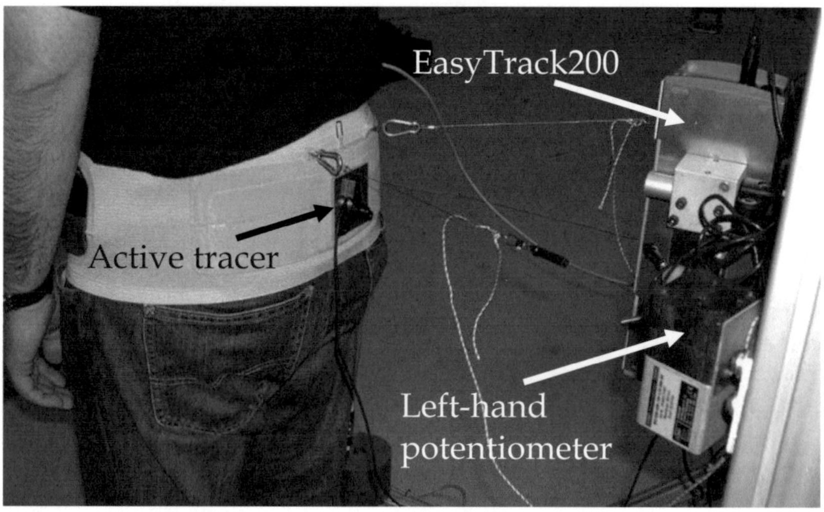

Fig. 14. Subject equipped for the measurement of pelvic movements.

Subjects then make two or three attempts at walking to familiarise themselves with the system. Then they repeat three series of measurements (1.4, 0.8 and 0.4m/s). A physiotherapist walking beside the patient governs the rate of travel, and WalkTrainer measures the effective speed. Several attempts may prove necessary before obtaining the desired walking speed. Each series takes place over a distance of around 20 metres and allows the acquisition of 15 walking cycles. The tracer's position relative to the pelvis is obtained through a calibration process.

The six degrees of freedom of the pelvis are thus measured, then processed with Matlab© using a graphic interface. Twenty people participated in the measuring campaign. These results will be used to generate trajectories for the pelvic orthosis based on a mathematical model including the walking speed and the patient's morphology, age, gender, etc. A typical vertical movement is shown in Fig. 15. The vertical line represents lifting of the right heel (~60% of the gait cycle). All the degrees of freedom are thus rapidly available in graphic form and in Excel© type files to facilitate analysis and exchange.

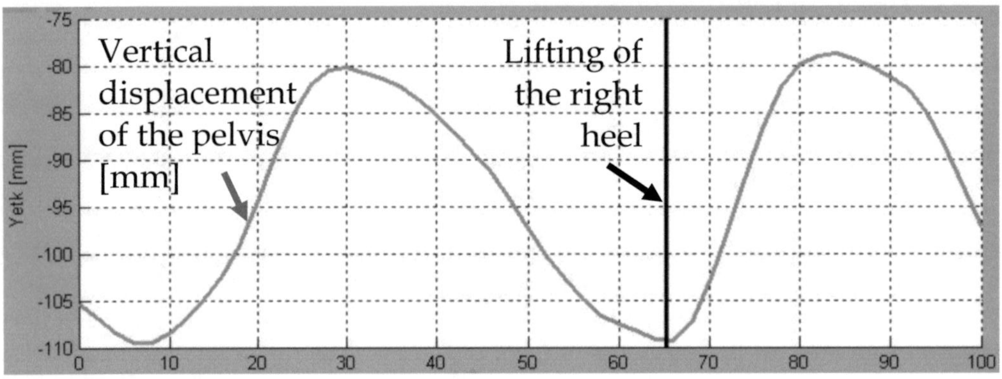

Fig. 15. Results of pelvic measurements, vertical displacement.

To enable the measurement of such movement it is essential to link WalkTrainer's position/speed to that of the subject by servo control. A special algorithm was developed for this task. It allows greater reactivity when necessary, while preventing the whole structure from following the slight oscillations of the pelvis according to the axis of advance.

5. WalkMaker™

5.1. Concept

WalkMaker™ will be a walk assisting cyberthosis using CLEMS type electrostimulation. The orthosis will serve as a mounting for the sensors required to control the electrostimulation, but will also have the function of helping and guiding the movements by active or passive actuators. It is intended for subjects who have not regained sufficient walking autonomy after exercising on WalkTrainer. These patients could benefit from WalkMaker to acquire a functional orthotic autonomous gait.

5.2 Challenges

The challenges in developing such a device are primarily mechanical. It has to provide sufficient rigidity to guide the limbs and pelvis, while also ensuring good compliance of certain degrees of freedom enabling smooth locomotion. The amount of guidance will be dependant on the neurological level of the lesion as well as the degree of paralysis.

The second challenge concerns the CLEMS electrostimulation which has to supply the basic energy of propulsion. The quality of control being directly linked to the quality of the muscular response obtained by training on MotionMaker and WalkTrainer, actuators mounted on the orthosis will probably have to filter the articular moments supplied by the muscles. Propulsion by the muscles and the use of a dynamic gait will permit reduced

energy consumption, be it electrical, pneumatic or other. Systems for recuperating energy during braking are also envisaged.
The final specification can only be established in terms of the results obtained with WalkTrainer. The main difficulty for this system is to propose an alternative at least as good as the wheelchair in functional terms, but also in terms of ease of use and implementation.

6. Conclusion

Cyberthosis brings a new approach to physical and neurological re-education. The patient regains his role as a protagonist in the movement, even if his voluntary mobility is reduced to nothing. This principle allows better emulation of the natural voluntary movements and so doing, places the patient in an ideal situation for relearning his motor patterns.
The first stage with MotionMaker has clearly shown the advantages of combining robotics and controlled electrostimulation to improve voluntary control. The activation of muscles in exercises of neurological re-education brings patients not only the recovery of muscle strength and joint mobility, but also the proprioceptive information essential for recovering the ability to activate by themselves their paralysed muscles. Training with WalkTrainer should allow one to go even further in the relearning of gait patterns by offering over-ground walking with controlled pelvic motion and muscle activity.

7. Acknowledgements

The Fondation Suisse pour les Cyberthèses would like to acknowledge the "Laboratoire de Système Robotique de l'Ecole Polytechnique Fédérale de Lausanne" as well as its associates for their scientific and technical support.
The FSC would also like to thank the "Loterie Romande" for its important financial help. The WalkTrainer™ project benefits from a grant made by the Swiss Innovation Promotion Agency, CTI Project N° 7485.2 LSPP-LS.

8. References

Arsenault, A.B., Winter, D.A. & Marteniuk, R.G. (1986). Treadmill Versus Walkway Locomotion in Humans: an EMG study. *Ergonomics*, Vol. 29, No. 5, 665-676

Belanger, M., Stein, R.B., Wheeler, G.D., Gordon, T. & Leduc, B. (2000). Electrical stimulation: Can it increase muscle strength and reverse osteopenia in spinal cord injured individuals? *Archives of Physical Medicine and Rehabilitation*, Vol. 81, No. 8, 1090-8.

Bohannon, R.W. & Smith, M.B. (1987). Interrater reliability of a modified Ashworth scale of muscle spasticity. *Physical Therapy*, Vol. 67, No. 2, 206-7

Dingwell, J.B., Cusumano, J.P., Cavanagh, P.R. & Sternad, D. (2001). Local Dynamic Stability Versus Kinematic Variability of Continuous Overground and Treadmill Walking. *Journal of Biomechanical Engineering*, Vol. 123, 27-32

Frischknecht, R. & Chantraine, A. (1989). Traitement de la spasticité par les agents physiques. *Annales de Réadaptation et de Médecine physique*, Vol. 32, 475-93

Fitzwater, R. (2002). A Personal View of FES Cycling. *Artificial Organs*, Vol. 26, No 3, 284-286

Goldfarb, M., Korkowsky, K., Harrold, B. & Durfee, W. (2003). Preliminary Evaluation of a Controlled-Brake Orthosis for FES-Aided Gait. *IEEE Transactions on Neural Systems and Rehabilitation Eengineering*, Vol. 11, No. 3, 241-8

Grundy, D., Tromans, A., Carvell, J. & Jamil, F. (2002). Medical management in the spinal injuries unit, In: *ABC of spinal cord injury*, Grundy, D. & Swain, A., 25-32, BMJ Books, London

Maury, M. (1981). *La paraplégie chez l'adulte et chez l'enfant*. Paris, Flammarion Médecine Sciences

Métrailler, P., Brodard, R., Frischknecht, R., Clavel, R. (2006a). Improvement of rehabilitation possibilities with the MotionMaker™. *Proceedings of Biobob2006, the first IEEE/RAS-EMBS international conference on biomedical robotics and biomechatronics*, Pisa, Italy

Métrailler, P., Brodard, R., Clavel, R., Frischknecht, R. (2006b). Closed loop electrical muscle stimulation in spinal cord injured rehabilitation. *Europa Medicophysica, Mediterranean Journal of Physical and Rehabilitation Medicine,* Vol. 42, 72-3

Postans, N.J., Malcolm, H.G., Hasler, J.P. & Douglas, J.M. (2003). FES augmented partial weight-gearing support treadmill training in acute incomplete SCI patients. *Proceedings of the 8th Conference of the International Functional Electrical Stimulation Society,* 135-37, Brisbane, Australia

Reikensmeyer, D.J., Emken, J.L., & Cramer, S.C. (2004). Robotics, Motor Learning, and Neurologic Recovery. *Annual Review of Biomedical Engineering*, Vol. 6, 497-525

Rushton, D.N. (2003). Functional Electrical Stimulation and rehabilitation – an hypothesis. *Medical Engineering & Physics*, Vol. 25, 75-78

Schmitt, C., Métrailler, P., Al-Khodairy, A., Brodard, R., Fournier, J., Bouri, M., Clavel, R. (2004a) The MotionMaker: a rehabilitation system combining an orthosis with closed-loop electrical muscle stimulation. *Proceedings of the 8th Vienna International Workshop in Functional Electrical Stimulation,* 117-20, Vienna, Austria

Schmitt, C., Métrailler, P., Al-Khodairy, A., Brodard, R., Fournier, J., Bouri, M., Clavel, R. (2004b). A study of a knee extension controlled by a closed loop functional electrical stimulation, *Proceedings of the 9th Conference of the International Functional Electrical Stimulation Society*, 135-37, Bournemouth, United Kingdom.

Sciavicco, L. & Siciliano, B. (2001) *Modelling and control of robot manipulators*, Springer-Verlag, New-York

Takahashi, C.D. & Reinkensmeyer, D.J. (2003) Hemiparetic stroke impairs anticipatory control of arm movement. *Experimental Brain Research*, Vol. 149, No 2, 131-40

Zäch, G.A. (2000) Espoir ou illusion. *Paraplégie N0 87*, Bulletin officiel de la Fondation Suisse pour la Paraplégie, Nottwil, 2-3

18

Haptic Device System For Upper Limb Motor Impairment Patients: Developing And Handling In Healthy Subjects

Tasuku Miyoshi[1], Yoshiyuki Takahashi[2], Hokyoo Lee[2], Takafumi Terada[3], Yuko Ito[4], Kaoru Inoue[4] & Takashi Komeda[1]
1. Shibaura Institute of Technology, JAPAN
2. Toyo University, JAPAN
3. Mitsubishi Precision Co. Ltd., JAPAN
4. Tokyo Metropolitan University of Health Sciences, JAPAN

1. Introduction

Based on an aging society with fewer children, an explosive increase in the number of older adults and patients with motor dysfunctions and a reduction in the number of caregivers are anticipated. Patients with motor dysfunctions can benefit from movement therapies. They may in some cases gain social independence and improvements in daily living and quality of life. When a stroke damages the motor pathways for the arm and leg, the prospects for functional recovery are better for the leg than for the arm. It has been reported that 25 of 33 individuals with spinal cord injuries learned to walk independently within 3 to 20 weeks (median 10.5) with partial body weight support treadmill training, known as Lauband therapy (Wernig & Muller, 1992). However, this treatment presents specific challenges for the therapist. The passive moving of a disabled person's legs is ergonomically difficult since the individual being treated cannot independently support and/or move his legs. In order to improve this therapy, a driven gait orthosis was developed for use on patients with varying degrees of paresis or spasticity for up to one-half hour (Colombo et al., 2000). For the sake of basic human movements, e.g., standing upright with stability or maintaining a steady gait, lower limb rehabilitation is an important aspect of regaining function.

From the viewpoint of assistance with daily activities, however, it is obvious that upper limb rehabilitation is also important, especially for stroke patients. There are several rehabilitation protocols: increased intensity of treatment (Lincoln et al., 1999), device-enhanced treatment (Sunderland et al., 1994; Feys et al., 1998), and specially focused sensorimotor activity for the affected limb, known as "constraint-induced movement therapy" (Miltner et al., 1999). In the case of constraint-induced movement therapy, a clinical trial with acute rehabilitation is feasible and is associated with less arm impairment at the end of treatment (Dromerick et al., 2000; Taub et al., 1993). In this respect, increased sensorimotor activity involving a paralyzed upper limb after a stroke leads to improved motor performance and enhanced activities of daily living.

Several groups are approaching upper limb rehabilitation with the use of robotics and information technology to control sensorimotor activity delivered to an upper limb paralyzed after a stroke. For example, MIT-MANUS (Aisen et al., 1997; Krebs et al., 2004) and Mirror Image Movement Enabler (Lum et al., 2006) are now well documented. To our knowledge, however, it is still unclear whether those kinds of applications are more effective for robotic rehabilitation than traditional methods. In addition, the effects of the assist/resist forces as subjects execute exercise protocols are still unknown, whereas robotic rehabilitation has some advantages in easily changing the intensity of rehabilitation exercises. To solve these problems, we designed a haptic device by applying virtual-reality technology as a robotic rehabilitation apparatus.

In this paper, we show our newly designed haptic device and some of its applications. We then demonstrate our preliminary experimental results achieved by healthy young subjects. Our goal was to apply the haptic device as a neurorehabilitation method with a reduction in the work load of the therapist. Therefore, in the last part of this paper, we describe the clinical relevance of using the haptic device in robotic rehabilitation. Parts of this research have been reported elsewhere (Takahashi et al., 2003; Lee et al., 2005).

2. Haptic device for upper limb motor rehabilitation

2.1 Concept behind the haptic device

We tried to develop a functional motor rehabilitation system using robotics and information technology. The haptic device was designed on the assumption that it is mainly used by patients alone or under the supervision of a therapist. In order to help the patients, this system is designed so that either the therapist or the patient can set up the personal data.

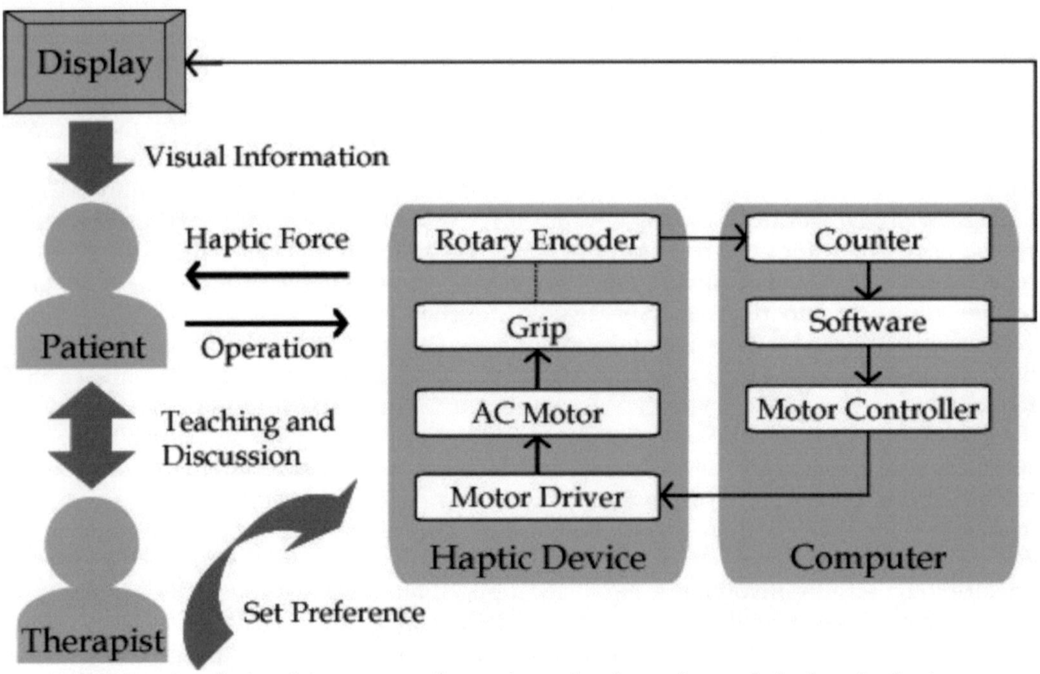

Fig. 1. Schematic relationships among the patient, the therapist, and the haptic device.

It is necessary for clinicians or therapists to make decisions with regard to safety and effective training, where the enhanced motor improvement results in the patients losing their concentration. Hence, a robotic rehabilitation system including a computer would record the training data and evaluate the level of recovery with regard to a motor dysfunction for further qualitative analysis.

The schematic relationships among patients, therapists, and the haptic device are shown in Fig. 1. Either the patients or the therapists select the training program shown on the monitor. The display shows both the selected program and the current status, while the patient conducts the training. After training, the patients and therapists discuss the outcome with regard to the day's activity and the progression of improvement. In addition, future directions and/or self-contemplation using the haptic device is discussed at this stage.

2.2 Design of the Haptic device

The haptic device consists of two servomotors with reduction gears and optical encoders, four link rods, a flat panel, and two man-machine interfaces; one is the monitor display, and the other one is the grip. Figure 2 is an overview of the haptic device.

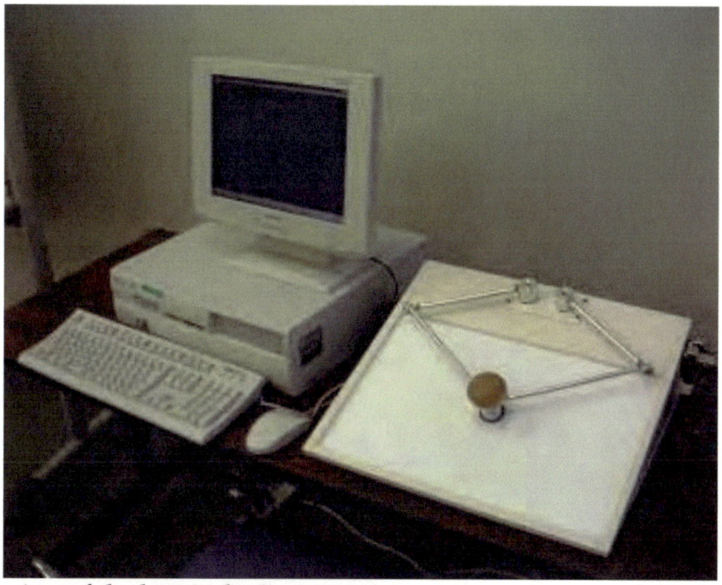

Fig. 2. An overview of the haptic device system.

The size of the haptic device is 430 mm in depth, 500 mm in width, and 190 mm in height. The moving range is 400 mm in the medio-lateral direction and 250 mm in the anterior-posterior direction. The length of the link rods is 190 mm for the motor side and 230 mm for the grip side. The grip and servomotors are connected by the link rods. Patients can move the grip on the surface of the flat panel and train their upper-limb movements in the planar horizontal plane. If the patient moves the grip of the haptic device, the cursor on the display moves simultaneously with the grip, and the patient can feel the virtual force applied to the grip. The current position of the grip can be calculated by the encoder pulse count and the length of the link rods. Figure 3 is a schematic figure of the haptic device used to calculate the current position of the grip (x, y) in a planar horizontal plane as follows,

$$\begin{bmatrix} x_c \\ y_c \\ x_d \\ y_d \\ s \\ t \\ x \\ y \end{bmatrix} = \begin{bmatrix} x_a - L_1\cos\theta_1 \\ y_a - L_1\sin\theta_1 \\ x_b - L_1\cos\theta_2 \\ x_b - L_1\sin\theta_2 \\ x_d - x_c \\ y_d - y_c \\ \frac{1}{2}\left(s - t\sqrt{\frac{4L_2{}^2}{s^2+t^2}} - 1\right) \\ \frac{1}{2}\left(t + s\sqrt{\frac{4L_2{}^2}{s^2+t^2}} - 1\right) \end{bmatrix} \tag{1}$$

where all of the symbols are followed in Fig. 3. The theoretical resolution of the grip position is 0.01 mm. The haptic device can deliver a maximum force of 30 N onto the hand grip in each direction. The 15-inch LCD is used for displaying the training program and the current position of the cursor. The aspect ratio of the display work field is in proportion to the actual flat panel.

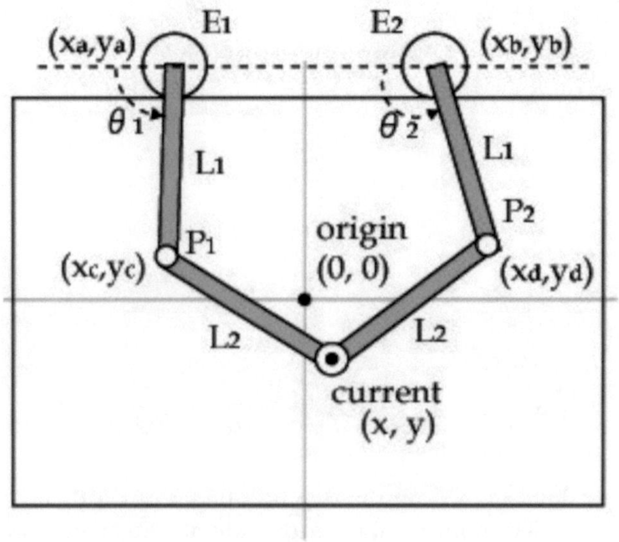

Fig. 3. A schematic figure of the haptic device in a planar horizontal plane. E1 and E2 denote the position of the axis of the servomotor; L1=190 mm; L2=230 mm; P1 and P2 denote the joint point between two link rods.

The haptic device provides six types of haptic force, as follows: load (Fl), assistance (Fa), spring (Fs), viscosity (Fv), friction (Ff), and special-effect force (Fe). The operator (usually the therapist) can change the types of haptic forces and their magnitudes according to the disorder levels of the users. The load/assistance forces were generated in the opposite/same direction of the grip velocity vector. The magnitudes of these forces increased in proportion to the distance between the current grip position and the target position. The load force Fl and the assistance force Fa are given as follows,

$$F_l = \begin{bmatrix} F_{lx} \\ F_{ly} \end{bmatrix} = K_l \left(\begin{bmatrix} x_0 \\ y_0 \end{bmatrix} - \begin{bmatrix} x \\ y \end{bmatrix} \right) \tag{2}$$

where the current grip position is (x, y), the target position is (x0, y0), and the gain is Kl. In the case of the assistance force, force Fa and gain Ka are applied instead of Fl and Kl. The spring force is generated in the direction of the initial grip position. The magnitude of this force increases in proportion to the distance between the current position and initial position of the grip. Spring force Fs is the same as (1), where gain Kl is replaced by Ks. The viscosity and the friction force are generated in the opposite direction of the grip velocity vector. The magnitude of the viscosity force increases in proportion to the velocity of the grip, whereas that of the friction force is constant. The viscosity force Fv and the friction force Ff are given as follows,

$$F_v = \begin{bmatrix} F_{vx} \\ F_{vy} \end{bmatrix} = K_v \begin{bmatrix} \dot{x} \\ \dot{y} \end{bmatrix} \tag{3}$$

$$F_f = \begin{bmatrix} F_{fx} \\ F_{fy} \end{bmatrix} = K_f \begin{bmatrix} \frac{\dot{x}}{|\dot{x}|} \\ \frac{\dot{y}}{|\dot{y}|} \end{bmatrix} \tag{4}$$

where the velocity of the grip is and the gain is Kv for the viscosity and Kf for the friction force. In order to provide special effects in some training programs, e.g., the contact force of the wall or the reaction force when hitting some objects, this special-effect force Fe was generated. The total haptic force on grip F was the summation of each force, as follows,

$$F = F_l + F_a + F_s + F_v + F_f + F_e \tag{5}$$

2.3 Implemented training programs

The haptic device is controlled with a PC/AT computer and implemented control software. The control software achieves the following functions: controlling the haptic device, displaying the training program and the current position of the cursor on the monitor, acquiring the training data for each patient, and evaluating the training results. Of course, the cursor on the display moves in synchronicity with the grip of the haptic device, and the system provides a haptic force that obeys Eq. (5). The data acquisition program stores the training data, such as the time and grip position. The stored data could be used for offline analysis in further quantitative assessment of the functional motor rehabilitation, since the evaluation program is now under construction.

The implemented training now available consists of five different basic training programs and two applied training programs. In the upper left column of Fig. 4, the point-to-point movement training program is shown. In this training, nine circles are shown on the display, and patients try to move the cursor from circle to circle. In the upper middle column of Fig. 4, the line drawing training program is shown. Nine small circles and lines that connect the circles are shown on the display, and patients try to move the cursor from circle to circle while staying on the lines.

In the upper right column in Fig. 4, the circle-drawing training program is shown. Four concentric doughnut rings are shown on the display, and patients try to move the cursor while staying on each doughnut ring. In the bottom left column in Fig. 4, the wave-drawing training program is shown. Two small circles and a sinuous wavy line are shown on the display, and the circles are connected with the wavy line.

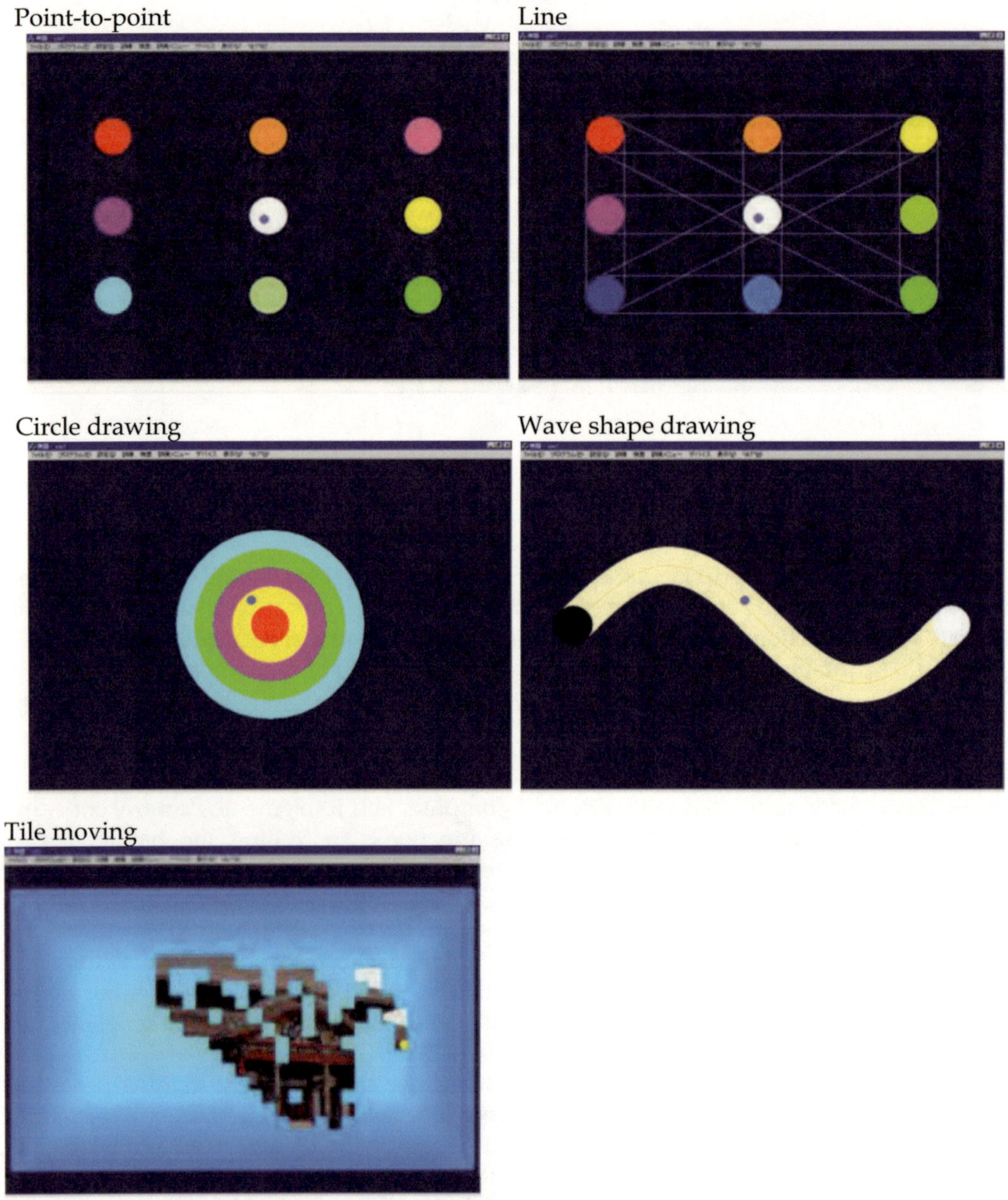

Fig. 4. Basic training programs displayed on the monitor.

Patients try to move the cursor from one circle to the other while staying on the line. In the bottom right column of Fig. 4, the tile-moving training program is shown. Square colored tiles are shown on the display, and patients try to move the cursor over all tiles. When the

cursor is over a tile, the color of the tile becomes clear, and a hidden picture appears. The displacement and the radius of the circles, the radius and the width of the doughnut rings, the amplitude and the cycle of the waves, the number of tiles, the magnitude and the direction of the virtual force, and the hidden picture are all changeable by the operators.
While the patients execute the basic training programs, some patients might become bored and lose their concentration on the training program. Therefore, we constructed further applied training programs involving hockey and maze games. These may help the patients not lose their motivation and maintain their concentration while training. On the left in Fig. 5, a hockey game is displayed on the monitor. The hockey game is similar to a table hockey game, and patients try to hit a puck and score against the computer program. Various haptic forces are delivered when moving the grip, e.g., impact, viscous, and spring forces. On the right in Fig. 5, a maze game is shown. Patients try to move the cursor from start to goal by going through a complex route. When the cursor hits the wall of the maze, patients feel the haptic forces and are not able to get over the wall. The velocity of the puck and the intensity and direction of the applied force are also changeable by the operators. These programs are effective for functional cognitive rehabilitation.

Hockey Maze

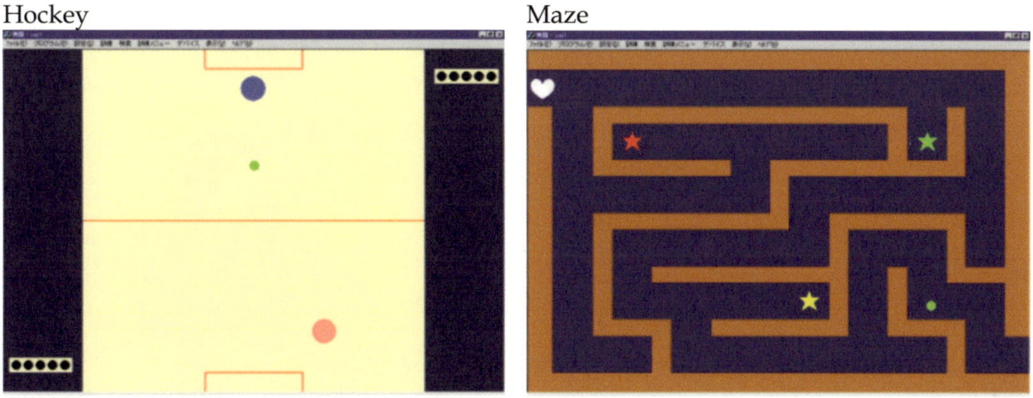

Fig. 5. Applied training programs displayed on the monitor.

3. Handling the haptic device in healthy subjects

3.1 Objective of the preliminary experiment

As reported in the Introduction, the effects of the assist/resist forces as the subjects execute their motor rehabilitation in a planar horizontal plane are still unknown. The virtual force relationships may play an important role in motor rehabilitation when making decisions on safe and effective robotic rehabilitation. Hence, the purpose of this preliminary experiment was to investigate the relationships between the assisting and the resisting force acting on the grip while subjects moved their grip from one point to another.

3.2 Methods

Nine healthy right-handed males (21 to 24 years of age) participated in this preliminary experiment. They had no known history of neurological disorders and gave informed consent approved by the local Ethics Committee of Shibaura Institute of Technology. Each subject was seated comfortably on a height-adjustable chair with his trunk immobilized by a strap and the wrist of his right forearm attached to the forearm support base with Velcro straps so that the elbow and shoulder rotation were in a horizontal plane. When the cursor displayed on the monitor was at the start position, the elbow joint angle was at 110 deg flexion (0 deg: full elbow extension), the shoulder angle was at 60 deg abduction and 35 deg medial rotation (0 deg: fundamental position), and the wrist and shoulder joints lined up straight in a horizontal plane. The subjects were then instructed to move the cursor from the start point to the mid-point (forward-motion phase) and from the mid-point to the goal position (backward-motion phase) along with the target line (30 mm width shown on the monitor) in a horizontal plane. The distance from the start to the mid-point was 200 mm; thus, the total travel distance was 400 mm in one cycle. In this preliminary experiment, the applied force was set at 2.5 N and was given constantly from the desired direction to the grip. Three force conditions (no-assist, anterior-to-posterior, and posterior-to-anterior; duration, 30 sec in each) were executed at random. On account of this, the anterior-to-posterior force condition became an assist force in the forward-motion phase and a resist force in the backward-motion phase. In fact, it showed opposite aspects in the posterior-to-anterior force condition. Figure 6 is a schematic figure for these preliminary experimental conditions with the direction of the applied force in light-gray arrows. These training sets were conducted 5 minutes per day and repeated for 5 days. All of the subjects carried out point-to-point movements at a self-determined comfortable speed each day. The number of the cycles per day varied day by day because the performance speeds tended to increase as training progressed.

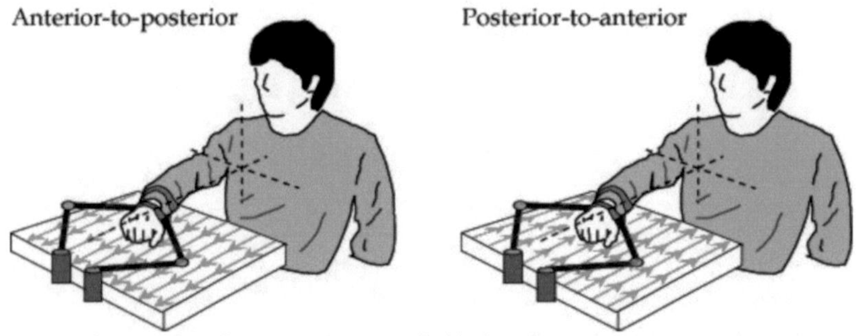

Fig. 6. Schematic figure for the experiment; (left) for the anterior-to-posterior applied force condition and (right) for the posterior-to-anterior applied force condition. The light-gray arrows denote the direction of the applied force.

On the first and last days, the surface EMG activities were recorded from the bellies of the biceps brachii (BB) and the triceps brachii (TB) muscles using pairs of Ag-AgCl electrodes (7 mm diameter; 3 cm inter-electrode distance). The EMG signals were amplified and band-pass-filtered (30 Hz - 5 kHz) with a bioelectric amplifier (AB-610J Nihon Kohden Co., Ltd.). All the data were stored in a personal computer at a sampling frequency of 100 Hz for both the current position (x, y) and the grip forces and 1 kHz for the EMG signals for off-line analysis. The EMG signals were then full-wave-rectified after subtracting the DC component. Both the forward- and backward-motion phases were expressed in relation to the 100% in each phase. The mean velocities and the positional errors, which were expressed as regression errors, for the forward- and the backward-motion phases were calculated from the cursor position data. Table 1 contains the details of the direction of the elbow and the shoulder joint movement and the expected EMG changes under the anterior-to-posterior/posterior–to-anterior applied force condition during the forward-/backward-motion phase.

	Elbow		Shoulder	Anterior-to-posterior		Posterior-to-anterior	
Forward	Extension	Agonist : TB	Inner rotation	Assist	BB : no change	Resist	BB : no change
		Antagonist : BB			TB : decrease		TB : increase
Backward	Flexion	Agonist : BB	Extorsion	Resist	BB : increase	Assist	BB : decrease
		Antagonist : TB			TB : no change		TB : no change

Table 1. Direction of the elbow and the shoulder joint angular displacement movements and expected EMG changes in anterior-to-posterior/posterior -to-anterior applied force condition during the forward-/backward-motion phase.

To investigate the effects of either the assist or the resist force to the EMG activities, the mean amplitudes of both the BB and the TB EMG activities under the no-assist condition in each phase were used to normalize the amplitudes under the two other conditions. EMG coordination between bi-articular muscles was indispensable for a smooth pedaling performance (Raasch and Zajac, 1999). In this respect, it was considered for the case of the upper limb movements that the smooth two-joint movement in a planar horizontal plane was achieved by the EMG coordination within the BB and the TB. In this paper, therefore, we defined the area under the subtracted two time-series of the BB and the TB EMG activities as EMG coordination in the forward-/backward-motion phase, as follows,

$$(\text{EMG Coordination}) = \left| \frac{\text{BB(i,t)}}{\text{RMS\_BB}} - \frac{\text{TB(i,t)}}{\text{RMS\_TB}} \right| \tag{6}$$

where BB(i,t) and TB(i,t) are the rectified EMG data in each phase, RMS_BB and RMS_TB are the root mean-squared EMG activities for the BB or the TB under the no-assist condition, and i denotes the forward- or the backward-motion phase. We then constructed a three-dimensional (3D) plot of the EMG coordination as a function of the mean velocity and the positional error. The EMG coordination can be expressed as a single plane on the 3D plot. When the positional errors increase and, as a result, EMG coordination decreases, the smoothness of the point-to-point movement is lost. In addition, the mean velocity and the positional error obey in a speed-accuracy tradeoff, also known as Fitt's law (Fitts, 1954). It will be demonstrated, however, that the EMG coordination is enhanced through training when the mean velocity increases rather than when there is an increase in the regression error and the EMG coordination. Namely, two slopes of each single plane, which were calculated as standardized partial regression coefficients using multiple regression tests, were used to quantify the contributions of the positional error and the mean velocity to the EMG coordination. One-way repeated analysis of variance was used to determine the significant differences among the no-assist, anterior-to-posterior, and posterior-to-anterior conditions. Levels were considered statistically significant at $P<0.05$.

3.3 Results

Figures 7-9 show a typical time series of the cursor positions on the XY-table, the cursor velocities, the EMG activities of the BB, and the TB under three different applied force conditions in one subject. It is clear that the movement velocity and the achievement periods were increased after training for the same duration. As for the movement velocities, their profiles became sharper than those before training, since both the acceleration and braking phases became steeper during both the forward- and backward-motion phases and showed a bell shape after training.

In the case of the levels of the EMG activities, the BB, which is the agonist muscle during the backward-motion phase, was enhanced under the anterior-to-posterior applied force condition. In addition, the TB EMG activities increased against the posterior-to-anterior applied force and decreased under the anterior-to-posterior applied force condition. These phenomena are shown more clearly in Figs. 10 and 11: when the subjects executed forward/backward motion, the EMG activities of the agonist muscles were enhanced against the resist force, whereas the levels of the antagonist muscles were decreased by the assist force compared with those under the no-assist condition.

The phasic EMG activities between the BB and the TB were shown more clearly after training, considering that the EMG coordination with the BB and the TB might correlate positively with the enhanced movement velocities. A three-dimensional (3D) plot of the relationship among the EMG coordination, positional error, and movement velocity in one subject (Fig. 12.) is shown in Fig. 7. In this case, the EMG coordination increased with the increase of the movement velocities, whereas the same tendencies for positional errors were not observed under all three conditions.

The contributions of the movement velocity and the positional errors to the EMG coordination are denoted by the two standardized partial regression coefficients of the single plane on the 3D plot (Fig. 13.). Under each condition, the EMG coordination was more dependent on the movement velocity than on the positional errors, since the standardized partial regression coefficient for the movement velocity was positive. In addition, the standardized partial regression coefficient under the posterior-to-anterior applied force condition was greater than that of either the no-assist or the anterior-to-posterior applied force condition. For the positional errors, the standardized partial regression coefficient was close to zero under the posterior-to-anterior applied force condition.

3.4 Discussion

The main objective of this preliminary experiment was to evaluate the efficacy of assist/resist applied force for upper limb muscle activities with a two-joint arm movement in the planar horizontal plane while using the haptic device. The extent to which our results can be generalized is questionable because they were based on data obtained from only healthy right-handed young subjects.

The muscle activation patterns responsible for initiating hand movements are processed in the central nervous system on the basis of a simple representation of movement orientation, without taking into account the specific dynamic effects of the motion (Karst and Hasan, 1991a, b). Recent studies, however, have demonstrated that the cortical motor activity is continuously modulated while performing drawing movements to accommodate changes in orientation and velocity of the arm end-effector trajectory (Schwartz and Moran, 1999; Scheidt et al., 2000). Our results demonstrated that the effects provided by an assist/resist force were different. In these respects, it was considered that the forward-/backward-motion phase against the resist force needs more positive recruitment of the central nervous system under the anterior-to-posterior and/or posterior-to-anterior applied force condition than under the no-assist condition and, as a result, EMG activities were enhanced. Simultaneously, the decreased EMG activities following the assist force suggested the negative recruitment of the central nervous system.

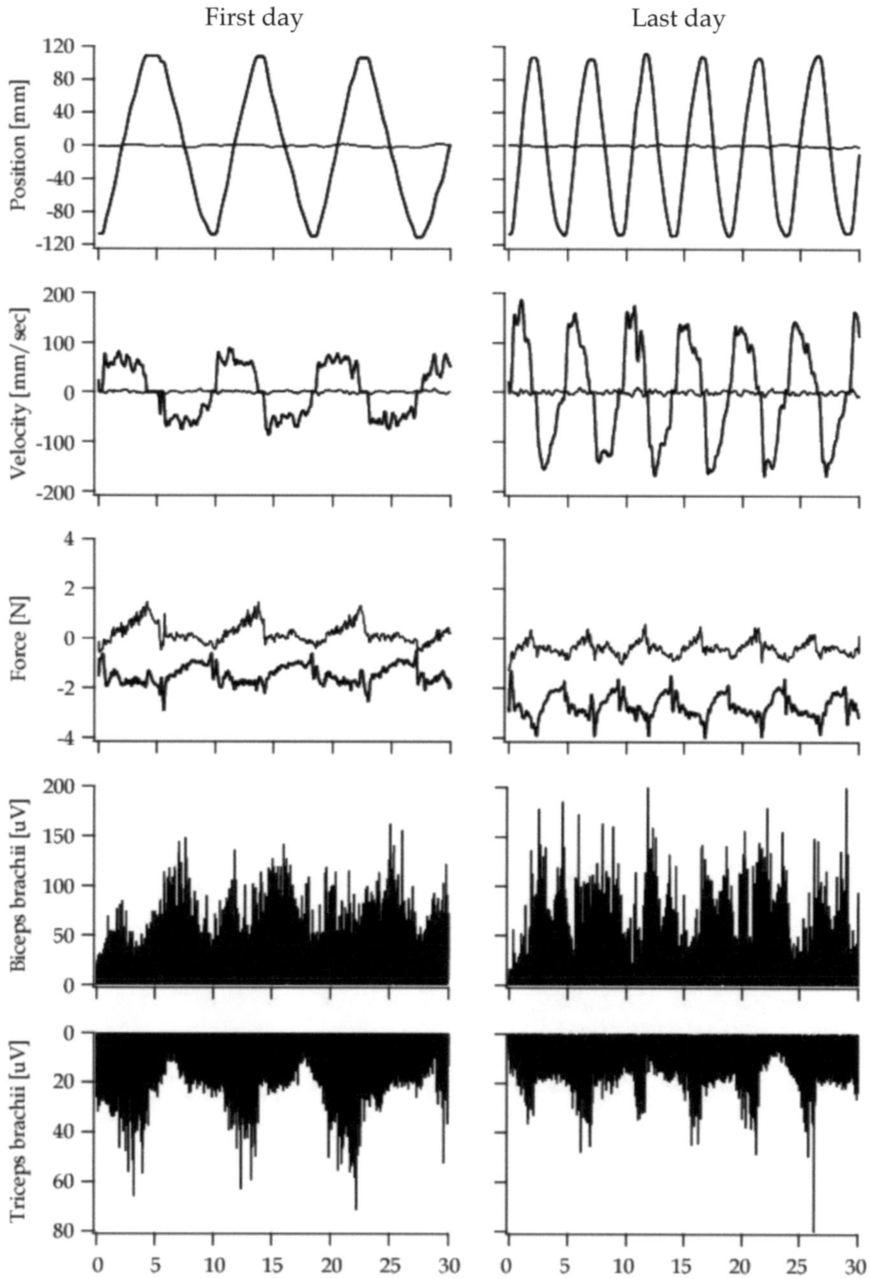

Fig. 7. The left panels show the typical time-series of the first-day waves under the no-assist condition; cursor positions (top column), velocities (middle upper column), force (middle column), and EMG activity of the BB (lower middle column) and the TB (bottom column) in one subject. The right panels show the last-day waves in the same subject. The thin lines denote x-axial variables of position, velocity, and force, and the thick lines denote the y-axial variables.

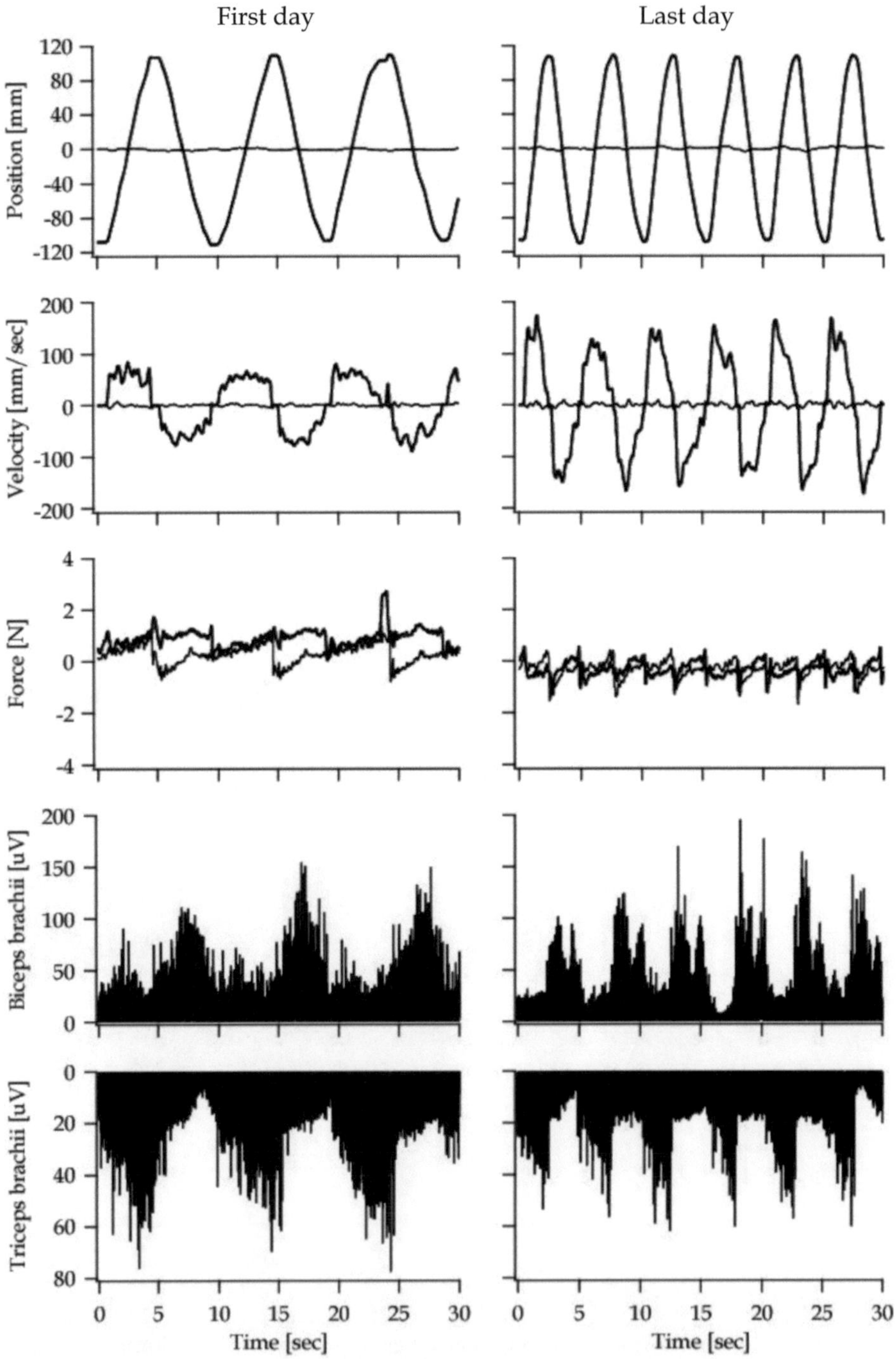

Fig. 8. Typical time-series under the anterior-to-posterior force applied condition in the same subject shown in Fig. 7. The orders of the panels and the lines are the same as those in Fig. 7.

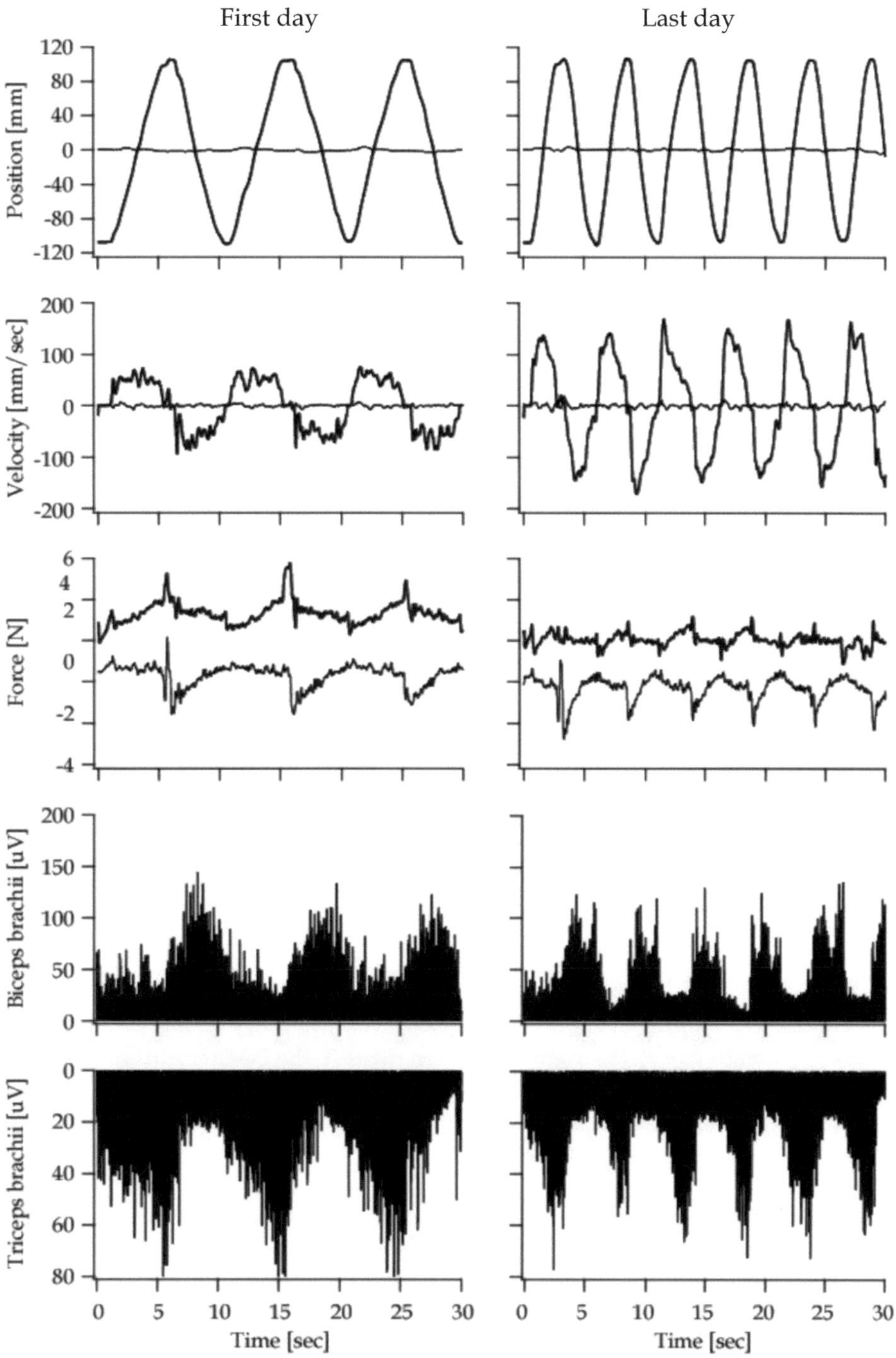

Fig. 9. Typical time-series under the posterior-to-anterior force applied condition in the same subject shown in Fig. 7. The orders of the panels and the lines are the same as those in Fig. 7.

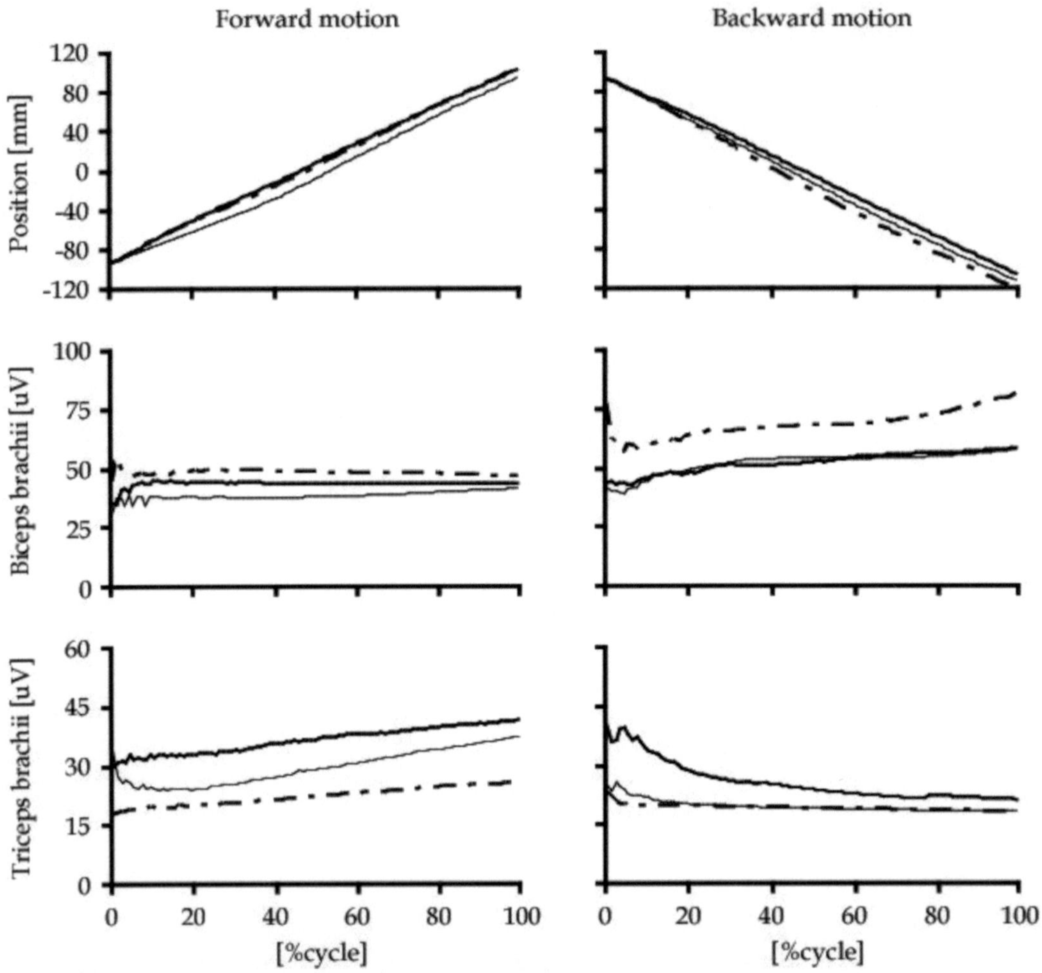

Fig. 10. The left panels show the ensemble-averaged waves in the forward-motion phases; cursor positions (top) and EMG activity of the BB (middle) and of the TB (bottom) in the same subject shown in Fig. 7. The right panels are those in the backward-motion phases. The thin lines denote the no-assist condition, the dashed lines show the anterior-to-posterior force applied condition, and the thick lines denote the posterior-to-anterior force applied condition.

In this study, we defined the EMG coordination as an index of the phasic relationships between agonist and antagonist muscles during the forward-/backward-motion phase. Thus, if the EMG coordination shows a large value, the effect to be provided by the agonist muscles is high against the demands of the movement task. The results suggest that the improvement in the movement speed after training was caused by the enhanced EMG coordination, since the contribution of the movement speed to the EMG coordination was significantly higher than that of the positional error.

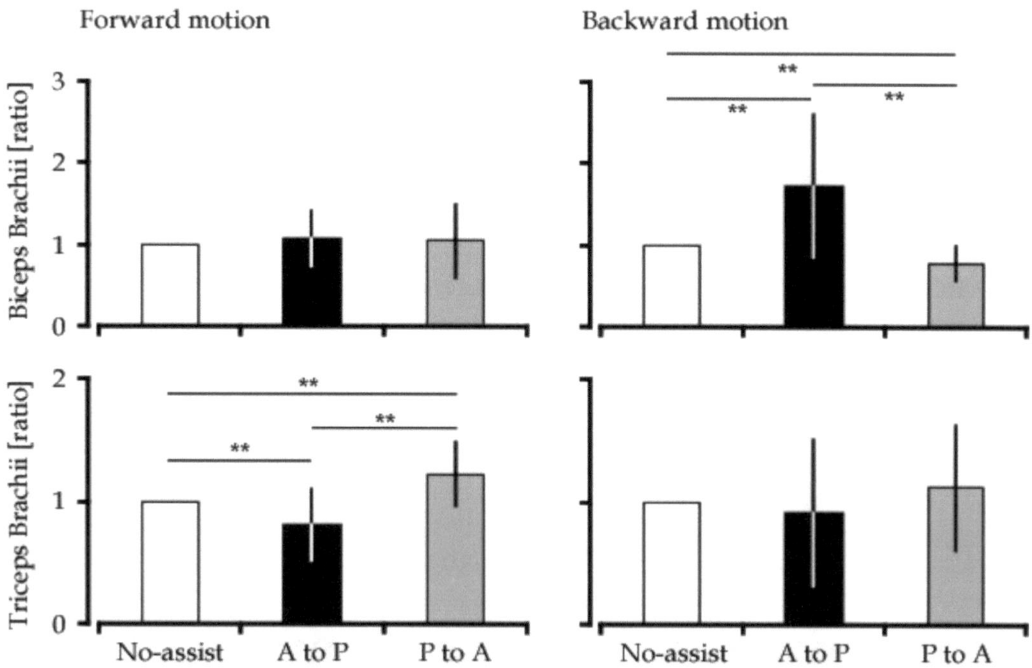

Fig. 11. Ratios of EMG activities of the BB and the TB under both the anterior-to-posterior and the posterior-to-anterior force applied conditions relative to the no-assist condition during the forward-motion phase (left) and the backward-motion phase (right). "A to P" means the anterior-to-posterior force applied condition, and "P to A" denotes the posterior-to-anterior force applied condition. (** : $P<0.01$).

4. Clinical relevance

Although the haptic device provided only 2.5 N force, the EMG activities increased or decreased depending on the adjustment and the direction of the force. These phenomena suggested that the application of only 2.5 N would have a training effect on the muscle force and the motor planning about trajectories of the wrist position. EMG data provided evidence of improved muscle activation patterns between agonist and antagonist muscles by the application of an assist/resist force as well as of improved EMG coordination. EMG coordination between bi-articular muscles was indispensable for a smooth pedaling performance (Raasch and Zajac, 1999). Therefore, the haptic device could improve upper limb EMG coordination, especially, for bi-articular muscles, such as the BB and the TB.

In general, rehabilitation methods for stroke patients, e.g., peg boards and sanding boards, are implemented by therapists. Although these methods keep the therapists' workload at a low level, it might be difficult to keep the patients' motivation and/or concentration until rehabilitation is achieved. Through the use of the haptic device, training programs could be transformed into computer games or other games that would attract the users and maintain their motivation. These programs might be effective for functional cognitive rehabilitation.

5. Conclusion

One critical question that should always be asked when considering rehabilitation methods is their duration, in other words, how long the training should last and/or whether the gains will persist for a significant period after training. In this respect, further studies are needed on the use of the haptic device as an upper limb rehabilitation method for stroke patients. EMG coordination would be an effective training index. Higher EMG coordination means the improvement of the upper limb movement at the neural control level, including the motor planning of the wrist position. Therefore, assessment of the improvement in the EMG coordination using the haptic device would indicate the length of effective training periods for the upper limb motor rehabilitation of stroke patients.

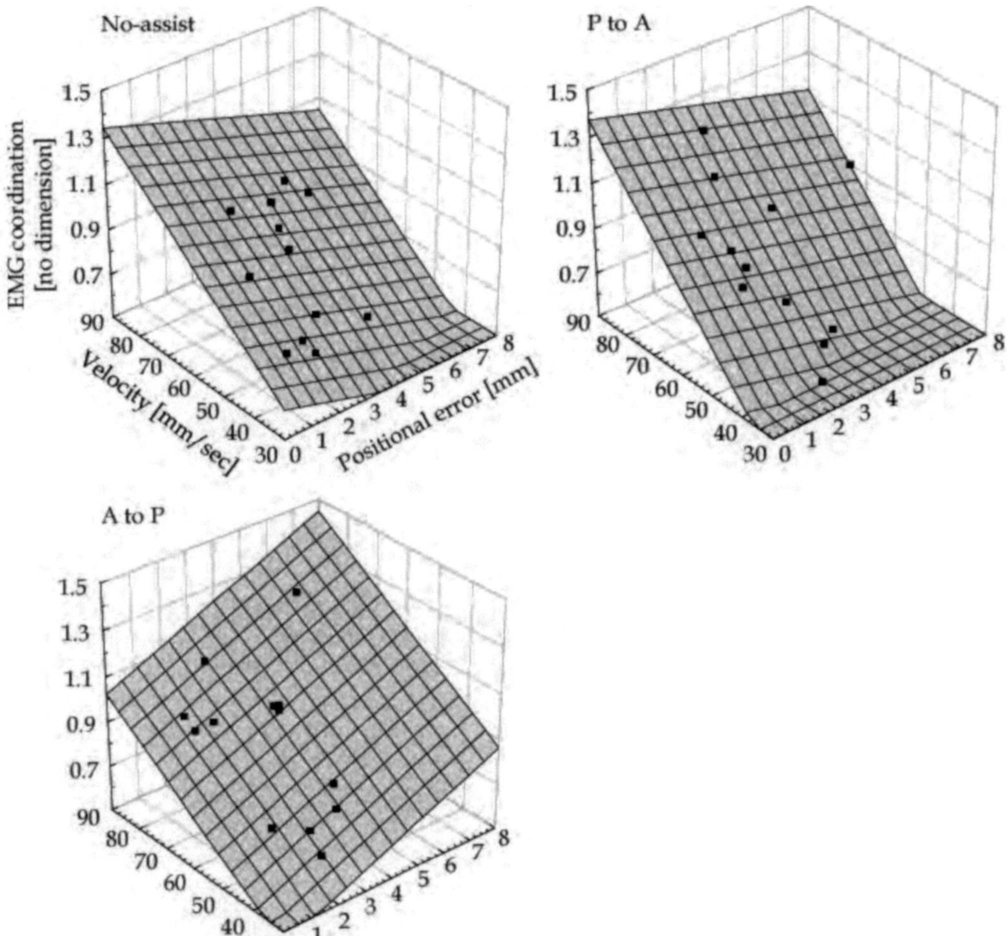

Fig. 12. Three-dimensional (3D) plots showing the relationship among the EMG coordination, positional error, and movement velocity in the same subject shown in Fig. 7. The left top 3D plot shows the no-assist condition; the left bottom denotes the anterior-to-posterior condition; and the right top shows the posterior-to-anterior force applied condition.

Another question is the intensity of the rehabilitation methods. This would depend on the remaining individual motor functions of each patient. In this regard, using the haptic device, the operators can easily change the magnitude and the direction of the virtual force. Namely, the haptic device could either induce the constraint movement using the large magnitudes of the virtual force or train against the resist force as the motor functions improve. In these respects, a robotic rehabilitation tool, specifically, the haptic device, would be an effective method for neurorehabilitation.

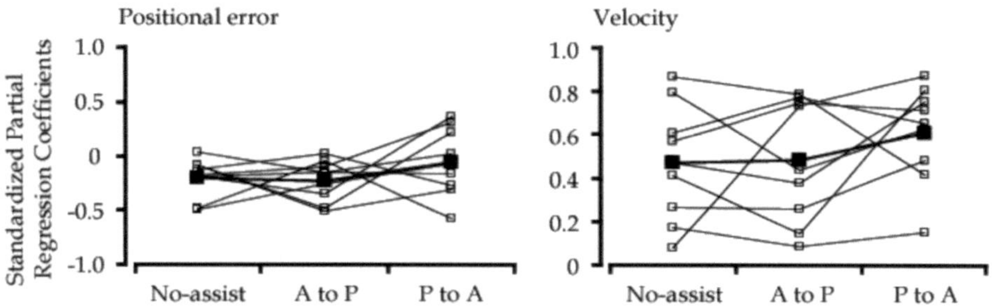

Fig. 13. Differences in sensitivity to both the positional error and the movement velocity. Although there are no significant differences in either of the standardized partial regression coefficients, the EMG coordination tends to increase with the posterior-to-anterior force applied in two-joint arm movements in a planar horizontal plane compared to those under the no-assist and the anterior-to-posterior force applied conditions. The open rectangles denote subject-to-subject changes, and the filled rectangles denote the grand averages.

In conclusion, we have developed the haptic device for upper limb motor rehabilitation, which can provide an assist/resist force on the grip. From the preliminary experimental results, the EMG data provided evidence of improved muscle activation patterns between the agonist and antagonist muscles by the application of the assist/resist force as well as of improved EMG coordination.

6. References

Aisen, M.L.; Krebs, H.I.; Hogan, N.; McDowell, F. & Volpe, B.T. (1997). The effect of robot-assisted therapy and rehabilitative training on motor recovery following stroke. *Archives of Neurology*, Vol.54, No.4, 443-446, ISSN: 0003-9942

Colombo, G.; Joerg, M.; Schreier, R. & Dietz, V. (2000). Treadmill training of paraplegic patients using a robotic orthosis. *Journal of Rehabilitation Research and Development*, Vol.37, No.6, 693-700, ISSN: 0748-7711

Dromerick, A.W.; Edwards, D.F. & Hahn, M. (2000). Does the application of constraint-induced movement therapy during acute rehabilitation reduce arm impairment after ischemic stroke? *Stroke*, Vol.31, No.12, 2984-2988, ISSN: 0039-2499

Feys, H.M.; De Weerdt, W.J.; Selz, B.E.; Cox Steck, G.A.; Spichiger, R.; Vereeck, L.E.; Putman, K.D. & Van Hoydonck, G.A. (1998). Effect of a therapeutic intervention for the hemiplegic upper limb in the acute phase after stroke: a single-blind, randomized, controlled multicenter trial. *Stroke*, Vol.29, No.4, 785-792, ISSN: 0039-2499

Fitts, P.M. (1954). The information capacity of the human motor system in controlling the amplitude of movements. *Journal of Experimental Psychology*, Vol.47, No.6, 381-391, ISSN:0022-1015

Karst, G.M. & Hasan, Z. (1991a). Initiation rules for planar, two-joint arm movements: agonist selection for movements throughout the work space. *Journal of Neurophysiology*, Vol.66, No.5, 1579-1593, ISSN: 0022-3077

Karst, G.M. & Hasan, Z. (1991b). Timing and magnitude of electromyographic activity for two-joint arm movements in different directions. *Journal of Neurophysiology*, Vol.66, No.5, 1594-1604, ISSN: 0022-3077

Krebs, H.I.; Ferraro, M.; Buerger, S.P.; Newbery, M.J.; Makiyama, A.; Sandmann, M.; Lynch, D.; Volpe, B.T. & Hogan, N. (2004). Rehabilitation robotics: pilot trial of a spatial extension for MIT-Manus. *Journal of Neuroengineering and Rehabilitation*, Vol.1, No.1, ISSN: 1743-0003

Lee, H.; Takahashi, Y.; Miyoshi, T.; Terada, T.; Inoue, K.; Ito, Y.; Ikeda, Y.; Suzuki, K. & Komeda, T. (2005). Basic experiments of upper limb rehabilitation using haptic device system, *Proceedings of the 2005 IEEE 9th International Conference on Rehabilitation Robotics*, pp. 444-447, ISBN :0-7803-9003-2, Chicago, 28 June - 1 July 2005, IEEE

Lincoln, N.B.; Parry, R.H. & Vass, C.D. (1999). Randomized, controlled trial to evaluate increased intensity of physiotherapy treatment of arm function after stroke. *Stroke*, Vol.30, No.3, 573-579, ISSN: 0039-2499

Lum, P.S.; Burgar, C.G.; Van der Loos, M.; Shor, P.C.; Majmundar, M. & Yap, R. (2006). MIME robotic device for upper-limb neurorehabilitation in subacute stroke subjects: A follow-up study. *Journal of Rehabilitation Research and Development*, Vol.43, No.5, 631-642, ISSN: 0748-7711

Miltner, W.H.; Bauder, H.; Sommer, M.; Dettmers, C. & Taub, E. (1999). Effects of constraint-induced movement therapy on patients with chronic motor deficits after stroke: a replication. *Stroke*, Vol.30, No.3, 586-592, ISSN: 0039-2499

Raasch, C.C., & Zajac, F.E. (1999). Locomotor strategy for pedaling: muscle groups and biomechanical functions. *Journal of Neurophysiology*, Vol.82, No.2, 515-525, ISSN:0022-3077

Scheidt, R.A.; Reinkensmeyer, D.J.; Conditt, M.A.; Rymer, W.Z. & Mussa-Ivaldi, F.A. (2000). Persistence of motor adaptation during constrained, multi-joint, arm movements. *Journal of Neurophysiology*, Vol.84, No.2, 853-862, ISSN: 0022-3077

Schwartz, A.B. & Moran, D.W. (1999). Motor cortical activity during drawing movement: population representation during lemniscate tracing. *Journal of Neurophysiology*, Vol.82, No.5, 2705-2718, ISSN: 0022-3077

Sunderland, A.; Fletcher, D.; Bradley, L.; Tinson, D.; Hewer, R.L. & Wade, D.T. (1994). Enhanced physical therapy for arm function after stroke: a one year follow up study. *Journal of Neurology, Neurosurgery, and Psychiatry*, Vol.57, No.7, 856-858, ISSN: 0022-3050

Takahashi, Y.; Terada, T.; Inoue, K.; Ito, Y.; Lee, H. & Komeda, T. (2003). Upper-limb rehabilitation exercises using haptic device system. *International Journal of Human-friendly Welfare Robotic Systems*, Vol.4, No.2, 18-22, ISSN:1598-3250

Taub, E.; Miller, N.E.; Novack, T.A.; Cook, E.W.3rd; Fleming, W.C.; Nepomuceno, C.S.; Connell, J.S. & Crago, J.E. Technique to improve chronic motor deficit after stroke. *Archives of Physical Medicine and Rehabilitation*, Vol.74, No.4, 347-354, ISSN: 0003-9993

Wernig, A. & Muller, S. (1992). Laufband locomotion with body weight support improved walking in persons with severe spinal cord injuries. *Paraplegia*, Vol.30, No.4, 229-238, ISSN: 0031-1758

19

Rehabilitation of the Paralyzed Lower Limbs Using Functional Electrical Stimulation: Robust Closed Loop Control

Samer Mohammed, Philippe Poignet, Philippe Fraisse & David Guiraud
LIRMM – CNRS/INRIA – Université de Montpellier II
France

1. Introduction

The reliability, the ease of donning and doffing and the robustness of controllers constitute the primary criteria to evaluate any control strategy based on Functional Electrical Stimulation (FES). This technique is used to excite muscles that are under lesions and no more controlled by paraplegic patients. Consequently, the patient could recover partially some of its lower limb functions, improving the cardiovascular system and bettering the whole quality of life. Many FES based studies; both open loop and closed loop control showed satisfactory results in movement restoration. Although open loop control strategy induces excessive stimulation of the main muscles and consequently fast muscular fatigue, it is still adopted in most clinics till now. This could be explained mainly by their relative simple implantation (Bajd et al., 1981). Actually closed loop control strategies still have several drawbacks, such as overwhelming the patient by sensors' feedback, tuning the parameters of the controllers and identification for every patient, the lack of understanding the muscle contraction phenomena, etc. Closed loop controllers in FES context have been reported in many studies (Riener & Fuhr, 1998); (Mulder et al., 1992); (Donaldson & Yu, 1996). Some authors use a simple PID controller (Wood et al., 1998), Knee Extension Controller KEC (Poboroniuc et al., 2003), a combination of feedback and feed-forward control or an adaptive approach (Ferrarin et al., 2001). Others use a first or a second order switching curve in the state space to control patient movements: The On/Off controller (Mulder et al., 1992) and the ONZOFF controller (Poboroniuc et al., 2002), in the so-called "controller-centered" strategies. The main advantage of these strategies is their low number of parameters to be tuned during stimulation. The so-called "subject centered" strategies, (PDMR: Patient-Driven Motion Reinforcement (Riener & Fuhr, 1998), CHRELMS: Control by Handle REactions of Leg Muscle Stimulation (Donaldson & Yu, 1996)), introduce the voluntary contribution of the upper body of the patient as an essential part of the control diagram. This latter is not yet adopted in clinical use because of the relative high number of parameters to be identified. In order to overcome these drawbacks, we have applied two robust control strategies that are, the High Order Sliding Mode (HOSM) controller (Fridman & Levant, 2002) and the Model Predictive Controller (MPC) also known as receding horizon controller (Allgöwer et al., 1999). These controllers have been evaluated in simulation to highlight i) their performance in terms of capability of tracking a pre-defined reference trajectory and ii) the robustness against force perturbation and model mismatch. Furthermore the MPC technique constitutes an adequate controller for nonlinear multivariable systems and enables us to incorporate explicitly constraints on inputs, outputs and system states. The performances of these controllers have also been compared with a classical pole placement controller. The originality of the presented study comes also from the fact that these control strategies rely on the use of a physio-mathematical based muscle model. In fact, few studies have treated the human muscle as an entire physiological element in a control scheme. Some authors used linear muscle models; others represent the muscle as a non-linear function of recruitment with dynamics activation, angle and angular velocity dependence (Riener & Fuhr, 1998); (Veltink et al., 1992). The muscle model used in this study has been recently published (El-Makssoud et al., 2004-a) and it is based on a complex physio-mathematical formulation of the macroscopic Hill and microscopic Huxley concepts reflecting the dynamic phenomenon that occurred during muscle contraction and relaxation. In this model, the number of recruited motor units increases as a function of both the intensity and the pulse width of the stimulus. This phenomenon is modeled by an activation model (representing the ratio of recruited fibers). The contraction dynamics is expressed by a set of nonlinear differential equations representing the mechanical model. The goal of the present study is to represent the interaction between a closed loop controller and a closely physiological muscle model matching.

In next section, the system modeling is presented; it includes the knee-muscle biomechanical model, its state space formulation and parameter identification based on experimental setup. In the third and fourth sections, simulation results for controllers based on HOSM and MPC are presented. A comparison study of the controller performance is presented in the fifth section.

2. System modeling

Since closed loop control of different muscles actuating the knee joint of a paraplegic patient constitutes a prerequisite step before any upward mobility such as: standing up, standing, walking, climbing stairs, etc., we limited, in this stage, the study to a small scale biomechanical system. It consists of two segments representing respectively the shank and the thigh connected to each other by a revolute joint of one degree of freedom. The thigh is supposed to be fixed with respect to the patient while the shank is free to move around the knee joint (Fig.1). Two agonist/antagonist muscles act on the knee, the quadriceps acts as an extensor muscle while the hamstrings are the flexor muscle group. As a result two forces F_q and F_h cause respectively the extension and the flexion of the knee.

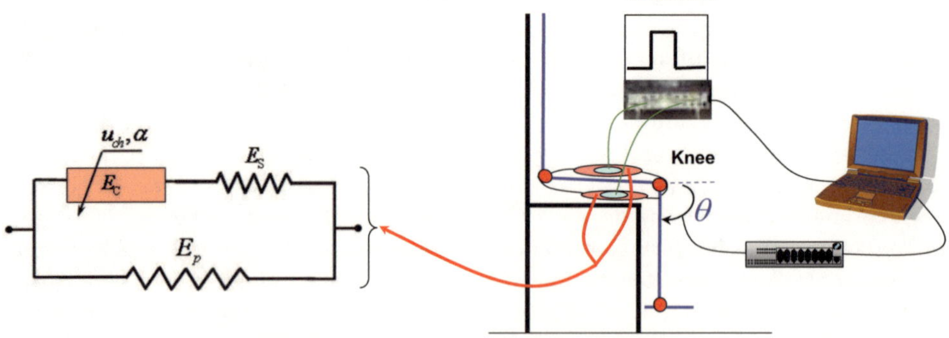

Fig. 1. Functional Electrical Stimulation applied to skeletal muscles.

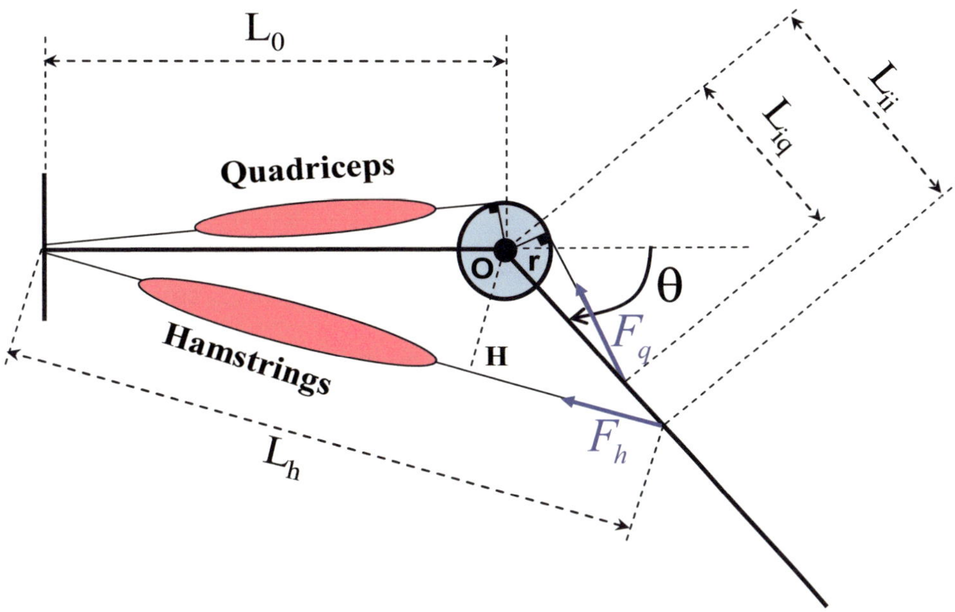

Fig. 2. Biomechanical model of the knee actuated by two groups of antagonistic muscles.

These forces are supposed to be constant along their directions on the whole corresponding muscle (Fig.2), (θ = 0 corresponds to full extension of the knee and θ = 90° represents the rest position). F_q and F_h are the inputs of the biomechanical model while the angle θ is the corresponding output. The geometric equations allow us to evaluate quadriceps length L_q depending on the knee angle variable theta:

$$L_q(\theta) = \sqrt{L_0^2 - r^2} + r\theta + \sqrt{L_{iq}^2 - r^2} \tag{1}$$

And the hamstrings length $L_h(\theta)$:

$$L_h(\theta) = \sqrt{L_0^2 + L_{ii}^2 + 2L_0 L_{ii} \cos(\theta)} \tag{2}$$

From the above equations, we can deduce the relative elongation of quadriceps and hamstrings.

$$\begin{aligned} \varepsilon_q(\theta) &= \frac{L_q - L_{0q}}{L_{0q}} = \frac{\sqrt{L_0^2 - r^2} + r\theta + \sqrt{L_{iq}^2 - r^2} - L_{0q}}{L_{0q}} \\ \varepsilon_h(\theta) &= \frac{L_h - L_{0h}}{L_{0h}} = \frac{\sqrt{L_0^2 + L_{ii}^2 + 2L_0 L_{ii}\cos(\theta)} - L_{0h}}{L_{0h}} \end{aligned} \tag{3}$$

L_{0q} and L_{0h} correspond respectively to the initial quadriceps and hamstrings lengths. Moment arm of the quadriceps is assumed to be constant and equal to the pulley radius r while the moment arm of the hamstrings depends on theta.

$$OH(\theta)=\frac{L_0 L_{ii}\sin(\theta)}{\sqrt{L_0^2+L_{ii}^2+2L_0 L_{ii}\cos(\theta)}} \tag{4}$$

From the equations (3), (4) and the equation of motion that is a nonlinear second order equation, we obtained the acceleration $\ddot{\theta}$ (Eq. 5) as a function of the inertia about the knee joint I, gravity, joint damping factor F_v and joint elasticity K_e.

$$\ddot{\theta}=\frac{1}{I}\left[rF_q-mg\cos(\theta)\beta L_1-K_e\theta-F_v\dot{\theta}-\frac{L_0 L_{ii}\sin(\theta)}{\sqrt{L_0^2+L_{ii}^2+2L_0 L_{ii}\cos(\theta)}}F_h\right] \tag{5}$$

Identifications of the above parameters were performed based on experiments and are presented in the next section.

2.1 Muscle model

In previous papers (El-Makssoud et al., 2004-a; b), a physiological skeletal muscle model has been proposed to describe the complex internal physiological mechanism controlled by FES. In order to develop strategies for simulation, motion synthesis and motor control during clinical restoration of movement, we have adopted this model. In (Fig.3) we show the muscle model with the parallel element E_p representing the passive properties of the muscle and two elements in series: the serial element E_s and the contractile element E_c. This model is controlled by two variables: u_{ch}, a chemical control input and α the ratio of recruited fibers. This model has been described by two sets of differential equations (Eq.6) where the outputs are K_c and F_c representing, respectively, the stiffness and force generated by the contractile element. K_0 and F_0 are the maximum values of K_c and F_c. These equations could be expressed as follow:

$$\begin{cases}\dot{K}_c=\left(s_0\alpha k_0-s_uK_c+s_vq\dfrac{s_0\alpha F_0-s_uF_c}{1+pK_c-s_vqF_c}K_c\right)u_{ch}-\dfrac{s_vaK_c}{1+pK_c-s_vqF_c}\dot{\varepsilon}\\ \dot{F}_c=\dfrac{s_0\alpha F_0-s_uF_c}{1+pK_c-s_vqF_c}u_{ch}+\dfrac{bK_c-s_vaF_c}{1+pK_c-s_vqF_c}\dot{\varepsilon}\end{cases} \tag{6}$$

$$s_u=sign(u_{ch})=\begin{cases}-1 & if\quad u_{ch}<0\\ +1 & if\quad u_{ch}>0\end{cases}\qquad s_v=sign(\dot{\varepsilon}_c)=\begin{cases}+1 & if\quad \dot{\varepsilon}_c>0\\ -1 & if\quad \dot{\varepsilon}_c<0\end{cases} \tag{7}$$

$$s_0=\frac{1+s_u}{2}\qquad a=\frac{L_0}{L_{c0}}\qquad b=L_0\qquad p=\frac{1}{k_s}\qquad q=\frac{1}{L_{c0}k_s}$$
$$\varepsilon_c=\frac{L_c-L_{c0}}{L_{c0}}\qquad \varepsilon_s=\frac{L_s-L_{s0}}{L_{s0}}\qquad \varepsilon=\frac{L-L_0}{L_0}\qquad L=L_c+L_s \tag{8}$$

Where s_u, and s_v are the sign functions related respectively to the control and velocities of the contractile element, L_c and L_s represent respectively the length of the contractile and the elastic elements. The ratio of recruited fibers α is considered as a global scale factor which gives the percentage of the maximal possible force that could be generated by the muscle.

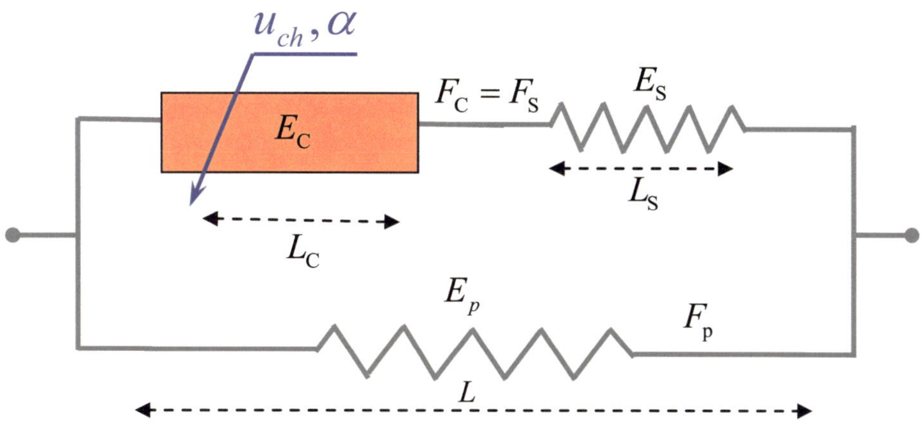

Fig. 3. Muscle model and particularity of E_c (El-Makssoud et al., 2004-a).

2.2 State space model of the muscles-knee

Let us consider the model of the muscles and knee joint as a non-linear state space model:

$$\dot{\mathbf{x}} = f(\mathbf{x}, \mathbf{t}, \mathbf{u}) \tag{9}$$

Where $\mathbf{x} = [x_1 \ldots x_6]^T = [K_{c_1} \quad K_{c_2} \quad F_{c_1} \quad F_{c_2} \quad \theta \quad \dot{\theta}]^T$ is the state vector while the control vector is expressed by $\mathbf{u} = [u_{q_{ch}} \quad \alpha_q \quad u_{h_{ch}} \quad \alpha_h]^T$. The variable θ represents the joint knee angle. The state variables K_{c1}, F_{c1}, u_{qch}, α_q and K_{c2}, F_{c2}, u_{hch}, α_h are respectively the state variables of the quadriceps and hamstrings. Consequently, the state representation of the biomechanical model (knee-muscles) could be expressed as:

$$\dot{x}_1 = \left(s_{0_1}\alpha_1 k_{0_1} - s_{u_1}x_1 + s_{v1}q_1 \frac{s_{0_1}\alpha_1 F_{0_1} - s_{u_1}x_3}{1 + p_1x_1 - s_{v_1}q_1x_3} x_1 \right) u_1 - \frac{s_{v_1}a_1x_1rx_6}{L_{01}\left(1 + p_1x_1 - s_{v_1}q_1x_3\right)}$$

$$\dot{x}_2 = \left(s_{0_2}\alpha_2 k_{0_2} - s_{u_2}x_2 + s_{v_2}q_2 \frac{s_{0_2}\alpha_2 F_{0_2} - s_{u_2}x_4}{1 + p_2x_2 - s_{v_2}q_2x_4} x_2 \right) u_2 + \frac{s_{v_2}a_2x_2L_0L_{ii}\sin(x_5)}{L_{02}\sqrt{L_0^2 + L_{ii}^2 + 2L_0L_{ii}\cos(x_5)}\left(1 + p_2x_2 - s_{v_2}q_2x_4\right)}$$

$$\dot{x}_3 = \frac{s_{0_1}\alpha_1 F_{0_1} - s_{u_1}x_3}{1 + p_1x_1 - s_{v_1}q_1x_3} u_1 + \frac{\left(b_1x_1 - s_{v_1}a_1x_3\right)rx_6}{L_{01}\left(1 + p_1x_1 - s_{v_1}q_1x_3\right)}$$

$$\dot{x}_4 = \frac{s_{0_2}\alpha_2 F_{0_2} - s_{u_2}x_4}{1 + p_2x_2 - s_{v_2}q_2x_4} u_2 - \frac{\left(b_2x_2 - s_{v_2}a_2x_4\right)L_0L_{ii}\sin(x_5)}{L_{02}\sqrt{L_0^2 + L_{ii}^2 + 2L_0L_{ii}\cos(x_5)}\left(1 + p_2x_2 - s_{v_2}q_2x_4\right)} \tag{10}$$

$$\dot{x}_5 = x_6$$

$$\dot{x}_6 = \frac{1}{I}\left(x_3r - x_4 \frac{L_0L_{ii}\sin(x_5)}{\sqrt{L_0^2 + L_{ii}^2 + 2L_0L_{ii}\cos(x_5)}} - mg\cos(x_5)\beta L_1 - K_ex_5 - F_vx_6 \right)$$

2.3 Model parameters identification

The parameters of the biomechanical system have been identified based on different protocols. The geometric parameters such as the insertion points, the muscle lengths, the moment arms, etc., were identified based on the Hawkins model (Hawkins & Hull, 1990) and using the Levenberg-Marquardt (Levenberg, 1944) algorithm. The knee joint dynamic parameters such as the joint stiffness and viscosity were identified through linear least square algorithm (Gautier & Poignet, 2002). Some muscle parameters such as the maximal muscle force and the force-length relationship were identified using non-linear interpolation. Other muscle parameters not yet identified on humans were taken from literature (El-Makssoud et al., 2004-a), basically the muscle stiffness and the contractile-elastic muscle length distribution.

2.3.1 Knee joint parameters identification

Kinematics data for the knee joint were measured through a motion analysis system and using the passive pendulum test. This test consists in recording the knee joint angle and velocity during a passive movement. The table 1 summarizes the identified knee joint parameters for a given subject. These parameters correspond respectively to the thigh length L_0, the quadriceps moment arm r and the two muscles insertion points L_{iq} and L_{ii} and their standard deviation. The hamstrings moment arm is position dependent (Eq. 4).

Parameter	L_0	r	L_{iq}	L_{ii}
Value (m)	0.3726	0.0397	0.0401	0.0648
Standard deviation (%)	0.335	3.230	3.138	0.441

Table 1. Knee joint parameter identification.

The parameters shown above, have been satisfactory identified and close to those found in literature (Kromer, 1994). The standard deviations were less than 4%. We can notice that the chosen movement trajectories excite sufficiently the unknown parameters. Figure 1 shows the muscle length computed by the Hawkins model and the model described above (Eq. 1, 2).

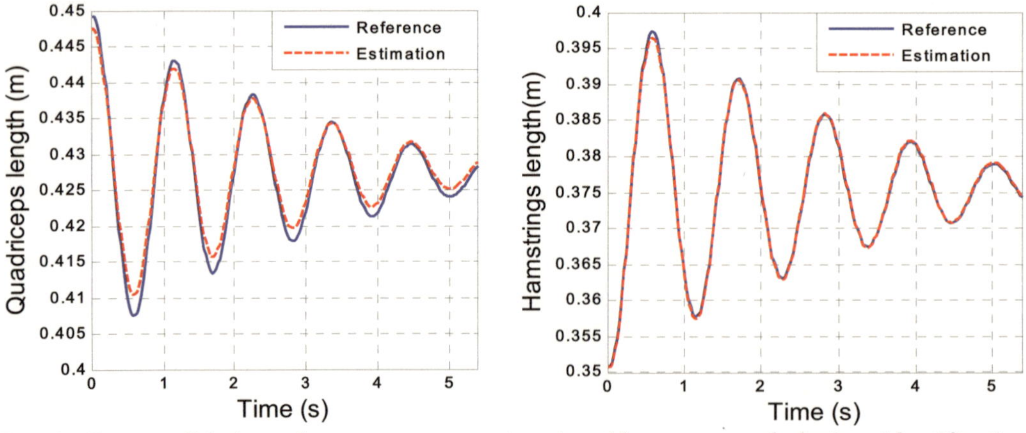

Fig. 4. Cross validation after parameter estimation (data not used during identification processing).

The dynamic parameters of the knee joint such as the knee stiffness and the knee viscosity were identified based on the following equation and using the linear least square method:

$$I\ddot{\theta} = -mgl\cos(\theta) - K_e\theta - F_v\dot{\theta} \tag{11}$$

We should notice that during a passive movement, the active moment produced by the muscles is equal to zero. Different subjects (healthy and paralyzed) have participated in the identification process. This latter was performed with the subject laying semi-supine with the lower legs hanging over the edge of a chair (Fig. 5). The operator raised the shank of the subject to given angle (about 45°) and leave the shank to swing freely until it reached the resting position (90°). The movement was recorded using a video based on motion analysis system (Vicon). Passive markers were fixed on the hip, knee and ankle (Fig. 5-b, 5-c). Kinematic data were acquired at 50 Hz sampling rate. In this application only three markers were sufficient to compute the knee joint angle and velocity. This system has the advantage to not overwhelming the subject by an external sensor that could affect the accuracy of the identification. Several tests were performed for each subject. The EMG signal analysis of the main muscles (quadriceps and hamstrings), serves only to identify any undesired voluntary muscle contractions and then reject the trial.

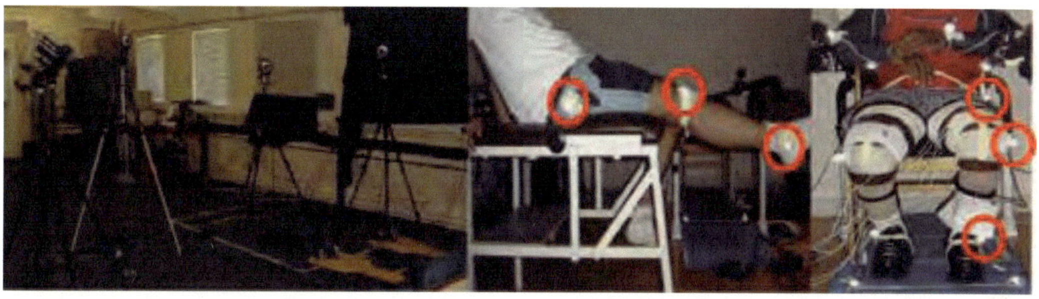

Fig. 5. a) Vicon system – b) Healthy subject - c) Paraplegic patient.

The anthropometric parameters such as the shank mass and inertia were estimated by using the regression equation proposed by DeLeva and Zatsiorsky (DeLeva, 1996), and by measuring the weight and the height of each subject. The anthropometric parameters of the subjects who participated in the identification are shown in table 2.

Subject	I ($Kg.m^2$)	m (Kg)	l (cm)
Healthy	0.1682	4.8852	19.46
Paraplegic 1	0.1536	4.5830	19.2
Paraplegic 2	0.2092	5.6162	20.26

Table 2. Estimation of the anthropometric parameters (Inertial moment, mass and length).

The dynamic parameters of the knee joint such as viscosity and stiffness were identified by means of linear least square methods (Gautier & Poignet, 2002). The knee angle position was extracted from the kinematic data, while velocity and acceleration were computed by numeric derivation using a low-pass filter. The identified parameters as well as their standard deviation (sd) are shown in table 3. These results could be compared to some results in literature (Ferrarin et al., 2001), computed in the same context.

Subject	F_v (N.m.s/rad)	sd (%)	K_e (N.m/rad)	sd (%)
Healthy	0.0838	6.4845	0.17	2.266
Paraplegic 1	0.0659	13.3589	0.1095	6.0050
Paraplegic 2	0.0897	10.6973	0.0529	10.1739

Table 3. Dynamic parameter identification.

2.3.2 Muscle parameters identification

The force-length relation (Riener & Fuhr, 1998) expressed by equation (Eq. 12) as well as the maximal isometric force that could be generated by a muscle were identified using a special experimental platform (Fig. 6)(Mohammed 2006). This latter is equipped by a force sensor, position sensor, a mechanical shank and foot blocking system, allowing force and position measurements during isometric stimulation tests.

$$F(L) = \exp\left[-\left(\frac{\overline{l}-1}{b_l}\right)^2\right] \tag{12}$$

Where $\overline{l} = \frac{L}{L_0}$, L is the muscle length and L_0 the muscle length at the rest position . b_l could be easily identified based on equation (Eq. 12).

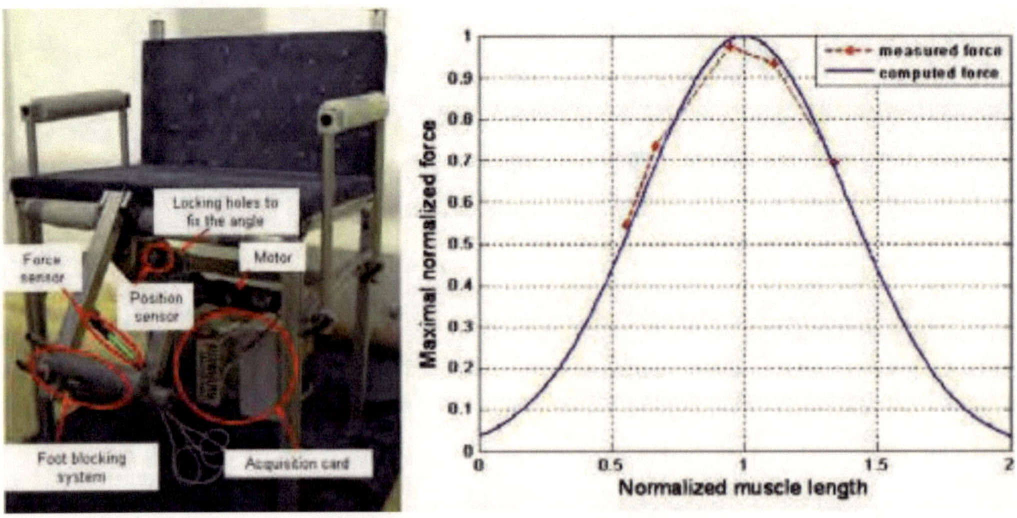

Fig. 6. Experimental platform and muscle parameter identification.

The muscle stiffness and the contractile-elastic muscle length distribution as shown in table (4), were taken from (El-Makssoud et al., 2004-a).

Muscle model parameters	Variable	quadriceps	hamstrings	Unit
Stiffness of the serial element E_s	K_s	1.10^4	1.10^4	N/m
Contractile element length E_c	L_{co}	41.10^{-2}	38.10^{-2}	m
Elastic element length E_s	L_{so}	8.10^{-2}	10.10^{-2}	m

Table 4. Parameters of both muscles: quadriceps and hamstrings

3. Sliding mode control

The nonlinearities of the muscle model and the required robustness regarding parameter variations and external disturbances lead us to adopt a controller relying on the sliding mode theory. This latter became recently widely used due to its high accuracy and robustness with respect to parameters' uncertainty and external disturbances. The control task is to keep a constraint, given by equality of a smooth function called sliding surface, equal to zero. The dynamic smoothness in the vicinity of the sliding surface represents the sliding order of the system. In this study, the goal was to control the muscles-knee biomechanical system under FES by means of high order sliding mode controller (HOSM) (Fridman, & Levant, 2002). The HOSM generalizes the basic sliding mode approach by acting on the higher order time derivatives of the sliding variable instead of influencing the first time derivative as it happens in the standard sliding mode control or first order sliding mode. Consequently, the discontinuity of the control vector does not appear in the first (r-1)th total time derivative (Eq. 13,14). The HOSM has the potential to provide greater accuracy and decrease the chattering phenomenon. A 2-sliding mode control may provide up to second order of sliding precision with respect to measurement interval. In this application, a state model of the knee with two antagonist muscles was derived. Here, the term antagonist will be used for muscles, whose moment in a two-dimensional system about a joint is in the opposite direction as the resulting joint moment. The antagonistic function of a muscle is not necessarily restricted to oppose motion but may give stability and stiffness to a joint. Unknown perturbations were added to the muscle forces generated in order to study the accuracy and robustness of the controller under external disturbances.

$$\frac{\partial s^{(i)}}{\partial \mathbf{u}} = 0, \quad (i = 1, 2, \ldots, r-1), \quad \frac{\partial s^{(r)}}{\partial \mathbf{u}} \neq 0 \tag{13}$$

$$s = \dot{s} = \ddot{s} = \ldots = s^{(r-1)} = 0 \tag{14}$$

Where s, r and **u** represent respectively the sliding surface, the relative degree and the resulting control vector.

3.1 Position control law strategy

The sliding surface used to constraint the dynamic behaviour of the biomechanical model is a first order differential equation chosen as:

$$s = \left(\dot{\theta}_d - \dot{\theta}\right) + \lambda\left(\theta_d - \theta\right) \tag{15}$$

Where $\dot{\theta}_d$ and θ_d are respectively the desired velocity and position, λ is a positive coefficient. Higher values of λ, lead to a faster convergence along the sliding surface to the zero point of the phase-plane. Let us consider the sliding surface (Eq. 15) in order to determine the relative order of the controlled system. We obtain the following result:

$$\frac{\partial \dot{s}}{\partial \mathbf{u}} = 0, \quad \frac{\partial \ddot{s}}{\partial \mathbf{u}} \neq 0 \tag{16}$$

Therefore, the relative degree of the sliding mode control is r = 2. Considering the step response case ($\ddot{\theta}_d$ = $\dot{\theta}_d$ = 0), the second order time derivative of the sliding surface can be written as:

$$\ddot{s} = -\ddot{x}_6 - \lambda \dot{x}_6 \tag{17}$$

The expression of the second order time derivative of the state variable x_6 is given by:

$$\ddot{x}_6 = \frac{1}{J}\left(\begin{array}{l} \frac{rS_{0_1}\alpha_1 F_{01}}{1+p_1x_1-s_{v_1}q_1x_3}u_1 - \frac{rs_{u_1}x_3}{1+p_1x_1-s_{v_1}q_1x_3}u_1 + r\frac{(b_1x_1-s_{v_1}a_1x_3)rx_6}{L_{01}(1+p_1x_1-s_{v_1}q_1x_3)} \\ -\frac{s_{0_2}\alpha_2F_{02}L_0L_{ii}\sin(x_5)}{(1+p_2x_2-s_{v_2}q_2x_4)\sqrt{L_0^2+L_{ii}^2+2L_0L_{ii}\cos(x_5)}}u_2 + \frac{s_{u_2}x_4L_0L_{ii}\sin(x_5)}{(1+p_2x_2-s_{v_2}q_2x_4)\sqrt{L_0^2+L_{ii}^2+2L_0L_{ii}\cos(x_5)}}u_2 \\ -\frac{(b_1x_1-s_{v_1}a_1x_3)rX_6L_0L_{ii}\sin(x_5)}{L_{01}(1+p_1x_1-S_{v_1}q_1x_3)\sqrt{L_0^2+L_{ii}^2+2L_0L_{ii}\cos(x_5)}} - x_4\frac{L_0L_{ii}x_6\cos(x_5)\sqrt{L_0^2+L_{ii}^2+2L_0L_{ii}\cos(x_5)}}{L_0^2+L_{ii}^2+2L_0L_{ii}\cos(x_5)} \\ -X_4\frac{L_0^2L_{ii}^2\sin^2(x_5)}{(L_0^2+L_{ii}^2+2L_0L_{ii}\cos(x_5))\sqrt{L_0^2+L_{ii}^2+2L_0L_{ii}\cos(x_5)}} + mg\beta L_1x_6\sin(x_5) - K_ex_5 - F_vx_6 \end{array}\right) \quad (18)$$

Inserting the expressions of $\dot{x}_6$ and $\ddot{x}_6$ within equation (Eq. 17) allows writing the second order time derivative of the sliding surface as:

$$\ddot{s} = \varphi(\mathbf{x},\mathbf{t}) + \gamma(\mathbf{x},\mathbf{t})\mathbf{u} \quad (19)$$

It is assumed that $|\varphi| \leq \Phi$, $0 < \Gamma_m \leq \gamma \leq \Gamma_M$ (Levant, 1993), where Γ_m, Γ_M and Φ are positive constants. We express the equation (Eq. 19) as:

$$\begin{cases} \dot{y}_1 = y_2 \\ \dot{y}_2 = \varphi(\mathbf{x},\mathbf{t}) + \gamma(\mathbf{x},\mathbf{t})\mathbf{u} \end{cases} \quad (20)$$

Where $y_1 = s$. In that case, the problem is equivalent to the finite time stabilization problem for a second order system.

3.2 Statement of the control algorithm

(Levant, 1993) presented a range of 2-sliding algorithms to stabilise second order uncertain nonlinear systems. In the current study we implemented the algorithm with prescribed law of variation of the sliding surface. This choice has been made based on criteria of relative robustness and finite time convergence (Fridman, & Levant, 2002). The general formulation of such a class of a sliding mode control algorithm is:

$$\dot{u} = \begin{cases} -u & if\ |u| > 1 \\ -V_M\, sign(y_2 - g_c(y_1)) & if\ |u| \leq 1 \end{cases} \quad (21)$$

Where V_M is a positive constant and g_c a continuous function (Fig. 7) as given by Eq. 22. Moreover, this function must verify some specific conditions (Fridman, & Levant, 2002).

$$g_c(y_1) = -\lambda_1 |y_1|^{\rho}\, sign(y_1), \quad \lambda_1 > 0, \quad 0.5 < \rho \leq 1 \quad (22)$$

The sufficient condition for the finite time convergence to the sliding manifold is defined by the following inequality:

$$V_m > \frac{\Phi + \sup[\dot{g}_c(y_1)g_c(y_1)]}{\Gamma_m} \quad (23)$$

Larger values of λ_1 accelerate the convergence to reach the sliding surface and provide better robustness and stability. A substitution of y_2 by Δy_1 is theoretically possible if y_2 is not available.

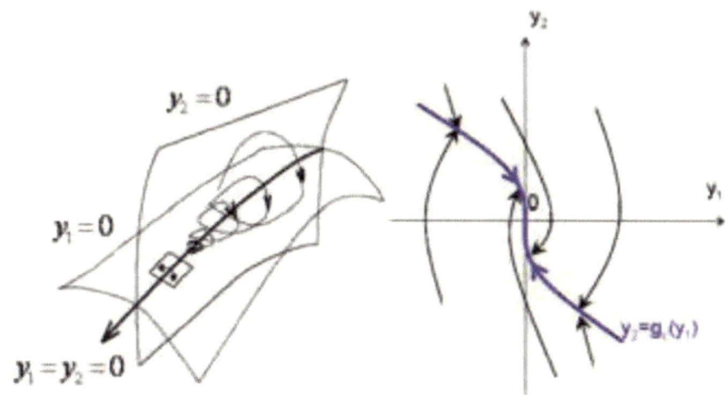

Fig. 7. Phase plot of the prescribed convergence law algorithm (Levant, 1993).

3.3 Simulation results

We have implemented the control algorithm defined by equation (Eq. 21) on the simulator of the knee-muscle biomechanical model (cf. Eq. 10). The components of the control vector **u** are the chemical inputs (u_q, u_h) and the ratio of the recruited fibers (α_q, α_h). These coefficients depend on sliding mode controller output. In our case, the knee joint is controlled by two muscle's groups: quadriceps and hamstrings. Consequently, there are two electrical currents, I_q and I_h as well as two Pulse Width Modulation values, PW_q and PW_h which have to be deduced from the sliding mode control variable u (Mohammed, et al. 2005). According to the sign of the resulting control variable at the output of the HOSM controller, we have chosen to stimulate either the quadriceps or the hamstrings (Eq. 25).

$$u = -\int V_M sign(y_2 - g_c(y_1))\,dt \qquad (\text{if } |u| \le 1) \tag{24}$$

$$\text{If } (u>0) \Rightarrow \begin{cases} I_q = \dfrac{u}{u_{nom}} I_{\max} \\ I_h = 0 \end{cases} \qquad \text{If } (u<0) \Rightarrow \begin{cases} I_q = 0 \\ I_h = \dfrac{u}{u_{nom}} I_{\max} \end{cases} \tag{25}$$

Where, u_{nom} and I_{max} represent respectively the nominal value of the sliding control variable u and the maximal value authorized to stimulate a muscle (around 200 mA). The current values for quadriceps I_q and hamstrings I_h and/or the Pulse Width, respectively PW_q and PW_h enable us to evaluate the required ratios of fibers to be recruited (α_q, α_h). The chemical inputs u_q and u_h are automatically activated when the electrical currents are respectively superior to zero. We have implemented this algorithm on a simulator built with the Matlab-Simulink environment. In the following simulations, we have applied two different knee desired positions, starting from the rest position, $\theta_d = 90°$ as:

$$\begin{cases} 1) \quad 1s < t < 4s : \theta_d = 130^\circ \\ 2) \quad 6s < t < 9s : \theta_d = 50^\circ \\ 3) \quad \text{Otherwise} : \theta_d = 90^\circ \end{cases} \tag{26}$$

The coefficients of the 2-sliding controller were chosen to verify the condition equations (Eq. 23). The following values have been used: $\lambda = 10$, $\lambda_1 = 20$, $\rho = 0.7$, $V_M = 1$. Figure 8-a shows the step response for different desired values. Desired and current angle curves match when sliding surface reaches zero. As we can notice, the dynamic of the system is constrained to the dynamic of the sliding surface. The finite time convergence of the sliding surface is about 1sec in knee flexion and extension (Fig.8-b). In Fig.9-a, we present the resulting stimulation currents for both quadriceps and hamstrings I_q and I_h. The control vector **u** computed by the equation (Eq. 24) is shown in Fig.9-b.

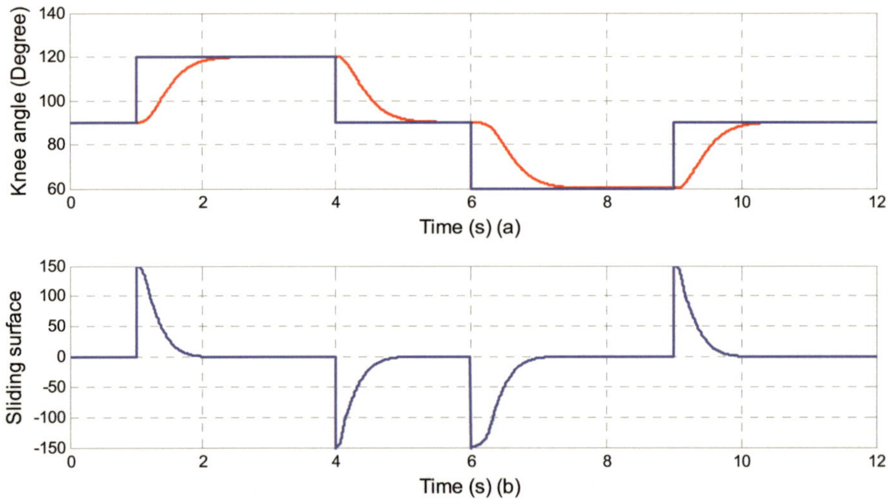

Fig. 8. a) Desired step and actual knee angle variation, b) Stabilization of the sliding surface.

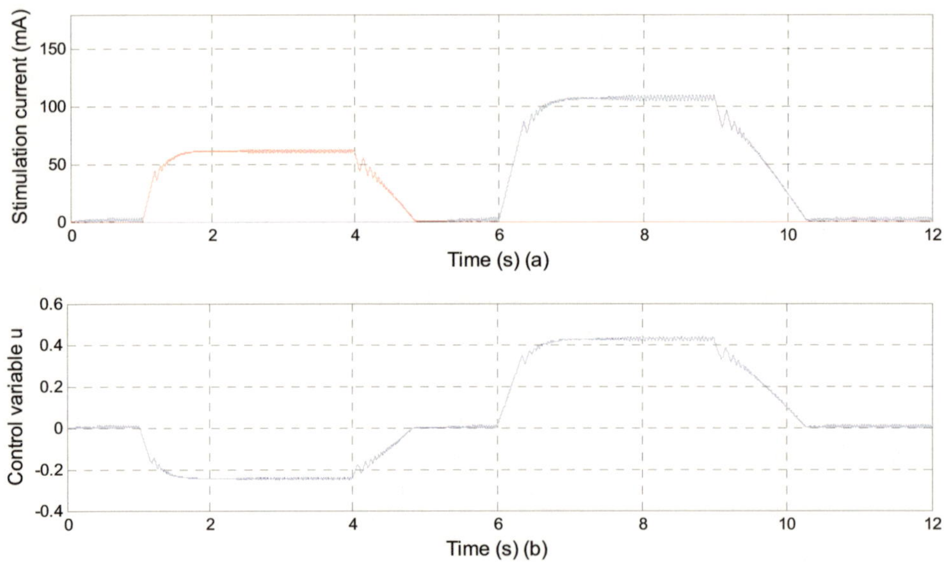

Fig. 9. a) Stimulation currents of both muscles, b) The control vector u.

4. Model predictive control MPC

The ability to handle nonlinear multi-variable systems that are constrained in states and/or control variables motivates the use of Model Predictive Control (MPC), (Allgöwer et al., 1999). This approach proved its efficiency in a large variety of industrial processes, especially in chemical processes. The MPC problem is usually stated as an optimization one subject to physical coherent constraints, and is solved with classical optimization algorithms. The MPC has been widely used in different applications due to their interesting properties (Camacho & Bordons, 1995). In our particular case, the nonlinearities of the muscle model, the constraints on the input stimulation current and on the output knee joint position lead us to adopt a controller relying on MPC. Few studies applied this technique to a musculoskeletal system. Some authors have used MPC with black-box models instead of continuous time physiological models (Schauer & Hunt, 2000).

4.1 Problem formulation

The MPC problem is usually formulated as a constrained optimization problem, (Allgöwer et al., 1999):

$$\min_{u_k^{H_p}} J(x_k, u_k^{H_p})$$

subject to:

$$\begin{aligned} u_{i|k} &\in U, \quad i \in [0, H_u] \\ x_{i|k} &\in X, \quad i \in [0, H_p] \end{aligned} \tag{27}$$

where

$$U := u_k \in \mathrm{R}^m \mid u_{\min} \le u_k \le u_{\max}$$
$$X := x_k \in \mathrm{R}^m \mid x_{\min} \le x_k \le x_{\max}$$

Internal controller variables predicted from time instance k are denoted by a double index separated by a vertical line where the second argument denotes the time instance from which the prediction is computed. $x_k = x_{0|k}$ is the initial state of the system to be controlled at time instance k and: $\hat{u}_k = \left[u_{0|k}, u_{1|k}, \ldots u_{H_u-1}, u_{H_u-1}, \ldots u_{H_u-1}\right]$ an input vector of dimension H_p (prediction horizon). At each sample, a finite optimal control problem is solved over the prediction horizon. We assume that we would like the controlled variables, y_k (Fig.10), to follow some reference trajectory r. Predictive control consists in computing the vector $\hat{u}_k$ of consecutive inputs $u_{i|k}$ over the control horizon H_u by optimizing the objective function J under given constraints (Eq. 27). The control signal is assumed to be constant after H_u samples over a horizon of $(H_p - H_u)$ dimension. When the solution of the optimal control problem has been obtained, the value of the first control variable in the optimal trajectory, $u_{k|k}$, is applied to the process. The rest of the predicted control variable trajectory is discarded, and at the next sampling interval the entire procedure is repeated (Kesson, 2003). These computations are updated at each sampling time.

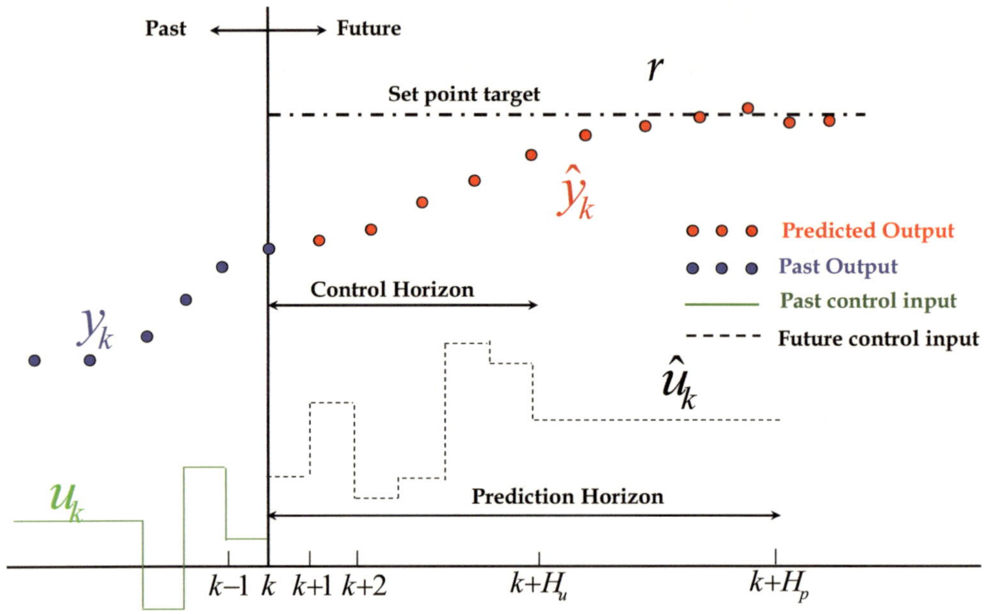

Fig. 10. Principles of the predictive control strategy design (Seborg et al., 2004).

The nonlinear equality constraint on the state represents the dynamic model of the system. Bounding constraints over the inputs $u_{i|k}$ and the state variables $x_{i|k}$ over the prediction horizon H_p are defined through the sets U and X (Eq. 27). The objective function J is usually defined as:

$$J(x_k, u_k^{H_p}) = \phi(x_{H_p|k}) + \sum_{i=0}^{H_u} L(x_{i|k}, u_{i|k}) \tag{28}$$

where Φ is a constraint on the state at the end of the prediction horizon, called state terminal constraint, and L a quadratic function of the state and inputs. The computation of the solution $u_k^{H_p}$ can be divided in two steps: firstly, computation of a solution satisfying the constraints (including the state terminal constraint), and secondly optimization. The first step involves bounding constraints (Eq. 27), and nonlinear constraints expressing the dynamic model of the system (Eq. 9). Simulations were performed in Matlab-Simulink environment using the "ode45" integration algorithm with variable step size. The simulation codes were adapted from MPCtools, (Kesson, 2003).

4.2 Model Linearization

The system (Eq. 9) is a nonlinear multivariable system. In a first step and in order to apply a linear predictive controller, we made some assumptions to the nonlinear system. The goal was to get a feasible solution before applying the controller to the non linear plant. Some hypotheses make this nonlinear system easier:

- We consider that the chemical control u_{ch} is a positive constant indicating a muscular fiber fusion. This hypothesis could be justified in our case by the fact that the stimulation frequency is much greater then the muscular fiber fusion.

Consequently, during stimulation, we have only contractions and no relaxations: $s_u = 1,\quad s_v = -1,\quad |u| = u,\quad |\dot{\varepsilon}_c| = -\dot{\varepsilon}_c$

- Only one muscle, the quadriceps has been taken into account in the following causing knee extension. When no extension, the gravity induces knee flexion to the rest position.
- We suppose that the stiffness of the serial element which represents the tendon is much greater than the stiffness of the contractile element. This hypothesis is true since we are performing only dynamic movements and no isometric stimulations were considered.

$$\dot{\varepsilon}_c = \frac{L_0}{L_{c0}}\dot{\varepsilon} - \frac{1}{L_{c0}K_s}\dot{F}_c$$

In the above conditions, the term $\frac{1}{L_{c0}K_s}\dot{F}$ is less than $10^{-3}\frac{L_0}{L_{c0}}\dot{\varepsilon}$

By taking into account the above assumptions, the plant model will have a reduced nonlinear form where $\mathbf{x} = [x_1\ x_2\ x_3\ x_4]^T = [K\ F\ \theta\ \dot{\theta}]^T$ is the state vector and $\mathbf{u} = \alpha$ is the control input. The plant model could thus be expressed by the following set of differential equations:

$$\begin{aligned}
\dot{x}_1 &= ax_1 + bx_1x_4 + cf_l(x_3)u \\
\dot{x}_2 &= dx_1x_4 + ax_2 + bx_2x_4 + ef_l(x_3)u \\
\dot{x}_3 &= x_4 \\
\dot{x}_4 &= fx_2 + h\cos(x_3) + lx_4
\end{aligned} \tag{29}$$

Where:

$$a = -u_{ch}, b = \frac{r}{L_{c0}}, c = u_{ch}K_0, d = -r, e = u_{ch}F_0$$

$$f = \frac{r}{I}, h = \frac{-mg\beta L_1}{I}, l = \frac{-F_v}{I}, f_l = \exp\left[-\left(\frac{\bar{l}-1}{b_l}\right)^2\right]$$

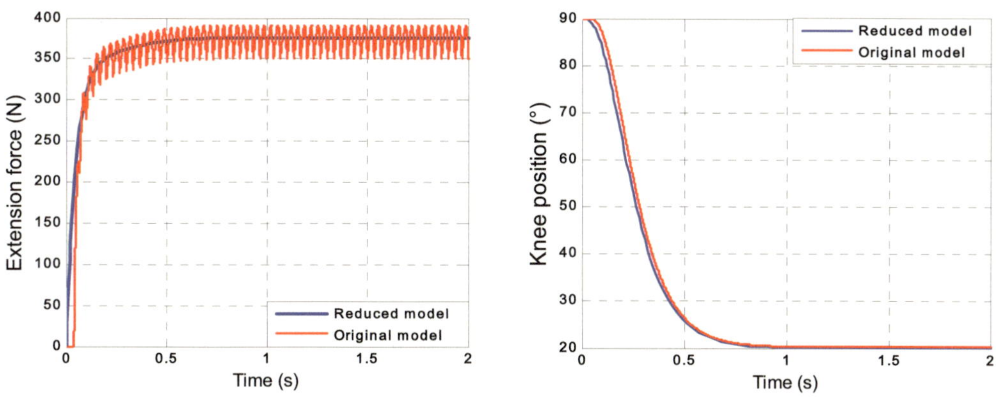

Fig. 11. Non linear models: original and reduced.

The above hypotheses were validated through simulations as shown in figure (11). This latter presents the responses of both, the original non linear model (Eq. 9) and the reduced non linear model (Eq. 29). On the left side, we show the force generated by both models. The original non linear model presents some oscillations reflecting the contraction-relaxation cycle. These oscillations results from the stimulation frequency. On the right side of figure (11), we present the knee position output of both models. We can notice that the linearized model fits well with the original one in terms of force generation as well as knee angular position. A linearization of this system around an arbitrary operating point $(\overline{\mathbf{x}},\overline{\mathbf{u}})$ has been computed using its Jacobian. The linear model could be formulated as follows:

$$\begin{cases} \dot{\mathbf{x}} = \mathrm{A}\,\mathbf{x} + \mathrm{B}\,\mathbf{u} \\ \mathbf{y} = \mathrm{C}\,\mathbf{x} + \mathrm{D}\,\mathbf{u} \end{cases} \tag{30}$$

Where:

$$\mathrm{A}=\begin{bmatrix} a+b\overline{x}_4 & 0 & c\overline{u}\dot{f}_l(\overline{x}_3) & b\overline{x}_1 \\ d\overline{x}_4 & a+b\overline{x}_4 & e\overline{u}\dot{f}_l(\overline{x}_3) & d\overline{x}_1+b\overline{x}_2 \\ 0 & 0 & 0 & 1 \\ 0 & f & -h\sin(\overline{x}_3) & l \end{bmatrix} \quad \mathrm{B}=\begin{bmatrix} c\overline{u}f_l(\overline{x}_3) \\ e\overline{u}f_l(\overline{x}_3) \\ 0 \\ 0 \end{bmatrix} \quad \mathrm{C}=\begin{bmatrix}0 & 0 & 1 & 0\end{bmatrix} \quad \mathrm{D}=0$$

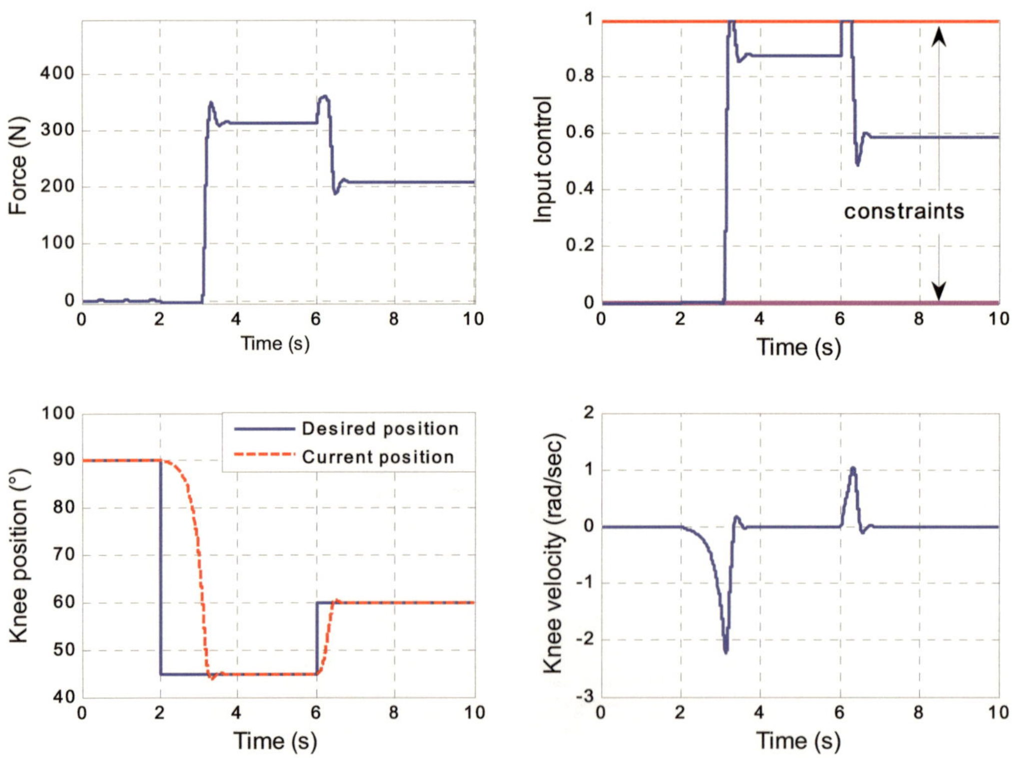

Fig. 12. Tracking knee joint trajectory and controller performance.

4.3 Simulation results (MPC)

Different simulation tests have been carried out. The sample period was set to 0.01 sec, the prediction and control horizon H_p and H_u were computed as a function of the system time constant: H_p =30 and H_u =10. The constrained input u = α was the recruitment variable. Since the recruitment function is static, the optimal pulse width or stimulation amplitude could be easily computed. The recruitment variable has been constrained to be between 0 and 1 representing respectively no fiber recruited and full recruitment. The controlled variable, which is the system output, was constrained to stay between θ = 0° (hyperextension) and θ = 90° (resting position). Only the knee angle was used as feedback to update the control input. Controller parameters were calculated offline. Simulation results are shown in figures 12, 13 and 14.

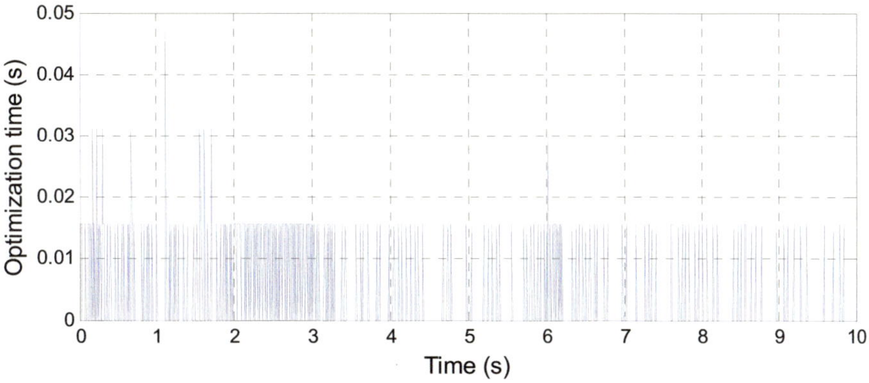

Fig. 13. Predictive control optimization time.

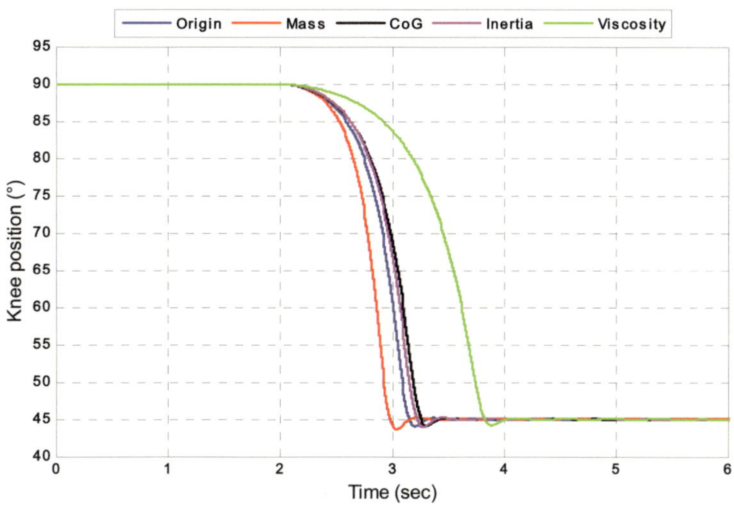

Fig. 14. MPC robustness: uncertainty on mass, position of the centre of gravity, inertia and viscosity.

In figure (12), initial conditions correspond to θ =90°, which means the knee joint is in the rest position. After 2 seconds, the desired trajectory was stepped to θ = 45° which corresponds to medial knee extension. The controller converges to the desired position in a finite time while maintaining the control input between its limits. At time = 6 s, we perform a 15° knee flexion inducing a muscle force and stiffness decrease. The controller managed to converge to the desired position and to fully compensate the position change without need for any feedback observer and respecting at the same time the constraints on input and output. Figure (13) shows the optimization time needed to perform the above simulation. It should be noticed that the muscle parameters used in these simulation relate to a healthy subject (Tables 2 and 3). The inaccuracy that may occur on these parameters when dealing with paraplegic patients could be compensated by the robustness of the (MPC) controller. In figure (14), we studied the controller robustness against parameter variations. In fact, the uncertainty could affect mainly the inertial parameters which have been estimated, based on statistical abacuses and regression equations (De Leva, 1996). Although the parameters uncertainties imposed were relatively important (20% - 25%) from the initial value, the MPC controller showed a satisfactory robustness regardless these uncertainties.

5. Controllers performance – comparative study

In this section, we have drawn a comparison between the controllers' performance (HOSM and MPC) in terms of input control and state regulation. These controllers were simulated under the same conditions. A classical linear controller based on poles placement (PP) serves as a reference controller.

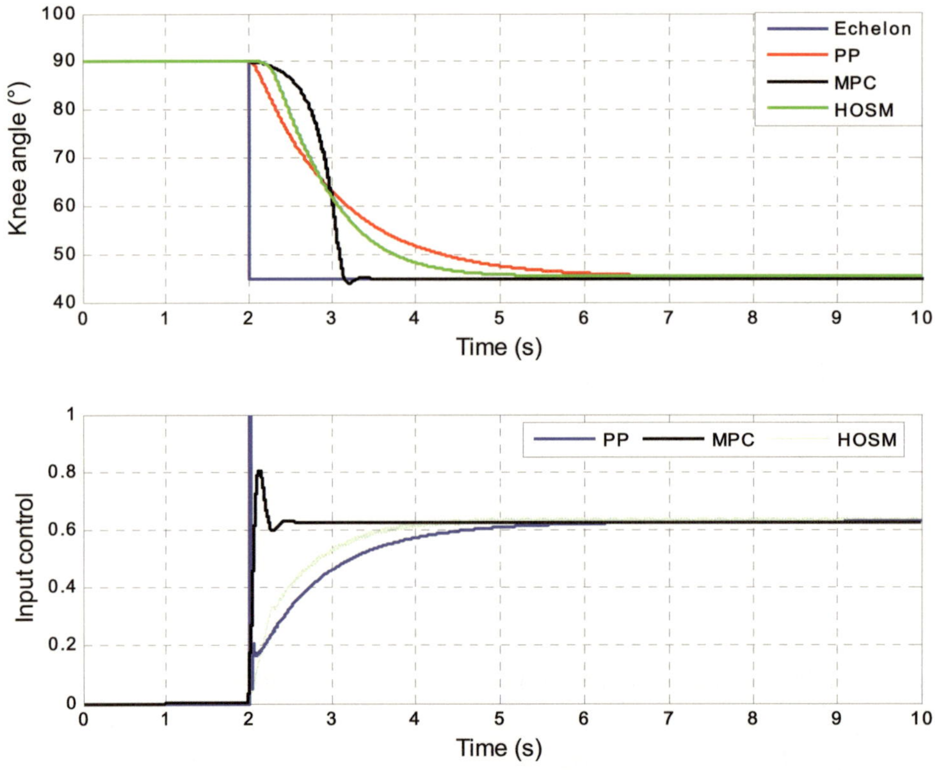

Fig. 15. Comparison of control strategies: desired position corresponds to 45° knee extension. PP for poles placement, MPC for predictive control and HOSM for high order sliding mode.

In figure (15), we have simulated a 45° knee extension by activating the quadriceps muscle. Unlike the PP controller which takes the longest time to converge to the desired position and presents at the same time an input saturation during the transient period, the MPC controller converged to the desired position in a relatively limited time. Saturation of the input control means an important rate of stimulation firing during the transient period. The HOSM controller shows a satisfactory performance in terms of time convergence and position regulation. We can notice that the system dynamics evolution is constrained to the sliding surface dynamic (Eq. 15). Input control does not show also any overshoot, and the chattering effect has been considerably reduced. In order to study the robustness of these controllers, we have induced a position perturbation that corresponds to a quick and limited knee flexion. In terms of position regulation figure (16) shows that the different controllers succeed to converge to the desired position. In terms of input control, the PP controller is very sensitive to this perturbation; the MPC controller is much less sensitive and finally the HOSM controller that showed the best performance against external perturbation.

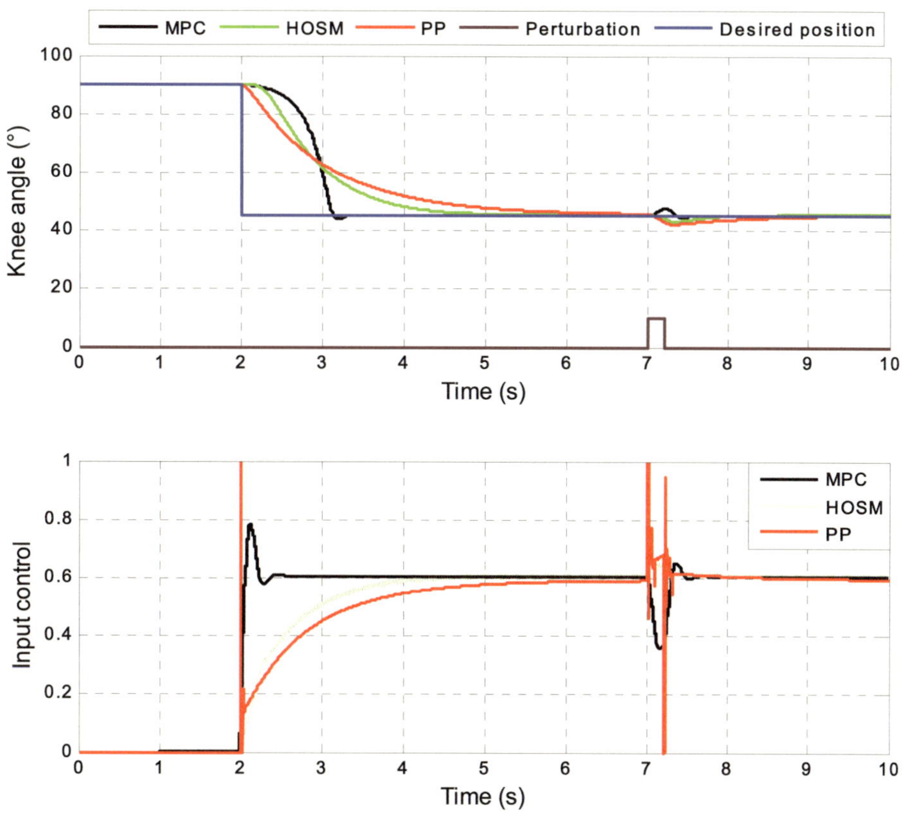

Fig. 16. Controllers behaviors against an external perturbation.

6. Conclusion

The main challenge that we face when applying FES to the paralyzed lower limbs is to avoid hyperstimulation and to defer the muscular fatigue as much as possible. Few studies have treated the human muscle as an entire physiological element in a closed loop system. Known by their robustness against unknown perturbation and their accuracy against model mismatch, we have used robust control techniques such as the High Order Sliding mode (HOSM) and the Model Predictive Control (MPC) in a closed loop control scheme. The MPC offers the possibility to integrate constraints on input, output and measured states explicitly in its formulation. These strategies have ensured, by simulations, a robust control and a safer movement of the paralysed lower extremities. The controllers were applied to a multi-scale muscle model developed within the *DEMAR* project and recently published (El-Makssoud et al., 2004 -a). It is based on internal physiological characteristics assembling two levels: the microscopic one, involving the sliding actin-myosin filaments and the macroscopic part represented by a contractile element and an elastic element. This highly non linear model has been described by a set of differential equations. We have made some realistic assumptions to the biomechanical model of the knee joint actuated by two groups of antagonistic muscles (quadriceps and hamstrings). As a result we obtained a simplified nonlinear version of the knee-muscle formulation. Dynamic and geometric parameters were identified based on experimental kinematics data recorded using a video based motion analysis. Different identification techniques were applied such as the least square, non-linear interpolation, regression equations, etc. We were able to control the quadriceps-hamstrings muscles for the knee flexion-extension in order to track a predefined position trajectory within a large range of movement. Satisfactory stability and tracking error were achieved after a finite time delay. The performance of the closed loop system has been assessed in the presence of external force perturbations. Controller responses to these perturbations vary from the most sensitive (PP) to the MPC controller and finally the HOSM controller which seemed to be the most robust against external perturbations. We should notice that the system dynamic was constrained to follow the sliding surface dynamics. The MPC had shown a better performance in terms of time response than the HOSM. The results show that we respect the constraints on input and output. We are trying to limit the computational effort which is a common deficit of the MPC design. Actually, the optimisation time obtained (Fig.13) is around 20 ms in Matlab environment which is quite encouraging for a real time implementation. Experiments are ongoing to validate the control scheme on paraplegic patients by using the multi-moment platform used during the identification protocol (Fig. 6).

7. References

Allgöwer, F.; Badgwell, T.A.; Qin, S.J.; Rawlings, J.B. & Wright, S.J. (1999). Nonlinear predictive control and moving horizon estimation - an introductory overview, *In: Frank, P.M (edt.), Advances in control: highlights of ECC'99*, Springer, (1999), p. 391-449.

Bajd, T.; Kralj, A.; Sega J.; Turk R.; Benko H. & Strojnik, P. (1981). Use of a two- channel functional electrical stimulator to stand paraplegics, In: *Physical therapy*, 61(4), p.526-7.

Camacho, E. & Bordons, C. (1995). Model Predictive Control in the Process Industry *Springer-Verlag New York, Inc.*

DeLeva, P., (1996) Adjustments to zatsiorsky-seluyanov's segment inertia parameters. *Journal of Biomechanics*, Vol.29, p.1223-1230.

Donaldson, N. & Yu, C. (1996). FES standing control by handle reactions of leg muscle stimulation (CHRELMS), *IEEE Transactions on rehabilitation engineering*, 4(4) p.280-284.

El-Makssoud, H.; Guiraud, D. & Poignet, P. (2004-a). Mathematical muscle model for Electrical Stimulation control strategies, *IEEE International Conference on Robotics and Automation*, p. 1282-1287.

El-Makssoud, H.; Guiraud, D. & Poignet, P. (2004-b). Enhancement of physiological and mechanical modelling of the skeletal muscle controlled by Functional Electrical Stimulation. *International Functional Electrical Stimulation Society (IFESS)*, Bournemouth, UK 6-9 September 2004.

Ferrarin, M.; Palazzo. F & Riener R. (2001). Model-Based Control of FES Induced Single Joint Movements, *IEEE Transactions on Neural systems and rehabilitation engineering*, 9(3), p.245-257.

Fridman, L. & Levant, A. (2002). High-Order Sliding Modes, *in: Sliding Modes Control in Engineering*, Ed. W. Perruquetti, J.P. Barbot, Marcel Dekker, Inc. New-York, p. 53-101.

Gautier, M. & Poignet P., (2002). Closed loop identification by inverse model of physical parameters of mechatronic systems. *Journal européen des systèmes automatisés*, Vol.36, No.3, p.465-480.

Hawkins, D. & Hull, M. (1990). A method for determining lower extremity muscle- tendon lengths during flexion/extension movements. *Journal of Biomechanics*, Vol. 23, p.487-494.

Kesson, J. (2003), Operator Interaction and Optimization in Control Systems, *P.hd thesis*, Department of Automatic Control Lund Institute of Technology.

Kromer, V. (1994). Analyse des forces musculaires au cours de la marche - Approche en corps rigide et simulation en mécanismes plans flexibles par éléments finis, *P.h.d. Thesis*, Institut national polytechnique de Lorraine (INPL).

Levant, A. (1993). Sliding order and sliding accuracy in sliding model control, *International Journal of Control*, Vol.58 No.6, p.1247-1263.

Levenberg, K. (1944). A method for the solution of certain problems in least square. *Quarterly applied Mathematics*, Vol. 2, p.164-168.

Mohammed, S.; Fraisse, P.; Guiraud, D.; Poignet, P. & H. El Makssoud, (2005-a). Robust Control Law Strategy Based on High Order Sliding Mode : Towards a Muscle Control, in: *IROS'05: International Conference on Intelligent Robots & Systems*, p. 2882-2887.

Mohammed, S. (2006), Contribution à la synthèse de movement et à la commande des muscles squelettiques sous Stimulation Electrique Fonctionnelle, *P.h.d. Thesis*, LIRMM-Université de Montpellier II.

Mulder, AJ.; Veltink, PH. & Boom, HB. (1992). On/off control in FES-induced standing up: a model study and experiments. *Medical and Biological Engineering and Computing*, 30(2), p. 205-212.

Poboroniuc, M.; Wood, D.; Donaldson, N.; Fuhr, T. & Riener R. (2003). Closed-loop control for FES-based restoration of standing in paraplegia, *2nd World Congress of the International Society of Physical and Rehabilitation Medicine-ISPRM*, Prague, Czech Republic, May 18-22, p.201-204.

Poboroniuc, M.; Fuhr, T.; Wood, D.; Riener, R. & Donaldson, N. (2002). FES-Induced Standing-Up and sitting down control strategies in Paraplegia", *FESnet Conference*. September 2nd-3rd, Glasgow, UK, p.1-3.

Riener, R. & Fuhr, T. (1998). Patient-Driven Control of FES-Supported standing Up: A simulation study, *IEEE Transactions on rehabilitation engineering*, 6(2), p.113-123.

Schauer, T. & Hunt, K.J., (2000). Nonlinear predictive control of knee-joint angle using FES, *International Functional Electrical Stimulation Society (IFESS)*, Aalborg, Denmark, p. 425-428.

Seborg, D.E.; Edgar, T. F. & Mellichamp, D. A., (2004) Process Dynamics and Control, 2nd edition, John Wiley and Sons, New York.

Veltink, P.H.; Chizeck, H.J.; Crago, P.E. & El-Bialy, A. (1992). Nonlinear joint angle control for artificially stimulated muscle. *IEEE Transactions on biomedical engineering*, Vol. 39 N.4, p. 368-380.

Wood, DE.; Harper, VJ.; Barr, FMD.; Taylor, PN., Phillips, GF. & Ewins, DJ. (1998). Experience in Using Knee angles as part of a closed-Loop Algorithm to control FES-Assisted Paraplegic Standing, *6th Vienna International Workshop on Functional Electrostimulation,* (Vienna, Austria), p.137-140.

20

Risk Evaluation of Human-Care Robots

Makoto Nokata[1] & Koji Ikuta[2]
[1]*Dept. of Robotics, Ritsumeikan University, Japan*
[2]*Dept. of Micro and Nano Systems Eng., Nagoya University, Japan*

1. Introduction

Human-care robots must be realized to nurse aged and disabled persons. These robots will need to work around elderly people and give them touches; therefore conventional safety strategies for industrial robots can not be applied to human-care robots. It is now necessary to make a new study of safety in the space where a human and a machine will exist together.

In this chapter, I carry out a Case Study of assessing several human-care robots according to ISO/TR 12100-1:1992 and ISO 14121:1999. Next, I propose a risk evaluation method of human-care robots and define evaluation measures which describe the degree of safety. Next, I apply my method to evaluate several safety design and control strategies, and then I prove the viability of my risk evaluation method. These proposed methods enable us to optimally distribute cost among several safety strategies, and to derive suitable approaching motion of a multi-link manipulator to a human. The validity and effectiveness of these methods are demonstrated by numerical analysis. As a result, the design and control to increase safety are successfully obtained.

2. Case Study on Safety of Human-care Robots

In general, the risk assessment and the risk reduction of machinery are carried out according to ISO/TR 12100-1 "Safety of machinery-Basic concepts, general principle for design" and ISO 14121:1999 "Safety of machinery-principles of risk assessment". I have carried out Case Study of assessing several human-care robots according to ISO/TR 12100-1:1992 and ISO 14121:1999. The aim of this case study is to clarify the key points of risk assessment and risk reduction for these robots. The following human-care robots are carried out case study of the risk assessment by use of block chart shown in Fig. 1 which is modified by ISO14971, that is "Medical devices: Application of risk management to medical devices".

Human-care robots

- ☐ Continuous passive motion device (CMP)
- ☐ Meal assistance robot
- ☐ Mobile ceiling lift
- ☐ Bed transfer
- ☐ Pet robot / Mental care robot.

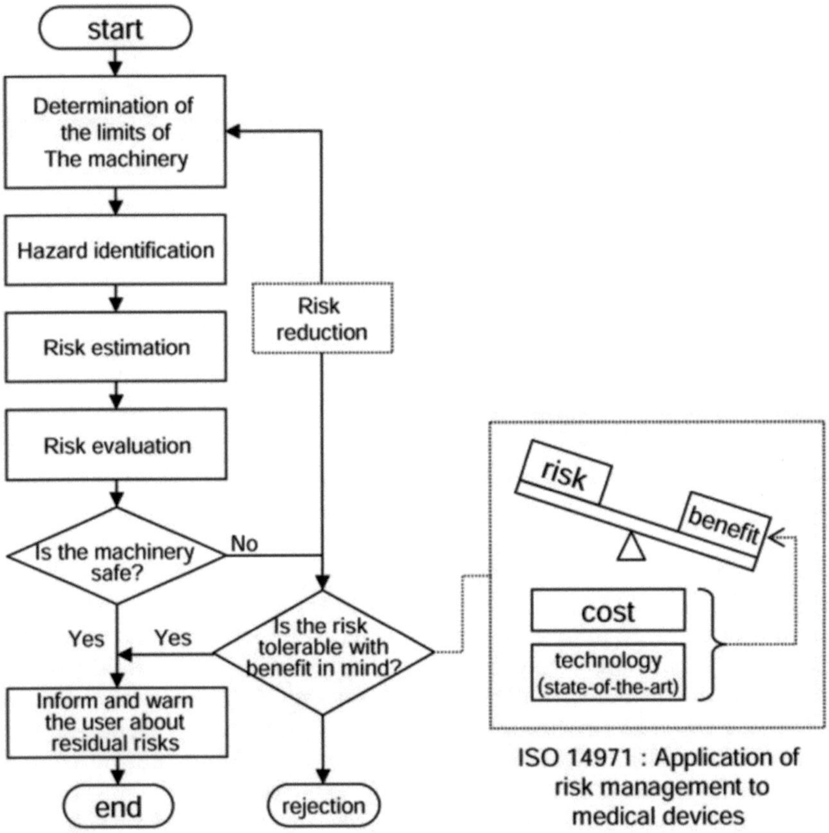

Fig. 1. The iterative process to achieve safety modified by ISO 14971.

Risk related to the considered hazard can be calculated by the following equation:

$$R = Q * F * C * N \tag{1}$$

R	:	risk related to the considered hazard
Q	:	probability of occurrence of harm
F	:	frequency and duration of exposure
C	:	severity of possible harm that can result from considered hazard
N	:	number of exposed people

Equation 1 has been used for estimating the risk of marketed human-care robots. However, this approach showed a lot of significant disadvantages. Some of them are briefly commented below:

(a) "R: risk related to the considered hazard " is influenced by the difference in a user and the body situation of cased person.

In case of in-home care, a caretaker or a cared person has to operate a human-care robot by himself / herself. Most of caretakers or cared persons are not familiar with their operation, the number of "Q: probability of occurrence of harm" becomes large caused by their

incorrect operation or misuse. Even though correct operation and movement, robots can injure the patient whose joint is stiff or whose bone is breakable such as osteoporosis, the Q number is so high.
As a result, risk of human-care robots is influenced by the difference in a user and the body situation of cased person. This is far different from a risk of machinery which can be estimated on the assumption that user is a specialist of operation and a person with a normal healthy body.

(b) The difference in the state of robot's work space greatly influences "R: risk related to the considered hazard ".
Stretcher and lifter have residual risk of the user's fall. The damage is dependent on a fall place. For example, the damage of falling to bed is low, but to rigid floor is high. Manipulator also gives user a risk of collision accident, the probability of accident is dependent on room space or user's position. As mentioned above, the difference in the state of robot's work space must be considered in estimating a risk of human-care robots.

(c) There is little judgment material for determining "Q: probability of occurrence of harm" and "C: severity of possible harm".
Compared with machinery, there are few statistics data about the accident report of human-care apparatus. The accident occurrence number of cases including a slight injury is unknown, so it is extremely difficult to determine "Q: probability of occurrence of harm". In addition, there is no method to calculate "C: severity of possible harm". In the present circumstances, these values are estimated experimentally or subjectively by the risk assessor.

(d) The risk cannot be expressed correctly by the multiplication of a risk element like Eq.1.
On the assumption that risk factors in Eq.1 have been independent mutually, risk level is calculated by multiplied each of them. However, there is a certain correlation between "F: frequency and duration of exposure" and "Q: probability of occurrence of harm" of human-care robots. No harm will come from only using Eq.1.

3. Proposal of Risk Assessment Guideline for Human-care Robots

This section proposes safety strategy for human-care robots according to results of case study mentioned above. Proposed guideline of risk assessment and risk reduction is shown in Fig. 2.
Fig.2 has similar structure to those, shown in Fig. 1. As a difference, the new structure is additionally improved:

- ☐ Determine limits: user, the extent of handicap, the condition of health, the ability of operation and so on
- ☐ The 3rd person who can do objective judgment with technical knowledge evaluates the contents of the carried-out risk assessment.

Judgments whether apparatus is introduced or not by carer, cared person and manager in consideration of benefit.

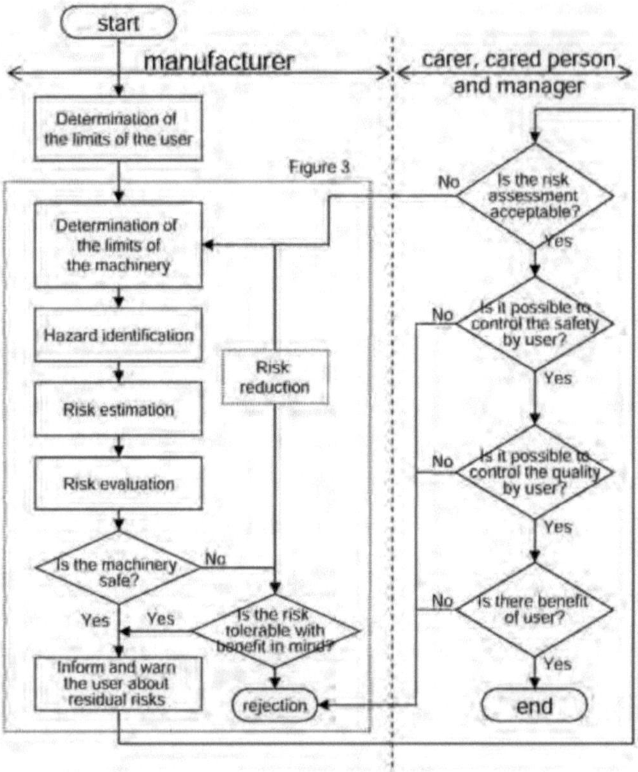

Fig. 2. Proposed guideline of safety strategy for human-care robots

4. Proposing Evaluation Measures of Risk

It is necessary to define "evaluation measures" for devising the general safety strategies of human-care robots. Evaluation measures enable us to compare the effect of each safety strategy on the same scale and to optimize the design and control of human-care robots.

In the field of information science, Dr. Shannon has defined information as the degree of entropy, he has there by advanced information theory remarkably. In the robotics field, Dr. Uchiyama and Dr. Yoshikawa defined the measure of manipulability, which has enabled us to compare the manipulation performance of various kinds of robot uniformly.

The former definition doesn't express enough about the quality of the information; the latter doesn't express various kinds of control performance completely. But I cannot deny their contribution to science and engineering. If I overcome some different opinions and define the risk evaluation measures of human-care robots, I will able to achieve similar effects.

First, I examined in detail the occurrence process of collision accidents. According to ISO 12100, some formulas for estimating the risk of machinery are proposed. A typical equation for risk related to the considered hazard is shown as Eq.1.

Many researchers have analyzed the "Q: probability of occurrence of harm" caused by human error, manipulation and so on. Their main topic is how to reduce the probability of accident and how to estimate it. The relation between the design and control of human-care robots and the dangerousness of injury has been paid little attention.

In the event of careless collision between robots and humans, the degree of "C: severity of possible harm that can result from considered hazard" can be expressed as Eq.2 by using only main factors such as design and control.

$$C = f\,(design) \cdot g\,(control) \tag{2}$$

In this research, I have been taking a stand on studying "what design or control can minimize human injury" at the occurrence of an accident. Put another way, the aim is to make quantitative evaluation of the effectiveness of safety design or control measures, and to minimize its dangerousness on condition that the Q: probability of occurrence is 1.
What should the evaluation measures be?
A human-care robot works around humans who move irregularly. I consider an appropriate safety strategy while adapting the classified design/control safety strategy mentioned previously. A safety design strategy is a means for reducing the injury to a human after an irregular collision. A safety control strategy is a means for minimizing the injury before a human-robot collision. It is important to estimate not the occurrence rate but the injury due to collision.
No matter what the cause of collision accident may be, the shock of mechanical injury depends on impact force, and the scar depends on impact stress. Namely I consider impact force and stress as evaluation measures.

5. Risk Evaluation Method Using Evaluation Measures

In this section, I propose a general quantitative method of evaluation using evaluation measures.
First, I define critical impact force F_c as minimal impact force that causes injury to human. Next, I define the danger-index α as the producible impact force F of robot against F_c in Eq.3.

$$\alpha = \frac{F}{F_c} \qquad (\alpha \geq 0) \tag{3}$$

Strictly speaking, the value of force F_c varies according to age, sex and body part. But I use one representative value for realizing the generality of risk evaluation. In exceptional cases such as eyes, where F_c is very low, these body parts are treated as a singular point. Another evaluation is needed for such points.
Next, I consider the overall danger-index provided by some safety strategies. I express the characteristic of safety strategies for minimizing the impact force by using a block chart, which is popular in the control field. For example, producible impact force is input, a safety strategy is a factor, its danger-index is transfer function, and injury to a human is output. The index is dependent on the transfer function. In this system, several factors are connected with each other in series. The characteristic of whole system can be expressed as the multiplication of each transfer function.
The total danger-index of whole robot α_{all} is expressed by the multiplication shown in Eq.4. This equation enables us to quantify the effect of safety strategies on the same scale:

$$\alpha_{all} = \prod_{i=1}^{n} \alpha_i \tag{4}$$

where "n" is the total number of safety strategies and "i" is the number of safe strategies.
As an example, I consider the case of reducing impact force by a perfect shock absorption material. Even if a robot collides with a human, the impact force to the human is qualitatively 0 because it is isolated by the material. The danger-index α_i about the shock absorption material is expressed as 0 by using the proposed risk evaluation method. The total danger-index multiplied by each index results in 0, so it is obvious to agree the usual.
Too many safety strategies reduce the ability of robot work or operation. This problem can be solved by devising a safety strategy on condition that required working ability is satisfied, or calculating the optimum solution between Eq.4 and efficiency of robot working. This is an advantage produced by a quantitative evaluation of dangerousness.
Defining impact force and the danger-index before improvement as F_0 and α_0 respectively, the improvement rate η can be calculated by Eq.5.

$$\eta = \frac{\alpha_0}{\alpha} = \frac{F_0}{F_c}\frac{F_c}{F} = \frac{F_0}{F} \tag{5}$$

F_c is cancelled in Eq.5, I can simply compare before and after safety strategies.
The algorithms of my risk evaluation method are the following:

1. Investigating the factor of damage to a human as evaluation measures.
2. Calculating the impact force F of each safety strategy.
3. Calculating the danger-index α from Eq.3.
4. Executing the risk evaluation by using the total danger-index.
5. Discussing the safety strategy from the result.

This method enables to evaluate the effect of each or all safety strategies.

6. Deriving Danger-Indexes of Safety Strategy

In this section, examples of safety design and control strategies will be given to show the practical derivation of a danger-index.

6.1 Safety design strategy

At first, I propose a linear approximate model of each safety strategy and solve it individually. The aim of approximation is in order to extract only the effect of a safety factor and remove the effects of other factor, as much as possible.
Usually, I make models and equations which satisfy all effects of boundary conditions at the same time. This method requires the reconsideration of them when the conditions are changed. If more phenomena are considered, it makes the equation complicated and increases unknown variables.
For evaluating and comparing safety strategies, it is necessary not only to consider all phenomena strictly but also to quantify the safety with the aim of wide use. As a result, I work out the danger-index of the safety strategy by using a linear approximate model individually.
This research supposes a collision accident between human and robot, and each safety strategy for reducing the damage from the collision is discussed. For example of a safety design measure, the reducing a robot weight in order to minimize the impact force is shown as follows. Impact force F is derived as Eq. 6 by Newton's equation of motion. This impact force *F* of robot against the critical one yields the danger-index α, Eq. 7.

$$F = ma \tag{6}$$

$$\alpha = \frac{ma}{F_c} \tag{7}$$

As an example, a danger-index is shown when robot material is changed from steel (density: 7.86 x 10^3[kg/m^3]) to aluminium (density: 2.69 x 10^3[kg/m^3]). When the robot moves at 1[m/s^2], the danger-index α is 0.34. Or if replaced with a plastic (density: 1.40 x 10^3[kg/m^3]), the index α is 0.18. In short, if the weight is reduced by half, α is half, too.
Similarly, it is possible to derive danger-indexes of several design strategies, such as absorbing impact force by soft cover, safety joint compliance, minimizing impact stress caused by shape, reducing surface friction and so on. The equations of these danger-indexes have been shown in References.

6.2 Safety Control Strategy

Danger-index equations of safety control strategy are derived in this research. If dynamical analysis or consideration of extra parameters is needed, the safety is evaluated by using some assumptions. For example of safety control strategy, "Effect of keeping distance" is shown as follows.
Sufficient distance between a human and a robot produces enough time to reduce impact force by braking, actions to avert collision, and so on. When the approaching speed of a robot (mass: m) is reduced at acceleration a from distance l. Time until collision Δt is obtained by Eq. 8, when v>0 and a>0.

$$l = v\Delta t - \frac{a\Delta t^2}{2} \quad \Delta t = \frac{v}{a} - \sqrt{\left(\frac{v}{a}\right)^2 - \frac{2l}{a}} \tag{8}$$

The collision speed becomes $v - a\Delta t$, and impact force F and danger-index α are expressed as in Eqs. 9 and 10. I assume that the impact force does not become a negative value.

$$F = m\frac{(v - a\Delta t) - v'}{dt} \tag{9}$$

$$\alpha = \frac{F}{F_c} = m\frac{(v - a\Delta t) - v'}{dt} \tag{10}$$

Here, I examine nursing motion by a multi-joint manipulator. First, "normalization technique of impact force" is introduced in order to pick up the effect of distance. In Eqs. 8 - 10, acceleration a has no influence on the effect of distance and differs between every robot. Velocity after collision v' cannot be specifically determined before the collision. These parameters are determined by the assumption that impact force is 1 [N] (normalized impact force). Therefore, unknown parameters in these equations, obtained from this technique, should be a=1[m/s^2], v'=0 [m/s], Δt =1.0 [s]. That is a normalization technique
I consider a concrete example of a robot with mass 10 [kg] approaching a human from a distance of 0.5 [m] at a velocity of 2[m/s]. The time until collision Δt, calculated from Eq. 8, is 0.27 [s]. Impact force F_0, obtained from Eq. 9, is 64.65 [N]. The critical impact force F_c is 490 [N] that is 10[%] of the force which the human head can withstand without injury. A safety factor of 10 on F_c is introduced on my own terms. Strictly speaking, F_c changes according to age, sex and body part. But I use 490 [N] as one representative value for

realizing the generality of risk evaluation. If another value of F_c is needed, the safety is evaluated by replacing just the equation of impact force F in Eq.3. Of course, exceptional cases exist, such as eye, where F_c is very low, these are treated as a singular point, and therefore another evaluation is needed for such points. The danger-index α_0 calculated from Eq. 10 is 0.13. When the robot is set up at 1.0 [m] apart from human, *dt*, *F* and α are 0.59[s], 24.15[N] and 0.049, respectively. The improvement rate η is 3.01. The result revealed quantitatively that the danger was decreased almost to 30[%].
Similarly, it is possible to derive danger-indexes of several control strategies, such as approaching safety velocity and safety posture so on. The equations of these danger-indexes have been shown in references.

7. Proposal of Design Optimization and Practical Examples

This section proposes a design and control optimization using my risk evaluation method.

7.1 Formulating the Design Optimization Method

First, I calculate the cost performance of safety methods. When the cost of safety method i (1,2,---,n) is Δy_i and the increased improvement rate is $\Delta \eta_i$, then the improvement rate for cost $\Delta \phi_i$ is expressed as Eq. 11.

$$\phi = \frac{\Delta \eta_i}{\Delta y_i} \tag{11}$$

Improvement rate η_i of safety method i is expressed as Eq. 12, which is increased improvement rate (invested cost $y_i \times \phi_i$) plus 1 (initial). 1 (initial) means an improvement rate before improving.

$$\eta_i = 1 + y_i \phi_i \tag{12}$$

Practical examples of optimizing the cost distribution are maximizing safety under fixed cost and minimizing total cost under fixed safety. These examples use three safety methods: decreasing weight, modifying shape and protective surfacing. The improvement rate per unit cost of each method is derived by my risk evaluation method.
The safety method, which is decreasing weight by replacing the stainless steel of a robot arm (100 x 80 x 300 [mm], $\rho_{sus} = 7.87$ [g/cm^3]) by duralumin ($\rho_{dur} = 2.80$ [g/cm^3]) is as follows. Danger-index can be expressed as Eq. 7, and improvement rate is derived by Eq. 13,

$$\eta = \frac{\alpha}{\alpha_0} = \frac{\rho_{sus} Va}{F_c} \frac{F_c}{\rho_{dur} Va} = \frac{7.87}{2.80} = 2.81 \tag{13}$$

where V is volume of material, a is acceleration at a collision.
The costs will come to $364, which consists of material expense of $64 plus wages of $300. The increase in the improvement rate is the value derived by Eq. 13 minus 1 (1 is value of the improvement rate before the improvement). As a result, the improvement rate per cost is expressed as Eq.14.

$$\phi_{weight} = \frac{2.81 - 1}{364} = 0.005 \tag{14}$$

By modifying the shape by planning off the four corners (*R5*), I obtain $\phi_{shape} = 0.0034$ ($\Delta\eta_{shape} = 0.67$, $\Delta y_{shape} = \$200$). A protective surfacing of soft material (thickness: 10[mm], E = 5.0[Mpa], 4 sides) gives $\phi_{shrface} = 0.0154$ ($\Delta\eta_{surface} = 2.16$, $\Delta y_{surface} = \$140$).

7.2 Maximizing Safety Under Fixed Cost

This section solves maximizing safety under fixed cost. The optimized cost distribution is obtained by satisfying total improvement rate $T_\eta \Rightarrow \max$ (Eq.15) and total cost Y=const (Eq. 16).

$$T_\eta = \left(1 + y_1^* \phi_1^*\right) \cdot \left(1 + y_2^* \phi_2^*\right) \cdots \left(1 + y_n^* \phi_n^*\right) : \max \tag{15}$$

$$y_1^* + y_2^* + \cdots + y_n^* = Y : const \tag{16}$$

If the total cost of improving one robot arm is \$500, each cost can be obtained by substituting the improvement rate per unit cost shown in above section for Eq.5 and Y=\$500 for Eq.16. The safety can be improved 9.76 times by distributing \$500 among decreasing weight \$227.05, modifying shape \$132.95 and protective surfacing \$140.00, specifically, replacing 62% iron with duralumin, chamfering 66% of corners and covering 100% of surface with rubber. As a result, it is possible to quantitatively determine the enforcement percentages of the safety method.

Another combination, such as decreasing weight \$360.00 (98%) and protective surfacing \$140.00 (100%) can increase safety 8.85 times, or decreasing weight \$300.00 (83%) and modifying shape \$140.00 (100%) can increase safety 3.91 times. These results clarify that the above combination is the best-optimized cost distribution.

As a result, this method enables us to quantitatively optimize safety design methods while considering cost and makes it easy to execute them efficiently.

7.3 A New Method of Calculate a Safe Approach Motion

This section proposes a new method for calculating a safe approach motion. The new method minimizes the total amount of danger index (Eq.17) considering the tolerant danger index.

$$\int \alpha(t)dt \to \min \quad 0 < t < T \tag{17}$$

This method chooses a safe path for which all danger indexes are below the tolerant danger index. The aim is to avoid the rise of the danger index.

I optimize the whole motion of a multi-link manipulator by using the new method, which is to minimize the total amount of danger index considering the tolerant danger index.

Fig. 3 shows the calculation result of safe motion when a human is stationed at 60[cm]. First, the tip joint moves, and then the whole part approach the human by stooping. The graph in Fig. 4 shows the danger index and the velocity of the optimized motion (Fig. 3). The maximum danger index is 0.251, and the tolerant danger index is 0.26. I can obtain a safe approaching motion in which the relative velocity is small and the posture is kept away from the human.

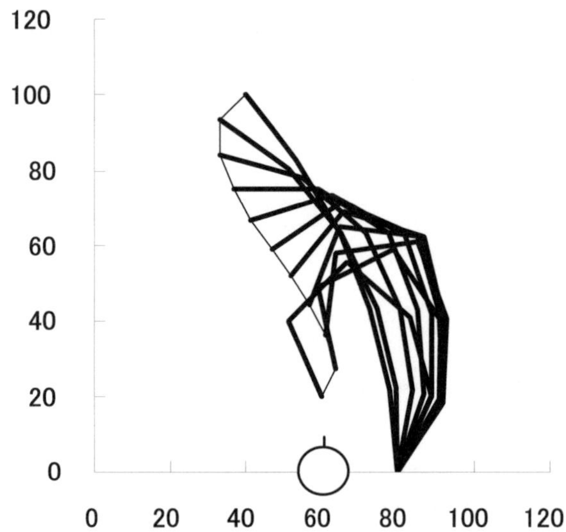

Fig. 3. Optimized approaching motion of multi-links manipulator; a human stays at 60[cm]. First, the tip joint moves, and then the whole part approach the human by stooping.

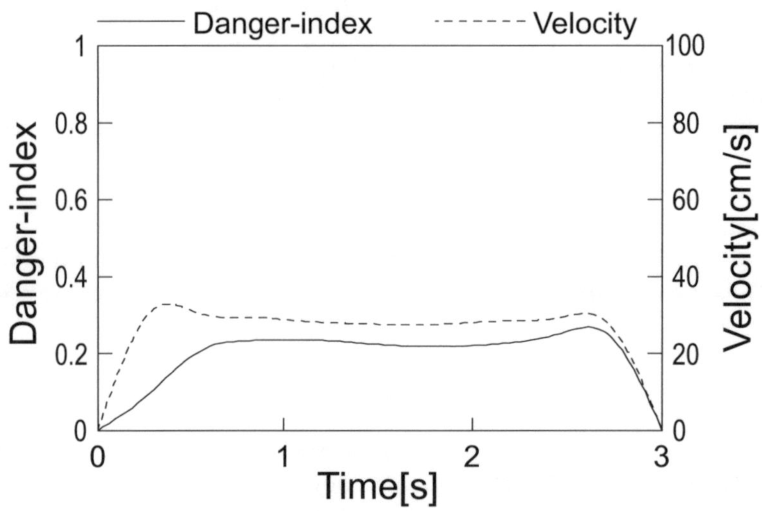

Fig. 4. Danger index and the velocity of the optimized motion shown in Figure 11.1. The maximum danger index is 0.251, the relative velocity is small.

Therefore, safety-optimized motion for any relationship between a human and a robot is achieved. To make good use of the safety-optimizing method, I ame now integrating the method into my special robot simulator for risk evaluation (Fig. 5). The robot simulator evaluates the designs and controls of various robots three-dimensionally, so this installation enables us not only to optimize practical robots but also to obtain various safety-optimized human-care motion.

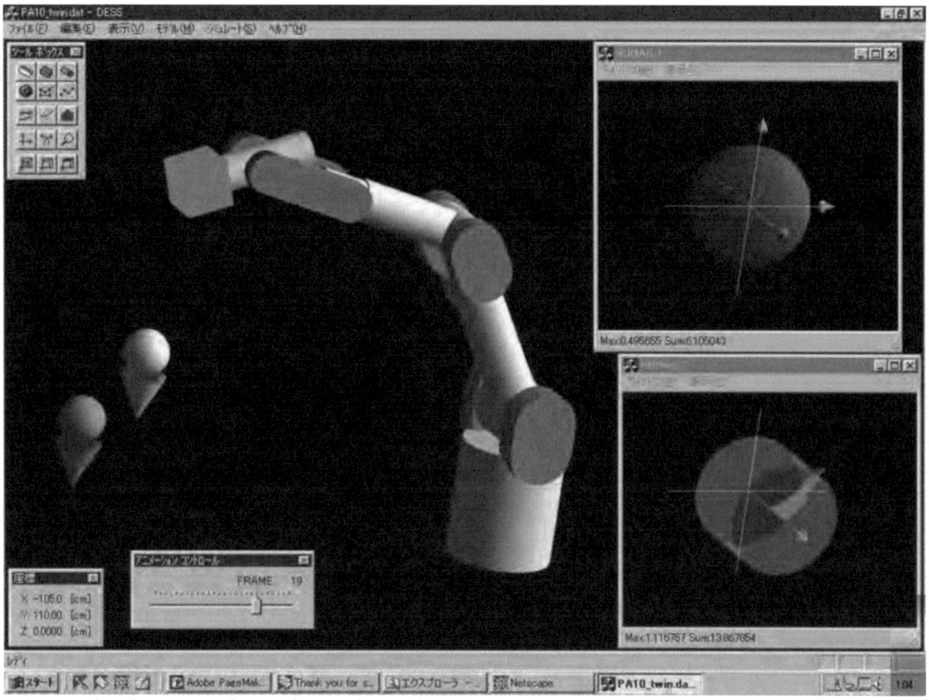

Fig. 5. Special robot simulator for risk evaluation.

8. Conclusion

This chapter presented the study of a safety strategy for human-care robots. Case study of assessing several human-care robots was carried out according to ISO/TR 12100-1:1992 and ISO 14121:1999. The problems of assessing these robots were discussed, a safety strategy for human-care robots has been proposed. Determine limits of special factors, judgments by certification system, benefit of robots for user have been added to the strategy.

I undertook a new study of safety in the coexistent space of human and machine in order to realize a human-care robot for the nursing of the aged or disabled. First, the human injury from robot and machine was investigated thoroughly, and I found that it was important to treat safety strategies in the light of mechanical injury. I grouped them as safety design and control strategy according to the difference in their contents. In order to take every safety strategy into consideration, impact force and stress were chosen as evaluation measures for quantifying risk. I proposed risk evaluation method and defined danger-index, improvement rate, and total evaluation index. Discussions of some general safety strategies proved the viability of my risk evaluation method.

Safety-optimizing method for human-care robot design and control was studied theoretically. A method of optimizing the safety design was proposed, and practical examples of optimizing the cost distribution were solved. I proposed a method of optimizing robot control and optimized the whole motion of a multi-link manipulator by minimizing the total amount of danger index while considering the tolerant danger index.

I will contribute my risk evaluation method to the overall safety performance of human-care robots.

9. References

Ikuta K, Kawahara A, Yamazumi S (1991). Miniature cybernetic actuators using piezoelectric device. Proc. of International Workshop on Micro Electromechanical Systems (MEMS'91), pp 131-135

Ikuta K, Makita S, Arimoto S (1991). Non-contact magnetic gear for micro transmission mechanism. Proc. of International Workshop on Micro Electromechanical Systems (MEMS'91), pp 125-130

Saito T, Sugimoto N (1997). A study on electro-rheological motion control using an antagonistic rotary actuator. Proc. the 6th Int. Conf. on ER-Fluids: ERMR '97

Suita K, et al. (1995). A failure-to-safety "Kyozon " system with simple contact detection and stop capabilities for safe human-robot coexistence. Proc. of IEEE Int. Conf. on Robotics and Automation, vol.3, pp 3089-3096

Dohi Takeyoshi (1996). Classification and safety of medical and human care robots. Proc. of JSME Annual Conference on Robotics and Mechatronics, pp 1181-1182 (in Japanese)

Saito Yukio et al. (1996). Research on safety operating of the assisting robot. Proc. of JSME Annual Conference on Robotics and Mechatronics, pp 1177-1180 (in Japanese)

Guidelines for the inclusion of safety aspects in standards, ISO/IEC GUIDE 51, 1990

Shannon C.E (1948). A mathematical theory of communication. Bell System Tech. J., vol. 27, pp 379-423

Yoshikawa T (1985). Manipulability of robotic mechanisms. The International Journal of Robotics Research, Vol.4, pp.3-9

Ikuta K, Nokata M (2001). Safety evaluation method of human-care robot design. Integration of Assistive Technology in the Information Age, IOS Press, pp 307-316

Ikuta K, Nokata M, Ishii H (2001). Safety evaluation method of human-care robot control and special robot simulator. Integration of Assistive Technology in the Information Age, IOS Press, pp 317-326

Nokata M, Ikuta K, Ishii H (2003). Optimizing method of human-care robot design and control for safety. Proc. Int. Conf. on Rehabilitation Robotics (ICORR'2003), pp 80-83

21

Robotic Exoskeletons for Upper Extremity Rehabilitation

Abhishek Gupta and Marcia K. O'Malley
Rice UniversityDepartment of Mechanical Engineering and Materials Science
Houston, Texas 77005 USA

1. Introduction

In 2003, 700,000 persons in the United States suffered a cerebral vascular accident (CVA), or stroke, with the total number of survivors estimated at 5.5 million. The total cost for rehabilitation and lost revenue in 2006 was 57.9 billion (Thom, Haase et al. 2006). Stroke commonly causes significant residual physical, cognitive, and psychological impairment (Gresham 1990). As the geriatric population increases and more effective therapies for acute stroke management emerge, there will be more survivors living with disabilities. In addition to greater numbers of survivors, there has been an increase in the number of more moderately affected survivors (Wolf, D'Agostino et al. 1992), which has increased the demand for stroke rehabilitation in an era of health care cost containment. Efforts to prevent stroke must, therefore, be balanced with pragmatic efforts to prevent disability and maximize quality of life for stroke survivors. Persons with hemiparesis following stroke constitute the largest group of patients receiving rehabilitation services in this country. The current consensus regarding rehabilitation of patients with some voluntary control over movements of the paretic limb is that they be encouraged to use the limb in functional tasks and receive training directed toward improving strength and motor control, relearning sensorimotor relationships, and improving functional performance (Gresham, Alexander et al. 1997). Given such recommendations, the research community has responded with efforts to improve the effectiveness of rehabilitative treatment of motor disability resulting from stroke.

1.1 Robotic devices for rehabilitation

A significant area of focus has been on the use of robotic devices for delivery of consistent and repeatable movement therapy. Indeed, the interest in rehabilitation applications for robotic devices, especially simple one- and two- DOF devices that focus on upper-extremity rehabilitation, has been increasing since the late 1980s and early 1990s (Erlandson 1992;

Reinkensmeyer, Dewald et al. 1996; Reinkensmeyer, Takahashi et al. 2000). For example, Khalili and Zomlefer suggested that a two joint robot system could be used for continuous passive motion and could be programmed to the particular needs of the patient (Khalili and Zomlefer 1988). Goodall et al. used two single degree-of-freedom (DOF) arms to stabilize sway in hemiparetic patients, and suggested the level of assistance could be withdrawn to encourage patients to relearn to balance on their own (Goodall, Pratt et al. 1987). White et al. built a single DOF pneumatically powered orthotic device for elbow flexion that could be used for continuous passive motion, to measure patient strength, and to assist elbow flexion (White, Scneider et al. 1993). Dirette et al. showed that a continuous passive motion (CPM) machine, when used regularly, can effectively reduce edema in the hands of flaccid hemiparetic patients (Dirette and Hinojosa 1994).

A more recent thrust of robotic assisted rehabilitation research has been to focus on the ability of the devices to assist limb movements and facilitate recovery of motor function in subjects with chronic hemiparesis due to stroke, such as with the Mirror-Image Motion Enabler - MIME (Burgar, Lum et al. 2000). In an initial study with MIME including twenty-eight subjects (two groups of 14), all had improved motor function as a result of therapy (Burgar, Lum et al. 2000). Preliminary data from these ongoing clinical efficacy trials suggest that robot-aided therapy has therapeutic benefits. Improvements have been demonstrated in strength and in the Fugl-Meyer (FM) assessment of motor function. Trends in the data suggest that the underlying mechanisms for these results may be increased strength, as well as more appropriate activation and inhibition of muscle groups.

The reader is referred to extensive reviews of robotic therapy for upper and lower extremity for a more complete discussion of the state of the field and results of ongoing clinical trials (Fasoli, Krebs et al. 2004; Hogan and Krebs 2004; Reinkensmeyer, Emken et al. 2004; Stein 2004; Riener, Nef et al. 2005; O'Malley, Ro et al. 2006). The MIME studies together with the cited related work support the conclusions that robotic manipulation of an impaired limb may favorably affect recovery following a stroke. An important additional finding is that improvements in motor control are possible beyond six months following a stroke.

Such findings with shoulder and elbow rehabilitation motivate the extension of robotic-assisted rehabilitation distally for the upper extremity, so that forearm pronation-supination, wrist flexion-extension, radial-ulnar deviation, and ultimately digital manipulation are enabled. Several devices have been presented in the literature to achieve at least a subset of these movements. For example, Charles et al. (Charles 2005) have developed an extension of the MIT-MANUS system to provide three rotational degrees-of-freedom for wrist rehabilitation. Hesse et al. (Hesse, Schulte-Tigges et al. 2003) have also extended the utility of their arm trainer to include wrist motion. In order to improve the applicability of the MIME system for full arm rehabilitation post stroke, the authors have developed a wrist rehabilitation robot, the *RiceWrist*, which interfaces with MIME and provides a variety of interaction modes for the therapist to select for the patient.

1.2 Haptic interfaces

Haptic or force-reflecting interfaces are a specific type of robotic device used to display touch- or force-related sensory information from a virtual or remote environment to the user (see, for example, surveys (Boman 1995; Burdea 1996; Lay and Day 2003). The ability to interact mechanically with virtual objects through incorporation of haptic feedback allows users to manipulate objects in the simulated or remote environment with ease when compared to a purely visual display. Added advantages of haptic simulators include increased repeatability, scalability, safety, and control over environmental conditions. It is also possible to simulate additional physical forces and fields, which may or may not be part of a natural environment, to convey information to the user. This makes a haptic display suitable for a variety of applications like remote operation in hazardous environments, simulators for surgical training (Basdogan, Ho et al. 2001; Feygin, Keehner et al. 2002; Carignan and Akin 2003), and rehabilitation research (Todorov, Shadmehr et al. 1997; Prisco, Avizzano et al. 1998; Jack, Boian et al. 2001; Sveistrup 2004). Physical therapy utilizing the resistance offered to a user's motion during haptic interaction can be used for rehabilitation of impaired arm movements in patients. Furthermore, research has shown that augmented feedback presented in virtual environments accelerates the learning of motor tasks (Todorov, Shadmehr et al. 1997). For these reasons, the authors have developed an arm exoskeleton that can be utilized for such training and rehabilitation applications.

1.3 Force feedback exoskeletons

In order to effectively interface with the distal joints of the upper extremity, many groups are turning towards exoskeleton-type robotic devices. Such ungrounded or wearable interfaces permit greater human movement during haptic interactions. However, the increased workspace for an ungrounded (Tsagarakis, Caldwell et al. 1999) device is achieved at the expense of design simplicity when compared to grounded (Bergamasco, Allotta et al. 1994) devices.

A force-feedback exoskeleton is a haptic device worn by the user. Arm exoskeletons can simulate large forces at the hand or arm, like the weight of an object that is held. This is achieved by providing feedback to the various joints of the arm—the shoulder, elbow, and wrist. Although worn by the user, the device itself may be grounded, in which case it restricts user mobility. In the mid 1960s and early 1970s, a group of researchers at Cornell University and later at General Electric developed some of the earliest master-slave teleoperation systems, the Handyman and Hardiman (Mosher 1967). The Hardiman was an anthropomorphic exoskeleton placed inside a larger slave robot, and was used to amplify human power output. Input commands from the user were obtained from both the arms and legs. These early exoskeleton haptic devices were hampered by limitations in actuation, computation, and control systems technology. The reader is encouraged to review (Burdea 1996) for an exhaustive discussion of the early stages of exoskeleton and haptic interface development. In recent years, improvements in sensing and actuation technologies, control systems, and computing resources have led to the development of many successful haptic interfaces.

Although there have been a large number of high-performance hand controllers, research in design of exoskeletons for other parts of the body is still in an early phase. The first modern exoskeleton arm/glove was designed and developed at ARTS laboratory for the replication of sensations of contacts and collisions (Bergamasco, Allotta et al. 1994). The ARTS arm, also known as the PERCRO exoskeleton, is a 7-DOF ungrounded device, attached to the operator's shoulder and torso. The operator holds onto the device with his/her palm. Hence, the device can only exert forces at the palm of the user. It uses DC motors with a cable transmission system for actuation. A 9-DOF under-actuated exoskeleton arm developed at the Korea Institute of Science and Technology (KIST) by Lee et al. addressed the workspace issues associated with the PERCRO exoskeleton. Their device allows for full reproduction of the human arm's workspace when operating the exoskeleton (Lee, Park et al. 1998). A revised exoskeleton device from the same group employs electrical brakes in place of pneumatic actuators for improved bandwidth (Kim, Lee et al. 2005). An alternate arm exoskeleton developed at KIST addresses the limited wearability issues of previous designs by using parallel mechanisms and pneumatic actuators (Jeong, Lee et

al. 2001). The wearable Salford arm addresses some of the issues and limitations of earlier designs (Tsagarakis, Caldwell et al. 1999). For example, nearly 90% of the human arm's workspace can be replicated with their device. Pneumatic muscle actuators (pMAs) were selected to power the robot due to their high power-to-weight ratio. A drawback of this choice is the highly nonlinear behavior and slow response of the pMAs, presenting additional control challenges.
In recent years, robotic exoskeletons are being developed specifically for rehabilitation applications, such as the ARMin system. This six-DOF device was designed to enable training for specific activities of daily living (Nef, Mihelj et al. 2006). Kousidou et al. have incorporated the Salford arm into the Rehab Lab system for virtual rehabilitation of complex three-dimensional trajectories in the workspace (Kousidou, Tsagarakis et al. 2006). Carignan et al. (Carignan and Liszka 2005) present a prototype five-DOF exoskeleton system currently under development that focuses on shoulder rehabilitation. Finally, Gupta et al. have incorporated their lower-arm exoskeleton device (Gupta and O'Malley 2006) into the MIME system, creating a full upper-extremity robotic rehabilitation system (Gupta, Patoglu et al. 2007). A review of exoskeleton devices for rehabilitation applications was compiled by Ruiz et al., and contains images of many of these devices (Ruiz, Forner-Cordero et al. 2006).

1.4 Exoskeleton control

Force control of arm exoskeletons is traditionally implemented under the assumption of pseudostatic operation (see, for example, (Bergamasco, Allotta et al. 1994)). In this approach, the robot Jacobian can be used to compute required actuator torques for some desired force at the end-effector. Recently, Rosen et al. presented some interesting results with the use of myosignals, command signals sent to the human muscles by the brain, in predicting human arm motion during operation of a single-DOF arm exoskeleton (Rosen, Brand et al. 2001). They demonstrated that the prediction of operator motion can be used to improve upon the force control and overall quality of the haptic device. The group has since expanded their design to include the full seven-DOF of the arm (Perry and Rosen 2006).

1.5 Exoskeleton design

Many exoskeleton interfaces attempt to optimize one or more of the following characteristics of the haptic system, namely power-to-weight ratio (Lee, Park et al. 1998; Tsagarakis, Caldwell et al. 1999; Jeong, Lee et al. 2001), workspace (Lee, Park et al. 1998), wearability (Jeong, Lee et al. 2001) or stability, and control bandwidth (Bergamasco, Allotta et al. 1994; Nakai, Oshashi et al. 1998; Williams II 1998). Individual designs, however, achieve these optimizations at the expense of other useful features, usually workspace (Bergamasco, Allotta et al. 1994; Nakai, Oshashi et al. 1998; Jeong, Lee et al. 2001) or control bandwidth (Lee, Park et al. 1998; Tsagarakis, Caldwell et al. 1999; Jeong, Lee et al. 2001). In this chapter, the authors present work towards the design of a high-quality haptic interface with a workspace comparable to that of human arm workspace. This is achieved at the expense of added weight and decreased mobility due to device grounding.

2. Design Challenges

Haptic feedback aids an operator to reliably complete a remote or virtual task. Primary requirements for such a system are the ability to convey commands to the remote or virtual plant and to reflect relevant sensory information, specifically forces in the remote or virtual environment, back to the operator. In essence, the dynamics of the device must not

interfere with the interaction between the operator and environment. An ideal haptic interface behaves as a rigid body, through which the user interacts with the environment, over the complete range of frequencies of forces in the virtual environment.
In practice, however, performance is limited by physical factors, such as actuator and sensor quality, device stiffness, friction, device workspace, force isotropy across the workspace, backlash, and computational speed. Force isotropy, which refers to the equality of force exertion capability of the device in all directions, is important to ensure consistent device performance across the workspace. The desired size and shape of the workspace itself is typically dependent on the target application, and serves as an important factor in determining the overall device size and mechanism. Increased workspace is only achieved at the expense of a larger and heavier device, since the force output requirements scale with the workspace size. Also of consideration in the design of haptic arm exoskeletons is the biomechanics of the human arm. The arm imposes a force/position constraint on the device, thus affecting the system behavior and performance. These design factors are discussed in detail in the following sections.

2.1 Biomechanics of Human Arm

A haptic arm exoskeleton places kinematic constraints on the human arm. The human arm has seven DOF: abduction/adduction and flexion/extension of the shoulder; rotation of the upper arm; flexion/extension of the elbow; rotation of the forearm; and radial/ulnar deviation and flexion/extension of the wrist. It is desirable that the haptic exoskeleton does not compromise the natural arm motion and workspace of the operator. The device should also have torque capabilities to match and enhance human abilities. Table I shows the workspace and torque capabilities of the human arm for reference.

2.2 Performance-Related Design Parameters

A high-quality haptic interface is characterized by stability robustness and transparency. The stability bandwidth refers to the range of frequencies of forces that can be reflected to the operator with the device, while ensuring stable system behavior. Research has shown that stability of a haptic simulation is related to the simulation rate, virtual wall stiffness, and device viscosity (Elllis, Ismaeil et al. 1996). Transparency is a measure of the degree of distortion between the force at the human-robot interface and the desired contact force as commanded through the virtual environment. Transparency can be degraded by such things as backlash, inertia, or friction in the haptic device, sensor resolution, and computational delay (Colgate and Brown 1994). Often with haptic interfaces, the quality of the device is characterized by the maximum virtual wall stiffness that can be stably displayed.

Joint	Human Isometric Strength (Nm)	Human Joint Workspace Limits (degrees)
Elbow Flexion/Extension	72.5	Flexion: 146 Extension: 0
Forearm Supination/Pronation	9.1	Supination: 86 Pronation: 71
Wrist Palmer/Dorsal Flexion	19.8	Palmer Flexion: 73 Dorsiflexion: 71
Wrist Abduction/Adduction	20.8	Adduction: 33 Abduction: 19

Table 1. Workspace and torque limits of human arm.

Research has shown that fairly low stiffness and force values are sufficient for object detection (O'Malley and Goldfarb 2002; O'Malley and Goldfarb 2004). Therefore, if a haptic exoskeleton is designed for teaching arm movements using virtual force fields, a low force output interface would suffice. In this case, as the authors intend for the device to be used as a general purpose training tool for arm movements, it is required that the device be able to simulate high-quality virtual surfaces. As a result, emphasis is placed on the design of a high-performance interface, which encompasses the human arm workspace. In addition, for rehabilitation applications, the ability to control feedback to individual human arm joints is desirable and has been addressed through this design.

2.3. Control-Related Design Parameters

As mentioned earlier, a haptic system applies trajectory-dependent forces to the operator's body. This is typically implemented in one of two modes—the impedance control mode or the admittance control mode. Impedance control techniques measure position at the human-machine interface and in turn adjust the commanded force at the human-machine interface depending on the virtual environment model to be displayed. It is desirable that an impedance-controlled haptic device allows free movement in response to the operator's motion commands, so that when the human is moving in free space (not in contact with any virtual objects), there is no resistance to motion. This requirement translates to a need for backdrivability in impendence-controlled haptic devices. In this control mode, it is also desirable for the device to have minimal inertia to facilitate maneuvering. Furthermore, low inertia and friction improve interface performance by reducing the forces required to compensate for device dynamics. Alternatively, admittance control methods rely on measurement of forces at the human-machine interface and controlled robot motion based on the virtual environment model. An admittance controlled haptic device should prevent movement of the robot in response to operator-generated forces to allow for consistent force measurement and motion control.

It is apparent that haptic exoskeleton design involves various tradeoffs, which limit the achievable performance of the device since, in all instances, stability must be maintained. To summarize these tradeoffs, mechanism design choices may limit or affect human motion abilities; sensor and actuator selection is directly related to device weight, force output range, system stability, and cost; and actuator placement and inclusion of transmissions affects the apparent inertia of the device. All of these design decisions are greatly influenced by the intended application for the device.

The MAHI exoskeleton, named for the Mechatronics and Haptic Interfaces Lab at Rice University, has been designed primarily for training and rehabilitation in virtual environments. These applications typically require the use of virtual force fields for guidance (Rosenberg 1993) or active assistance (Gillespie, O'Modhrain et al. 1998; O'Malley and Gupta 2003). The exoskeleton device must therefore allow natural human arm movements, with minimal reduction in workspace of the human arm. Because the device is to be worn, special care must be taken to ensure safety of the wearer. Furthermore, mobility of the interface is not normally a requirement for such a system. Hence, the device can be grounded to support excessive weight, and gravity compensation can be implemented through the controller. Additionally, the low accelerations and velocities associated with human movements ensure that the inertia of the device plays a small role in its operation (Shimoga 1992; Bergamasco, Allotta et al. 1994). Therefore, when designing the MAHI exoskeleton, the kinematic design of the robot was given prime consideration.

3. MAHI arm exoskeleton

3.1 Basic Mechanism Design

The basic kinematic structure of the 5-DOF MAHI exoskeleton is depicted in Fig. 1. The exoskeleton is comprised of a revolute joint at the elbow, a revolute joint for forearm rotation, and a 3-revolute-prismatic-spherical (RPS) serial-in-parallel wrist.

The 3-RPS platform, mentioned by Lee and Shah (Lee and Shah 1988), consists of a base plate, three extensible links l_1 , l_2 , and l_3 , and a moving platform, as shown in Fig. 2. The moving platform houses the end-effector that is affixed to the operator during operation. The moving platform is connected to the three extensible links by means of spherical joints spaced at 120° along the circumference of a circle of radius r. The other end of the links connects to the base platform via revolute (pin) joints, which are also spaced 120° along a circle of radius R. The axes of rotation of the revolute joints are oriented along the tangents to the circle of radius R. Linear actuators placed along the link are used to change the link length, thereby moving the top platform. It should be noted that the platform has limited movement transverse to the vertical axis through the base and no singularities for $\theta_i \in (0, \pi)$ (Lee and Shah 1988).

The choice of a parallel mechanism for the design of the exoskeleton wrist over a serial mechanism was motivated primarily by the compactness of the parallel mechanism. Furthermore, use of a parallel mechanism allows for higher torque output, stiffness, and decreased inertia compared to a similar serial mechanism. During operation, the robot is worn so that the axis elbow joint of the robot aligns with the operator's elbow joint, and the top plate of the wrist of the robot aligns with the wrist joint of the operator. This configuration aids in preserving natural arm movements by aligning the robot's kinematic structure with that of the human arm. Velcro strapping and an ergonomic palm splint are used to maintain this alignment. The mapping between the robot configuration and arm position is further simplified by the use of the 3-RPS kinematic structure for the robot. The equivalence between the human wrist joint angles and the xyz Euler angle representation for the orientation of the platform is shown in Section 3.4.

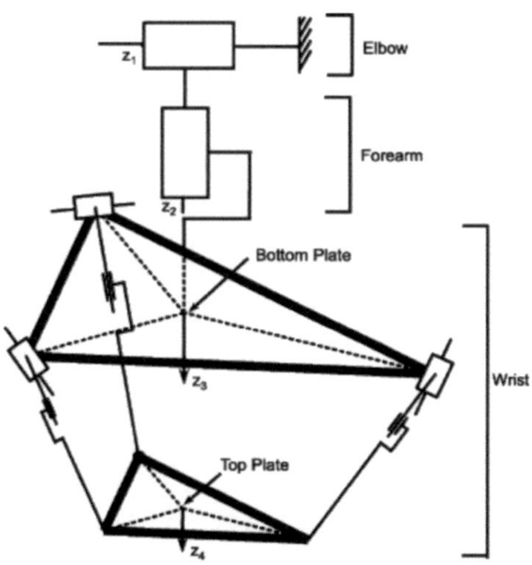

Fig. 1. Exoskeleton mechanism: A 3-RPS platform is used as the wrist of the robot. Joints R1, R2, and R3 and B1, B2, and B3 are located at vertices of equilateral triangles.

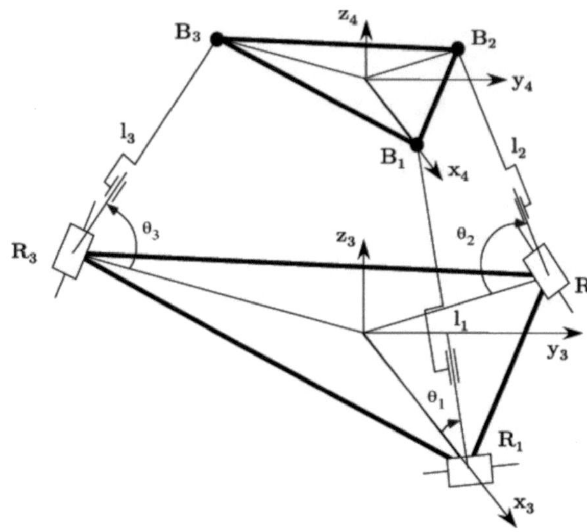

Fig. 2. 3-RPS platform, adapted from (Lee and Shah 1988).

3.2 Sensing and Actuation

Sensor Selection Sensor resolution affects the range of frequencies of forces that can be displayed by the haptic interface (Colgate and Brown 1994). Consider, for example, the simulation of a thin virtual wall. If the sensor resolution or the computational speed is not high enough, then there exists a possibility that the human can pass his/her arm through the wall without feeling the force. Furthermore, during simulation of stiff virtual surfaces, reduction in sensor resolution increases the delay in sensing the human's actions in the virtual environment, and this delay can decrease system stability. With these considerations, high resolution optical encoders were selected for the device.

Actuator Selection The actuators for a haptic device determine the range of magnitude and frequencies of forces that can be displayed with the interface. To reproduce real-life environments, it is desirable that the device be able to display forces in a large range of magnitudes as well as frequencies. In general, the use of high-power actuators is accompanied with an increase in weight, thereby increasing the inertia of the device. Thus, high power-to-weight ratio and high bandwidth are desirable qualities for actuators used in a haptic interface. The bandwidth refers to the dynamic response of the actuator; a low-bandwidth actuator fails to display high-frequency forces to the operator, reducing system transparency in such situations. This gains importance in that human kinesthetic/proprioceptic sensing bandwidth is 20-30 Hz and tactile sensing bandwidth is 0-400 Hz (Shimoga 1992).

No single actuator technology provides the benefit of both high power-to-weight ratio and high bandwidth. Pneumatic actuators are inexpensive and provide the benefit of high power-to-weight ratio. However, pneumatic actuators have a low bandwidth, which limits their utility as actuators for haptic interfaces. Tsagarakis et al. used pMAs for their exoskeleton (Tsagarakis, Caldwell et al. 1999). However, these actuators have highly nonlinear dynamics in addition to low bandwidth, making them unsuitable for application in haptic devices. Hence, electrical actuation was chosen for the MAHI exoskeleton. Electrical actuators have a lower power-to-weight ratio than pneumatic actuators but have very high bandwidth. This increases the weight of the device but allows for better force reflection through the interface.

Transmission and Actuator Placement A transmission can be used to increase the torques or forces delivered by the device, but at the expense of speed of operation. The bandwidth of human motor output, which represents the ability of the hand and fingers to exert forces, is 10-15 Hz (Shimoga 1992), thus making the use of a transmission in haptic interfaces advantageous. Furthermore, use of a transmission allows the actuators themselves to be placed closer to the base of the robot, reducing rotational inertia. Use of transmissions, however, is associated with tradeoffs like backlash, nonlinear dynamics, and complex cable routing. For example, gears introduce backlash into the system, whereas belt drives introduce nonlinearities. Friction, backlash, backdrivability, and size were key considerations in designing the transmission. A cable drive, which, by design is backdriveable and free of backlash, is used as the transmission for elbow and wrist. In contrast, the forearm joint is direct drive actuated. For the elbow joint, a large cable drive with an approximate 10:1 transmission ratio was used, allowing backlash-free motion that is fully backdriveable (See Fig.3). High torque rotary electric motors with a cable-driven mechanism are employed for the robot wrist (Fig. 4), whereas the forearm joint is directly driven using a frameless electrical motor.

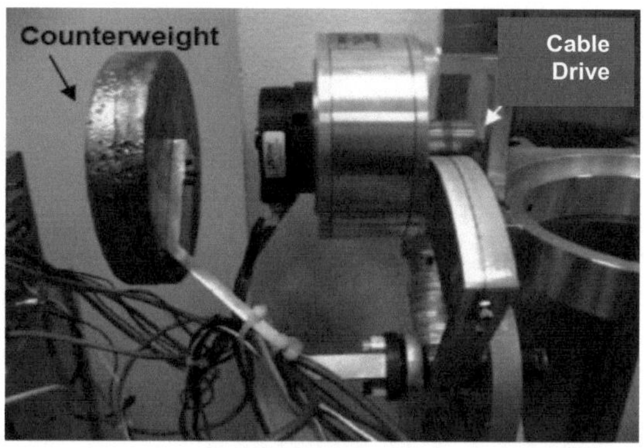

Fig. 3. Elbow joint with a cable drive and counterweight for gravity compensation.

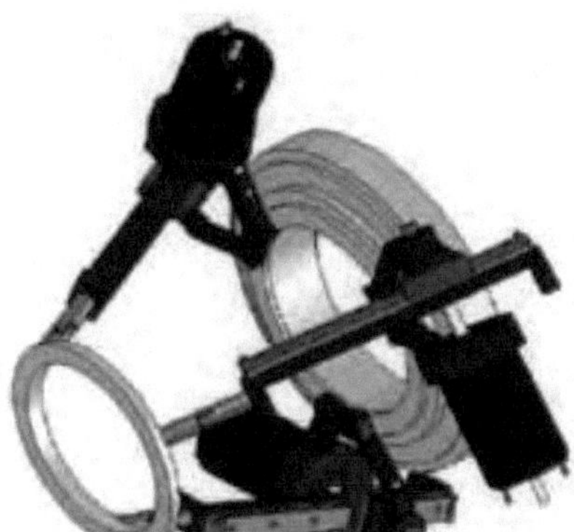

Fig 4. Wrist component of the MAHI arm exoskeleton employing electrical motors with a cable drive.

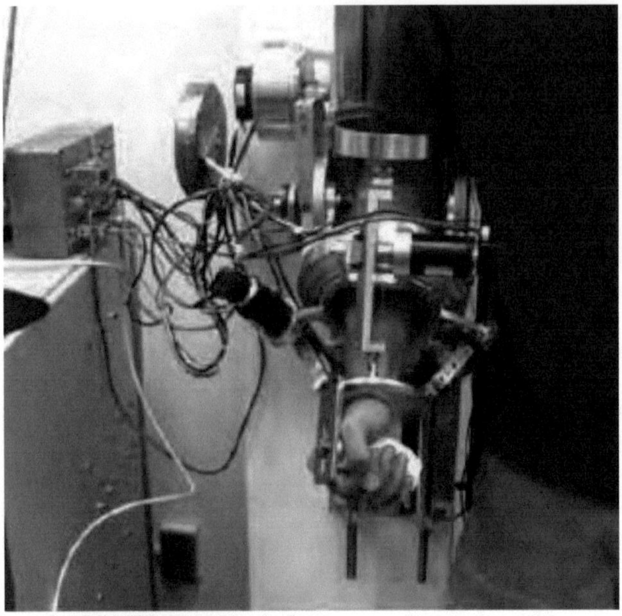

Fig. 5. User operating the MAHI arm exoskeleton.

3.3 Mechanical Design of MAHI Exoskeleton

Fig. 5 depicts a user operating the MAHI arm exoskeleton. The forearm joint employs a frameless brushless DC motor with direct actuation. Due to the use of frameless actuators, the amount of material required for construction was minimized thus reducing the weight of the device. The wrist platform is actuated through high torque rotary electric motors and a cable drive transmission. The range of motion of the spherical joint at the movable plate of the platform limits the workspace of platform. Equations developed by Lee and Shah were used to compute the range of rotations required from the spherical joint in order to meet our workspace criteria (Lee and Shah 1988). It was found that commercially available spherical joints do not suffice to meet the workspace requirements. Hence, the spherical joint was replaced by a 4 DOF spherical joint between the top plate of the platform and the corresponding linear joint links. This joint consisted of a universal-joint attached at either end to the link and the moving platform via rotary joints. This adds redundancy to the system and permits larger rotations. For the purpose of kinematic analysis, the redundancy does not affect any of the geometric relations or equations. Mechanical stops at workspace limits, soft software stops and an emergency stop switch are employed to ensure operator safety. For a detailed discussion of the design of the exoskeleton, the reader is referred to (Gupta and O'Malley 2006; Sledd and O'Malley 2006).

3.4 Kinematic Properties of MAHI Arm Exoskeleton

Table 2 shows the workspace for the MAHI arm exoskeleton in terms of the range of motion about each of the three primary degrees of freedom and corresponding human joint workspace limits. The device is singularity-free and the forward and kinematics of the device have a unique solution within the workspace. For a detailed discussion of the kinematics of the robot refer to (Gupta and O'Malley 2006).

Joint	Peak Torque Output Limits (Nm)	Joint Workspace Limits (degrees)
Elbow Flexion/Extension	55	Flexion: 90 Extension: 0
Forearm Supination/Pronation	5.08	Supination: 90 Pronation: 90
Wrist Palmer/Dorsal Flexion	5.26	Palmer Flexion: 45 Dorsiflexion: 45
Wrist Abduction/Adduction	5.26	Adduction: 45 Abduction: 45

Table 2. Workspace and torque output limits of MAHI arm exoskeleton.

The workspace of the MAHI arm exoskeleton is 100% of the average human joint range of motion except for palmar flexion and dorsiflexion where it is 60%. As shown in Fig. 6, compound movements of the wrist remain singularity-free, albeit with some reduction in the range of motion similar to the case of a human wrist. Thus the MAHI arm exoskeleton provides adequate range of motion for a human operator. It should also be noted that the device is backlash- free due to the use of direct-drive and cable-driven actuation and is highly backdriveable. Furthermore, the 3-RPS platform allows for compact design, centered on the human arm, which increases wearability and maximizes the achievable workspace of the exoskeleton.

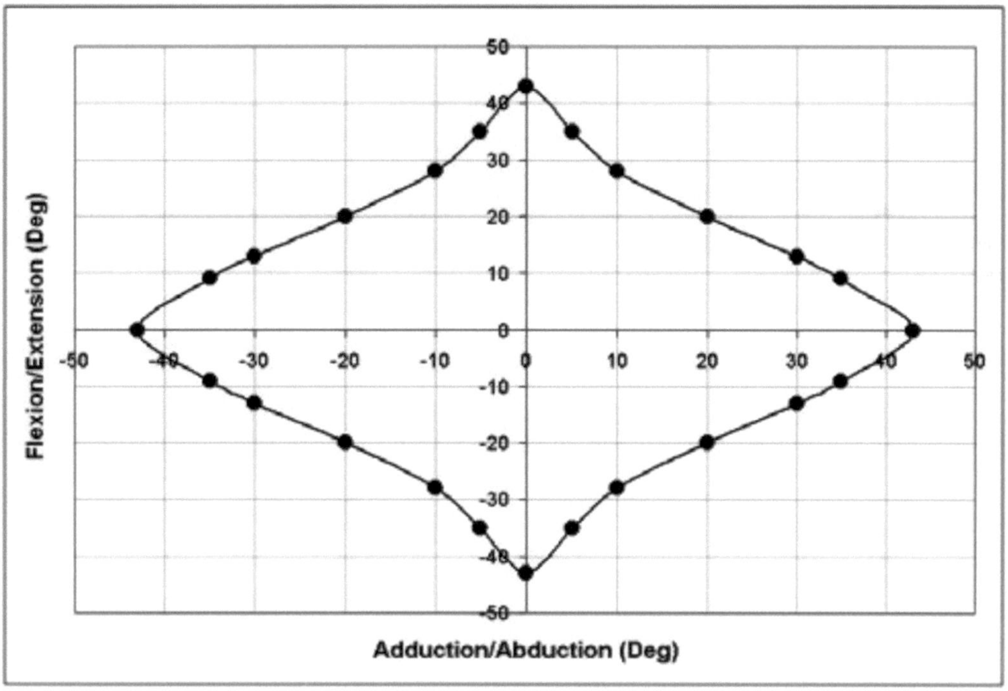

Fig. 6. Range of motion of MAHI arm exoskeleton wrist.

Fig. 7 shows the manipulability of the MAHI arm exoskeleton measured as the absolute determinant of the inverse Jacobian (Yoshikawa 1985). Manipulability of a robot is a quantitative measure that captures the ease with which the device can arbitrarily change position and orientation from a given posture. For the MAHI arm exoskeleton, the manipulability measure is greatest in the center of the workspace, with the wrist at 0° of abduction/adduction, (a) and flexion/extension, (b). Manipulability, as expected, is low at the extents of each joint range of motion, although more so during flexion/extension. For the tasks of rehabilitation and training, it is expected that most useful interactions via the haptic device will take place away from the joint limits, and so manipulability should not limit device performance.

Measurement of Human Motion A simplified kinematic model of the human lower arm and the wrist is shown in Fig. 8. Notice that axes x_4 of the platform (see Fig. 2) and z_2 of the human wrist joint coincide when the exoskeleton is worn by an operator. Similarly, axes y_4 of the platform and z_3 of the arm coincide for any rotation, α, of the top plate of the platform about x_4, or of the human wrist about z_2 (Fig. 8). Furthermore, {3} of the platform has a fixed orientation with respect to {1} of the human arm.

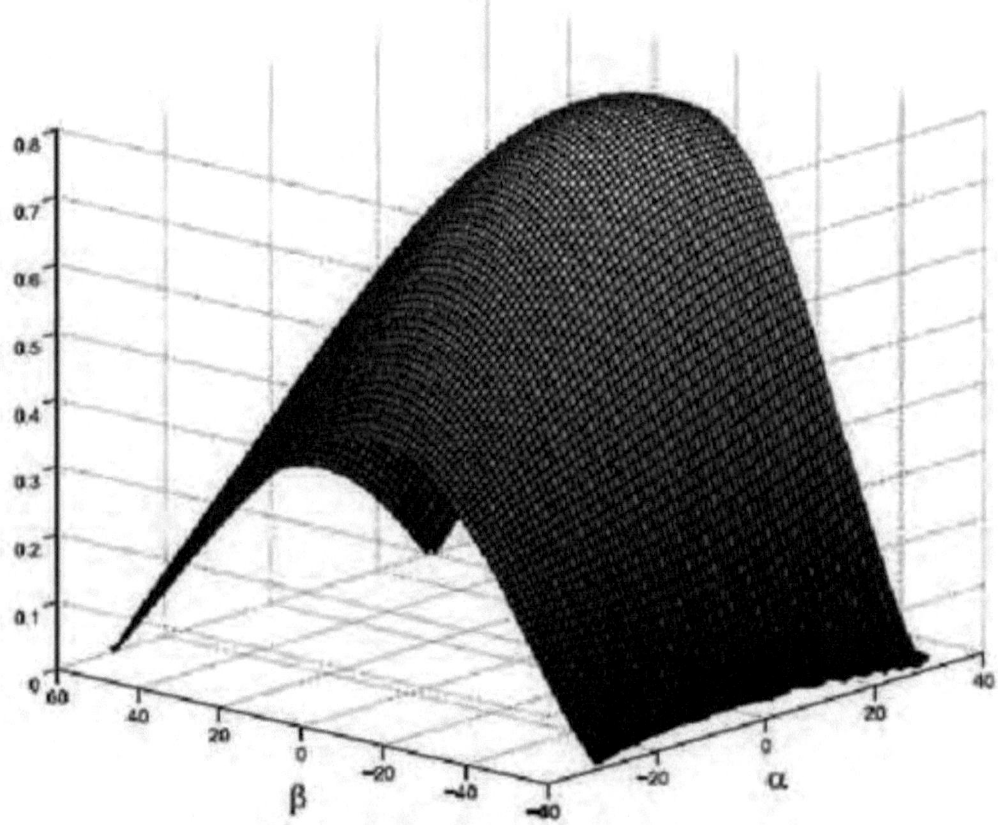

Fig. 7. Manipulability of the wrist mechanism.

Hence, a rotation of the top plate of the platform about axis x_4 (Fig. 2) followed by another rotation about axis y_4 (Fig. 2), is equivalent to a transformation from {3} to {1} of the arm. This implies that with the top plate of the platform centered at the operator's wrist joint, the measurement of the orientation of the top plate with respect to the base of the platform in terms of xyz-Euler angles corresponds to measurement of the flexion/extension and abduction/adduction of the human wrist joint. Thus, the Euler angle of rotation α about axis x_4 corresponds to abduction/adduction of the wrist while the rotation angle β about y_4 corresponds to flexion/extension. With the forearm joints of the robot and human being coincident, the measurement of position of operator's elbow and forearm from robot coordinates and vice versa is trivial.

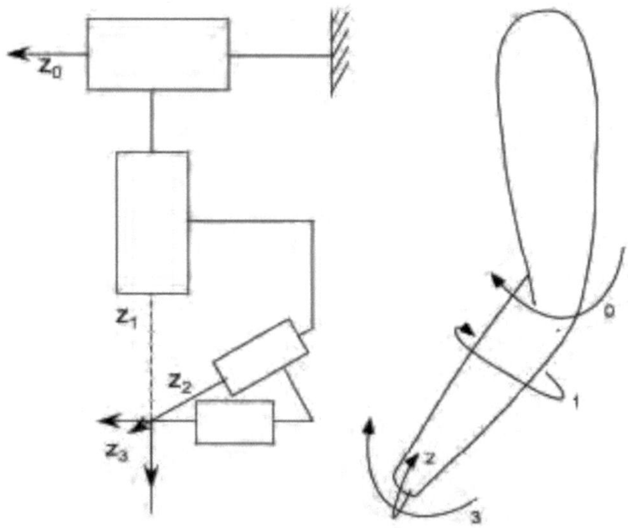

Fig. 8. Simplified kinematic model of the human arm: Other axes have not been shown for clarity. Axes 0 through 3 represent elbow rotation, forearm rotation, wrist adduction/abduction and wrist flexion/extension respectively.

4. Control and Dynamic Performance

The MAHI arm exoskeleton is controlled via a 3.2 GHz Pentium 4 PC with 2GB of RAM. The hardware is controlled through the MATLAB Real Time Workshop Toolbox from Mathworks, and WinCon from Quanser Consulting. All data I/O is handled by the Q8 board from Quanser. Position and force controllers were designed for the elbow, forearm and the wrist platform. Separate joint-space and task-space controllers were designed and tested for the wrist platform. Note that the task-space of the wrist platform refers to the three degrees of freedom corresponding to flexion/extension and abduction/adduction of the wrist, and the height of the platform. The following sections describe controller design in detail.

4.1 Controller Implementations

Joint level control for the MAHI exoskeleton is implemented via a joint-space proportional derivative (PD) trajectory controller. In addition, an inverse kinematics based task-space position controller was designed for the wrist, as shown in Figure 9. The commanded task-space positions and velocities were used to generate reference commands for the aforementioned joint-space controller. The performance of the device under joint-space position control was verified through step responses, set joint control and trajectory following control.

A task-space PD position controller for the wrist platform was also implemented as shown in Figure 10. As compared to the inverse kinematics based controller described in the previous section, this controller allows for independent control of wrist degrees of freedom, namely abduction/adduction, flexion/extension, and platform height. This is critical as during operation it is desirable to constrain the height of the platform to be a constant dependent upon the length of the subject's forearm. Furthermore, this provides the ability to selectively provide guidance and/or feedback to individual human wrist joints. The performance of the controller is discussed in Section 4.2.

Force control for the exoskeleton is implemented as a task-space impedance force controller, as shown in Fig. 10. It is assumed that the velocities of motion are small enough to ignore the dynamic terms in the equations of motion of the device. It should be noted that in the case of the elbow and forearm, the task-space and the joint-space are the same and hence, the impedance controller is simply a joint-space controller. The results of force control are discussed in Section 4.2 through haptic display of virtual walls.

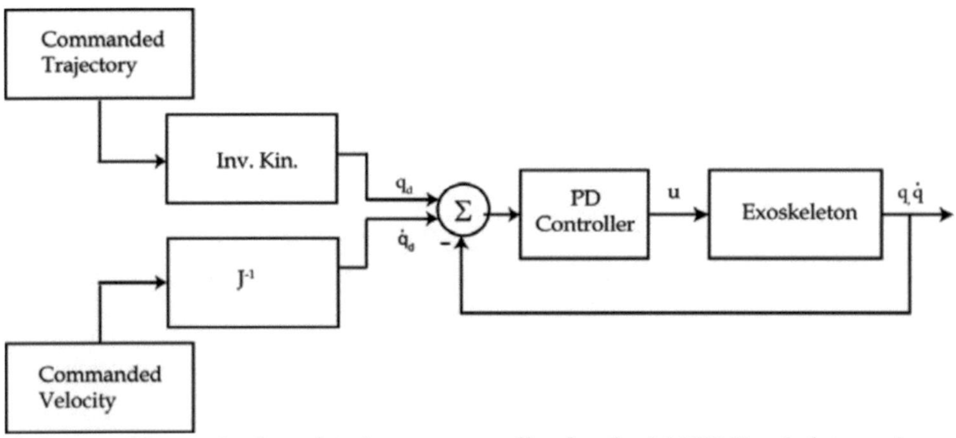

Fig. 9. Inverse kinematics based trajectory controller for the MAHI Exoskeleton where, J is the Jacobian of the device; q_d, $\dot{q}_d$ are the desired joint position and velocities; q, $\dot{q}$ are the current joint position and velocities; and u is the control input.

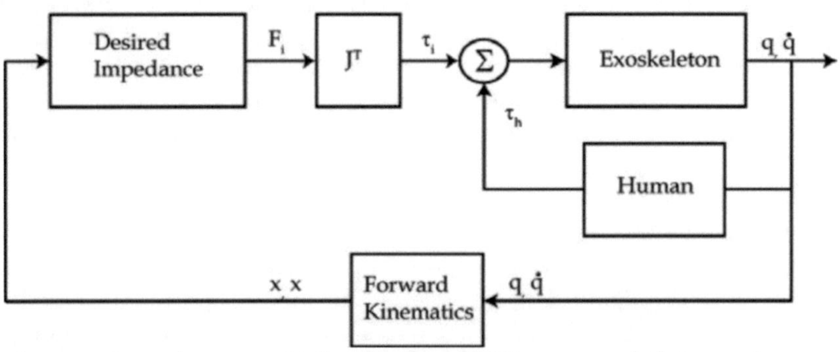

Fig. 10. Task-space impedance controller for the MAHI arm exoskeleton, where, q, $\dot{q}$ are the current joint position and velocities; x, $\dot{x}$ are the current task-space position and velocities; F_i is the desired environment force; J is the Jacobian of the MAHI exoskeleton; τ_i is the desired joint torques; and F_h is the human induced joint torque.

4.2 Dynamic Performance

Tables 1 and 2 list the human isometric strength and the peak torque output capabilities of the MAHI arm exoskeleton for the corresponding joints, respectively. The torque capabilities lag behind human abilities due to practical considerations owing to the power-to-weight characteristics of electrical actuators. Coulomb friction was measured to be 0.041 Nm and 1.134 Nm in the forearm and wrist joints respectively. Viscous friction was found to be negligible.

Position Control As described in Section 4.1, the position control for the wrist and forearm was implemented through a PD controller. Figure 11(a) shows the closed loop step response of the forearm. It can be easily seen that the device reaches steady state position of 1 rad in less than 1 s with no overshoot or oscillations. There is a small steady state error (< 1%) in position due to friction in the bearings, motor cogging and the gravitational torque acting on the joint. The steady state error can be eliminated with the use of a PID controller instead of the PD controller employed. The trajectory following behavior of the forearm tracking a sinusoidal reference signal at a frequency of 4 rad/s is depicted in Figure 11(b). This further verifies that the bandwidth of the controller is over 4 rad/s and matches human actuation bandwidth. Similar results were obtained for the wrist controller.

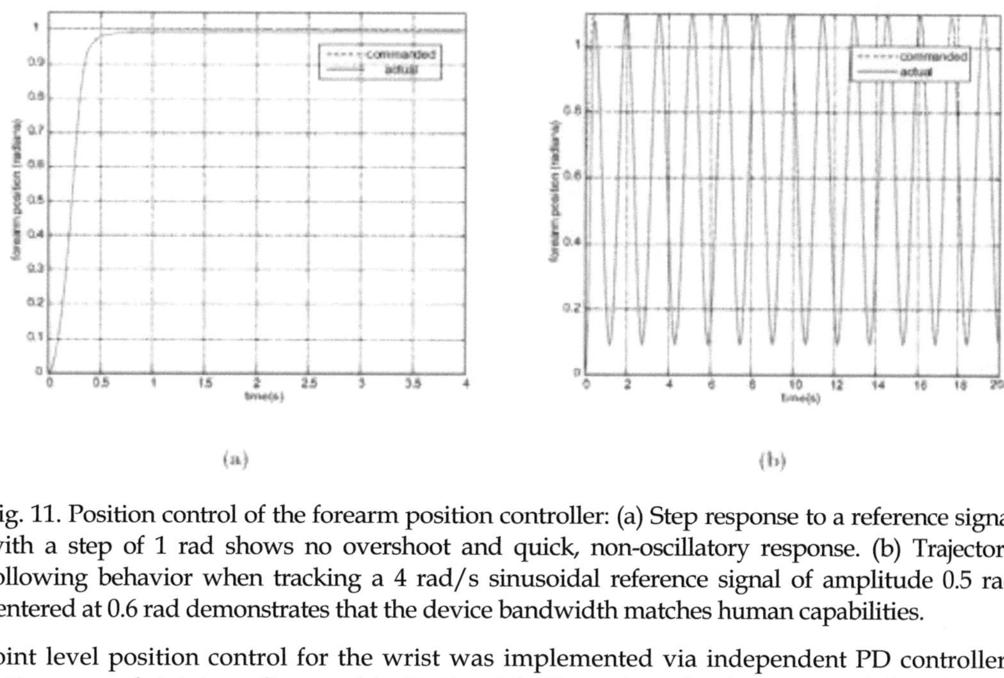

(a) (b)

Fig. 11. Position control of the forearm position controller: (a) Step response to a reference signal with a step of 1 rad shows no overshoot and quick, non-oscillatory response. (b) Trajectory following behavior when tracking a 4 rad/s sinusoidal reference signal of amplitude 0.5 rad centered at 0.6 rad demonstrates that the device bandwidth matches human capabilities.

Joint level position control for the wrist was implemented via independent PD controllers acting on each joint, as discussed in Section 4.1. Control results demonstrated that there is negligible structural coupling between the actuated joints. The low structural coupling between the linear joint axes also serves to verify the mechanical design process showing that the axes could be independently controlled as theoretically predicted. A task space PD controller for the wrist platform was also implemented as described in Section 4.1. Trajectory following behavior of the task-space controller tracking sinusoidal trajectories in abduction/adduction and flexion/extension at 4 rad/s is shown in Figure 12. Note the quick system response with little overshoot when tracking sinusoidal trajectories of amplitude 0.15 rad at a frequency of 4 rad/s. Note that the platform height was constrained when testing responses in abduction/adduction and flexion/extension as we start at the boundary of the workspace where it is not possible to change orientation of the top plate of the platform without changing platform height. Trajectory following capability is useful for guidance during training or rehabilitation. These results also serve to verify adequate system performance throughout the workspace of the wrist. For a detailed discussion of the performance of the device under position control please refer to (Gupta, Patoglu et al. 2007).

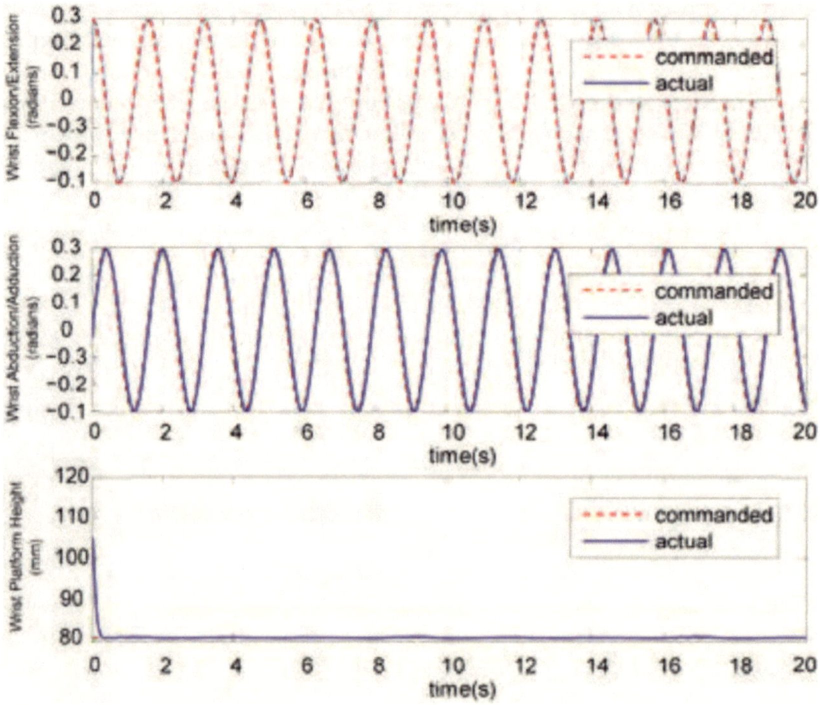

Fig. 12. Task space trajectory tracking control of the wrist platform (reference: height- 80 mm; abduction/adduction and flexion/extension - sinusoids of amplitude 1.5 rad at 4 rad/s).

Force Control As described in Section 4.1 force control for the exoskeleton was implemented through an impedance controller. Figure 13 depicts a subject's interaction with a virtual wall at the forearm joint, implemented as a spring-mass system of stiffness 150 Nm/rad and damping of 10 Nm/rad/s, located at 1 rad. Regions (a), (b) and (c) demonstrate the approach, steady contact and penetration into the wall, respectively. Note that due to torque limitations of the forearm motor, the user can overcome the wall force, thereby saturating the motor. Larger motor output is desired for simulating stronger walls, but device torques that exceed human limits could compromise user safety.

Figure 14 depicts a typical user interaction with two virtual walls located at a rotation of 0.2 rad in flexion/extension and abduction/adduction respectively. The virtual wall was implemented as a spring-damper system. Although slight chattering is noticed upon contact, the device successfully constrains the operator. Upon decreasing the wall gain, it is noted that chatter occurs at larger user penetration depths into the wall. The platform torque output does not match the limits of the human joints and hence, the human operator can saturate the motor output. We believe this actuator saturation along with the low stiffness of the cable drive transmission to be responsible for the chatter.

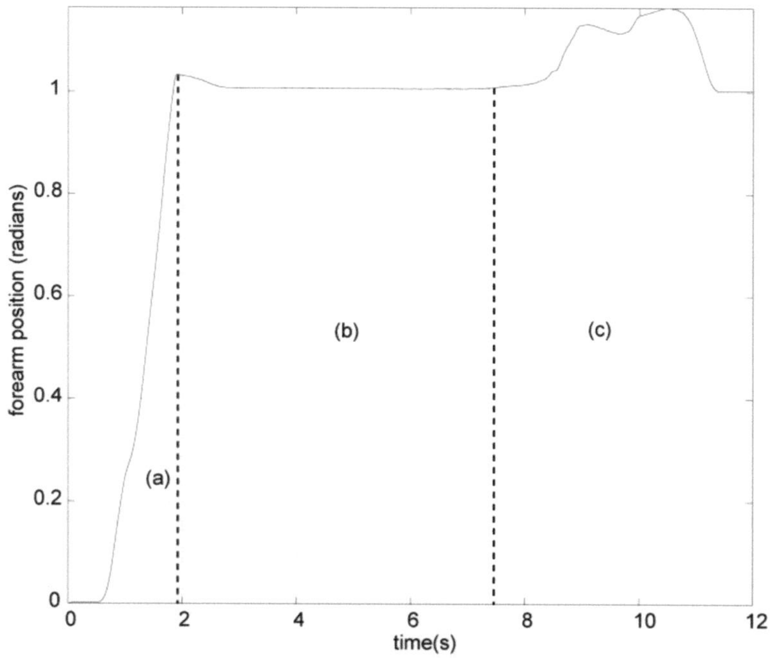

Fig 13. User interaction with virtual wall located at 1 rad for the forearm joint. Regions (a), (b) and (c) demonstrate the approach, steady contact and penetration into the wall. 0.5 mm from their initial position. This demonstrates that there is negligible structural coupling between the actuated joints. The low structural coupling between the linear joint axes also serves to verify the mechanical design process showing that the axes could be independently controlled as theoretically predicted.

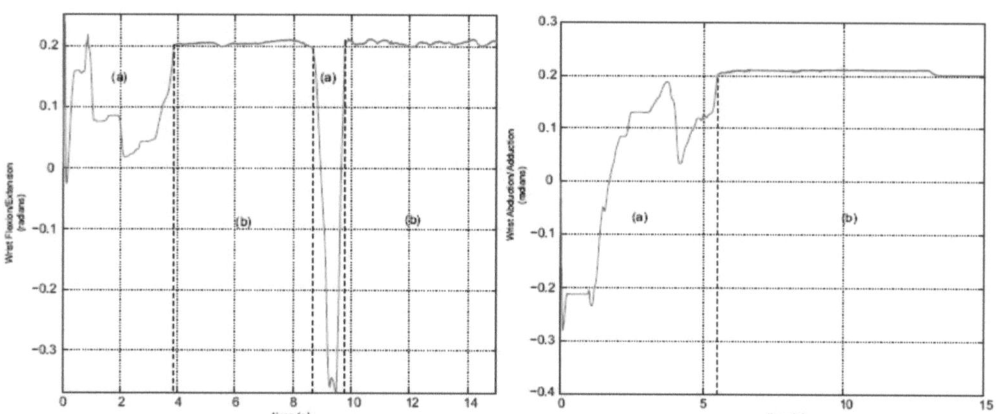

Fig. 14. (a) A virtual wall located at 0.2 rad wrist flexion/extension; (b) A virtual wall located at 0.2 rad wrist abduction/adduction.

5. Integration of MAHI exoskeleton with MIME

Prior work has studied the ability of a device (Mirror-Image Motion Enabler – MIME) (Burgar, Lum et al. 2000) to assist limb movements and facilitate recovery of motor function in subjects with chronic hemiparesis due to stroke. MIME incorporates an industrial robot and operates in three unilateral modes and one bimanual mode. In unilateral operation, passive, active-assisted, and guided movements against a resistance are possible. The bimanual mode enables the subject to practice bilateral, coordinated movements with rate and range under his or her control.

In the current version of MIME, subjects are seated in a wheelchair modified to improve seating support and reduce movements of the upper body. They can sit close to either the front or rear of an adjustable height table. A PUMA-560 robot is mounted beside the table. It is attached to a wrist-forearm orthosis (splint) via a 6-axis force transducer, a pneumatic breakaway overload sensor set to 20 Nm torque, and a quick-release coupling mechanism. The subject's arm is strapped into the splint with the wrist in neutral position. Robot/forearm interaction force and torque measurements from the transducer are recorded and archived by a personal computer. The control program monitors these data and the motion of the robot in order to prevent potentially hazardous situations from occurring. Switches and mechanical stops are strategically placed to permit rapid de-activation of the robot, if necessary.

Preliminary data from clinical efficacy trials using MIME suggest that robot-aided therapy has therapeutic benefits. Improvements have been demonstrated in strength and in the FM assessment of motor function. Trends in the data suggest that the underlying mechanisms for these results may be increased strength, as well as more appropriate activation and inhibition of muscle groups (Burgar, Lum et al. 2000).

Such findings with shoulder and elbow rehabilitation motivate the extension of robotic-assisted rehabilitation distally for the upper extremity, so that forearm pronation-supination, wrist flexion-extension, radial-ulnar deviation, and ultimately digital manipulation are enabled. The MAHI exoskeleton wrist (*RiceWrist*) has been integrated with the Mirror-Image Motion Enabler (MIME) (Burgar, Lum et al. 2000) system (see Figure 15). Velcro strapping and a molded splint are used to attach the subject's arm to the device. MIME and *RiceWrist* communicate through the serial port. Communication is mainly for synchronization of start and end of trials.

5.1 MIME-*RiceWrist* Rehabilitation Setup

Figure 16 shows the overall setup for the MIME-*RiceWrist* rehabilitation system. The therapist maintains high level supervisory control over the therapy session. The therapist can customize the physical therapy sessions according to the needs of individual patients. The *RiceWrist* extends the three unilateral operation modes of MIME to include forearm supination and pronation, wrist flexion and extension, and radial and ulnar deviation.

The three unilateral modes of MIME are:

- Passive mode: the robot guides the user to a predetermined goal position.
- Active-assisted mode: similar to passive mode, but the robotic assistance does not begin until the patient overcomes some preset force threshold.
- Constrained mode: the patient moves his/her arm against a viscous field to a goal position. A moving virtual wall prevents the patients from retracting their arm.

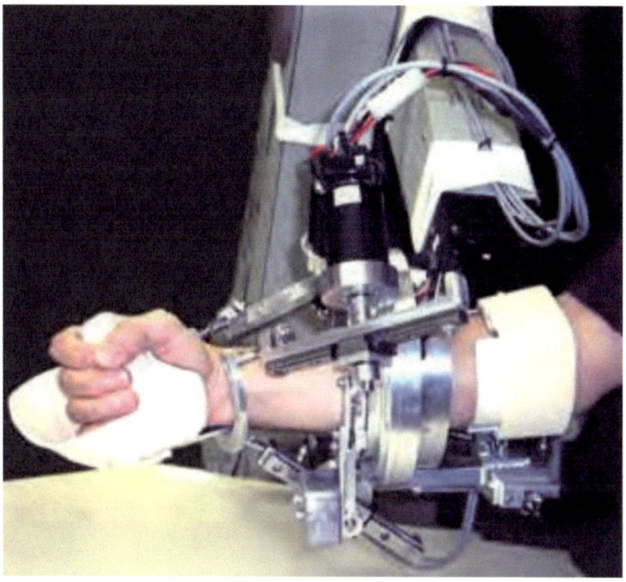

Fig. 15. Subject operating the integrated MIME-*RiceWrist* System.

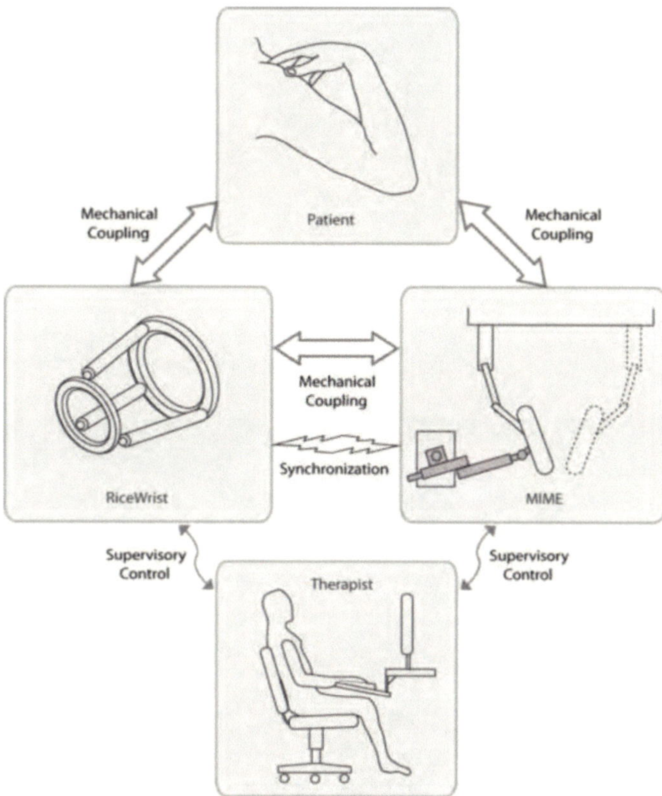

Fig. 16. MIME-*RiceWrist* rehabilitation system setup.

A graphical user interface (GUI), as shown in Fig. 17, is provided to the therapist to facilitate customization of the sessions. The GUI provides an interface to record patient information and individual session details. Prior to a therapy session, the therapist can record the joint limits of the patient to plan the desired start and end positions for reaching movements. This information is also stored on a local file for future reference and updates. For each trial, the therapist can then choose the desired trajectory by selecting start and end positions, number of repetitions and the speed of travel. Three different modes of operation – passive, triggered and constrained – are implemented on the system. Through the GUI, the therapist can also select the mode of operation and associated parameters.

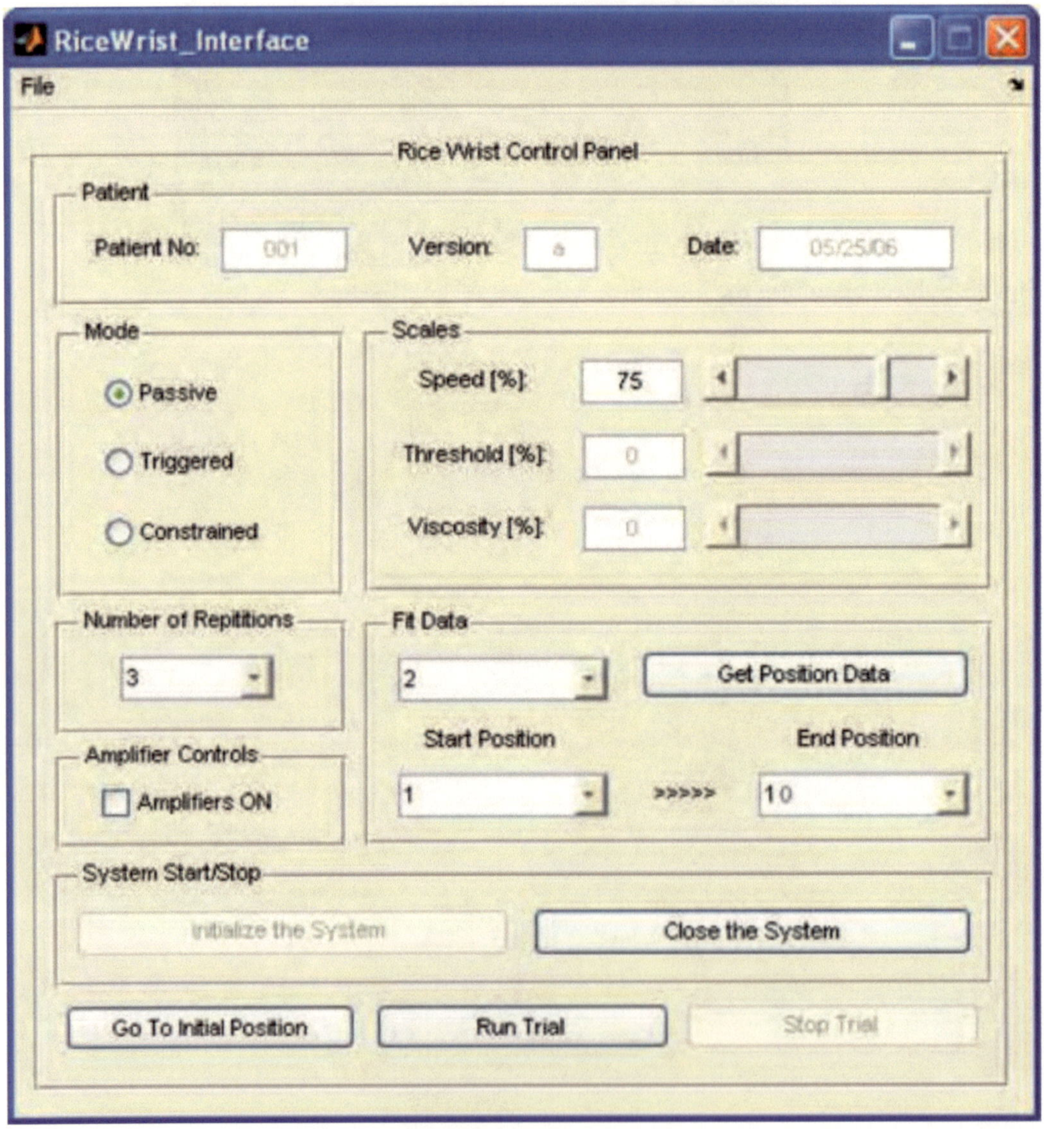

Fig. 17. Graphical user interface for the therapist

5.2 Control Modes

Three control modes that match the control modes of the MIME system – passive, triggered or constrained, have been implemented on the *RiceWrist*. Figure 18 depicts the structure of the controller for the MIME-*RiceWrist* system. The system has five modes of operation, three of which are the aforementioned control modes. The other modes are GoTo and Wait. When operating in the GoTo mode, the system moves to an initial position, which is specified by the therapist. On reaching the desired position, the system switches to the Wait mode, in which a virtual fixture is used to restrict arm movement, until the therapist initiates or resumes the trial. Following the command from the therapist, the system switches to one of the three control modes until the desired end position for the trial is reached. Upon reaching this position, the system switches back to the Wait mode until the therapist commands to initiate the return motion. This process can be repeated for the desired number of repetitions. The **GoTo mode** is implemented as a joint-space trajectory controller, as described in section 4.1. The desired trajectory is computed through linear interpolation using the current and specified initial positions. The **Wait mode** is implemented as a task-space impedance force controller. A high stiffness virtual wall prevents arm motions until a new mode is activated. **Passive** and **Triggered** modes are also implemented through joint-space controllers, whereas the **Constrained mode** is implemented as a task-space impedance force controller as used for the Wait mode. Unlike the Passive and Triggered modes, which are passive, this is an active mode where the patient is required to actively move his arm to the end position. Once movement has been initiated along the trajectory motion reversal is restricted by implementation of a virtual wall in that direction. Resistive impedance can also be displayed to the patient along the trajectory to provide strength training.

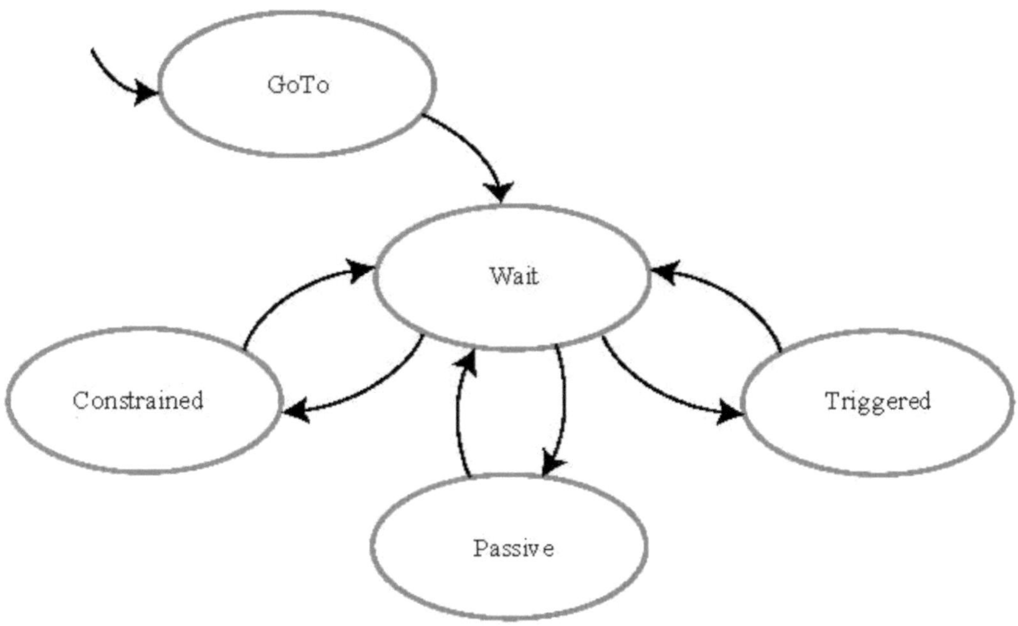

Fig. 18. Structure of the switching controller for the MIME-*RiceWrist* System.

5.3 Controller Performance of the *RiceWrist*

Figure 19 presents the experimental results when the *RiceWrist* is operating in the Passive Mode. Subfigures 19 (a)—(d) depict the trajectories for the four different joints, namely the wrist axes I, II, III, and forearm. Passive mode employs decoupled joint level trajectory controllers for each actuated axis. The solid lines in the figures represent the desired (commanded) trajectories, which are computed through linear interpolation between the specified initial and final joint positions. The dashed lines represent the experimentally recorded trajectories when the *RiceWrist* is operating freely. Finally, the dotted lines represent the experimentally recorded trajectories when the *RiceWrist* is worn by a human subject. The close match among the desired and experimentally observed trajectories imply adequate disturbance rejection characteristics of the implemented controllers.

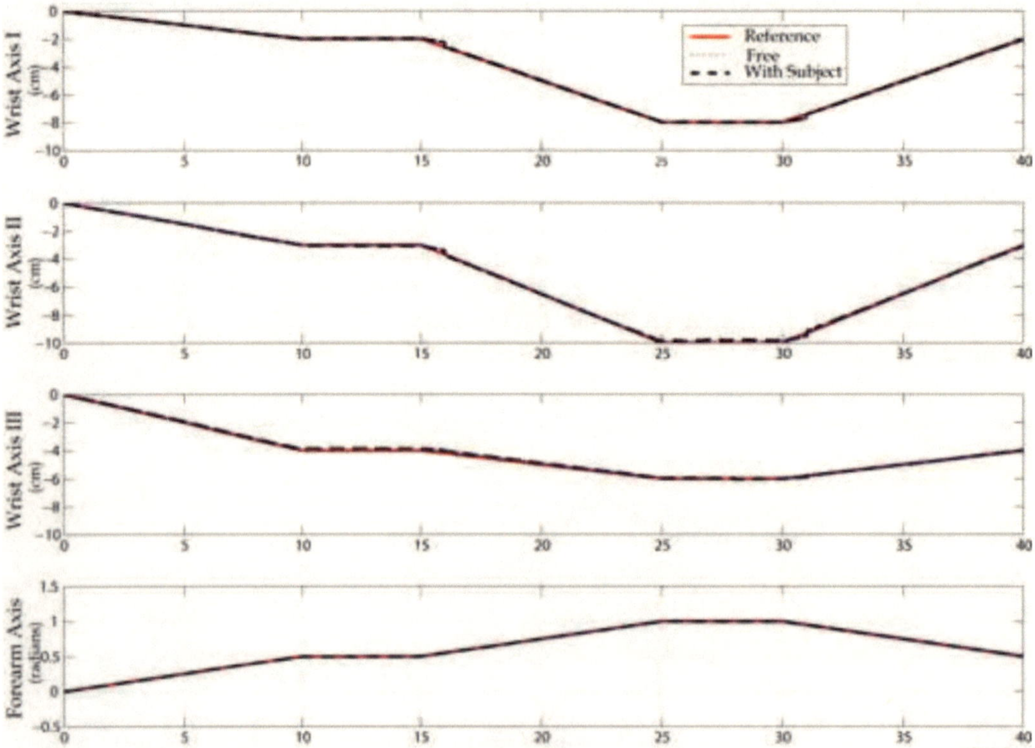

Fig. 19. Experimental results for the *RiceWrist* operating in the Passive mode.

6. Conclusions and Future work

This chapter has presented an overview of existing arm exoskeleton robotic devices, with a focus on those aimed at upper-extremity rehabilitation. The design and control of the MAHI arm exoskeleton was presented as a case study in exoskeleton design for rehabilitation applications. The device is compact, low-friction and backlash-free with high manipulability in the workspace of interest. Additionally, the MAHI exoskeleton allows unconstrained human arm movements over a large workspace and provides for easy measurement of elbow, forearm and wrist joint angles. The device exhibits excellent behavior under position control with a fast response time, very small oscillations, little overshoot and small steady state errors. Furthermore, there is little structural coupling between various controlled degrees-of-freedom of the device (forearm rotation, wrist flexion/extension and wrist abduction/adduction). The ability of the device to independently provide accurate guidance or kinesthetic feedback to individual human joints is critical during motor learning. It is demonstrated that the device is able to simulate sufficiently stiff virtual surfaces although, the quality of the surface is limited by maximum torque output of the robot.

The chapter concludes by presenting the *RiceWrist*, a sub-set of the MAHI exoskeleton identical in design yet lacking the elbow joint, which has been integrated with the Mirror-Image Motion Enabler (MIME). The *RiceWrist* extends the three unilateral operation modes of MIME to include forearm supination and pronation, wrist flexion and extension, and radial and ulnar deviation. Currently, preliminary trials with healthy patients are underway in order to tune the experimental protocols of the MIME- *RiceWrist* system. Future work will focus on clinical trials with hemiparetic stroke patients to study the efficacy of the approach in forearm/wrist rehabilitation. The device will also be used as a test bed for studying mechanisms of human motor learning and development of training methodologies.

7. References

Basdogan, C., C.-H. Ho, et al. (2001). “Virtual Environments for Medical Training: Graphical and Haptic Simulation of Laproscopic Common Bile Duct Exploration.” *IEEE/ASME Trans. Mechatron.* **6**(3): 269-285.

Bergamasco, M., B. Allotta, et al. (1994). *An Arm Exoskeleton System for Teleoperation and Virtual Environment Applications*. IEEE Int'l Conf. Robot. Automat.

Boman, D. K. (1995). “International Survey: Virtual-Environment Research.” *Computer* **28** (6): 57-65.

Burdea, G. C. (1996). *Force and Touch Feedback for Virtual Reality*, John Wiley Inc.

Burgar, C. G., P. S. Lum, et al. (2000). “Development of Robots for Rehabilitation Therapy: The Palo Alto VA/Stanford Experience.” *Journal of Rehabilitation Research and Development* **37**(6): 663-673.

Carignan, C. and M. Liszka (2005). *Design of an arm exoskeleton with scapula motion for shoulder rehabilitation*. IEEE Conference on Advanced Robotics.

Carignan, C. R. and D. L. Akin (2003). Using Robots for Astronaut Training. *IEEE control syst. mag.* **23:** 46-59.

Charles, S. K. K., H. I.; Volpe, B. T.; Lynch, D. & Hogan, N. (2005). *Wrist Rehabilitation Following Stroke: Initial Clinical Results*. International Conference on Rehabilitation Robotics.

Colgate, J. E. and J. M. Brown (1994). *Factors Affecting the Z-Width of a Haptic Display*. IEEE Int'l Conf. Robot. Automat.

Dirette, D. and J. Hinojosa (1994). “Effects of Continuous Passive Motion on the Edematous Hands of Two Persons with Flaccid Hemiplegia.” *American Journal of Occupational Therapy* **48**(5): 403-409.

Elllis, R. E., O. M. Ismaeil, et al. (1996). “Design and Evaluation of a High-Performance Haptic Interface.” *Robotica* **14**: 321-327.

Erlandson, R. F. (1992). "Applications of Robotic/Mechatronic Systems in Special Education, Rehabilitation Therapy." *IEEE Trans. Rehab. Eng.* **3**(1): 22-34.

Fasoli, S. E., H. I. Krebs, et al. (2004). "Robotic Technology and Stroke Rehabilitation." *Topics in Stroke Rehabilitation* **11**: 11-19.

Feygin, D., M. Keehner, et al. (2002). *Haptic Guidance: Experimental Evaluation of a Haptic Training Method for a Perceptual Motor Skill.* Int'l Sympo. Haptic Interfaces for Virtual Environ. Teleop. Syst.

Gillespie, B., S. O'Modhrain, et al. (1998). *The Virtual Teacher.* ASME Int'l Mech. Eng. Congress Expo.

Goodall, R. M., D. J. Pratt, et al. (1987). "Enhancing Postural Stability in Hemi-Plegics Using Externally Applied Forces." *Intl. J. of Rehab. Research (suppl 5)* **10**(4): 132-140.

Gresham, G. E. (1990). "Past Achievements and New Directions in Stroke Outcome Research." *Stroke* **21 (9 Suppl):II**: 1-2.

Gresham, G. E., D. Alexander, et al. (1997). "Rehabilitation." *Stroke* **28**(7): 1522-1526.

Gupta, A. and M. K. O'Malley (2006). "Design of a Haptic Arm Exoskeleton for Training and Rehabilitation." *IEEE/ASME Trans. Mechatron.* **11**(3).

Gupta, A., V. Patoglu, et al. (2007). "Design, Control and Performance of RiceWrist: A Force Feedback Wrist Exoskeleton for Rehabilitation and Training." *Int'l J. Robot. Research.*

Hesse, S., G. Schulte-Tigges, et al. (2003). "Robot Assisted Arm Trainer for the Passive and Active Practice of Bilateral Forearm and Wrist Movements in Hemiparetic Subjects." *Archives of Physical Medicine and Rehabilitation* **84**(6): 915-920.

Hogan, N. and H. I. Krebs (2004). "Interactive Robots for Neurorehabilitation." *Restorative Neurology and Neuroscience* **22**: 349-358.

Jack, D., R. Boian, et al. (2001). "Virtual Reality Enhanced Stroke Rehabilitation." *IEEE Trans. Neural Syst. Rehab. Eng.* **9**(3): 308-318.

Jeong, Y., Y. Lee, et al. (2001). *A 7 DOF Wearable Robotic Arm using Pneumatic Actuators.* Int'l Symp. Robot.

Khalili, D. and M. Zomlefer (1988). "An Intelligent Robotic System for Rehabilitation of Joints and Estimation of Body Segment Parameters." *IEEE Trans. Biomed. Eng.* **35**(2): 138-146.

Kim, Y. S., J. Lee, et al. (2005). "A force Reflected Exoskeleton-Type Masterarm for Human-Robot Interaction." *IEEE Trans. Syst., Man, Cybern. A* **35**(2): 198-212.

Kousidou, S., N. Tsagarakis, et al. (2006). *Assistive Exoskeleton for Task Based Physiotherapy in 3-Dimensional Space.* IEEE/RAS-EMBS International Conference on Biomedical Robotics and Biomechatronics.

Lay, S. D. and A. M. Day (2003). "Recent Developments and Applications of Haptic Devices." *Comp. Graph. Forum* **22**(2): 117-132.

Lee, K. M. and D. K. Shah (1988). "Kinematic Analysis of a Three Degrees-of-Freedom in-Parallel Actuated Manipulator." *IEEE Trans. Robot. Automat.* **4**(3): 354-360.

Lee, S., S. Park, et al. (1998). *Design of a Force Reflecting Master Arm and Master Hand using Pneumatic Actuators.* IEEE Int'l Conf. Robot. Automat.

Mosher, R. S. (1967). From Handyman to Hardiman, SAE paper no.670088.

Nakai, A., T. Oshashi, et al. (1998). *7DOF Arm Type Haptic Interface for Teleoperation and Virtual Reality Systems.* Int'l Conf. Intell. Robots Syst.

Nef, T., M. Mihelj, et al. (2006). *ARMin – Robot for Rehabilitation of the Upper Extremities.* IEEE International Conference on Robotics and Automation.

O'Malley, M. K. and M. Goldfarb (2002). "The Effect of Force Saturation on the Haptic Perception of Detail." *IEEE/ASME Trans. Mechatron.* **7**(3): 280-288.

O'Malley, M. K. and M. Goldfarb (2004). "The Effect of Virtual Surface Stiffness on the Haptic Perception of Detail." *IEEE/ASME Trans. Mechatron.* **9**(2).

O'Malley, M. K. and A. Gupta (2003). *Passive and Active Assistance for Human Performance of a Simulated Underactuated Dynamic Task.* Int'l Sympo. Haptic Interfaces for Virtual Environ. Teleop. Syst.

O'Malley, M. K., T. Ro, et al. (2006). "Assessing and Inducing Neuroplasticity with TMS and Robotics." *Archives of PMR, Special Issue on Neuroplasticity and Neuroimaging in Acquired Brain Injury: Measurements, Concepts, and Applications.*

Perry, J. C. and J. Rosen (2006). *Design of a 7 Degree-of-Freedom Upper-Limb Powered Exoskeleton.* IEEE Conference on Biomedical Robotics and Biomechatronics.

Prisco, G. M., C. A. Avizzano, et al. (1998). *A Virtual Environment with Haptic Feedback for the Treatment of Motor Dexterity Disabilities.* IEEE Int'l Conf. Robot. Automat.

Reinkensmeyer, D. J., J. P. A. Dewald, et al. (1996). "Robotic Devices for Physical Rehabilitation of Stroke Patients: Fundamental Requirements, Target Therapeutic Techniques, and Preliminary Designs." *Technology and Disability* **5**: 205-215.

Reinkensmeyer, D. J., J. L. Emken, et al. (2004). "Robotics, Motor Learning and Neurologic Recovery." *Annual Reviews in Biomedical Engineering* **6**: 497-525.

Reinkensmeyer, D. J., C. D. Takahashi, et al. (2000). "Design of Robot Assistance for Arm Movement Therapy Following Stroke." *Advanced Robotics* **14**(7): 625-637.

Riener, R., T. Nef, et al. (2005). "Robot-Aided Neurorehabilitation of the Upper Extremeties." *Medical and Biological Engineering and Computing* **43**: 2--10.

Rosen, J., M. Brand, et al. (2001). "A Myosignal-Based Powered Exoskeleton System." *IEEE Trans. Syst., Man, Cybern. A* **31**(3): 210--222.

Rosenberg, L. (1993). *Virtual Fixtures: Perceptual Tools for Telerobotic Manipulation.* IEEE Int'l Symp. Virt. Reality.

Ruiz, A. F., A. Forner-Cordero, et al. (2006). *Exoskeletons for Rehabilitation and Motor Control.* Biomedical Robotics and Biomechatronics, 2006. BioRob 2006. The First IEEE/RAS-EMBS International Conference on.

Shimoga, K. (1992). *Finger Force and Touch Feedback Issues in Dexterous Telemanipulation.* NASA-CIRSSE Int'l Conf. Intel. Robot. Syst. for Space Expl.

Sledd, A. and M. K. O'Malley (2006). *Performance Enhancement of a Haptic Arm Exoskeleton.* Int'l Sympo. Haptic Interfaces for Virtual Environ. Teleop. Syst.

Stein, J. (2004). "Motor Recovery Strategies after Stroke." *Topics in Stroke Rehabiliation* **11**: 12-22.

Sveistrup, H. (2004). "Motor Rehabilitation using Virtual Reality." *J. NeuroEng. and Rehab.* **1**(10).

Thom, T., N. Haase, et al. (2006). "Heart disease and stroke statistics-2006 update: a report from the American Heart Association Statistics Committee and Stroke Statistics Subcommittee." *Circulation* **113**(6): e85-151.

Todorov, E., R. Shadmehr, et al. (1997). "Augmented Feedback Presented in a Virtual Environment Accelerates Learning of a Difficult Motor Task." *J. Motor Behav.* **29**(2): 147-158.

Tsagarakis, N., D. G. Caldwell, et al. (1999). *A 7DOF Pneumatic Muscle Actuator Powered Exoskeleton.* Int'l Workshop Robot and Human Interact. Commun.

White, C. J., A. M. Scneider, et al. (1993). *Robotic Orthosis for Stroke Patient Rehabilitation.* IEEE Intl. Conf. Eng. Med. Biol.

Williams II, Robert L.; Murphy, Mark A.; North, Debra; Berlin, James & Krier, Michael (1998). *Kinesthetic Force/Moment Feedback via Active Exoskeleton*. Image Society Conf.

Wolf, P. A., R. B. D'Agostino, et al. (1992). "Secular Trends in Stroke Incidence and Mortality: The Framingham Study." *Stroke* **23**: 1551--1555.

Yoshikawa, T. (1985). "Manipulability of Robotic Mechanisms." *Int'l J. Robot. Research* **4**(2): 3-9.

22

Upper Limb Rehabilitation System for Self-Supervised Therapy: Computer-Aided Daily Performance Evaluation for the Trauma and Disorder in the Spinal Cord and Peripheral Nerves

Kengo Ohnishi, Keiji Imado**, Yukio Saito* & Hiroomi Miyagawa**
*Okayama Prefectural University, *Tokyo Denki University, **Oita University*
Japan

1. Introduction

With the serious impact on life caused by the disability after cerebrovascular accidents and other serious trauma of the nervous system, prevention strategies and survivors' rehabilitation programs are one of the social needs in many countries. As in super-graying society with low death and birth rate like Japan, an approach of just fostering aid personnel with necessary expertise will not be satisfactory to ensure the quality of the care services. Research in therapeutic technique needs to be paralleled by technology development to reduce the load on the care givers and medical staffs, as well as the development of devices that directly assists the survivors' independent living. Furthermore, advanced efforts are made in Japan to generally decentralize healthcare from clinics to homes and local communities. The escalating healthcare service need to be halted, and strategies such as shortening the patient's hospital stay by reducing the time spent in bed and maximizing the time spent for rehabilitation with the support of technology. To meet our goals, further scientific research is required to understand the factors for enhancing the rehabilitation effects. This will reduce the hands-on one-on-one treatment so that the therapy programs can be provided in homes and local clinics without full-time supervision. With the promising achievements in rehabilitation robotics, we believe further studies on sensor-based assessments and motion control with intelligent systems can support reliable advancements of the therapy programs.
In this chapter, our work on developing a rehabilitator system for cervical spinal cord injured clients is presented. Our main aim is to provide post-hospital-discharge clients with opportunity for voluntary training and to assist self-supervised therapy. Automatic recording, adaptive exercise control, and multilateral analysis are the key technology that we target for recruiting and assisting the client's rehabilitation and medical staff's interest in using the device.

2. Target Population and Rehabilitators

2.1 Cervical Spinal Cord Injury and Therapy

The incidence of Spinal Cord Injury (SCI) lies between 10.4 and 83 per million inhabitants per year by (Wyndaele et al., 2006). One-third of the patients with SCI are tetraplegic and

50% of patients with SCI have a complete lesion. The mean age of patients sustaining their injury is 33 years-of-age, and the sex distribution is 3.8 male per female. Shingu and Sumida (Shingu et al., 1995; Sumida et al., 2001) report the characteristics of Japan. The incidence is 40.2 per million inhabitants per year, which yeilds 5,000 new people per year and 80,000 patients are alive. The statistics on the age of injury for SCI in Japan is different from those with single-peak distribution of the European countries and USA. The Japanese figure is a bimodal distribution with peaks at the age of 20 and 59. From the same statistics, the number of Cervical Spinal Cord Injuries (CSCI) out numbers the thoracic and lumber spine injuries after the age of 40. Furthermore, the rate of CSCI goes up to 88% for those aged over 65. From these figures, it is clear that rehabilitation programs are needed for the new patients at greater age. Another problem is seen in the senior CSCI clients that 15 to 20 years had passed after their injury (Takaoka et al., 1999). Their functional ability declines due to muscular weakness, being easily-fatigued, and pain which are age-related. These clients need nearly full nursing care. And with lower activity, secondary medical condition can be developed to complicate their condition more and restrict the participation to rehabilitation program.

From these facts, rehabilitation for the senior clients is as critical as those for the young injured clients in Japan. The major problems for the senior population are insufficient amount of medical rehabilitation for the acute clients, and strong depression that weakens the motivation to the participation to rehabilitation program for the chronic clients (Takaoka et al., 1999). We believe that both group would benefit from using an easy-to-use therapy device to retrain or maintain their physical ability. As (Lenze et al., 2004) reports, if senior patient's good participation in physical and occupational therapy shortens the length of stay in the hospital, it would be favourable for the clients to use a device during their stay and then take home the same system. That way, the program will be consistent and the clients would have a better understanding of how to use the device and know how to assess their performance after the discharge. Furthermore, if a regular exercise regime would help to control pain as (Latimer et al., 2004) reports, recordings of the exercise session may help the medical professional to gain further understanding of the pain symptom and other comorbidity of SCI.

2.2. Rehabilitators

Many upper limb rehabilitation devices applying robotics and mechatronics technology are developed. Just to name a few devices, they are Massachusetts Institute of Technology Manus (Krebs et al., 1998), Mirror Image Motion Enabler (Shor et al., 2001), Assisted Rehabilitation and Measurement Guide (Kahn et al.; 2001), GENTLE/s (Amirabdollahian et al., 2001; Coote et al., 2003), and Exercise Machine for Upper Limb (Furusho et al., 2003),. These rehabilitators are designed to mainly treat stroke patients' hemiparetic proximal upper limb by passively or partially assisting the motion of the subject (Reinkensmeyer, 2003; Reinkensmeyer et al., 2000). Prange reports on a systematic survey on the clinical results of these rehabilitators (Prange et al., 2006). Due to the limited number of participants in the reviewed papers and their follow up studies, it is still difficult to draw a firm conclusion of the impact of the rehabilitators. However the results show better positive improvements compared to conventional methods in many cases.

These systems with robot assisted rehabilitation enables to provide services with accuracy and repeatability, while recording the performance with quantitative measure. However, robotic system faces difficulty of implementing safety feature requirements to properly use the robot's movability. To reduce the risk at operation, skilled operator needs to be at site to observe the proper process flow and to react on emergency. In addition, further research is necessary to discuss the control method and appropriate set up for the robotic arm to assist the motions and forces to satisfy positive effect of use which a trained therapist will normally do in their program. For robotic rehabilitation, Hogan states based on their research results that 1) muscle strengthening offers no advantage over movement training, 2) passive movements is insufficient and active participation is required, and 3) progressive training based on measures of movement coordination yields substantially improved outcomes (Hogan et al., 2006). Moreover, space, cost, and usability are the decisive factors of purchasing such systems to be used in local clinics or homes. Financial aid as well as technical aids will be needed to have such device widely used.

In addition, the applicant of rehabilitation robot is currently focused on stroke patients. SCI is also known to cause a major physical disability from nerve damage. Peripheral nerve damage in upper limb also strongly affects the hand function and paralyses the digit movements. The lesion of the stroke patient is in the cortical area where the plasticity of the brain will play an important role in the recovery of the functional ability, whereas the lesion of the spinal cord and peripheral nerves are damage to the signal transmission line network. Recovery such as nerve regeneration and reinnervation process may need surgical procedure and will take longer time to regain the function. Therefore, the outcome and methodologies of the stroke rehabilitation may not be fully applied to the rehabilitation strategies for the SCI. Studies on Functional Electrical Stimulation (Popovic et al., 2002; Haugland et al., 1999) for the SCI is also a field where researches are ongoing to obtain joint movements in the upper limb. Their results and other exercise therapy assessment methods should be mutually beneficial. Assessment is one area that all fields can have good information exchange and new assessment technique will contribute in understanding the observable fact in multifaceted approach.

3. Method

3.1 Design Concept and System Structure

Our objective is to develop a device that CSCI clients and medical professionals can use to do the routine exercise at home or neighbouring local clinic, and to evaluate the momentary and temporal changes of the performance. The first goal was to create a prototype hardware and a test-bed training program to run a small field test. Our objective for this study was to confirm whether the device can be used in local clinics without engineer or technician at site, and whether the therapists can recruit outpatients to use the device by themselves on regular bases. With few steps of modification, the device has assisted to encourage a subacute CSCI patient and a chronic CSCI patient with severe depression to use the device to prepare themselves to restart the therapy which they were first a poor participant. Also, a young peripheral nerve injured patient was keen to use the device almost every day over 6 months period. With these small but encouraging successful experiences and constructive data, our next and current goal is to propose an evaluation method that is easy to understand and capable of encouraging the subjects to maintain their exercising routine. Our device had encouraged the subject to work out when the subjects where in a stage where they were still very physically and mentally weak and unprepared for regular therapy programs. However, as the subjects became more active and less physically limited, the exercise and performance scores were unchallenging, monotonous, and unattractive. A more sensitive measure such as feature extraction method that can analyse the data multilaterally with minimum processing load is in need. The ambition of the future system is to automatically or interactively feedback the performance data to the program parameters as in video games and enhance the training effect. This will be our future goal which are discussed later.

3.2 Hardware, Software and Operation

The system consists of a liquid crystal display, a personal computer, interface peripherals, and a joystick-type controller (See Fig. 1). The first prototype controller consists of a grip, joystick module, buttons. The controller has a plastic stage that can be fitted on the laptop of a subject sitting on an adult-size wheelchair or on the device's computer desk. The second prototype is redesigned to be used on desktop and the buttons are omitted by modifying the software to run and respond to conditions automatically. The joystick is a stiff rod and does not have tilt angle as in video game joystick controllers. A tri-axial load cell is developed and installed in the joystick to measure the exerted force. The strain gauge is mounted on the load cell and the amplifier circuit is installed in a case under the stage. Amplified signals from the strain gauges are scanned by 12-bit A-D converter board (Interface Co., Model: PCI- 3171A, Japan). The sampling frequency is 5 kHz. This is conditioned to reduce the rag of marker movements on screen while smoothing the signal with moving-average method. Each of the sampled signals in the horizontal plane is integrated and compared with the initial condition values. Then the differences are assigned to a quadratic function to compute the marker travel distance, dX, dY. The marker travel distance for dZ, which is shown as a floating bar on the screen, is processed in proportion to the difference value.

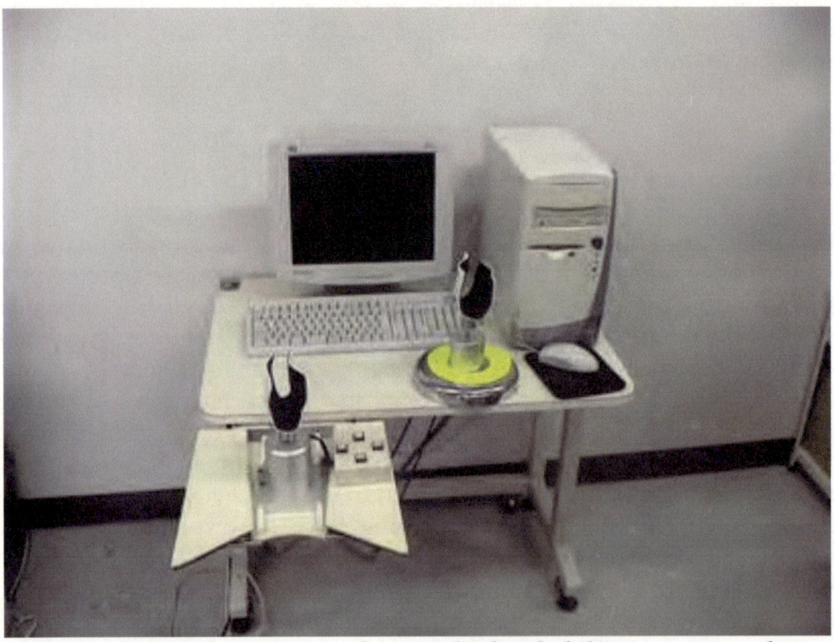

Fig. 1. The first and second prototype of upper limb rehabilitation system for spinal cord and peripheral nerve injury. The first prototype in the front left is mounted on a stage to place on the laptop. The second prototype is for desktop use.

The system operation is like a video game. A circle and a flower shape trajectory are arranged for exercise and evaluation menu (See Fig. 2). Sagittal plane is set as the Y-axis (vertical axis) on the trajectory, and the frontal plane as the X-axis (horizontal axis). A red circle target and a green square marker are presented on the screen. The target on the trajectory moves at a constant angular speed, counter-clockwise from the initial position on the positive X-axis. The subject's goal is to maintain the marker within minimum distance to the target center. The subject controls the marker by applying force to the joystick based on the visual information of the trajectory and target-marker distance. The system diagram of the operation is shown in Fig.3. The exercise session is followed by a one-minute presentation of the performance result. The locus of the marker and score are computed from the recorded performance data and presented on the screen.

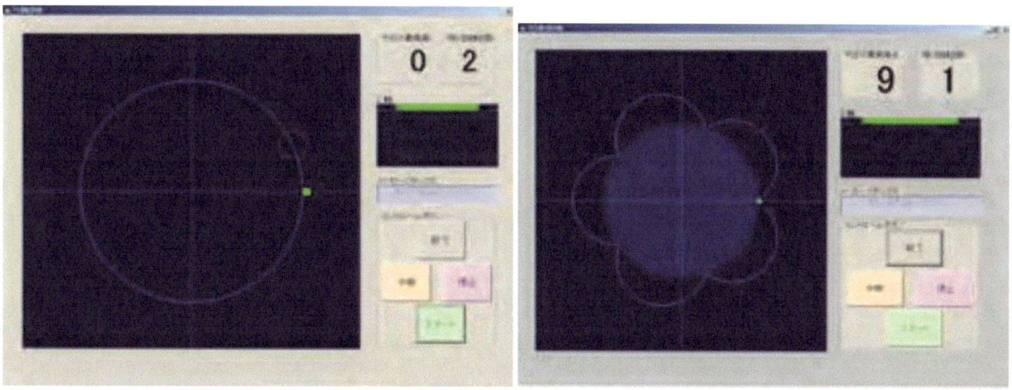

Fig. 2. Two trajectory, circle and flower shape, are created for the exercise screens. The red small circle on the trajectory is the target which is followed by the green square marker that the subject operates. Forces applied to the joystick in sagittal and frontal plane propels the marker in X-Y coordinate. The bar in the middle right represent the force applied to the vertical axis and moves like a floating stick with buoyancy.

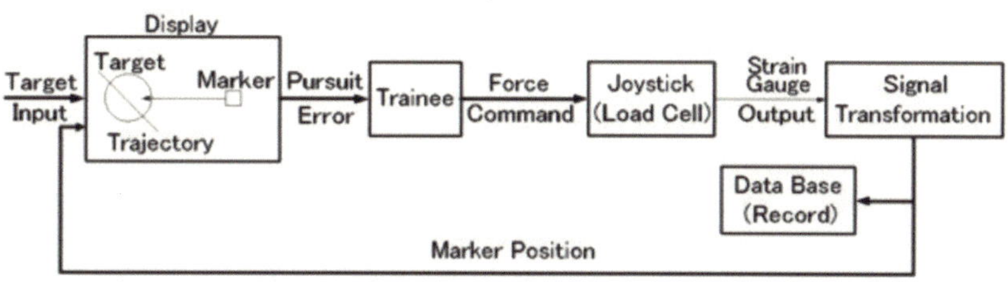

Fig. 3. The system diagram of the operation scenario.

3.3 Performance Indices

Many performance indices are proposed to evaluate the recorded upper limb operation data. Krebs' group reported their two categories of performance indices based on the type of human-machine interaction, with and without robot assistance (Krebs et al., 2001). Hand path displacement, lateral deviation of subject's movement from a straight line connecting the targets, and other 4 indices are calculated as the unconstraint indices. Mean force, speed, and power are calculated during the robot assistance as the constraint indices. Furusho's group uses positioning deviation in time series to discuss their subject's performance changes as the training proceeds (Furusho et al., 2003). Takahashi's group described the subject group's characteristics by describing the data in relation of the time required for the task to the sum of square of error distance (Takahashi et al., 2003). Chelette's group compared the sensitivity of time domain parameters and phase plane parameters as metrics of performance. The time domain parameters showed usefulness in distinguishing subject ability groups, however they recommend error phase plane parameters because of their higher sensitivity to the effect of special force reflection (Chelette et al., 1995). Ide's group proposed four phases in cursor operation; response time, approaching time, adjusting time, and switching time (Ide et al., 1995). With total time, number of inching operation, and the four indices, they described the characteristic of the CSCI patients' joystick operation. Murayama developed a system that uses a stylus pen and a monitor with a built-in digitizer to evaluate the performance of drawing circular trajectory (Murayama, 2002). For analysis, he proposed mean velocity, acceleration, and power spectrum of the squared residual error to characterise the difference of the subjects and the effect of rehabilitation.

As in these earlier studies, we also used residual error distance in time domain as our main evaluation index. The marker locus $\boldsymbol{M}$ is calculated by summing dX and dY in time sequence, as in Equation (1). The error distance is calculated as the distance of the marker position $\boldsymbol{M}$ and the target position $\boldsymbol{T}$ as in Equation (2).

$$X_M(t)=\sum_{n=0}^{t} dX(n)+X_0, \quad Y_M(t)=\sum_{n=0}^{t} dY(n)+Y_0 \tag{1}$$

$$E(t)=\sqrt{\{X_T(t)-X_M(t)\}^2+\{Y_T(t)-Y_M(t)\}^2} \tag{2}$$

$\{\boldsymbol{M} \mid X_M(t), Y_M(t)\}$: Marker position,
$\{\boldsymbol{T} \mid X_T(t), Y_T(t)\}$: Target position,
$E(t)$: Error distance
t: sampled time

Since our target tracking scenario exercises a steady amplitude force generation in all circumference direction, the distribution of the control signal is also assessed. By plotting the forces in F_x-F_y coordinate and discussing the density of the plotted points, the result in the early stage of the experiment showed wider distributed pattern, whereas the latter were congregated to a relation of sum of $|F_x|$ and $|F_y|$ being constant.

As mentioned previously, the momentary target-marker distance is a common measure for discussing the performance. This error in time series describes the subject's continuous positioning error which is an accumulated response delay. Therefore, the result is strongly influenced by the response at the starting point and the ratio between target speed and the gain of marker displacement. The result is influenced by the feedfoward characteristic during the learning curve which will diminish when the target speed is constant. The performance characteristic can be further studied by presuming a control system and identifying the parameters in a model-based approach. Furthermore, the performance can be studied in space, frequency or non-dimensional domain instead of discussing it in time or time-space domain. In this study we chose to model the geometrical characteristic to discuss the precision. Since our target trajectory is based on circles, we implemented a method used in measuring the roundness to discuss the position error as next.

When considering the target trajectory as a perfect circle, the marker locus can be presumed as distorted circle. That is, the marker locus can be identified as a sinusoidal waveform with distortion component that can be expressed as periodic function. Consequently, harmonic analysis (Nakata, 1972) is implemented to model the performance locus. On identification, the center of target trajectory coordinates O is set as the center of roundness measurement. When the marker locus is described as K and the center of the target trajectory as O, a norm circle M is computed. M is a circle with an center O′ and radius a_0. See Fig. 4 for their relation. By describing the displacement of center O′ in polar coordinates as (c_1, ϕ_1), locus K is expressed as Equation (3) through (7). The coefficient of the right end term in Equation (3) is insignificant when n is significant, and consequently, n can be agreed as a finite number. In our algorithm n = 24 is applied, therefore 24 equally divided harmonic analysis is used to calculate the norm circle's eccentric relation (c_1, ϕ_1) and a_0. Here, the compared distortion $\varepsilon(\theta)$ is the subtraction of the norm circle M from the locus K, as Equation (8). We equally divided the circle in 24 segments so the compared distortion is computed as ε_p at the selected 24 point on the circle.

$$K:\ k(\theta) = a_0 - E + a_1 \cos\theta + b_1 \sin\theta + \sum_{n=2}^{\infty}(a_n \cos n\theta + b_n \sin n\theta) \quad (3)$$

$$a_0 - E = \frac{k_1 + k_2 + \cdots + k_{23} + k_{24}}{24} \quad (4)$$

$$a_1 = \frac{k_1 \cos(\pi/24) + k_2 \cos(\pi/12) + \cdots + k_{23}\cos(23\pi/24) + k_{24}}{12} \quad (5)$$

$$b_1 = \frac{k_1 \sin(\pi/24) + k_2 \sin(\pi/12) + \cdots + k_{23}\sin(23\pi/24)}{12} \quad (6)$$

$$c_1 = \sqrt{a_1^2 + b_1^2}\ ,\ \varphi_1 = \tan^{-1}(-b_1/a_1) \quad (7)$$

$$\varepsilon(\theta) = \varepsilon_p = k_p - \{a_0 + a_1\cos(p\pi/24) + b_1 \sin(p\pi/24)\} \quad (8)$$

$$\because p = 1, 2, \cdots, 24$$

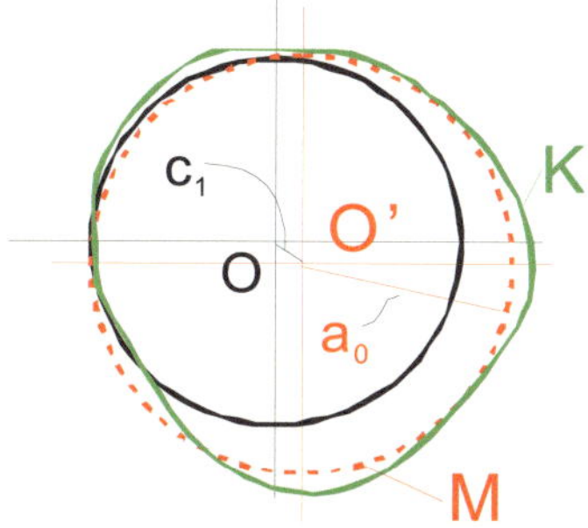

Fig. 4. Diagram of the norm circle and parameters in the harmonic analysis.

The recorded data is calculated offline into the four variables c_1, ϕ_1, a_0, and ε_p. First, the marker locus ***L**:[x,y]* is computed by summing the marker displacements for unit time, Δx_t and Δy_t, and then transformed to polar coordinate L_p: *[k,θ]*. The radius of the target trajectory E is normalized (= 1), and the marker locus K is transformed accordingly. On selecting the k_p from the converted marker locus data, the value corresponding for θ with the closest acceptable approximation to n_p (= 0, 15, 30, …, 360 degrees) is chosen. We used 0.5 degrees in the algorithm for processing the locus that is virtually a circle. When no candidate is found, acceptable range is expanded. The algorithm will halt with an error in case where the marker locus does not close as a circle and forms a C-shape. This occurs when the subject drops greatly behind the target and the final position of the marker does not come near to the starting point before the unit session time is up. In such case, the value for the θ closest to 360 degree is chosen to fill in the data. Furthermore, the marker locus over wraps when the marker over runs the target and reverses. In such locus, k_p is chosen from the most neighboring value to n_p.

4. Field Test and Evaluation Results

All subjects were tested following informed consent. Twelve able-bodied subjects □8-male and 4-female, average age 22.6, Std. Dev. 0.99□participated in the pilot test for creating the database and to confirm the validity of the index and algorithm. The two CSCI subjects' data was then applied to computation. These data was collected after approval of the study from the Institutional Review Board of each hospital that the subjects were receiving their medical treatment. Informed consent was given from the therapist before the test. The first subject was a senior male ambulatory patient and the trials were made at his presence to the clinic on his pace. This subject was paresis and capable of walking but had numbness in both arms at the beginning of the test. The numbness had decreased to a level that there was no discomfort when the subject withdrew from the test. The second subject was a senior male hospital patient. He was a quadriplegic and both arms were very weak and the voluntary ranges of motion of the upper limb joints were limited to minimal. He had strong depression and needed personal care for all activity at the beginning of the test, but regained partial strength in the shoulder by the end of first 4 weeks of the test. Both patients had returned to the clinic reporting decrease in their upper limb sensory-motor function and to reapply for a treatment.
The target speed was set to 1.0 rpm. The controller was set on the side table and the hand position was adjusted to suit each patient. The first CSCI subject had four sets of each circle and flower-pattern trajectory pattern as routine exercise session and the second CSCI subject had two of each pattern. Testing began after the patient understood how to control the marker on the screen by practicing on the demonstration mode and the gains in the controller were adjusted for each subject at the beginning of the test. No modifications were made to the condition through the whole trials.
Ten days of data was recorded between a 49-days period for the first subject, and 18 days of data was recorded between an 85-days period. The first and tenth day's data of both subjects were evaluated with the proposed indices. The marker loci of the two subject's last trial in their session are shown in Fig. 6. The target-marker error distance are described in Fig. 7.

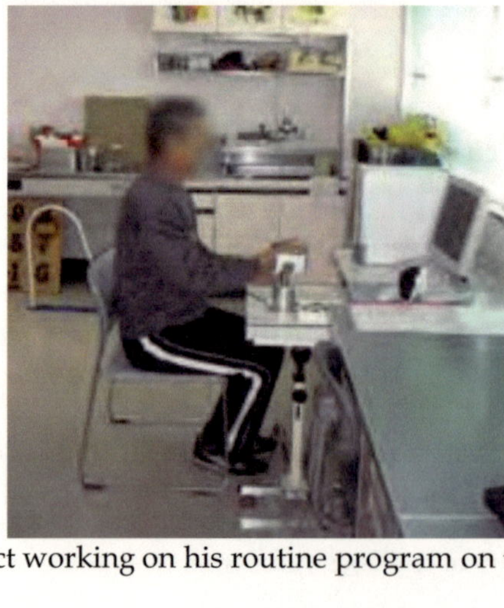

Fig. 5. The first CSCI subject working on his routine program on the device.

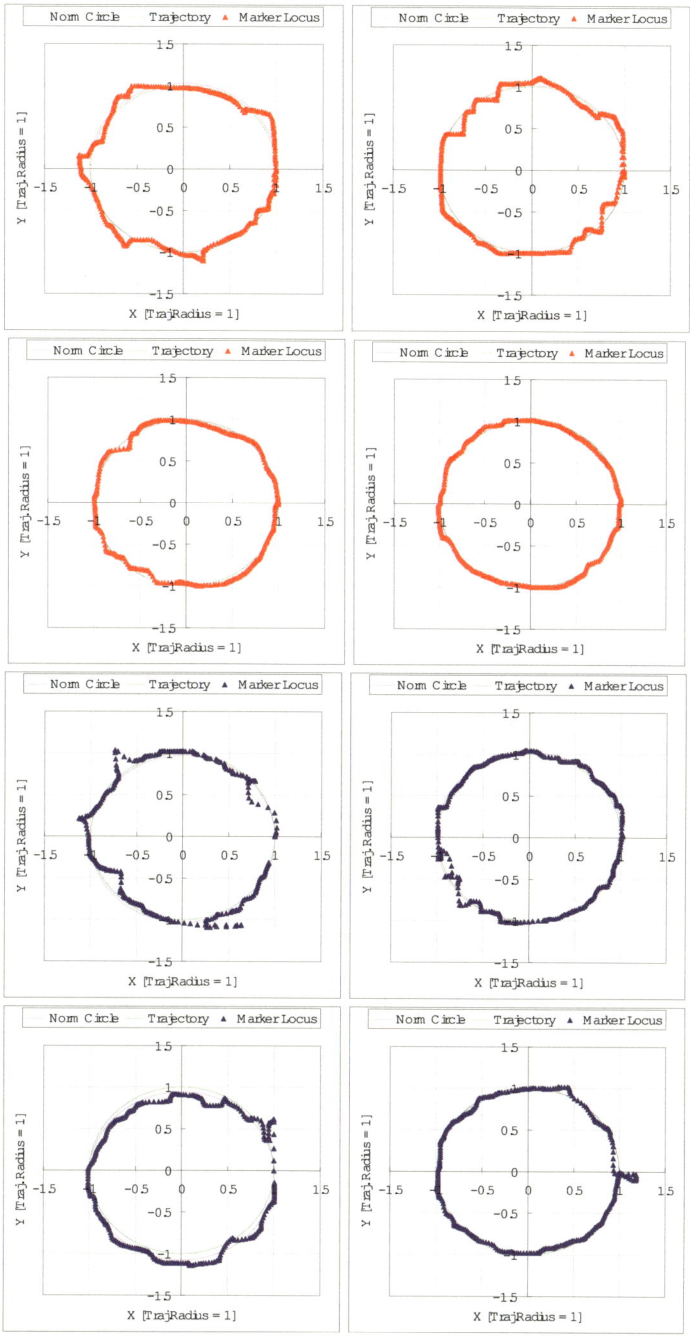

Fig. 6. The diagram of the 1st (top 4) and 2nd (bottom 4) CSCI subject's marker loci and norm circles of each trial. The 1st and 3rd row are their 1st day's, and 2nd and 4th row are their 10th day's data. The graphs in the left column are the first and the right column are their last trials of each day.

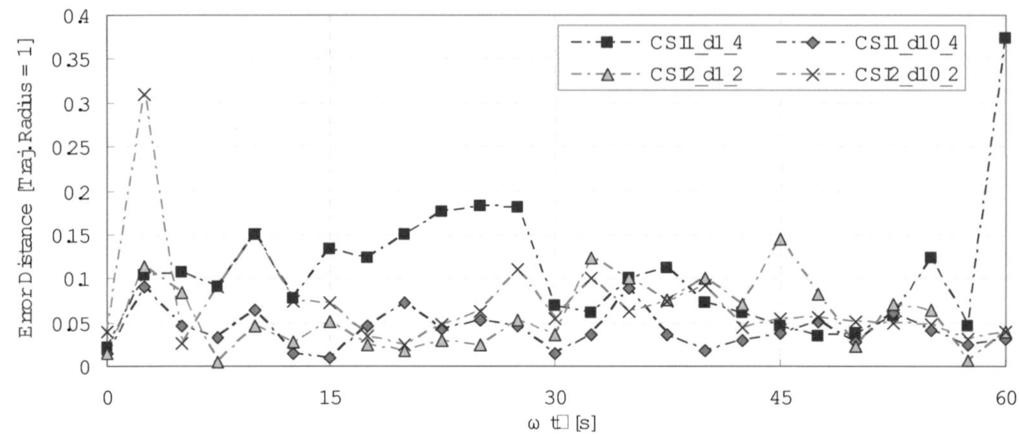

Fig. 7. The variance of error distances in time series. The first and second CSCI subject's data are presented as CSI1 and CSI2, accordingly. The 1st day's data is shown as d1 and 10th day's data as d10. The data are all last trials of the day.

5. Discussion

The first CSCI subject's performance on the first day is shown at the top row of Fig. 6. As seen in the right diagram's locus, the track is relatively square. This illustrates that the direction of the marker was only changed in a while. The error distance for this session's result drawn in Fig. 7 are higher then the other 3 results. When interpreting these information from the graphs, you can picture that the subject was having difficulty following the target. However, it is difficult to comment the major cause of the error was whether he was running behind the target or off the trajectory. Also the upsurge at the end of the trial in Fig. 7 cannot be found on the locus of top right diagram of Fig. 6. For the second subject the dislocation at the start on the tenth day's locus in the bottom right diagram of Fig. 6 can be confirmed as the peak at the left end in Fig. 7. The immediate decrease of error distance in Fig. 7 shows that subject had instantly caught up to the target. However, there is another rise of error around 30s in Fig. 7. For the first day, the cause is running off the trajectory seen as the wavering in the diagram of Fig. 6. However, since no major wavering of the locus is seen in the bottom right diagram of Fig. 6, it is assumed that the cause of the 10th day's result is delay.

To confirm the error in space domain, the variables c_1, ϕ_1 , a_0, and ε_p are computed. The results of a_0 are described in Fig. 8, the eccentric relation in Fig. 9, and ε_p in Fig. 10. It is shown in Fig.8. that all error of the norm circle radius is less than 2% of the target trajectory's radius. Furthermore, the variations of the radius within a day are smaller on the tenth day for both subjects. From Fig. 9, it shows that the majority of the dislocated center remain within the 2% range of the c_x-c_y coordinates. Compared with this, the second subject's first session's result are located exceedingly to the negative side in the c_y direction. Furthermore, both CSCI subject's results show that the distance from the center had decreased in their tenth day's session. In Fig. 10, the maximum distortion had decreased in the 10th day's data for both subjects. These diagrams interpret the strategies of following the target in a quantitative manner. The points inside the 0 describes that the subject is taking a shorter path and moving the marker with reduced effort to track the target. If the error distance is small and the distortion is negative as in the top-left area (t = 15-30 s, n = 6-12) of the second-subject's first-day data, the subject is presumed to be relaxed and composed of following the target. In contrast, when the error distance is large and distortion is negative as in the bottom-left area (t = 30-45 s, n =12-18) of the second-subject's tenth-day's data, the subject is presumed to have difficulty following the target and learned to take a shorter path to compensate the delay. Consequently, the geometrical information is quantitatively comparable and feature are extracted with these indices for further understanding of the performance.

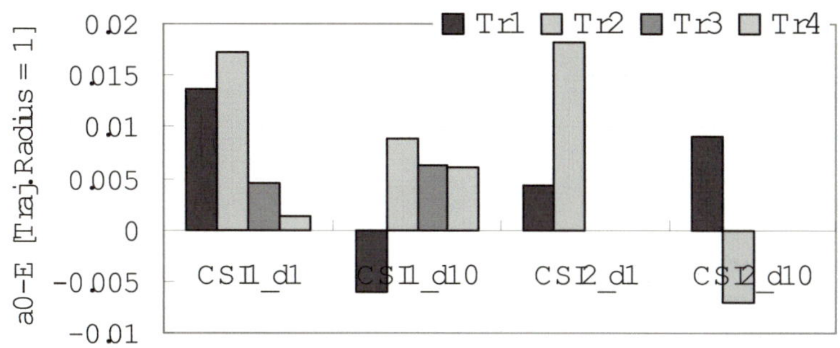

Fig. 8. The error of the norm circle's radius to the target trajectory's radius in each exercise session of the CSCI subjects. Left two are the first subject's and right two are the second subject's results. The d1 in the figure are for the 1st day's data and d10 are for the 10th days data. Tr1 through Tr4 are the order of the exercise session in each day.

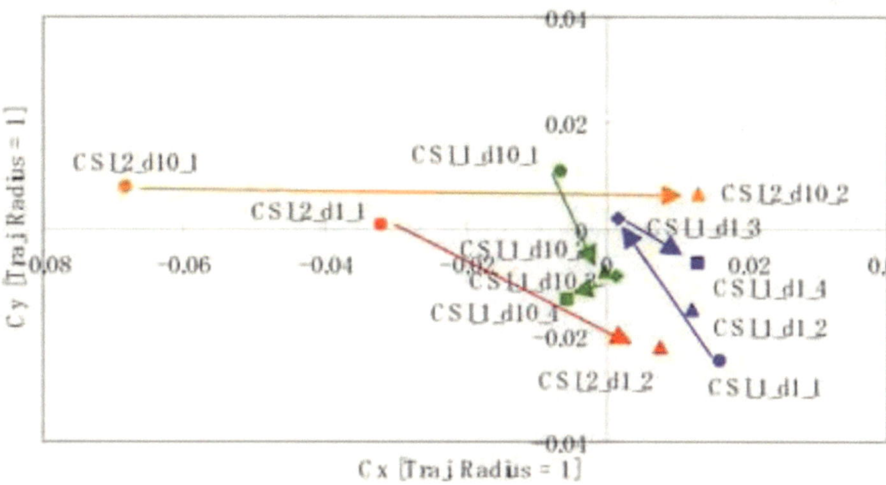

Fig. 9. The eccentric relation of the norm circle in each exercise session. The arrows describe the time variance of the norm circle center within the session. The first and second CSCI subject's data are presented as CSI1 and CSI2, accordingly. The 1st day's data is shown as d1 and 10th day's data as d10. The trials are described as _1 to _4.

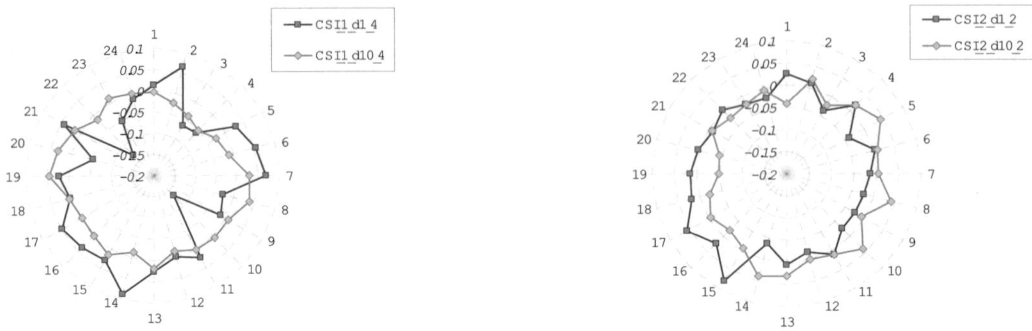

Fig. 10. The distortion of the marker trajectory to the norm circle. Left is the result of the first CSCI subject and the right is the result of the second CSCI subject. The numbers 1 to 24 describes the points in 15- degrees increment from the starting position around the target trajectory.

6. Future Research

Based on our experience with our subjects the scores presented after each unit session strongly affect the subject's motivation. The subjects were first very pleased with the scores being higher then they expected. However, our simple scoring algorithm based on the error distance rating was not sensitive to the gradual performance changes they were making. The mismatch of the score and what they sensing on their performance improvement has caused less interest of continuing the exercise. The computational results show that indices of harmonic analysis can extract feature of the subject's performance quantitatively. Therefore, these indices may help to set an adequate goal for the subjects to attempt. As an example, matching the norm circle radius to the target trajectory can be a short time goal to begin with, and then the eccentric relation. If we gain further understanding of the exercise effect on the neuromuscular function, the goals can be established based on previous successful rehabilitation cases or target tasks that the subject aims of achieving. As an example, a participant who joined the test earlier commented that the training helped him to regain stability of driving with a steering wheel. An exercise scenario can be created to reinforce such task accomplishment.

To enhance further understanding of the recovery of the upper limb function in spinal cord and peripheral injuries, utilizing electromyogram (EMG) recordings in parallel with the joystick device will be useful. Calacie's group showed that EMG recording was more accurate for predicting contractile force within multiple muscle groups at both acute and chronic stages following spinal cord injury. And with the EMG recording system, they had found that recovery of voluntary contraction in motor-incomplete injury tends to occur after 5 week post-injury, which are post hospital discharge (Calacie et al., 2004). The disadvantage of the EMG method is that the system is expensive and requires time consuming setup. With these conditions, it is unlikely to be used at home or local clinics, therefore easier method such as our system to confirm the timing of recovery will be beneficial. Further study to correlate the EMG activities with force-based positioning will be needed.

Further research is needed for developing an automatic adjustment function in the exercise scenanrio. Target speed and marker's response to the applied force should be automatically

tweaked based on feeding back performance score. In our testing setups, the marker's response to the force, i.e. marker gain, was adjusted to the individual with trial and error. By applying Jacobs' result in (Jacobs et al., 2004) , where the peak and mean power loading differed from the level of injury and the subject's body mass, it would be superior to create a database to automate or ease the selection in the initial adjustment. Method based on evidence should be more reasonable for the medical staffs and would be a better interface than numerically or graphically setting the parameters. Furthermore, it would assist the evaluation with proper bias on comparing the data with different level of functional disability.
Further study on advanced method for robust multidimensional data analysis is needed for these devices to be more useful in the clinical condition where the subjects have wide variety of disability and neuromuscular function is unstable. A methodology with higher accuracy and sensitivity without adding additional cost for the diagnosis will be an indispensable requisites to develop such device at a suitable scale. We believe Mahalanobis-Taguchi System will be one of the key tools to implement (Kanbayashi et al., 2006). This evaluation method creates an unit distance scale from the similarity among the ideal or healthy data constellation. Mahalanobis distance is computed as an level of anomalousness or the degree of severity. When the result is larger than a single unit on the scale, the distance from the center is presented as the tested data's abnormality. Therefore, the prominent the abnormal condition is the greater the computed distance will become. To implement this method, data from an able-bodied subjects are collected to create the scale. Then the different level of CSCI and peripheral nerve disorder subject's should be evaluated to correlate the scale with the functional limitation. By discussing the distribution of the subjects' performance score of the clinically distinctive level and equivocal level, the accuracy and sensitivity can be verified.

7. Conclusion

The research backgrounds and the design concepts of a simple take-home system for upper limb rehabilitation of the cervical spinal cord and peripheral nerve injured subjects are presented. A force-based target tracking task is selected for application. A method for evaluating the performance on a circular locus is presented and the result of implementing the algorithm is described. Using the harmonic analysis method quantifies the geometric character of the locus and adds sights to understand subject's performance in a quantitative manner. Our result are limited due to small number of subjects and further experiments are needed. Further work is needed to create a exercising program scenario based on quantitative and subjective indices and clinical testing.

8. References

Amirabdollahian, F.; Loureiro, R.; Driessen, B. & Harwin, W. (2001). Error correction movement for machine assisted stroke rehabilitation, In: *Integration of Assistive Technology in the Information Age*, Mokhtari, M. (Ed.), 45-59, IOS Press, ISBN1-58603-171-6, Amsterdam

Calancie, B.; Molano, M.R. & Broton, J.G. (2004). EMG for assessing the recovery of voluntary movement after acute spinal cord injury in man, *Clinical Neurophysiology*, 115, 1748-1759, ISSN 1388-2457

Chelette, T.L.; Repperger, D.W. & Phillips C.A. (1995). Enhanced metrics for identification of forearm rehabilitation, *IEEE Transactions on Rehabilitation Engineering*, Vol. 3, No. 1, 122-131, ISSN1063-6528

Coote, S.; Stokes, E.; Murphy, B. & Harwin, W. (2003). The effect of GENTLE/s robot-mediated therapy on upper extremity dysfunction post stroke, *Proceedings of the 8th International Conference on Rehabilitation Robotics*, 59-61, ISBN89-88366-09-3, Daejeon, Korea, Apr., 2003, HWRS-ERC, Daejeon

Furusho, J.; Koyanagi, K.; Ryu, U.; Inoue, A. & Oda, K. (2003). Development of rehabilitation robot system with functional fluid devices for upper limbs, *Proceedings of the 8th International Conference on Rehabilitation Robotics*, 31-34, ISBN89-88366-09-3, Daejeon, Korea, Apr., 2003, HWRS-ERC, Daejeon

Goto, E.; Ohnishi, K.; Miyagawa, H. & Saito Y. (2005). Field test of a force control rehabilitation system for quantitative evaluation of the disorder in the upper extremities, *Proceedings of the 2005 IEEE 9th International Conference on Rehabilitation Robotics*, 82-85, ISBN0-7803-9004-0, Chicago, IL, USA, June, 2005, Omnipress

Haugland, M.; Lickel, A.; Haase, J. & Sinkjær, T. (1999) Control of FES thumb force using slip information obtained from the cutaneous electroneurogram in quadriplegic man, *IEEE Transactions on Rehabilitation Engineering*, Vol. 7, No. 2, (June) 215-226, ISSN1063-6528

Hogan, N; Krebs, H.I.; Rohrer, B.; Palazzolo, J.J.; Dipietro, L.; Fasoli, S.E.; Stein, J; Hughes, R; Frontera, W.R.; Lynch, D. & Volpe, B.T. (2006). Motions or muscles? Some behavioural factors underlying robotic assistance for motor recovery, *Journal of Rehabilitation Research & Development*, Vol. 43, No. 5, (Aug./Sept.) 605-618, ISSN 0748-7711

Ide, M.; Fujiie, K; Mitarai, K. & Kurosu, K. (1995). Operational characteristics of joystick with single-speed floating action on cervical injuries, *The Japanese Journal of Ergonomics*, Vol. 31, No. 2, 141-149

Jacobs, P.L.; Johnson, B.M.; Mahoney, E.T.; Carter, A.B. & Somarroba, G.A. (2004). Effect of variable loading in the determination of upper-limb anaerobic power in persons with tetraplegia, *Journal of Rehabilitation Research & Development*, Vol. 41, No. 1, (Jan./Feb.) 9-14, ISSN 0748-7711

Kahn, L.E.; Averbuch, M.; Rymer, W.Z. & Reinkensmeyer, D.J. (2001). Comparison of robot-assisted reaching to free reaching in promoting recovery from chronic stroke, In: *Integration of Assistive Technology in the Information Age*, Mokhtari, M. (Ed.), 39-44, IOS Press, ISBN1-58603-171-6, Amsterdam

Kanbayashi, Y.; Saito, Y.; Yano, H. & Ohnishi, K. (2006). Evaluation study of an arm training system for patients with cervical spinal cord injuries, *Quality Engineering*, Vol. 14, No. 3, (June 2006) 69-74 (in Japanese)

Krebs, H.I.; Hogan, N.; Aisen, M.L. & Volpe, B.T. (1998). Robot-aided neuro-rehabilitation, *IEEE Transactions on Rehabilitation Engineering*, Vol. 6, No. 1, 75-87, ISSN1063-6528

Krebs, H.I.; Volpe, B.T.; Palazzolo, J.; Rohrer, B.; Ferraro, M.; Fasoli, S.; Edelstein, L. & Hogan, N. (2001). Robot-aided neuro-rehabilitation in stroke: interim results on the follow-up of 76 patients and on movement performance indices, In: *Integration of Assistive Technology in the Information Age*, Mokhtari, M. (Ed.), 45-59, IOS Press, ISBN1-58603-171-6, Amsterdam

Latimer, A.E.; Martin Ginis, K.A.; Hicks, A.L. & McCartney N. (2004). An examination of the mechanisms of exercise-induced change in psychology well-being among people with spinal cord injury, *Journal of Rehabilitation Research & Development*, Vol. 41, No. 5, (Sept./Oct.) 643-652, ISSN 0748-7711

Lenze, E.J.; Munin, M.C.; Quear, T.; Dew, M.A.; Rogers J.C.; Begley, A.E. & Reynolds III, C.F. (2004). Significance of poor patient participation in physical and occupational therapy for functional outcome and length of stay, *Archives of Physical Medicine and Rehabilitation*, Vol. 85, (Oct) 1599-1601, ISSN 0003-9993

Murayama, N. (2002). Technical approach for rehabilitation medicine: development of a quantitative analysis system for voluntary movement functions in the upper limb, Japanese Journal of Rehabilitation Medicine, Vol. 39, No. 11, 735-743 (in Japanese)

Nakata, T. (1972). *Engineering Analysis*, Ohm, Tokyo (in Japanese)

Ohnishi, K. ; Goto, E.; Ikeuchi, H.; Imado, K.; Miyagawa, H. & Saito, Y. (2005). Development testing of a force control rehabilitation system for disorder in the upper extremities, *Proceedings of the First International Conference On Complex Medical Engineering*, 504-509, ISBN4-9902522-0-9, Takamatsu, Japan, May, 2005

Ohnishi, K.; Goto, E.; Sugiki, F.; Imado, K.; Ikeuchi, H.; Kito, N.; Miyagawa, H. & Saito, Y. (2004). Home-use upper limb rehabilitation device for cervical spinal cord injured patients, In: *Computers helping people with special needs*, Miesenberger, K.; Klaus, J.; Zagler, W. & Burger, D. (Eds.), 880- 888, Springer-Verlag, ISBN3-540-22334-7, Berlin Heidelberg.

Ohnishi, K.; Miyagawa, H.; Negoto, H. & Saito, Y. (2003). Rehabilitation system for arm-eye coordination of the palsy arm, *Proceedings of 6th Japan-France Congress on Mechatronics and 4th Asia-Europe Congress on Mechatronics*, 117-122, Hatoyama, Saitama, Japan, Sept, 2003

Popovic, M.R.; Popovic, D.B. & Keller, T. (2002) Neuroprostheses for grasping, *Neurological Research*, Vol. 24, (July) 443-452, ISSN0161-6412

Prange, G.B.; Jannink, M.J.A.; Groothuis-Oudshoorn, C.G.M.; Hermens, H.J. & IJzerman M.J. (2006). Systematic review of the effect of robot-aided therapy on recovery of the hemiparetic arm after stroke, *Journal of Rehabilitation Research & Development*, Vol. 43, No. 2, (Mar./Apr.) 171-184, ISSN 0748-7711

Reinkensmeyer, D.J. (2003). Chapter 35 Rehabilitators, In: *Standard handbook of biomedical engineering & design*, Kutz, M. (Ed.), 35.1-35.17, McGraw-Hill, ISBN0-07-135637-1, New York

Reinkensmeyer, D.J.; Hogan, N; Krebs, H.I.; Lehman, S.L. & Lum, P.S. (2000). 38 Rehabilitators, robots, and guides: new tools for neurological rehabilitation, In: *Biomechanics and neural control of posture and movement*, Winters, J.M. & Crago, P.E. (Eds.), 516-533, Springer-Verlag, ISBN0-387-94974-7, New York

Shingu, H.; Ohama, M.; Ikata, T.; Katoh, S. & Akatsu, T. (1995). A nationwide epidemiological survey of spinal cord injuries in Japan from January 1990 to December 1992, *Paraplegia*, Vol. 33-4, 183-188, ISSN 0031-1758

Shor, P.C.; Lum, P.S.; Burgar, C.G.; Van der Loos, H.F.M.; Majmundar, M. & Yap. R. (2001) The effect of robotic-aided therapy on upper extremity joint passive range of motion and pain. In: *Integration of Assistive Technology in the Information Age*, Mokhtari, M. (Ed.), 79-83, IOS Press, ISBN1-58603-171-6, Amsterdam

Sumida, M.; Tokuhiro, A.; Magara, A.; Toyonaga, T. & Uchida, R. (Eds.), (2001). *Clinical outcome of spinal cord injury*, Ishiyaku Publishers, ISBN4-263-21125-1, Tokyo (In Japanese)

Takahashi, Y.; Terada, T.; Inoue, K.; Ito, Y.; Lee, H. & Komeda, T. (2003). Upper-limb rehabilitation exercises using haptic device system, *International Journal of Human-friendly Welfare Robotic Systems*, Vol.4, No.2, 18-22

Takaoka, T.; Wakabayashi, H. & Ito, T. (1999). Rehabilitation for home-bound elderly disabled with spinal cord injury, *Journal of Clinical Rehabilitation*, Vol. 8, No. 10, 943-950 (In Japanese)

Wyndaele, M. & Wyndaele, J-J. (2006) Incidence, prevalence and epidemiology of spinal cord injury: what learns a worldwide literature survey? *Spinal Cord*. Vol. 44-9, 523–508, ISSN 1362-4393

23

PLEIA: A Reconfigurable Platform for Evaluation of HCI acting

Peralta H., Monacelli E., Riman C., Baklouti M., Ben Ouezdou F., Mougharbel I. 1 , Laffont I.[2] & Bouteille J.[2]

LISV, Engineering Systems Laboratory of Versailles, Versailles Saint Quentin en Yvelines University, France.

[1]Lebanon University, Lebanon

[2]New Technologies Platform, Raymond Poincaré Hospital France

1. Introduction

For people with severe motor disabilities, it is difficult or sometimes impossible to use standard interface devices (mouse, keyboards, joysticks, trackballs, etc …). The evaluation of their capabilities, the education or re education of abilities and the compensation of their deficiencies is essential. Nowadays, the performance of a person is only determinated by the observation of the trajectory followed by the cursor during the exercises and to facilitated people's accessibility to computer and electrical devices, few exist. Standard test and reliable indicators would bring a better evaluation of the use of peripheral interfaces for motor handicapped people. Two ways of research have been developed: some researchers have focused on defining new peripheral devices, others have focused their works on new rehabilitation process and algorithms to adapt commands. We assume that we are able to associate on the same study of pointing task: computer, wheelchair and environment control.

2. Problem

For the handicapped person, the use of interface controls could be a very complex task. The systems for aiding the person are controlled by an interface. It is founded on the relation between the Human Computer Interactions (HCI). The most important problem in the Human interaction is the adequacy between the user and the interface: computer, wheelchair, remote control… Moreover, the wide range of motor disabilities makes impossible the development of standard solutions. In most cases, a customized interface device is developed to fit to the deficiency of person. Some laboratories focused their researches on the design and the development of a personalized and adjustable Human-Computer Interface (HCI). However, for motor disabilities, few studies based on the interface tasks and quantitative evaluations were conduced. Nowadays, there are few works that present simple and reliable indicators (Buaud A.,2003)(Kadouche R, 2004) for evaluating the performance of impaired users. Usually this task is achieved by a qualitative evaluation led by the therapist (fig. 1). There are some methods for evaluating the dexterity. For example, the method used today by the occupational therapist is based on the functional evaluation by a direct analysis of the other activity acting as operator (cinesiologic analysis):

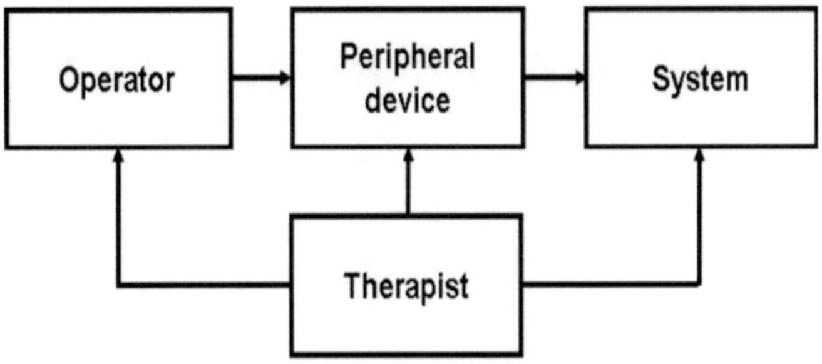

Fig. 1. Evaluation scheme for normal therapy session.

The therapist acts on the operator, the peripheral device and the system. This system can be a personal computer, an external system such as powered wheelchair or a toy. The feedback used by the therapist is qualitative. The therapist is able to adapt the device changing internal parameters (such as sensibility, position, as well as, the configuration of system). These corrected actions are done following the therapist expertise.

3. Objective

PLEIA (Peralta H., 2006) software can be integrated into the evaluation scheme (fig. 2) as assistive system for the therapist.

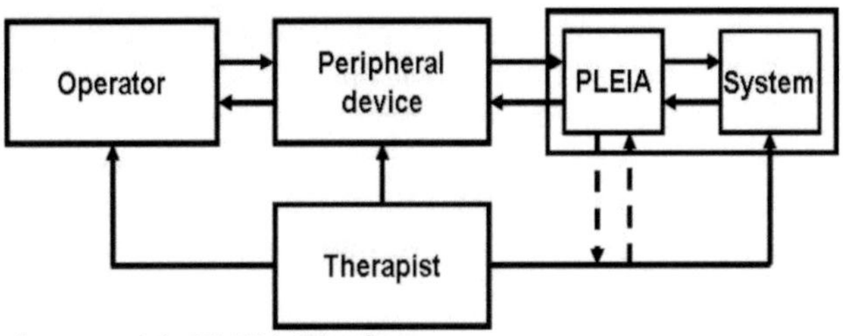

Fig. 2. Evaluation scheme with PLEIA Platform.

PLEIA gets information from the peripheral device. The therapist can access to these information. Then he can act on PLEIA, on the peripheral device or on the system. The evaluation of their capabilities by the interface capabilities is essential. Today in the scope of adaptation and quantitative measures of capacity, few evaluation standard methods exist. The evaluation are oriented to handicap, but the information measured just allow to determinate delay and trajectory by basic indicators. Therefore, it is necessary to find new methods to evaluate the peripheral devices by computers processing's mean. The monitoring of the user capability is useful for determining the diagnostic information. The plan for the rehabilitation could be also based on evaluation result (Dipietro, L. 2003). Thus, it is necessary to have a set of quantitative criteria, a therapy methodology and common tools to be applied by the occupational therapist.

The objective is then to define suitable exercises associated with quantitative criteria in order to evaluate the adaptation between the user and the peripheral (fig. 3). It includes performance but also handling evaluation at a time and on a period training.

4. Related Research

4.1 Evaluation studies

There are studies to determine analytical evaluation from the pointing devices with the user interaction. The first work about the hand movement is the Fitt's Law which is based on a model of human psychomotor behavior developed in 1954. It gets the measure of a Movement Time (MT) index. This is the result of the relationship between movement time, distance, and accuracy. Many works about the evaluation of movement and Human Computer Interaction (HCI) are based on this law.

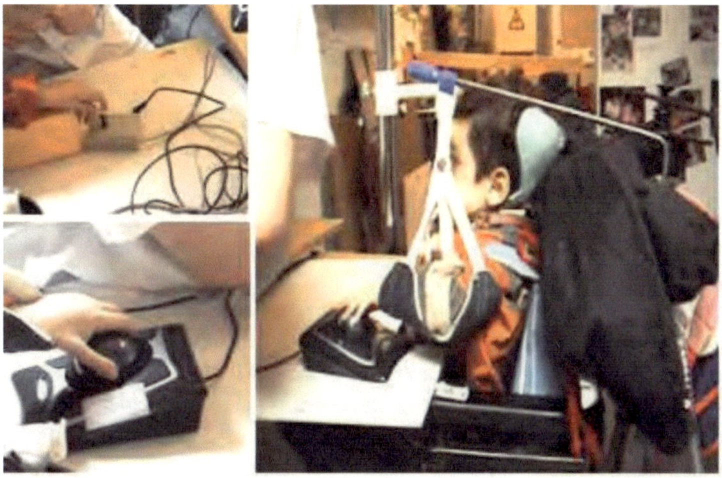

Fig. 3. Examples of peripheral device.

The main interest in this law is that it can be applied to pointing and dragging using a mouse, trackball, joystick, and touch screen (Keates, S., 2002) (Soukoreff, R. 2004). Mackenzie (MacKenzie, I., 2001) proposed seven new accuracy measures to evaluate computer pointing devices. The measures are intended to elicit subtle differences among devices through an analysis of the cursor movement along the cursor path. The ISO standard to assist evaluation of pointing devices is ISO 9241: "Ergonomic design for office work with visual display terminals (VDTs)." The part 9 is "Requirements for non-keyboard input devices". In (ISO 9241-9) are included mouse, joysticks, track ball, tablets and overlays, touchpad, touch sensible screens. The standard specifies the quality of the input devices in terms of performance criterion: "it is considered useable, if users can achieve a satisfactory level of performance on a given task and maintain an acceptable level of effort and satisfaction".

4.2 Methods to improve the mobility with pointing systems

If the interface is correctly adapted to the abilities of user, there are many solutions to improve it. Some solutions have been developed for accessibility and mobility. These solutions are based on command sensor adaptation processing. For example, "smart wheelchair", "adaptive interfaces" and "adaptive commands" (Thieffry, R., 2005) develop assistive methodology in order to reduce the physical, perceptual, or cognitive skills necessary to operate with safety a powered wheelchair or another system (walker or computer pointing system). Other works on assistive robotic wheelchair system improve the acting by the design of specific sensor interfaces like in the Wheelesley (Yanco, H., 2002). (Kang, S., 2004) shown one joystick for a system like an electric wheelchair. This system helps to drive easily and safety. Another system was experimented. (Jeong, H. 2004) proposed a new Human-Computer-Interaction (HCI) method for a quadriplegic, which is controlled by clenching teeth. Two clenching patterns, did seven instructions including rest, up, down, left and right as well as click and double click actions are made for the control of a pointing device. The control source is EMG[1]. An experimental system of voice interface is presented in (Tellex, S., 2005). It is an alternative controlled manner. The system "understands" natural language motion commands. The works show the possibility to compensate and improve the user mobility. The big parts of such systems use a pointing interface as command access. The questions are then: How could the users have the right peripheral device? It is convenient for his proper abilities? Can another interface improve his development on the control of his system? A step of evaluation with different interfaces is necessary.

4.3 Evaluation platforms

Platforms for improving the HCI acting based on exercises have been developed (Shimizu, H., 2006) for re-educational therapy. Today, the computer applications include graphical interfaces. Actions as "click", "displace", "drag and drop" are essential to handle a computer. There are many software, for handicapped persons that basically are centered on learning. For example, Judy Lynn Software, Inc. offers different categories of software for different patient (depending upon age and symptom), these work to improve certain activity as visual tracking, cause effect, hand - eye coordination, etc. We can find similar software of many companies as: Marblesoft, Simtech publication, Widget software. In conclusion, the exercises proposed by these softwares have an educational interest but they do not include a performance evaluation of user acting. Adeprio Diffusion proposes to save the results of patient acting. Efficasouris (Adameczek, A., 2005) is a software developed to evaluate the pointing capabilities of patient with the mouse, saving the performance. The designers have built four modules: 1) The game module, 2) The statistical module to save the performance data of patient, 3) Diagnostic or User identification and personal perception (this module is a questionnaire model, used to know qualitative the point of view on test and software) and the last one, 4) Virtual Keyboard, serves to design a virtual keyboard adapted to the patient from the analysis data. The last module is the objective of efficasouris. The medical team realizes subjective analysis (based on a questionnaire) and objective analysis which are made directly (observation of the interaction with the user during the test) and indirectly (using cameras and record data performance). The software has three indexes: task time, task error, and clicks number (accuracy). Another example is Catch Me™ by lifetool. It is evaluation software with interesting properties as creation of exercises, tuning of exercises and parameters configuration as mouse speed, colors, forms, wallpapers, volume. The analyzed results are: game time, right actions number, wrong actions number and average time by action. This does not include information on the user handling.

The following section explains the main idea for therapy methodology on PLEIA software.

---

[1] Electromyogram (EMG)

5. PLEIA

5.1 Description of Software Platform for Interface & Interface Evaluation (PLEIA)

The PLEIA software platform (by French acronymic) is our specialized evaluation platform. The PLEIA proposes an open methodology (fig.4) to evaluate the user's dexterity with the pointing devices using different peripheral computer devices at the end of the process. It allows to adapt these devices to characteristic of user using different feedback modes (light, sound, haptic, etc...) dedicated to occupational therapist. PLEIA tools allow to elaborate specific exercises based on functional systems: from computer interface to wheelchair command.

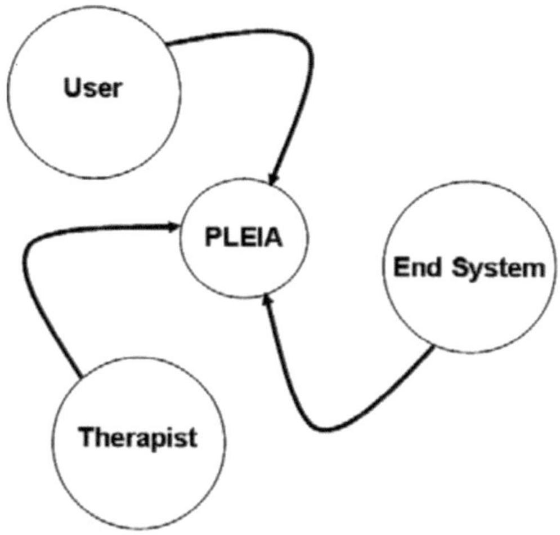

Fig.4. PLEIA as centre of the evaluation, assistance and compensation process.

The therapy session could be oriented on different goals: function learning (especially for the young children), evaluation of dexterity with different peripheral and generalization for other systems like wheelchair command. PLEIA is composed on three blocks with the same functionalities:

- **PLEIA evaluation**: This module was programmed to evaluate the dexterity through 5 main tests: 1) Reach Target, 2) Drag and drop, 3) Follow path, 4) Click Targets, 5) Exploration screen zones. This chapter is centered on this module.
- **PLEIA functional awaking**: This module allows user to act on real object (robots, toys, etc.). It is dedicated for the young children. The same evaluation could be done.
- **PLEIA functional**: This module is dedicated to evaluate handling of a powered wheelchair (often goal of the therapy).

PLEIA is a program that allows therapist to create specific exercises with scenarios. It could be connected to different peripheral interfaces (joystick, trackball, mouse, keyboard, etc.) and act on devices as robot (khepera™), toys and electric wheelchair. All information and performance data (time, errors, coordinates, etc ...) are analyzed. The patient tests different peripheral devices. The therapist evaluates which is more adequate for pointing systems. Different analytic indexes have been developed (see section 6). The therapist could create suitable configurations of exercise (named scenarios) with different tuning parameters such as cursor speed, sound, cursor and objects dimensions and appearance. This platform can be connected for remote experiment with other medical centers. Basically, PLEIA includes different exercises. The proposed test could include different elements, such as obstacles, objectives to reach, object to take, trajectories, cursor. These elements are shown in (fig. 5).

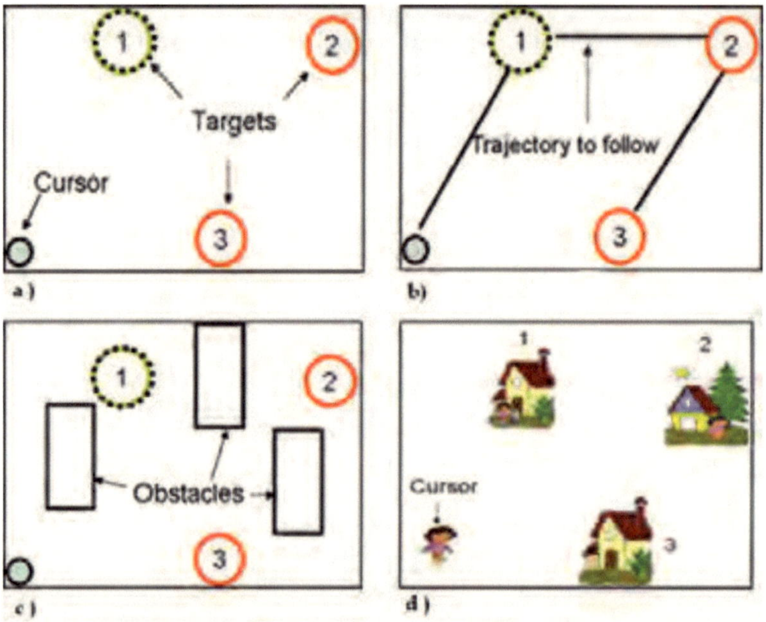

Fig. 5. Exercise models on PLEIA Software with the same scenario: a) Reach the targets, b) Follow path, c) Avoid the obstacles, d) Mode tuned.

Reach the targets (fig 5a), the aim of this test is to evaluate a displacement. The trajectory is shown by sequence of object. The dotted circle is the next objective to reach. The (fig. 5b) shows the same configuration of target, with path constraint. The next scenario (fig. 5c) is used when the patient present uncontrolled movements. The trajectory includes targets and obstacles to avoid. The (fig. 5d), shows the same test with different images. The therapist uses them to improve the attention of children. Fig. 9 present other example of PLEIA test.

5.2 PLEIA Functionalities

The functionalities that PLEIA offers are:

- Exercise configuration assistance:

The configuration of exercise is based on a wizard processing in order to be user friendly.
The medical team is able to choose the suitable exercise for evaluating the patient performance. We suggest five main model exercises: (1) Reach target: reaching certain objects on the computer screen. (2) Drag and drop: It refers to the capacity to hold a button and at the same time do the displacement. (3) Follow path: It evaluates the capacity of following a track. (4) Click on the targets: this test has been thought to measure the user accuracy, with different target sizes. (5) Exploration screen zones: this exercise evaluates work reachable space. It is very important to mention that the objects designed by the therapist on the scenario (trajectories, obstacles, wallpapers, etc) can be simple or complex depending upon the type of exercise. The decision is taken by the therapist.

- Patient test information:

PLEIA memorizes user actions (see section 6).

- Performance indexes as trajectory length, errors, clicks used in the exercise, accuracy, time delay, and command analysis.
- Assistance Mode:

To compensate the patient disability, We used feedback such as visual, audio, or vibration associated to test conditions (ex. Impact with the obstacle) to inform the user. Specific assistance like sensitive attraction could be used in the execution.

6. Method evaluation

6.1 Participants.

We present in this section, two children evaluations, Claudia and Robert. Each participant was identified as "child with disability" by the medical team. They can not use mouse, basic joystick or trackball because of their limitation in the mobility and muscular weakness. The fatigability is another factor to take into account. The test must take a few minutes (1 to 2 min), and the session has a 45 min duration at the worst case fro the good results.
Claudia is four years old child. She suffers from myopathy. She uses minitrack stick. She handles it with the left index finger. Special technical adaptations are required (fig. 6).
Robert is seven years old child. He suffers from myopathy, uses a mini joystick HMC™ with InfraRed connection. Robert uses the left thumb finger to handle his medical aid.
We have then introduced new indicators that could help the therapists to evaluate the performance of each patient.

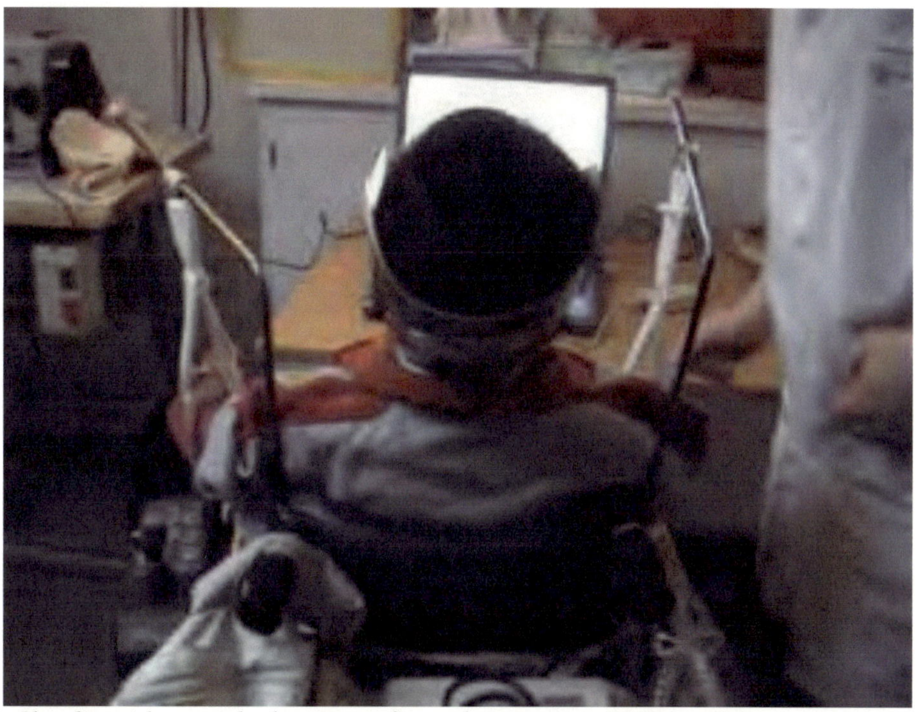

Fig. 6. Claudia with special adaptations for makes a test on PLEIA software.

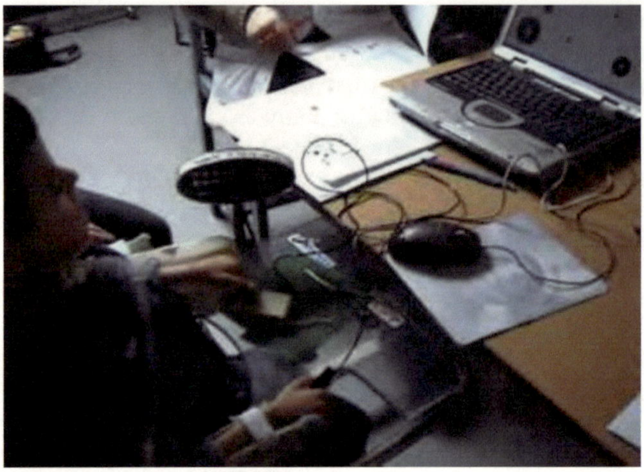

Fig. 7. Robert in therapy session with PLEIA.

These indicators have been implemented in a software platform (PLEIA). It is developed in collaboration with the Raymond Poincare Hospital and Saint Maurice Hospital (Paris Hospital).
PLEIA include user information. It includes the data of test, date, disabilities of patient, and other information of patient.
The patient is placed in front of monitor (between 0.60 m to 0.80 m). The computer's devices are installed in the best condition of comfort and functionality for the patient. This last condition depends upon the deficiency and the position of the patient (fig. 8).

6.2 Measurement and performance indexes

The indicator based on a set of performance focus the peripheral adaptation problem. In other words, they allow quantifying the realization of pointing tests and to appreciate the choice and the configuration of the peripheral device. They carry out comparisons to appreciate the evolution of the results of one user or relative to different classes of users.

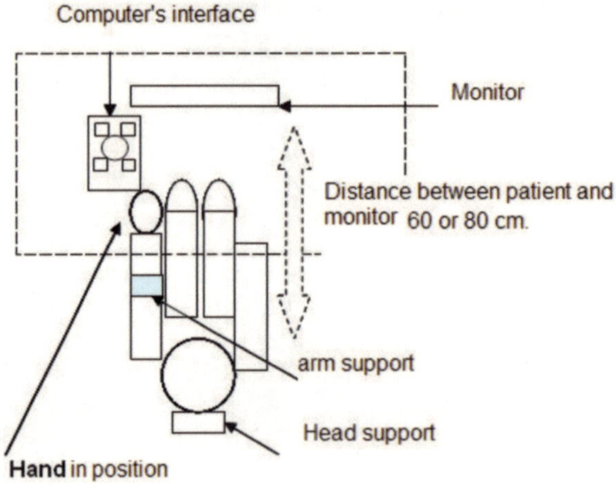

Fig. 8. Localization of patient.

We defined two groups of indicators: (a) task indicators which use direct results of the test execution, (b) comfort indicators which are centered on the behavior of the patient.

1) Task indicators: The indicators of tasks are the first order indicators which give a direct classification of the performances of the user. Based on tests, we retained three basic measurements:

- **Total time of exercise (TT)**: It is the time to finish the exercise.
- **The Covered Distance (CD):** It is the addition of all cursor displacement.
- **The collision (C) or Failure (F)** is a problem occurrence in the test: collision with obstacle, target unreachable.

2) Comfort indicators: The indicators of comfort have been introduced to evaluate user easiness in manipulating the device. The proposed indicators are:

- **Pause Rate (PR):** This indicator calculates the ratio of cursor stop delay in the exercise. This indicator expresses the "fatigue" of the user on a specification test with peripheral.

$$PR = \frac{PT}{TT} \tag{1}$$

PT: Pause time
TT: Test time.

- **User Action (UA).** This indicator estimates the number of user action on the peripheral interface.

$$UA = \sum_{i=0}^{TT} \left[(K_1 \Delta I_1)_i^2 + (K_2 \Delta I_2)_i^2 \right] \tag{2}$$

ΔI_1, ΔI_2: Peripheral inputs variation (between two sequential inputs).
TT : Test Time
i : Sample time in the test.
K_1,K_2: Normalization gains

- **Command Load (CL):** This indicator estimates the interface action number of the user versus a reference user.

$$CL_{user} = \frac{UA_{user}}{UA_{ref}} \tag{3}$$

UV_{ref} : User action variation (Valid person).
UV_{user}: User action variation (User)

- **Efficient Coefficient (EC).** It estimates the efficiency of user commands. An inefficiency is defined as the user actions that tend not to optimize the result of the test

$$EC = \sum_{i=0}^{TT} \left[\left((K_1 I_1)_i^2 + (K_2 I_2)_i^2 \right) * K_3 \Delta Gd_i \right] \tag{4}$$

ΔGd_i : Goal distance variation on the sample i

ΔI_1, ΔI_2: Peripheral inputs variation.
TT : Test Time
i : Sample time in the test.
K_3,K_1,K_2: Normalization gains

- **Efficient Load (EL)**. This ratio estimates the user efficiency between the Reference Efficient Coefficient (EC) getting of valid user and the User Efficient Coefficient, multiplied by the Rate Time. This Ratio Time is defined as reference total time (time to finish the test by the Reference User) and the user total time.

$$EL_{user} = \frac{EC_{ref}}{EC_{user}} * \left(\frac{TT_{ref}}{TT_{user}} \right) \quad (5)$$

EC_{ref} : Efficient Coefficient (Valid user).
EC_{user} : Efficient Coefficient (user).
TT_{ref} : Test Time reference (Valid user)
TT_{user} : Test Time reference (user)

7. Experimentation

The exercise designed for the children by the occupational therapist (fig. 9) is a sequence of 12 targets.

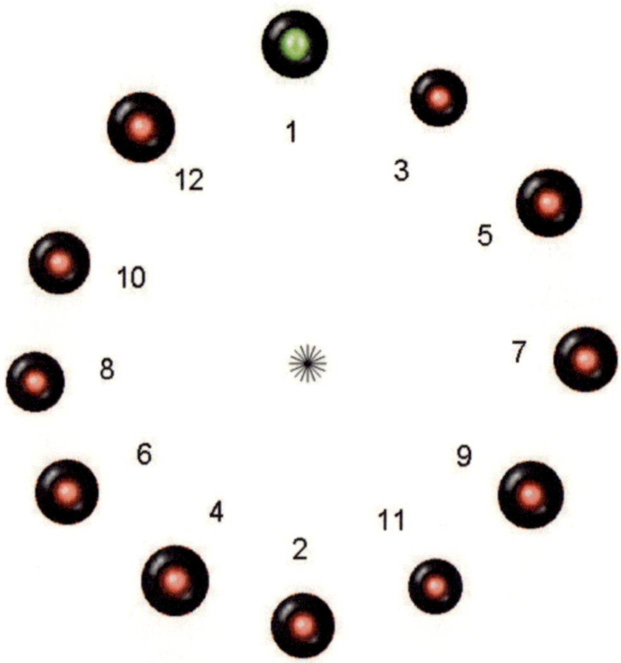

Fig. 9. Exercise designed for the Children

For a best understanding, PLEIA (configured by the therapist) displays sequentially only the next target, and hides the others. When the next target is reached, it is cleared and another appears. One sound can be also associated (feedback configuration, target reaching). This exercise does not have obstacles avoidance and the aim is the evaluation of dexterity.

o Experimentation with the abilities of Claudia.

Claudia knew PLEIA in November 2006. Her mobility and understanding were limited and difficult. This child had trouble with the test "follow path". This child could not avoid obstacles and the movements sometimes were without control. Then, the therapist proposed a test without obstacles and path. At first time it was only a simple test with one target. She practiced the test many times. After, the therapist proposed an exercise more complex. Test with 12 targets to reach. This article is based on two evaluations done in February 2007, November 2006 with the same 12 target test (fig.10 and 11) and the same technical aide and settings. Before , she practiced the model test proposed by the therapist without data saved. The therapist explained and practiced with her the activity and movements wanted. The therapist says when the patient has understood the activity, then, the data are saved.

The first session, Claudia made four practical test, the data were saved after (fifth test). The total test in the first session was eight. Trajectories at the beginning were sometimes uncontrolled.

The second session, the practical test number, was increased, because, the therapist saw that the patient did the test without difficulty, the test number in this session was nine. We can see that the movements in the second test are more optimized. The understanding about the aim of the exercise is better. She has a tactic to reach the target: when she goes to reach the next target, the displacement is very fast and exceeds the position of the target, then, she comes back to the target with circular and controlled slowly movement.

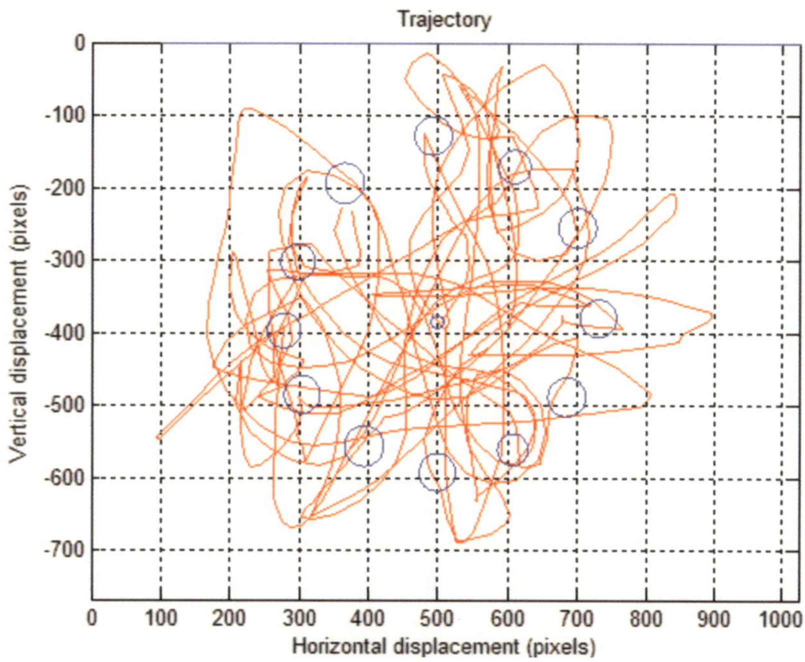

Fig.10. Trajectory of Claudia in November 2006.

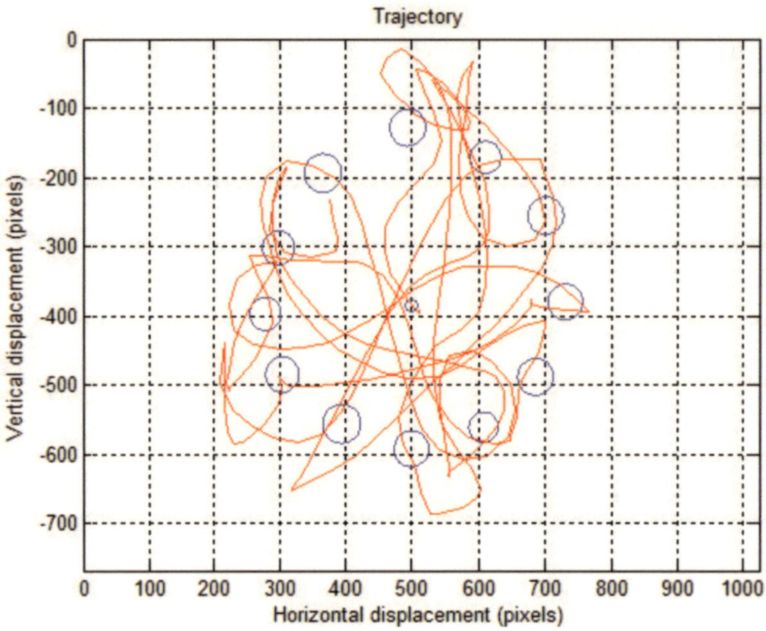

Fig.11. Trajectory of Claudia in February 2007.

The fig.12. Shows the evaluation phases distance in time (ms) for the two exercises. The scope of the first curves (noted (a)), is longer than the second (noted (b)). The displacement in the first exercise is slower than in the second test. The user action index (UA) represent user action on the peripheral device, this index is a function of the energy cost that the user must employ to realize the test. This index gives information to the adaptation between the user and his peripheral.

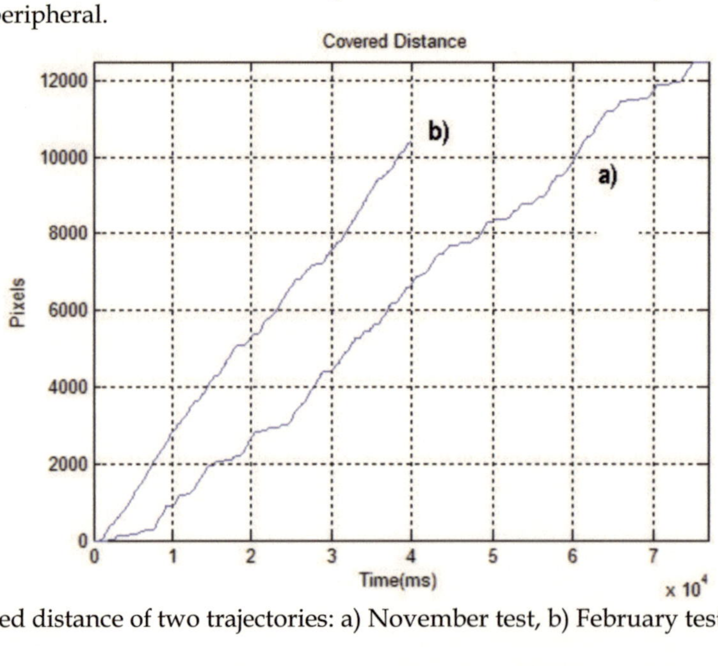

Fig. 12. Covered distance of two trajectories: a) November test, b) February test.

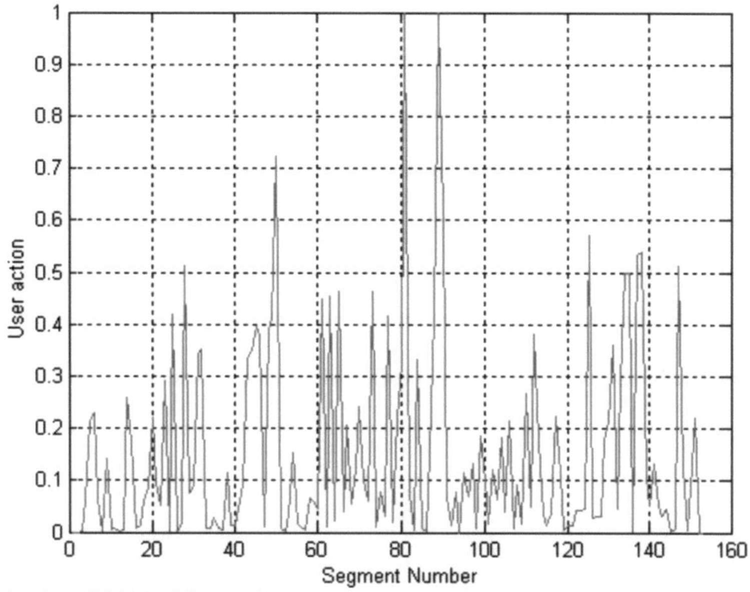

Fig. 13. User Action (UA) in November.

The Command Load (**CL**), shows the rate between the Action User versus a Reference User. Claudia acts more on the peripheral in the first test (2.43 on **CL**) . The efficiency Load (**EL**) is different (8 to 27 %). In fact Claudia had understood the test because the **RP** was lower (13.65 to 2.5). It is not an adaptation of peripheral but an adaptation of Claudia (a cause of training). She was more ready for the evaluation test (see table 1).

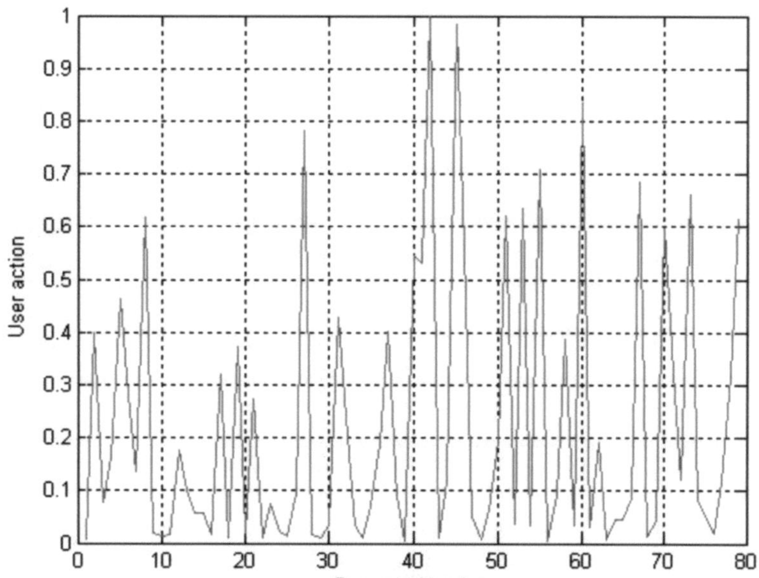

Fig. 14. User Action (UA) in February.

Sample	Test Time (TT) (ms)	Covered Distance (CD) (pixels)	Rate of Pause (RP) (%)	**Command Load** (CL)	Efficient Load (EL) (%)
Nov2006	76900	12500	13.65	2.43	8
Feb2007	39900	10500	2.5	0.89	27

Table 1. Claudia results.

- Experimentation with Robert

The first contact of Robert with PLEIA was in May 2006. The test shows, were made in November 2006. He has a good control on the technical aid but he acts slowly. The same exercise was used, in similar conditions.
Fig. 15 and 16 show two trajectories. We can notice that he has a good control on his technical aid. The trajectories are "cleaner" and very specific, He has a little problem with the diagonal trajectory, but the straight lines are good.

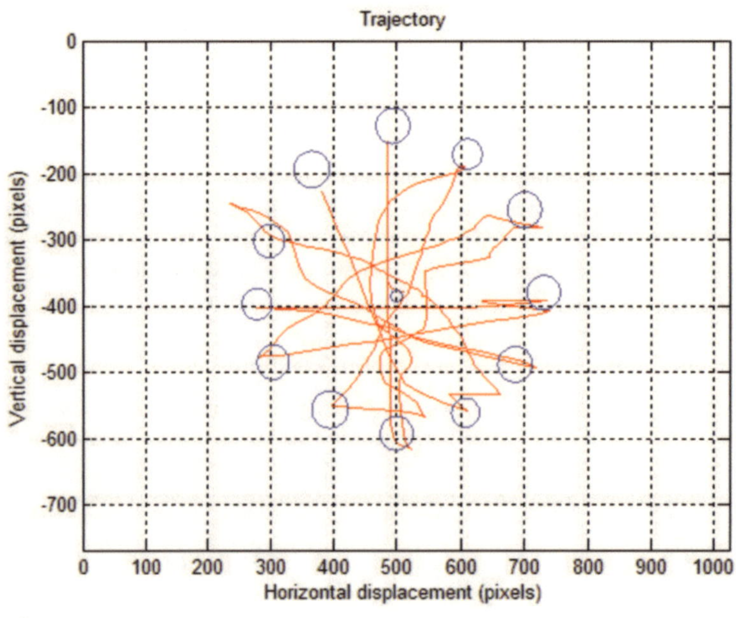

Fig. 15 Robert first trajectory

The occupational therapist observes that when Robert reaches the target, he makes a little pause. He is planning a few seconds the best trajectory to reach the next target. He has employed more time in the test 1 that the test 2 (10 %).
Between the two test, Robert has increase the number of actions (CL = 1.14 to 1.58 %) with some benefit (TT decrease of ~10%). However, he increases his efficiency (EL from 53 to 97%), see table 2.
In fact, in comparison with Claudia, the behavior is similar however he has a biggest pause rate (16.80). It means that Robert is more cerebral and he takes advantage from pause to stratify the next actions. Claudia is more reactive on peripheral. The result is that Robert acts more efficiently that Claudia.

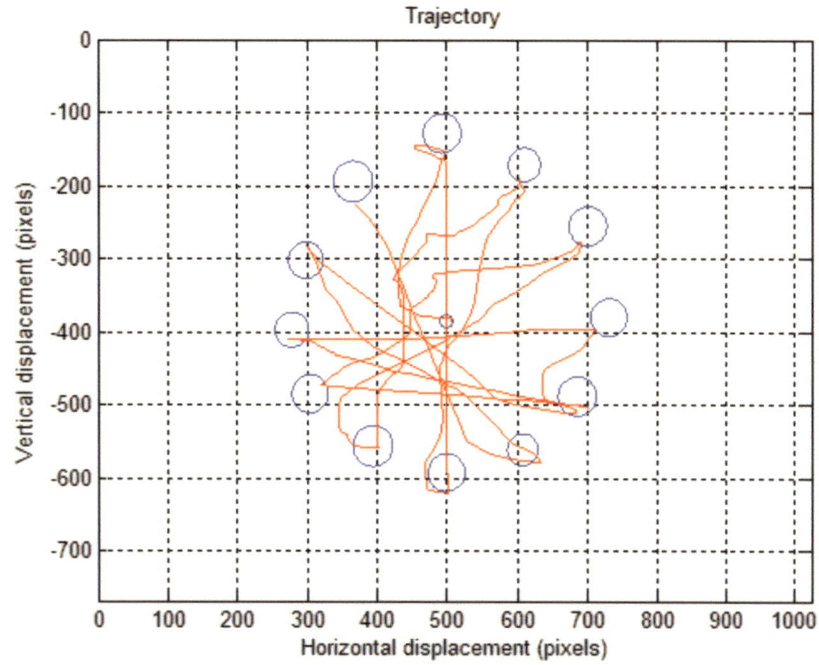

Fig. 16. Robert second trajectory.

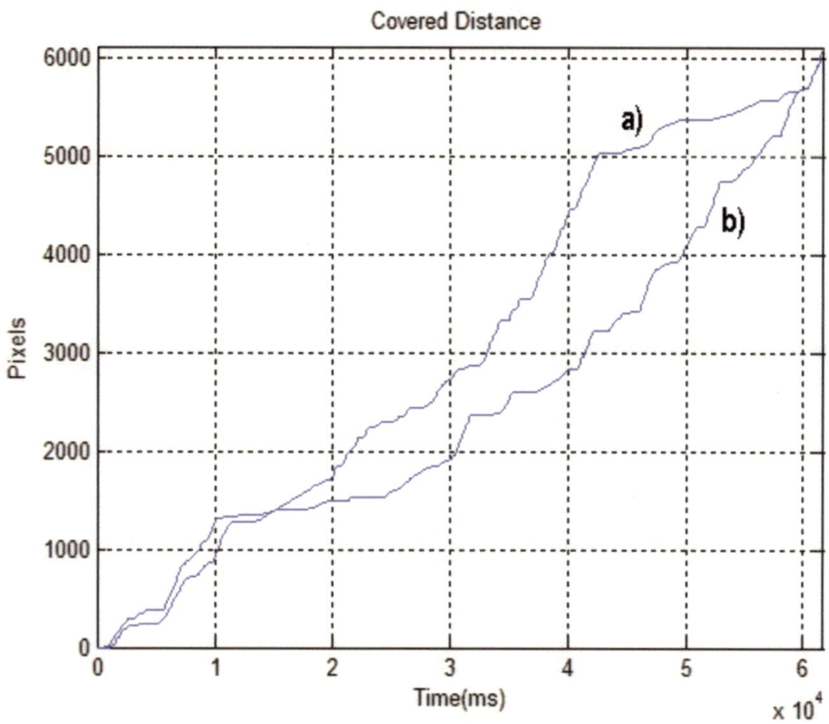

Fig. 17. Robert Covered Distance (first test (a) and the second test (b)).

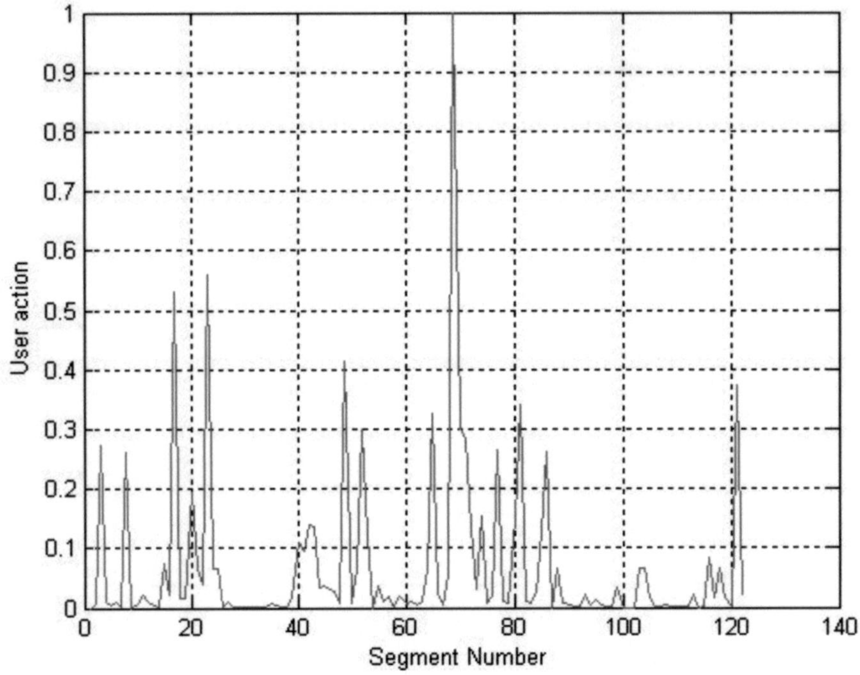

Fig. 18. User Action (UA) in the Robert first test.

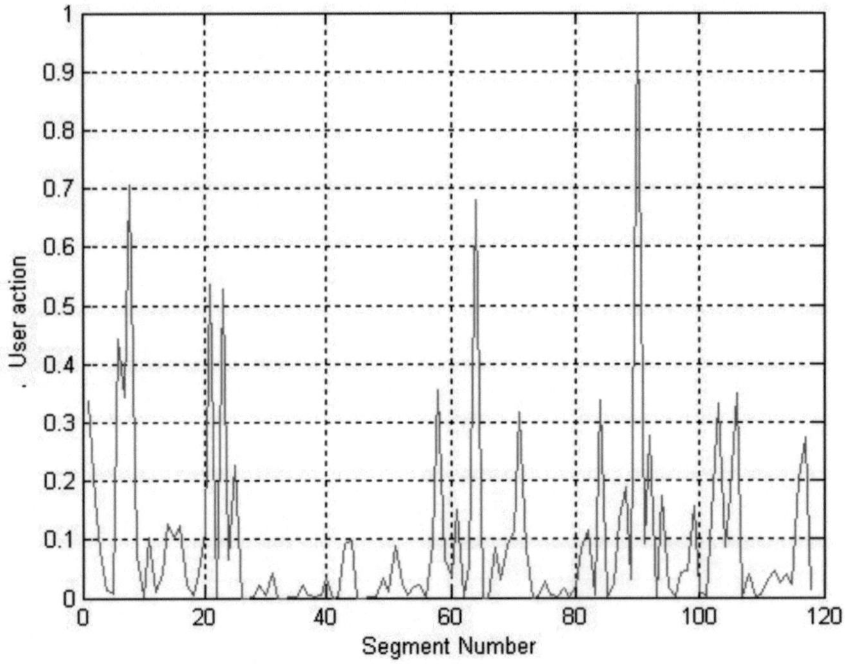

Fig.19. User Action (UA) in the Robert second test.

Sample	Test Time (TT) (ms)	Covered Distance (CD) (pixels)	Rate of Pause (PR) (%)	Command Load (CL)	Efficient Load (EL) (%)
Test1	61800	6125	14.56	1.14	53
Test2	59500	5690	16.80	1.58	97

Table 2. Robert results.

8. Conclusion

Today the methods used by the medical team and occupational therapist are often qualitative. PLEIA software can be employed as a tool to evaluate the pointing user's capabilities.
We proposed the new indexes to improve the classical evaluations methods that use the common factors as distance, time, errors and trajectory.
The index command load shows the energy that the user employs to act on his technical aid. This energy could be not to be in direct relation with the efficiency, when the user realizes a task.
PLEIA's capacities can be expanded as rehabilitation platform, telerehabilitation and experimentation platform for HCI systems with different haptic devices.
The experiments are based on the real evaluation cases.
In two cases, we evaluated the initial capabilities. The occupational therapist conclusions were: interface difficulties, some uncontrolled movements and the technical aid needs a best adaptation. The trajectories and indicators showed clearly this behavior. Claudia has a good interest with the exercises of PLEIA. The therapist detects that she has the same behavior as she rides her electric wheelchair.
We start test PLEIA with the other modules in order to evaluate children with robots and wheelchair. In these modules, all indicators are included. We will compare evaluation tools.

9. Acknowledgments

We thank Medical team and all occupational therapists of Raymond Poincare Hospital (Brezin unit 4), the Specialized Educational Center (Champigny France) and the Informatics' Unit of National Saint Maurice Hospital for his assistance in all experimentations in PLEIA.

10. References

Adameczek A. & Choquet T., & Huynh, Lefur .2005. Efficasouris: Outils pour les Ergothérapeutes et Clavier Virtuel. Report of project of studies, DESS HANDI, Nouvelles Technologies et Handicaps Sensori-moteurs, Paris ,France. March 2005.

Buaud, A., Roussel D.,. Truchot B,(2003). Evaluation process based on user's need: ergonomic evaluation of multimedia games for visually impaired children. AAATE 2003, Dublin, Ireland, September 2003. IOS Press, Craddock G., McCormack L., Reilly R., Knops H., Amsterdam, The Netherlands, pp. 237-241.

Dipietro,L. Sabatini, A. Paolo,D. (2003). Evaluation of an Instrumented gloved for hand movement acquisition. Journal of Rehabilitation Research and Development Vol. 40, No. 2 ,(March/April 2003),pp 179-190.

ISO/DIS 9241-9 Ergonomic requirements for office work with visual display terminals, non keyboard input device requirements. International Organisation for Standardisation, 1998.

Jeong, H. & Kim J. Choi, J. Lecture Notes in Computer Science (LNCS), Spring Berlin, ISBN 978-3-540-22312-2

Kadouche, R.,& Abdularazak B., Mokhtari, M .(2004). Designing an evaluation method for computer accessibility for people with severe disabilities. Proceding of 9th International Conference on Computers Helping People (ICCHP) with Special Needs, Springer, pp. 845-848, ISBN:3-540- 22334-7, Paris, France, July, 2004.

Kang, P. J. K. (2004). A Hand Gesture Controlled Semi-autonomous Wheelchair. Proceeding of 2004 IEEE/RSJ International Conference on Intelligent Robots and Systems, Vol.. 4 No. 2, pp.3565 - 3570, September 28 - October 2, 2004 , Sendai, Japan.

Keates, S., Hwang, F., Langdon, P., Clarkson, P.J., Robinson, P. (2002). Cursor Measures for Motion impaired Computer users. Proceedings of the ASSETS 2002 ACM Fifth ACM Conference on Assistive Technology-, New York, pp. 135-142, ISBN 1-58113-464-9, Edinburgh, Scotland

MacKenzie, I.S. & Kauppinen T., Silfverberg, M.(2001). Accuracy Measures for Evaluating Computer Pointing Devices. CHI '01: Proceedings of the SIGCHI conference on Human factors in computing systems, ACM Press, pp. 9-16.ISBN 1581133278, Seatle Washington, 31 march-5 april.

Peralta , H. & Riman, C., & Monacelli, E., A reconfigurable Evaluation and Assistance Platform for Handicapped People. Interational Conference on Intelligent Robots and Systems IROS 2006, IEEE, Beijing , Chine, October 9-15, 2006

Shimizu H, C. S. M. (2006). Programmed Instruction to teach pointing with a computer mouse in preschoolers with developmental disabilities. Research in Developmental Disabilities, Vol.27 ,No.(2), Mar-Apr 2006, pp. 175-189, PMID: 15970426.

Soukoreff R.W., Mackenzie I. S. (2004). "Towards a standard for pointing device evaluation, perspectives on 27 years of Fitts' law research in HCI." Int. J. Human-Computer Studies: 751–789.

Tellex, S., and Roy, D. (2006). Spatial routines for a simulated speech-controlled vehicle. Proceedings of the 1st ACM SIGCHI/SIGART conference on Human-robot interaction, 2006,pp. 156--163, ISBN: 1-59593-294-1, Salt Lake City, Utah, USA. March 02 - 03, 2006 ACM Press

Thieffry, R., Monacelli ,E. Laplace S. (2005). Adaptative Command and Generalization to Locomotion Aid Systems. Proceedings of the 2005 IEEE International Conference , ICRA, pp. 2643 - 2648, April 18-22, Barcelone, Spain.

Yanco, H. A. (2002). Evaluating the Performance of Assistive Robotic Systems. Performance Metrics for Intelligent Systems, NIST, Gaithersburg, MD, August 2002

Internets Sites

(Adeprio diffussion) http://www.adeprio.com

(Judy Lynn) http://www.judylynn.com/

(Marbesoft) http://www.marblesoft.com/

(Simtech publication) http://www.hsj.com/products.html

(Widgit software) http://www.widgit.com/

24

Facial Automaton for Conveying Emotions as a Social Rehabilitation Tool for People with Autism

Giovanni Pioggia, Maria Luisa Sica, Marcello Ferro, Silvia Casalini, Roberta Igliozzi[1], Filippo Muratori[1], Arti Ahluwalia, Danilo De Rossi
Interdepartmental Research Center "E. Piaggio", University of Pisa, Italy
[1]Scientific Institute Stella Maris (IRCCS), Pisa, Italy

1. Introduction

The terms Autistic Spectrum Disorders (ASD) and pervasive developmental disorders refer to a wide continuum of associated cognitive and neuro-behavioral disorders, including, but not limited to, three core-defining features: impairments in socialization, impairments in verbal and nonverbal communication, and restricted and repetitive patterns of behaviors. Although autism was first described over 50 years ago, our improved understanding of this complex disorder has emerged over the past two decades. Despite recent intense focus on autism, its study continues to be an art and science in fast evolution. There is marked variability in the severity of symptomatology across patients, and level of intellectual function can range from profound mental retardation through the superior range on conventional IQ tests. In ASD we can find: marked impairment in the use of multiple nonverbal behaviors, such as eye-to-eye gaze, facial expression, body posture, and gestures to regulate social interaction. The communication impairments seen in the autistic spectrum are far more complex than presumed by simple speech delay and share some similarities with the deficits seen in children with developmental language disorders or specific language impairments. Young autistic children, even if verbal, almost universally have comprehension deficits, in particular deficits in understanding higher order complex questions. Deficits in pragmatics, the use of language to communicate effectively, are almost universally present too. Another core characteristic of ASD is the presence of stereotyped behaviors and circumscribed/unusual interests, which encompass qualitative deficits in several aspects of behavior. It is moreover well documented that individuals with autism have impairments in processing of social and emotional information, as evident in tasks assessing face and emotion recognition, imitation of body movements, interpretation and use of gestures and theory of mind [Baron-Cohen 1994, Davies 1994, Dawson 1998, Smith 1994]. Typically developing infants show preferential attention to social rather than inanimate stimuli; in contrast, individuals with autism seem to lack these early social predispositions [Spelke 1995, Maestro 2002]. This hypothesis was recently substantiated in a neurofunctional study [Schultz 2000] of face perception in autism, in which adequate task performance was accompanied by abnormal ventral temporal cortical activities, which in turn suggested that participants had treated faces as objects. Klin et al. [Klin 2002] created an experimental paradigm to measure social functioning in natural situations, in which they used eye-tracking technology to measure visual fixations of cognitively able individuals with autism. When viewing naturalistic social situations, people with autism demonstrate abnormal patterns of social visual pursuit consistent with reduced salience of eyes and increased salience of mouth, bodies and objects. In addition, individuals with autism use atypical strategies when performing such tasks, relying on individual pieces of the face rather than on the overall configuration. Alongside these perceptual anomalies, individuals with autism have deficits in conceiving other people's mental states or "mindblindness" [Baron-Cohen 2000]. The cognitive theory of mindblindness [Baron-Cohen 1997] suggests that individuals with autism have difficulty in conceiving of people as mental agents and cannot adequately perceive another persons mental state. This often leads to typically inappropriate reactions or behaviours in a variety of social encounters. Recent studies have shown that individuals, particularly those with high functioning autism, can learn to cope with common social situations if they are made to enact possible scenarios they may encounter. By recalling appropriate modes of behavior and expressions in specific situations, they are able to react appropriately. There are now a number of highly structured therapeutic approaches based on emotion recognition and social skill training using photographs, drawings, videos or DVD-ROMs (for example Mind Reading, produced by Human Emotions, UK). Currently, these treatment approaches suggested the use of robotic systems in order to encourage children with autism to take initiative and to interact with the robotic tools.

The use of the robotic technology aimed to help autistic subjects in everyday life began in 1976 with the work of Sylvia Weir and Ricky Emanuel [Weir 1976]. They used a mobile turtle-like robot, LOGO, able to interact with a patient within a highly structured environment. More recently François Michaud [Michaud 2003, Michaud 2002] and his research team at the University of Sherbrooke, investigated the use of mobile robots as a treatment tool. They tested several robots, different in shape, color and behavior, in order to study the main characteristics that may capture the attention of people with autism. They obtained important insights for the comprehension of human-robot interaction in autism sustaining the robot hypothesis as useful. People with autism focus their attention on single details, but the interaction with a robot may allow an autistic subject to concentrate herself/himself on the limited number of communication modalities of the robot. In addition, while the stress of the learning with a teacher can be detrimental, the interaction with a robot, which often the young patients associate with media and/or cinema characters, can reduce the emotional pressure allowing the child to better learn from the environment.

A more structured approach to the use of autonomous robots is AURORA (AUtonomous RObotic platform as a Remedial tool for children with Autism) [Dautenhahn 2002a, Dautenhahn 2002b]. AURORA represents the first systematic study on a therapeutic approach of robots in autism. People with autism are invited to interact in coordinated and synchronized social actions with the robots and the environment. In AURORA, behavior-based architectures for the use of different robotic platforms such as mobile and humanoid robots (Robota developed by Aude Billard [Billard 2002]) were developed.

Recently the development of emotional cognitive architectures allowed the interaction to be based on empathy, e.g. the KISMET [Breazeal 2001] project developed by Cynthia Breazeal at the Robotic Life Group of MIT Media Lab, INFANOID or KEEPON [Kozima 2004, Kozima 2002] developed by Hideki Kozima at the National Institute of Information and Communications Technology (NICT) of Japan. INFANOID is an upper-torso child-like robot, capable of pointing, grasping, and of expressing a variety of gestures, while KEEPON is a simple yellow snowman-like robot, both equipped by eye-contact and joint attention functions.

FACE (Facial Automaton for Conveying Emotions) [Pioggia 2004, Pioggia 2005] on the other hand follows a biomimetic approach. In FACE the biological behaviour is mimicked by means of dedicated smart soft materials and structures, intelligent control strategy, algorithms and artificial neural networks. It is part of an innovative android-based treatment which focuses on core aspects of the autistic disorder, namely social attention and the recognition of emotional expressions. FACE is a social believable artifact able to interact with the external environment, interpreting and conveying emotions through non verbal communication. FACE captures expressive and psychophysical correlates from its interlocutor and actuates behaviours with kinesics, a non verbal communication conveyed by body part movements and facial expressions. In the framework of A social therapy, FACE can act as an interface between a patient and a trained therapist in a specially equipped room. Both physiological and behavioural information is acquired in real time by means of an unobtrusive sensorized wearable interface from the patient during the treatment. This approach provides a structured environment that people with autism could consider to be "social", helping them to accept the human interlocutor and to learn through imitation. On the basis of a dedicated therapeutic protocol, FACE is able to engage in social interaction by modifying its behaviour in response to the patient's behaviour. Following an imitation-based learning strategy, we hope to verify that such a system can help children with autism to learn, interpret and use emotional information. If such learned skills can be extended to a social context, the whole FACE system will serve as an invaluable therapeutic tool for ASD, which we call FACE-T (T as in "therapy"). The FACE-T system consists of FACE itself, a sensorised life-shirt and the therapeutic protocol.

2. Social interaction and communication

Since the first days of our lives we are social beings. Children meet people's gaze, turn towards a voice, catch mom or dad's fingers and smile, but children affected by ASD show difficulties in taking part in such daily social interaction and communication with others. Children affected by ASD have impairment in the use of multiple nonverbal behaviors, such as eye-to-eye gaze, facial expression, body posture, and gestures. Young autistic children, even if verbally skilled, almost universally have comprehension and language communication deficits, i.e. they lack skilful use of language to communicate effectively. The presence of stereotyped behaviors and circumscribed interests can be also underlined. Meltzoff argued that an underdevelopment of the social communication can be explained in terms of imitation impairment [Meltzoff 1995]. Children usually imitate the behaviour of an interlocutor, children with autism do not; causing serious consequences. Early imitation is one of the most important instruments for the social learning, as well as innate to humans [Rizzolatti 1999]. An essential prerequisite for imitation is a connection between the sensory systems and the motor systems such that percepts can be mapped onto appropriate actions. This mapping is a difficult computational process as visual perception takes place in a different coordinate frame from motor control. This process is also more complex than pure object recognition since it requires integration of multiple objects (i.e., several limbs), their spatial relations, their relative and absolute movements, and even the intention of these movements.
The possible connection to imitation, however, came with the discovery of the mirror neurons [Rizzolatti 1999], a new class of visuomotor neurons recently discovered in the monkey's premotor cortex (F5 area). These neurons respond both when a particular action is performed by the recorded monkey and when the same action, performed by another

individual, is observed [Pellegrino 1992]. From imaging and transcranial magnetic stimulation studies, there is also a great deal of evidence that a similar mirror system exists in humans [Decety 1994, Fadiga 1995, Decety 1996]. Surprisingly, this system seems to involve the Brocas area [Rizzolatti 1998], a brain region normally associated with speech production. The possible homology of F5 in monkey and Brocas area in humans led some authors [Rizzolatti 1998] to speculate that the ability to imitate actions and to understand them could have subserved the development of communication skills. This idea is consistent with Meltzoff and Moores [Meltzoff 1995] works and interpretations. Gallese and Goldman [Gallese 1998] suggest rather that mirror neurons participate in mind reading, a process accomplished by using ones own mental apparatus to predict the psychological state of others through mental simulations.

Rizzolatti pointed out that the process of imitation plays a crucial role in distinguishing between actions arising from within or actions induced by others [Rizzolatti 1999]. Imitation paves the way to the comprehension of the intentions of others establishing a reciprocal non verbal communication process in which the roles of imitator and model are continuously exchanged [Nadel 2004a, Nadel 2004b]. Moreover, in the early years, imitation plays a fundamental role for the emergence of proprioception, of the perception of the external world and of the ability to act our own actions. Enhancing the imitation skills of children through specifically designed treatments based on imitation may yield to an improvement in social development. Recently it has been proposed that the characteristic impairments of ASD, including deficits in imitation, theory of mind and social communication, can be caused by a dysfunction of the mirror neuron system [Dapretto 2005].

However, what strategy can be used to control and enhance the emergence of human-android imitation? As a first step, our idea was the realization of a structure capable of creating its own representations of the surrounding environment. It is an associative memory through which it may be possible to navigate within a behavioural space. These characteristics are typical of some areas of the central nervous system. This led us to abandon the idea of realising a controller based solely on a group of neurons in various states of connection. Furthermore, preformism impedes the topological and geometrical structure from developing in an adaptive manner. As a first approach, we used the model developed by Izhikevich [Izhikevich 2003] and a learning model based on the Theory of Neuronal Group Selection (TNGS) of G. Edelman [Edelman 1993]. As a first approach the learning process in FACE is based on imitating predefined stereotypical behaviours which can be represented in terms of FAPs (Fixed Action Patterns) followed by a continuous interaction with its environment. FAPs can be classified as belonging to action schemes, partly fixed on the basis of physical constraints and sensory-motor reflexes, partly subjected to a specialization on the basis of the experience. FACE is therefore able to continually learn, to adapt and evolve within a simplified behavioural space as a function of the environment and to maintain spontaneous activity open to any innovative and intelligible behaviours arising which may then be interpreted.

3. Non verbal communication and autism

Non verbal communication is usually understood as the process of sending and receiving wordless messages. Such messages can be communicated through gesture; body language or posture; facial expression and eye contact; prosodic features of speech such as intonation and stress and other paralinguistic features of speech such as voice quality, emotion and speaking style. Non verbal communication can occur through any sensory channel sight, sound, smell, touch or taste. Also, non-verbal communication comes in many forms at the same time. For example, a person's dress, tone of voice, attitude, and movement all contribute to the communication going on in a certain situation. The communication problems of autism vary depending on the intellectual and social development of the individual. Some may be unable to speak, whereas others may have rich vocabularies and are able to talk about topics of interest in great depth. Despite this variation, the majority of autistic individuals have little or no problem with pronunciation. Most have difficulty effectively using language. Many also have problems with word and sentence meaning, intonation, and rhythm. Those who can speak often say things that have no content or information. For example, an autistic individual may repeatedly count from one to five. Most autistic individuals do not make eye contact and have poor attention duration. They are often unable to use gestures either as a primary means of communication, as in sign language, or to assist verbal communication, such as pointing to an object they want. For many, speech and language develop, to some degree, but not to a normal ability level. This development is usually uneven.

4. Instruments of diagnostic observation

At the present time no "objective" procedure exists for the diagnosis of autism. Clinicians must, accordingly, rely on their clinical judgement, aided by guides to diagnosis such as DSM-IV (APA, 1994) and ICD-10 (World Health Organization, 1993), as well as by the results of various assessment instruments such as checklists, interviews, rating scales and observation schedules. Thus, an important help for all mental health operators that work with this disorder is given by standardised instruments that can facilitate in "communicating" to one another from a similar "point of view" during the diagnostic process. Besides this, these are very useful instruments that can create comparability across clinicians and researchers, as well as instruments that can individuate more homogeneous groups for research: Autism Diagnostic Interview - Revised (ADI-R) [Lord, Rutter & Le Couter, 1994] and Autism Diagnostic Observation Schedule - Generic (ADOS-G) [Lord, Risi, Lambrecht, Cook, Leventhal et al. 2000] are complementary instruments currently defined as the "gold standard" diagnostic instruments.

ADI-R is a standardised, semi structured, investigator-based interview for caregivers of autistic individuals, which provides a diagnostic algorithm for the ICD-10 and DSM-IV definition of autism. The focus is upon obtaining detailed descriptions of real behaviours and then establishing typicality and pervasiveness for diagnosis of autism. We find three sections about specific areas related to the diagnosis of autism: Communication and language (with different questions about verbal and non-verbal aspects of communication); Social development and play (in which interviewer asks about the presence, for example, of shared behaviours, emotional reciprocity, etc); and repetitive and stereotyped behaviours and unusual interests.

ADOS-G is an instrument that collects standard information about a child's behaviour in response to a predetermined schedule of activities. Activities and behaviours are taken from empirical research in autism and child development and refer to social and communicative features.

The CARS scale (Childhood Autism Rating Scales) [Schopler, et al., 1988] was developed in order to aid in the diagnostic process but it is also used to assess changes in autistic symptomatology at two/three years, at one year and at 6 month intervals. More recently it has been used also in shorter longitudinal studies. The CARS scale is subdivided in 15 items, relative to the main behavioural areas; it is assigned a variable score from 1 to 4 to every item; the score 1 indicates a behavior appropriate to the age, while a score 4 indicates an abnormal behavior. The total score obtained after the CARS test has an undeniable diagnostic and clinical usefulness. Inquiring the score of the single items of the test it is however possible to characterize other patient behaviors.

5. FACE, the biomimetic social interactive machine

The realisation of a social interactive machine entails critical requirements for its body, its sensory perception system, its mobility and its ability to perform tasks. The human mind responds and modifies itself with respect to the real world enabling the body to perceive, to act and to survive; human intelligence arises primarily from the interpretation of the body's needs. For this reason we preferred to follow a mind-body monism, i.e. an embodied mind able to perform the processing phase taking into account the domain of experiences where the machine is placed; such processes influence and are influenced by its own presence.
Dynamic interaction mechanisms are needed in order to place the android inside its environment: FACE is provided with extrinsic perception in order to interiorize the external world and to be able to suitably react. It possesses body structures as a support to the intrinsic perception (proprioception) and motor activity. The formation of a relationship domain close to a human context underlies the need of a high degree of believability in the FACE robot. Furthermore the robot has a space-time capability for both egocentricity and allocentricity, taking into account the actuation of preprogrammed behaviours as well as an imitative learning strategy.
The android FACE consists of a passive articulated body equipped with a believable facial display system based on biomimetic engineering principles. The latest prototype of the FACE robot is shown in Figure 1. Its head consists of an artificial skull covered by an artificial skin which is a thin silicone-based mask equipped with sensory and actuating system. The mask is fabricated by means of life-casting techniques and aesthetically represents a copy of the head of a subject, both in shape and texture. An artificial muscular architecture and servomotors allow FACE to express and modulate the six basic emotions (happiness, sadness, surprise, anger, disgust, fear) in a repeatable and flexible way. This process can be controlled thanks to an artificial skin consisting of a 3D latex foam equipped with a biomimetic system of proprioceptive mapping described in section 6.1. This structure allows the expression required to be achieved by means of a trial and error process. The artificial skin covers an artificial skull which is equipped with an actuating system.

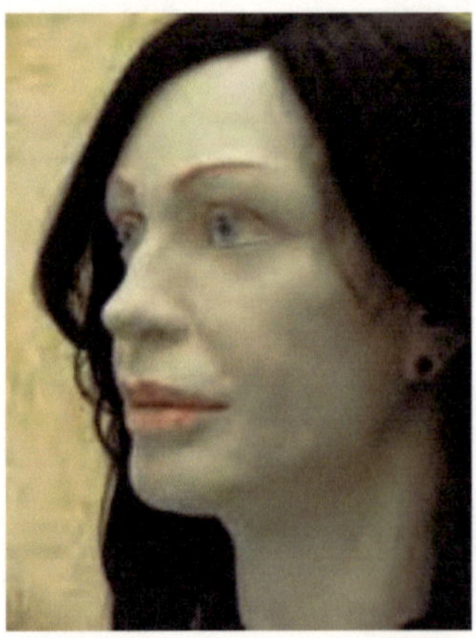

Fig. 1. The latest prototype of FACE.

FACE can enable real-time acquisition of both physiological and behavioural information by means of an unobtrusive sensorized wearable interface from the interlocutor. It is able to analyse the emotional reactions of individuals through optical analyses of facial expressions, to track a human face over time and to automatically store all data (described in section 6.2). The robot's eyes are realised using animatronic techniques and their expressiveness is achieved through an artificial muscular structure surrounding the orbital region. It sees differently from man, using stereoscopic vision over frequency rather than over space. A three-dimensional contouring apparatus, equipped with a section for data analysis, rebuilds an internal representation of a portion of the world before it. Currently FACE surveys the curvature of the three dimensional scene once per second. We adopted a neural approach to allow FACE to recognize the expression of a subject. A dedicated process detects a number of points (markers), which are used to divide the human face into four main areas (left eye, right eye, nose and mouth). The data of each area are processed by a hierarchical neural-network architecture based on Kohonen self organizing maps and a multi-layer perceptron.

6. Perception and learning of the human behavior

In human-machine social interaction, the intersection between biology and engineering needs a context which enables the conditions for the development of adapting dynamics. Perception and learning of the dynamics of human-machine interactions play an important role in social verbal and nonverbal communication. In order to enable continuous learning and adaptation within a simplified behavioural space, a social robot must be provided with extrinsic perception in order to interiorize the external world, it must also possess an intrinsic perception system and an imitative learning strategy must be adopted. The process of imitation is innate to humans and plays a crucial role in distinguishing between actions arising from within or actions induced by others, as well as the expression of emotions. Imitation paves the way to the comprehension of the intentions and emotional expressions of others establishing a reciprocal non verbal communication process in which the roles of the imitator and of the model are continuously exchanged. Moreover, in the early years of the life, imitation plays a fundamental role for the emergence of proprioception, of the perception of the external world and of the ability to act our own actions. This is especially evident considering the imitation of emotional expression.

In designing a biomimetic android such as FACE the relationship between mind and body must also be considered. As mentioned, in the previous section, FACE must have an embodied mind, and an interactive relationship with its environment to enable imitative learning and proprioception.

6.1 The intrinsic perception system

The FACE artificial sensing skin is a 3D latex foam, under which lies a sensing layer. The sensing layer responds to simultaneous deformations in different directions by means of a piezoresistive network which consists of an Conductive Elastomer (CEs) composites rubber screen printed onto a cotton lycra fabric. CE composites show piezoresistive properties when a deformation is applied and can be easily integrated into fabrics or other flexible substrates to be employed as strain sensors. They are elastic and do not modify the mechanical behaviour of the fabric. CEs consist in a mixture containing graphite and silicon rubber. In the production process of sensing fabrics, a solution of CE and trichloroethylene is smeared on a lycra substrate previously covered by an adhesive mask. The mask is designed according to the desired topology of the sensor network and cut by a laser milling machine. After the deposition, cross-linking process of the mixture is obtained at high temperature. Furthermore, by using this technology, both sensors and interconnection wires can be smeared by using the same material in a single printing and manufacturing process.

From technical viewpoint, a piezoresistive sensing fabric is a system whose local resistivity is a function of the local strain. In a discrete way, it can be thought of as a two dimensional resistive network where single resistors have a non-linear characteristic that depends on the local strain. The integral impedance pattern is a function of the overall shape of the sensorized fabric and allows mapping between the electrical space and the shape space. For the characterisation of the sensors in terms of their quasi-static and dynamic electromechanical transduction properties sensors were serially connected. In this case, a current is superimposed in the circuit and high impedance differential voltages are acquired from each sensor. Two multiplexers allow a sensor to be selected and the relative signal is acquired by a differential amplifier. A microprocessor drives the whole system, performs the analogous/digital conversion and exchanges data via an usb interface. The device is provided with an automatic calibration subsystem which allows gain and offset to be tailored to each sensor.

6.1 The extrinsic perception system

FACE-T can enable real-time acquisition of both physiological and behavioural information by means of an unobtrusive sensorized wearable interface from the interlocutor. FACE itself is able to analyse the emotional reactions of individuals through optical analyses of facial expressions, to track a human face over time and to automatically store all data (Pioggia et al., 2004). The neuro-computational pre-processing strategy adopted to perceive a subject's face is based on Kohonen Self Organizing Maps (KSOMs). Each KSOM represents a portion of the subject's face (left eye, right eye, nose and mouth) and data of a zone is input to only one map; in this way, each KSOM is trained with the purpose of clustering data coming from the respective zones. The outputs of the KSOMs are used to form the input pattern for the multimodal sensory fusion system.

A wearable interface (life-shirt) for the acquisition of physiological signals from human subjects has been developed at our research labs and integrated into the FACE-T system. The life-shirt approach consists in the integration of smart sensors in a handy garment, together with the integrated electronic devices and the on-body pre-processing of the acquired signals. From a general point of view, the main innovation of this technology lies in the combination of wearable technologies (sensorized garments, electronic sensors, tailored algorithms, on-body computing) together with the user feedback.

The life-shirt within FACE-T collects heterogeneous physiological signals from the human interlocutor of FACE. Acquired signals are transmitted to a server workstation which performs the processing tasks. The life-shirt is based upon three key points: a network of smart sensors, i.e. electrodes and connections embedded on fabric; a wearable acquisition and processing framework equipped with wireless communication systems; a model for data classification, correlation and prediction. Electrodes and connections are woven in the garment, using natural or synthetic fibers containing conductive yarns. A suitable positioning of the electrodes allows physiological signals such as the ECG and the skin electric conductance to be acquired. CE composites rubber screen printed onto fabric have been used to transduce the respiration rhythm. The output of the life-shirt is pre-processed as input vector patterns for the multimodal sensory fusion system, described in the following section.

6.3 Multimodal sensory fusion

A framework for the management and synchronization of data and processes arising from the global FACE-T system has been developed within FACE-T. The framework core and the application processes are interfaced to the sensor array through a framework I/O interface. The framework I/O interface has been developed in order to act as a buffer for the flow of information from the sensors to the application process. Signals coming from different sensor arrays are gathered in parallel and are encoded following a standard protocol. The encoded information is received by a dedicated filter for each sensor, which then sorts them to framework I/O interface. Figure 2 shows the flow of information to and from the framework core.

Communication channels are established as connections between application processes. The domain of data flowing through connections and the flow chart of the application processes can be properly designed according to a specific application. Processes and connections are managed at run time and they can be manipulated under request. The presence of dynamic structures implies a configurable resource management, so the framework offers an optimised interface for enumeration and direct access requests. A spatial definition of the entities involved in the framework can moreover be supplied, making this information available to the control system for subsequent processing. To guarantee the execution of real-time applications an inner synchronization signal is provided from the framework core to the processes and to the framework I/O interface, enabling to gain time-space correlation.

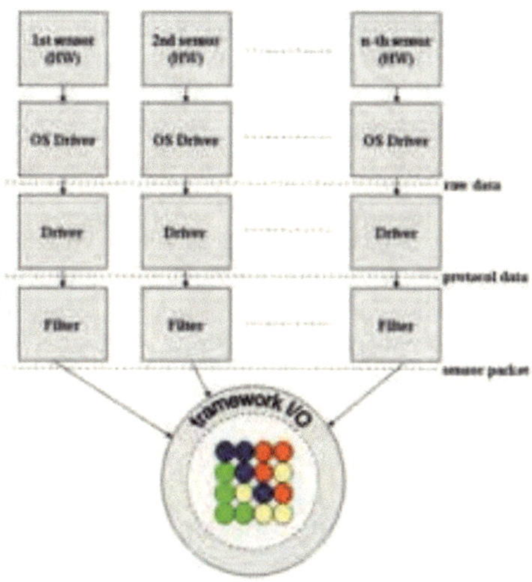

Fig. 2. Framework for the management and synchronization of data and processes.

The framework architecture has been designed as a hierarchical structure whose root is a manager module. It is realised as a high-level container of generic modules representing the environment in which process modules and I/O filtering interfaces are placed. Communication channels are realised as connections in specific topologies. All modules are realized as running processes while their control and synchronization is managed by the framework. A real-time approach for data analysis takes advantage of the framework capability to manage interconnected modules through efficient communication channels. In this way the application is able to control all the modules of the processing chain, including analysis protocol management and sensor array interfaces. Connections are delegated to

dispatch synchronization information and user-defined data. The filtering interface modules are able to drive the transducer hardware and to dispatch information to process modules. All base modules manage dynamic structures and they are designed to maintain data consistency while the environment state may change. This behaviour permits the execution of dynamic and real-time parallel distributed processing while synchronization and data flow are managed by the environment.
This multimodal sensory fusion system manages data and signals from all elements of the FACE-T network allowing dynamic integration of different codes.

6.4 A neural network for the classification of the behavior of the interlocutor

In order for the FACE-T system to codify the behavior of the interlocutor, and so interactively adapt FACE to the patient's reactions, a powerful neural network has been implemented.
The complexity of a biological neuron may be reduced by using several mathematical models. Each of these reproduces some of the functionalities of real neurons, such as the excitability in response to a specific input signal. E. Izhikevich (Izhikevich 2003) recently developed a simple model for an artificial neuron which is able to reproduce almost all the functionalities of biological neurons. The model takes 13 FLOPs to simulate one millisecond of neuron activity and it is based on a top-down approach, using two differential equations with four parameters. The computation efficiency and the introduction of axonal delays show the possibility of creating a neural network able to perform real-time classification and prediction tasks (Izhikevich 2005). In this work the Spike-Timing-Dependant Plasticity (STDP) rule (Izhikevich et al. 2004), which permits the implementation of a real time learning rule based on signals which continuously flow from the framework I/O, has been adopted according to the Theory of Neuronal Group Selection (TNGS) of G. Edelman on selection as the basis for the learning process (Edelman 1993).
The TNGS suggests a novel way for understanding and simulating neural networks. The time variable is taken into account in the learning task, so that neural groups may raise from a selection process. The correspondence between synaptic weights and axonal delays exists as a result of the neuron behavior. One neuron can belong to many groups, and the number of groups is usually higher than the number of the neurons in the map. This guarantees a memory capability which is higher than the capability reached by classical artificial neural networks. The classical approach in artificial neural networks simulation takes into account the modulation of the action potential rhythm as the only parameter for the information flowing to and from each neuron. Such a strategy seems to be in contrast with novel experimental results, since neurons are able to generate action potentials which are based on the input spike timings, with a precision of one millisecond. The spike-timing synchrony is a natural effect that permits a neuron to be activated in correspondence with synchronous input spikes, while the neuronal activation of the post-synaptic neuron is negligible if pre-synaptic spikes arrive asynchronously to the target neuron. Axonal delays usually lie in the range [0.1 - 44] milliseconds, depending on the type and location of the neuron inside the network. Such a property becomes an important feature for the selection of the neural groups. The selection of neural groups is the result of the variation of synaptic connection according to the STDP rule. If a spike coming from an excitatory pre-synaptic neuron causes the firing of the post-synaptic neuron, the synaptic connection is reinforced since it is given the possibility to generate another spike in order to propagate the signal. Otherwise the synaptic connection is weakened. The values of the STDP parameters are chosen in order to permit a weakening that

is greater than the reinforcement. Such a strategy permits the progressive removal of unnecessary connections and the persistence of the connections between correlated neurons.
The network design is inspired by the anatomical structure found in the mammalian cortex. With respect to the total number (N) of neurons, a percentage equal to 80% consists of excitatory neurons, while the remaining 20% are inhibitory neurons. Cortical pyramidal neurons showing a regular spiking behaviour have been adopted for the excitatory subsection, which correspond to appropriate values for the Izhikevich neuron model. Inhibitory neurons have been simulated adopting the model of the cortical interneurons which exhibit fast spiking properties. Each neuron is connected to M different neurons in order to obtain a connection probability (M/N) equal to 0.1, but inhibitory neurons are connected only to excitatory neurons. Moreover, the synaptic weights of the connections arising from the inhibitory neurons remain unchanged during the learning process, while those regarding the connections from the excitatory neurons change according to the STDP rule. Axonal delays are fixed in the range between 1 millisecond and 20 milliseconds. The time resolution has been set to 1 millisecond. The training phase has been carried out for more than 8 hours.
As the application starts, all the connections have the same synaptic weight. The network needs many seconds to get stabilised through depression and strengthening of the synaptic weights. During this first phase, the network shows the presence of a high amplitude rhythm, with frequency in the range between 2 Hz and 4 Hz (delta waves).
After a few hours of network activity the spiking rhythm becomes uncorrelated and frequency in the range between 30 Hz and 70 Hz appear (gamma waves). The appearance of such rhythms is called PING (Pyramidal-Interneuron Network Gamma) and seems to be related to the spikes of the pyramidal cells which excite the inhibitory interneurons. Such interaction allows a mutual inhibition which temporarily switches-off the network activity. As the network becomes stable, the oscillation rhythm is assessed in the frequency range between 2 Hz and 7 Hz and the training phase is ended. The presence of a large number of neural groups can be noted, each able to perform a reproducible spike sequence with a precision of one millisecond. The test phase consists in recording neural group activity in response to predefined FAPs. A labeling procedure allows association of a specific FAP to a neural group. Each FAP is able to select one group inside the network, showing that the network is able to perform classification tasks. Such classification is realised by a memory capability which is far greater than the number of entities involved into the network.
In our opinion, the current neural models do not include the role of glia cells and in particular those of the astrocytes. As has been recently demonstrated, the glia modulates neural communication achieving a two-dimensional continuum in which calcium ion waves influence synaptic communication. The glia cells are the centre of spontaneous activity induced by the continuous rhythm of the oscillations of ions at specific frequencies which influence the coordination and control of neural cells. The complex and dense branching which extends from each astrocyte defines a three-dimensional space, thereby defining an anatomical domain of influence. In the future it is our intention to consider the group of the domains of influence as a single continuous domain, as first suggested by Beurle [Beurle 1956], equipping FACE with a controller, or neurocontroller, made up of groups of neuro-entities placed inside a continuous volume of connected astrocyte cells within an epigenetic topology.

7. Actions: a behavior-based approach

Behavior-based control draws inspiration from biology, and tries to model how animals deal with their complex environments and thus forms the basis of FACE's control architecture. The components of behavior-based systems are called behaviors: these are observable patterns of activity emerging from interactions between the robot and its environment. Such systems are constructed in a bottom-up fashion, starting with a set of simple behaviors which couple sensory inputs to robot actions. Behaviors are added to provide more complex capabilities. New behaviors are introduced into the system until their interaction results in the desired overall capabilities of the robot. Behavior-based systems and reactive systems share some similar properties: both are built incrementally, from the bottom up, and consist of distributed modules. However, behavior-based systems are fundamentally more powerful, because they can store representations, while reactive systems cannot do so. As mentioned above, an essential prerequisite for imitation is a connection between the sensory systems and the motor systems such that percepts can be mapped onto appropriate actions. In a behavior-based system, the sensing and action oriented behaviors use the same mechanisms and operate on a similar time-scale and representation, enabling the perception of relative and absolute movements, and even the intention of these movements.

7.1 The cognitive architecture

The cognitive architecture of FACE is shown in Figure 3. The external world is sensed by FACE and the different stimuli are extracted in terms of neural group activities. In the Perception System, these activities are bound by threshold controlled processes that encode the current set of beliefs about the internal and external state of the android and its relation to the world. The result is a set of response-specific thresholds that serve as antecedent conditions for specific behavioral responses.

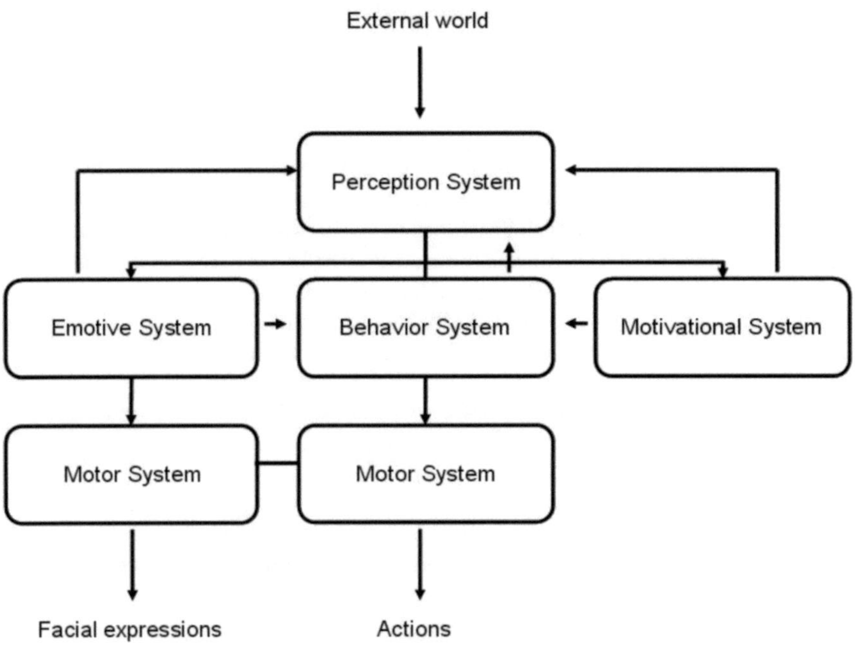

Fig. 3. The cognitive architecture.

The Emotive System sends a feed-back to the Perception System in order to participate in the evaluation of the stimulus, to the Behavior System in order to participate in the selection of the behavior selection and to the Motor System to activate the facial expression consistent with the emotion. The Motivational System is aimed at influencing the behavior selection. The behaviors participate in the evaluation of the stimulus and they are activated by the Motor System.

7.2 The perception system

The perception system analyzes and interprets information from the senses about the outside world. Without a perception system, an individual would be oblivious to any stimuli present in the environment. The perception system is a critical link in making sense of incoming information. It processes the stimuli creating a representation of the surrounding environment on the basis of the following percepts:

- S1 : percept pertinent people's presence
- S2 : percept pertinent physiological data
- S3 : percept pertinent dangerous interaction
- S4 : percept pertinent gaze direction

Activation/deactivation of each percept is represented by means of Boolean values. S1 is activated in case a person is present in the room. S2 is activated when life-shirt is connected. S3 is activated in case of a dangerous interaction with the interlocutor, such as rapid movements of the subject close to FACE. Finally, S4 indicates the occurrence of eye-contact with the subject.

7.3 The motivational system

The "needs", or drives, of a machine necessarily influence the behavior selection. They also provide a functional context (i.e. the aim, namely which need the android tries to address) that influences the behavior and perception, as well as the android affective state. Thus, they can also indirectly bias the behavior through the emotion system. Since the drives operate on a slower time scale than the emotions, they contribute to the long-term affective state (or mood of the android) and its expression. The motivational system is based on the following drives corresponding to the first levels of Maslow's Hierarchy of Needs:

- P1 : physiological needs
- P2 : safety needs
- P3 : social needs
- P4 : esteem needs

7.4 The emotive system

Several theorists argue that a few select emotions are basic or primary: they are endowed by evolution because of their proven ability to facilitate adaptive responses to the vast array of demands and opportunities a creature faces in its daily life (Ekman & Friesen 1992, Ekman 1992). The emotions of anger, disgust, fear, joy, sorrow, and surprise are often supported as being basic from evolutionary, developmental, and cross-cultural studies (Ekman 1992). Each basic emotion serves a particular function (often biological or social), arising in particular contexts, to prepare and motivate a creature to respond in adaptive ways. They serve as important reinforcers for learning new behavior. In addition, emotions are refined and new emotions are acquired throughout emotional development. Emotions seem to be centrally involved in determining the behavioral reaction to environmental (often social) and internal events of major significance for the needs and goals of a creature (Izard 1993). The emotive system of FACE is based on the following emotions:

- E1 : enjoyement
- E2 : sadness
- E3 : anger
- E4 : disgust
- E5 : fear
- E6 : surprise

7.5 The behaviors

Every behavior is modelled as a separate goal-directed process. In general, both internal and external factors are used to compute their relevance (whether or not they should be activated). The behavior system allows FACE to respond to a stimulus and to fulfil the aim. Once the stimulus is evaluated by the perception, motivational and emotive systems, the expected behavior, present in the following list, must be activated on the basis of the aim, of the environment and on the security needs:

- B1 : self preservation
- B2 : quite
- B3 : gaze
- B4 : joint attention
- B5 : communication (imitation)

B1 is devoted to the security needs. It can be activated on the basis of an evaluation of the motivational system and/or on the basis of emotive system. B2 indicates a warning. B3 and B4 activate respectively the eye contact and the joint attention. B5 enables the imitation task.

7.5 The motor system

The motor system directly implements the following actions in FACE:

- A1 : attention
- A2 : rest
- A3 : quite expression
- A4 : ocular movements
- A5 : head movements
- A6 : facial expressions

Each action is a collection of motor primitives that directly drives each motor by applying voltage pulses. During the pulse application the selected motor applies an increasing force, while, during the rest phase the motor is floating.

8. Experimental results

A block schema of the experimental set-up for the FACE-T system is shown in figure 4. It consists of a specially equipped room, provided with two remotely orientable video cameras, in which the child, under the supervision of a therapist, can interact with FACE by means of a liquid crystal screen, a keyboard and a mouse. Both FACE and the interactive

module are connected to a computer. The subject wears the life-shirt for recording physiological data. The database also contains data from the audio visual recording system present in the room. Other therapists or Hidden Observers compile evaluation sheets during sessions, and the data scanned from these will also be added to the database and used for successive analysis.
In order to obtain a preliminary evaluation of the behavior of children affected by ASD when exposed to FACE, we set up an experimental session in which the reactions of 4 subjects (3 male and 1 female), between 7 and 20 years old, were monitored and compared. The children with autism had been diagnosed using ADI-R and ADOS-G, two specific diagnostic instruments, as high functioning autism, and are currently under treatment at the Stella Maris Institute (IRCCS) in Pisa, Italy.

Subjects	Age	IQ
S1	10y6m	105
S2	9y6m	87
S3	8y11m	85
S4	20y6m	52

Table 1. Autism rating scale for the selected subjects.

Experiments were carried out in order to study the interaction with FACE during twenty minute sessions. We studied:

- both spontaneous behavior of the participants and their reactions to therapist presses in correlation with the time course of the physiological and behavioural data
- the focusing of the attention towards FACE's eye movements
- the spontaneous ability of imitation of gesture and expressions of the android

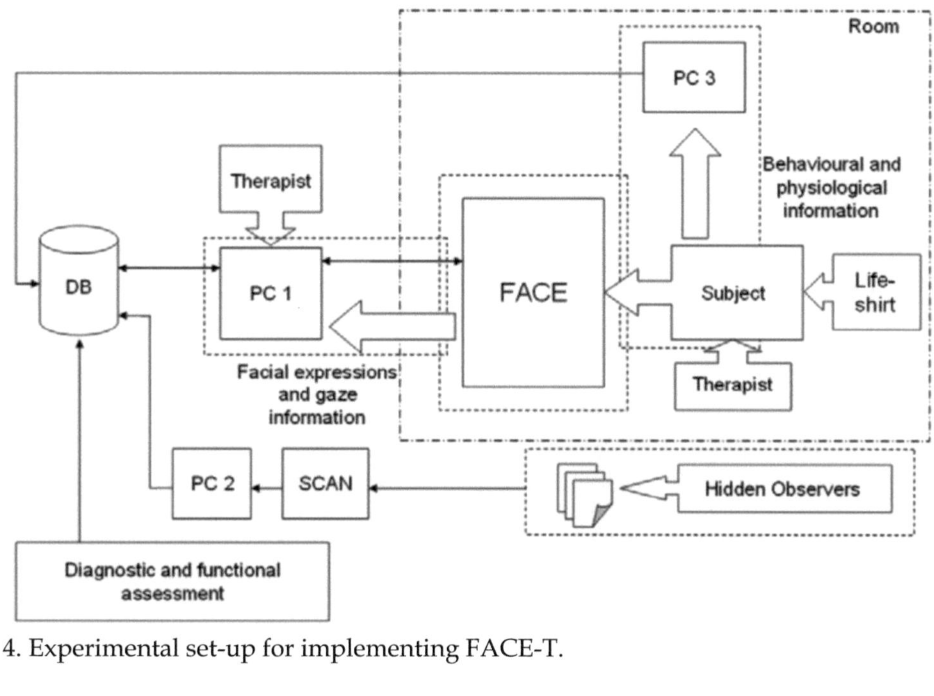

Fig. 4. Experimental set-up for implementing FACE-T.

The evaluation of the treatment effect was performed using 8 relevant items from the CARS scale.

Figures 5, 6, 7 and 8 supply a graphical comparison between the score obtained in items of CARS scale in previous interactions during psychological treatments and the one obtained with FACE. In particular, we observed that the CARS score decreased or remained the same for all items as regards subjects 2 and 3 after the therapy session. Only subject 4 (the oldest, with lowest IQ and highest ADOS rating) showed an increase of 0.5 points for listening, fear and verbal communication. More importantly, all the subjects demonstrated a decrease in the score of emotional response in the CARS scale of between 1 and 0.5 points, and imitation in 3 out of 4 children, so implying a marked improvement in these areas after interacting with FACE. Even though these are the first set of clinical trials, it is clear that the presence of FACE in a therapeutic environment can lead to improvements in the areas of social communication and imitation. As shown in figure 9, the cardiac frequency of the patient increases after his attention is focused on the robot, and remain fairly high till he is forced to focus on his emotional relationship with FACE.

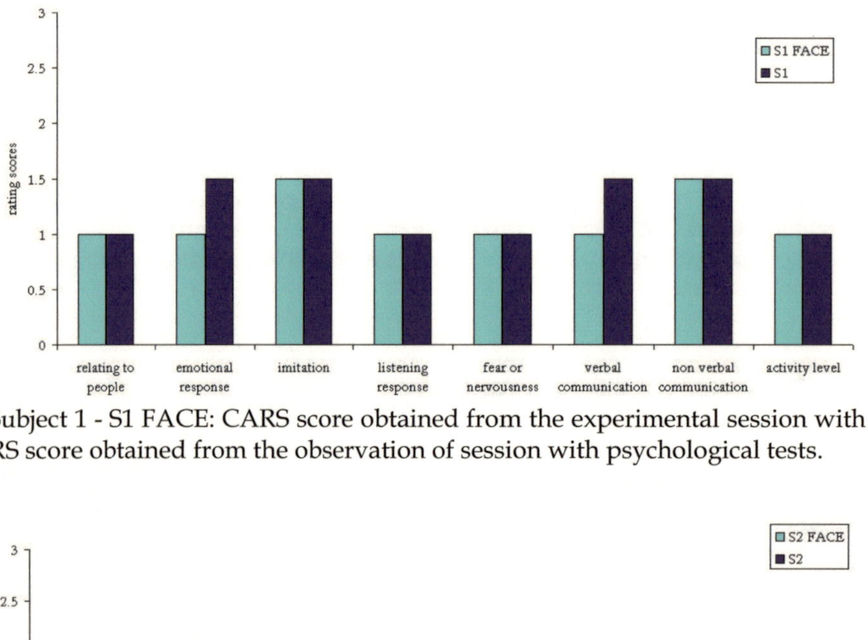

Fig. 5. Subject 1 - S1 FACE: CARS score obtained from the experimental session with FACE. S1: CARS score obtained from the observation of session with psychological tests.

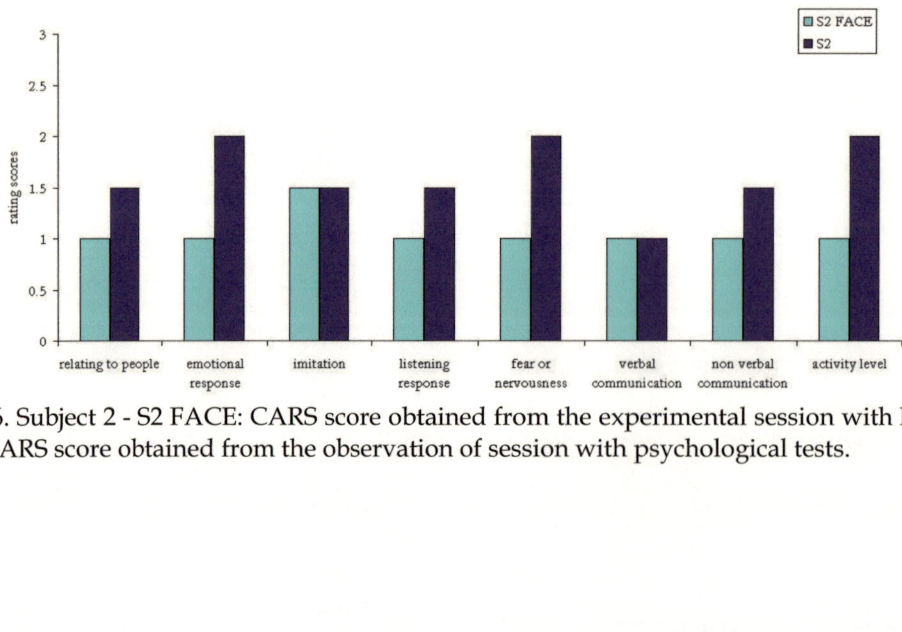

Fig. 6. Subject 2 - S2 FACE: CARS score obtained from the experimental session with FACE. S2: CARS score obtained from the observation of session with psychological tests.

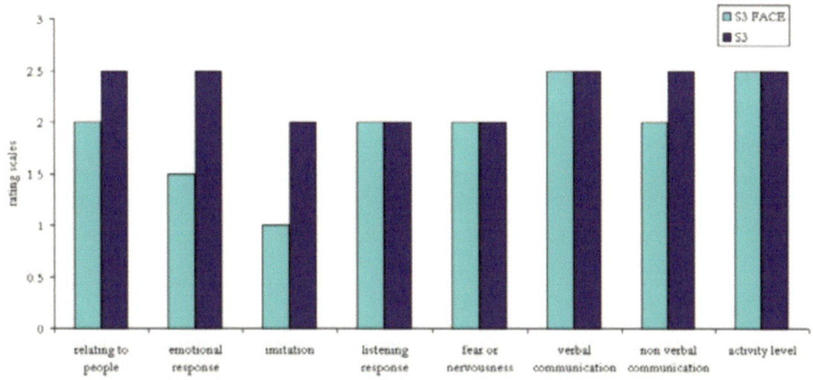

Fig. 7. Subject 3 - S3 FACE: CARS score obtained from the experimental session with FACE. S3: CARS score obtained from the observation of session with psychological tests.

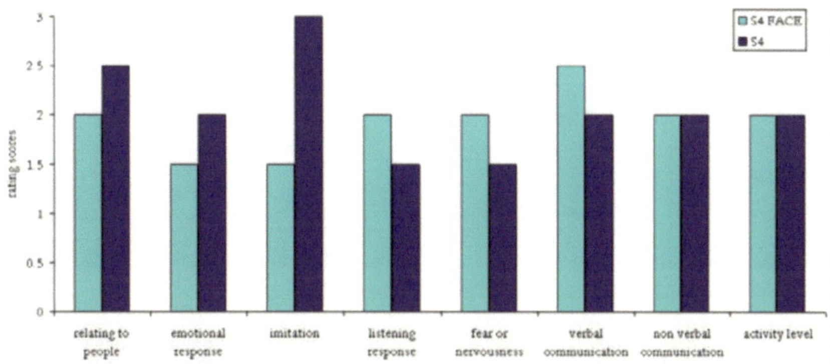

Fig. 8. Subject 4 - S4 FACE: CARS score obtained from the experimental session with FACE. S4: CARS score obtained from the observation of session with psychological tests.

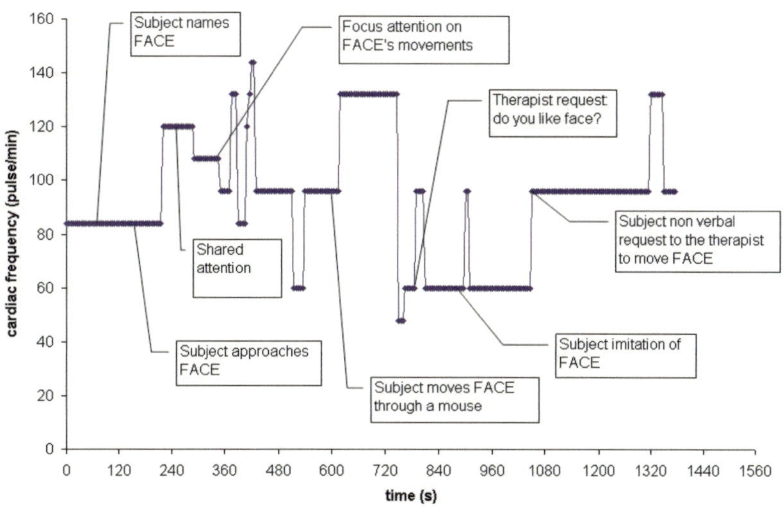

Fig. 9. Typical trace of a subject's heart rate during the treatment.

Figures 10, 11 and 12 show snapshots of an experimental session. In figure 10 the subject shows is shown to completely focus his attention on FACE. In figure 11 a spontaneous approaching of the subject for eye contact with FACE is shown. While figure 12 shows the non verbal requesting of the subject through a conventional gesture (a wink).

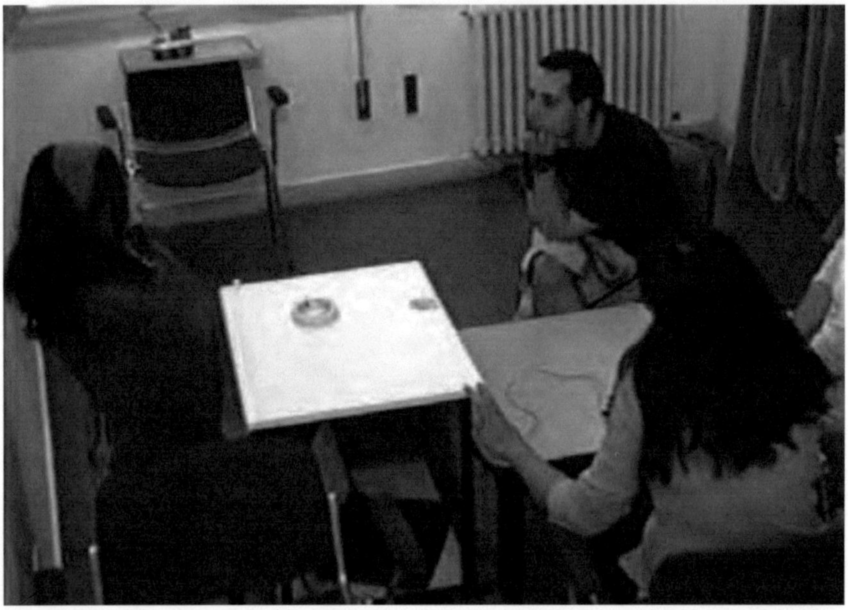

Fig. 10. Experimental session: focus of attention on FACE (S4).

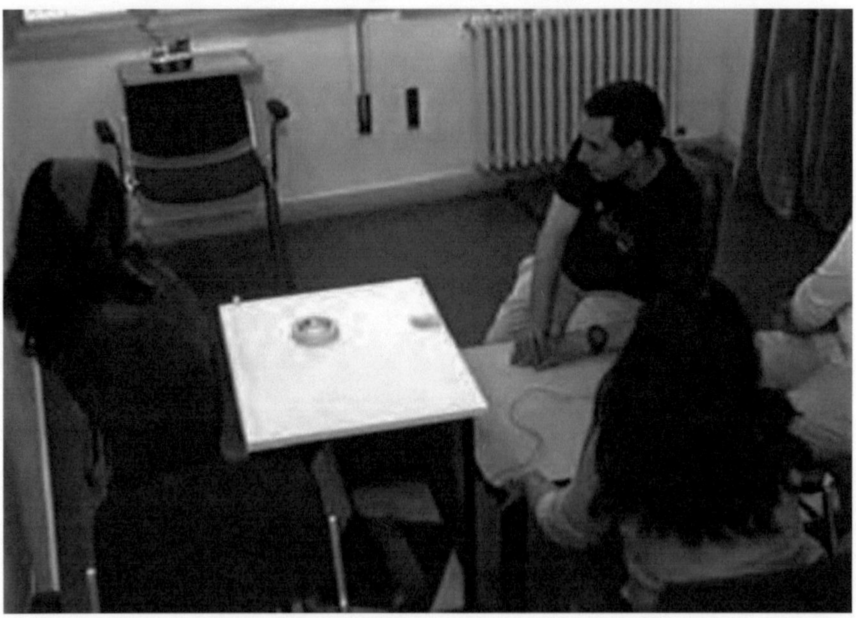

Fig. 11. Experimental session: spontaneous approaching for eye contact with FACE (S4).

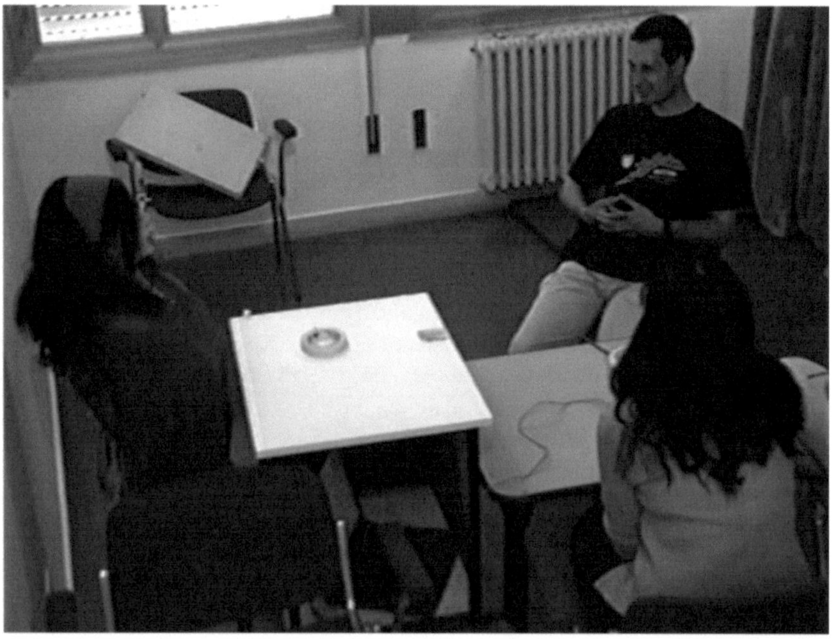

Fig. 12. Experimental session: non verbal requesting through conventional gesture (S4).

The therapeutic trails are still in preliminary phases. Nevertheless, all 4 subjects as well as controls show no fear in the presence of FACE, and all autistic subject showed same improvement in CARS scores, particularly as regards imitation, communication and emotional response.
Future work in this direction will focus on identifying specific criteria for evaluation the subject response, on conducting a larger range of trails, and on repeating treatment monitor signs of progress in patients. These initial results illustrate the validity of the android based FACE-T approach in social and emotive treatments in ASD. We believe that its potency lies in the fact that FACE is based primarily on learning by imitation while deficits in imitation are implicated in ASD.

9. Conclusion

The aim of FACE-T is to act as a human-machine interface for non verbal communication. The learning process in FACE is based on imitating predefined stereotypical behaviours which can be represented in terms of FAPs followed by a continuous interaction with its environment. At present FACE is applied to enhance social and emotive abilities in children with autism. The experimental sessions allowed us to collect preliminary data in terms of therapeutic treatment for patients with disorders in the autistic spectrum. However, what is behind FACE? There is the application of the smart soft matter, algorithms and robotics, there is the attempt to understand the complexity of biological behaviour, there are people with autism. During a test, little M., following the movements of FACE's eyes, noticed that FACE looked at him again and a little bit surprised, upon a request of the therapist to give a meaning to this situation, said "I exist too and therefore I'm important". What is behind FACE?.

10. Acknowledgments

Authors would like to thank the Academy of Fine Arts of Carrara, Italy, http://www.accademiacarrara.it, in the persons of Director Baudinelli and Prof. Marchetti for the work performed on the latest prototype of FACE.

11. References

American Psychiatric Association (1994). Diagnostic and statistical manual (4th ed.). Washington, DC: Author.

Baron-Cohen, S.; Ring, H.; Bullmore, E.; Wheelwright, A.C. & Williams, S.C.R. (2000). The amygdala theory of autism. Neuroscience and Behavioral Reviews. 24, 355-364.

Baron-Cohen, S. (1997). Mindblindness: An Essay on Autism and Theory of Mind. Cambridge, MA: MIT Press.

Beurle, R.L. (1956). Properties of a mass of cells capable of regenerating pulses. Phil. Trans. R. Soc. A240, 5597.

Billard, A. (2002). Play, Dreams and Imitation in Robota. In K. Dautenhahn, B. Edmonds and L. Canamero (eds), Socially Intelligent Agents, Kluwer publisher, 165-173.

Breazeal (Ferrell), C. & Scassellati, B. (2000). Infant-like Social Interactions Between a Robot and a Human Caretaker in Special issue of Adaptive Behavior on Simulation Models of Social Agents, guest editor Kerstin Dautenhahn.

Dapretto, M.; Davies, M.S.; Pfeifer, J.H.; Scott, A.A.; Sigman, M.; Bookheimer, S.Y. & Iacoboni, M. (2005). Understanding emotions in others: mirror neuron dysfunction in children with autism spectrum disorders, Nature Neuroscience 9, 28 – 30.

Dautenhahn, K. (2002a). Design Spaces and Niche Spaces of Believable Social Robots. Proceedings IEEE Ro-man 2002 International Workshop on Robot and Human Interactive Communication, September 25-27, Berlin, Germany, pp. 192-197, IEEE Press.

Dautenhahn, K.; Werry, I.; Rae J. & al., (2002b). Robotic playmates: analysing interactive competencies of children with autism playing with a mobile robot. In Dautenhahn K, Bond A, Canamero L et al, eds. Socially intelligent agents creating relationships with computers and robots. Kluwer Academic Publishers. 117-124.

Davies, S.; Bishop, D.; Manstead, A.S.R. & Tantam, D. (1994). Face Perception in children with autism and Aspergers Syndrome. Journal of Child Psychology and Psychiatry, 35, 1033-1057.

Dawson, G.; Meltzoff, A.; Osterling, J. & Rinaldi, J. (1998). Neuropsychological correlates of early symptoms of autism. Child development, 69, 1277-1285.

Decety, J.; Perani, D.; Jeannerod, M.; Bettinardi, V.; Tadary, B.; Woods, R.; Mazziotta, J.C. & Fazio, F. (1994). Mapping motor representations with positron emission tomography. Nature, 371, 600-602.

Decety, J. (1996). Do imagined and executed actions share the same neural substrate? Cognitive Brain Research, 3, 87-93.

Edelman, G.M. (1993). Bright Air, Brilliant Fire: On the Matter of the Mind. Basic Books; Reprint edition.

Ekman, P. (1992). Are there basic emotions? Psychological Review 99 (3), 550-553

Ekman, P. & Friesen, W. (1982). Measuring facial movement with the facial action coding system, In: Ekman, P. (Ed.), Emotion in the Human Face. Cambridge University Press, Cambridge, UK, pp. 178-211.

Fadiga, L.; Fogassi, L.; Pavesi, G. & Rizzolatti, G. (1995). Motor facilitation during action observation: A magnetic stimulation study. J. Neurophysiol., 73, 2608-2611.

Gallese, V. & Goldman, A. (1998). Mirror neurons and the simulation theory of mind-reading, Trends in Cognitive Sciences Vol . 2, No. 12.

Klein, A.; Warren Jones, BA.; Schultz, R.T.; Volkmar, F.R. & Cohen, D. (2002). Visual Fixation Patterns During Viewing of Naturalistic Social Situations as Predictors of Social Competence in Individuals with Autism. Arch Gen Psychiatry. 59: 809-816.

Kozima, H.; Nakagawa, C. & Yano, H. (2004). Can a robot empathize with people?, International Journal Artificial Life and Robotics Vol.8, pp.83-88.

Kozima, H. (2002). Infanoid: A babybot that explores the social environment, K. Dautenhahn, A. H. Bond, L. Canamero, B. Edmonds (eds.), Socially Intelligent Agents: Creating Relationships with Computers and Robots, Amsterdam: Kluwer Academic Publishers, pp.157-164.

Izard, C. (1993). Four systems for emotion activation: cognitive and non cognitive processes, Psychological Review 100, 68-90

Izard, C. (1977). Human Emotions, Plenum Press, New York, NY.

Izard, C. (1994). Cognition is one of four types of emotion activating systems, In: Ekman, P., Davidson, R. (Eds.), The Nature of Emotion. Oxford University Press, New York, NY, pp. 203-208.

Izhikevich, E.M. (2003). Simple model of spiking neurons. IEEE transaction on neural networks, vol. 15, n° 6.

Izhikevich, E.M. (2005), Polycronization: computation with spikes. Neural Computation.

Izhikevich, E.M.; Gally J.A. & Edelman G.M. (2004). Spike-timing dynamics of neural groups. Cerebral Cortex, 14:933-944

Lord, C. ; Rutter, M. & Le Couter, A. (1994). Autism Diagnostic Interview-revised: A revised version of a diagnostic interview for caregivers of individuals with possible pervasive developmental disorders. Journal of Autism and Developmental Disorders 24, 659-686.

Lord, C.; Risi, S. ; Lambrecht, L. ; Cook, E.H. ; Leventhal, B.L. & al. (2000). The Autism Diagnostic Observation Schedule-Generic: A standard measure of social and communication deficits associated with the spectrum of autism. Journal of Autism and Developmental Disorders, 30, 205-223.

Maestro, S.; Muratori, F.; Cavallaro, M.C.; Pei, F.; Stern, D.; Golse, B. & Palacio-Espasa, F. (2002). Attentional skills during the first 6 months of age in autism spectrum disorder. J Am Acad Child Adolesc Psychiatry, 41(10):1239-45.

Mataric, M. (2002). Situated Robotics, Encyclopedia of Cognitive Science, Nature Publishers Group, Macmillian Reference Ltd.,

Michaud, F.; Duquette, A. & Nadeau, I. (2003). Characteristics of mobile robotic toys for children with Pervasive Developmental Disorders. Proceedings IEEE Conference on Systems, Man, and Cybernetics.

Michaud, F. & Théberge-Turmel, C. (2002). Mobile robotic toys and autism. In Dautenhahn K, Bond A, Canamero L et al, eds. Socially intelligent agents creating relationships with computers and robots. Kluwer Academic Publishers, 125-132.

Meltzoff, A.N. & Moore, M.K. (1995). Infant's understanding of people and things: From body imitation to folk psychology. In J. L. Bermúdez, A. Marcel, & N. Eilan (Eds.), The Body and the Self (pp. 43-69). Cambridge, MA: MIT Press.

Meltzoff, A.N. & Moore, K.M. (1997). Explaining Facial Imitation: A theoretical Model, Early development and Parenting, Vol 6, 179-192.

Nadel, J. ; Revel, A. ; Andry, P. & Gaussier P. (2004a). Towards communications: first imitation in infants, children with autism and robots. Interaction Studies. 1, 45-75.

Nadel, J., (2004b). Early imitation and the emergence of a sense of agency. Proceedings of the Fourth International Workshop on Epigenetic Robotics, Genova, Italy.

O'Reilly, R.C. & Munakata Y. (2000). Computational Exploration in Cognitive Neuroscience: Understanding the Mind by Simulating the Brain. Bradford Book, MIT Press, Cambridge.

Pioggia, G.; Ahluwalia, A.; Carpi, F.; Marchetti, A.; Ferro, M.; Rocchia, W. & De Rossi, D. (2004). FACE: Facial Automaton for Conveying Emotions. Applied Bionics and Biomechanics. 1(2), 91-100.

Pioggia, G.; Igliozzi, R.; Ferro, M.; Ahluwalia, A.; Muratori, F. & De Rossi, D. (2005). An Android for Enhancing Social Skills and Emotion Recognition in Autistic patients. IEEE Transaction on Neural System and Rehabilitation Engineering. 3(4), 507-515.

Rizzolatti, G.; Fadiga, L.; Fogassi, L. & Gallese, V. (1999). Resonance behaviors and mirror neurons. Archives of Italian Biology. 137, 85-100.

Rizzolatti, G. & Arbib, M.A. (1998). Language within our grasp. Trends Neurosci., 21, 188-94.

Schopler, E.; Reichler, R.J. & Renner, B.R. (1988). The Childhood Autism Rating Scale. Los Angeles: Western Psychological Services.

Smith I. M., Bryson S.E. Imitation and action in autism: A critical review. Psychology Bulletin, 1994, 116, 259-273.

Spelke, E.S.; Phillips, A. & Woodward, A.L. (1995). Infants Knowledge of objects motion and human action. In: Sperber D., Premack D., Premack AJ., eds causal Cognition: A Multidisciplinary Debate. Oxford, England: Oxford University Press; 44-78.

Schultz, R.T.; Gauthier, I.; Klin, A.; Fulbrigth, R.; Anderson, A.; Volkmar, F.R.; Skudlarski, P.; Lacadie, C.; Cohen, DJ. & Gore, J.C. (2000). Abnormal ventral temporal cortical activity among individuals with autism and asperger syndrome during face discrimination. Arch Gen Psychiatry. 57: 331-340.

Tager-Flusberg, H. & Cohen, D.J. (1994). Understanding other minds: Perspectives from autism. New York: Oxford University Press.

Weir, S. & Emanuel, R. (1976). Using Logo to Catalyse Communication in an Autistic Child. D.A.I. Research Report, University of Edinburgh.

World Health Organization (1993). International classification of diseases. (10th ed., Draft version). Geneva.

25

Upper-Limb Robotic Rehabilitation Exoskeleton: Tremor Suppression

J.L. Pons, E. Rocon, A.F. Ruiz, J.C. Moreno
Bioengineering Group, Instituto de Automática Industrial - CSIC
Spain

1. Introduction

The interest of the scientific community in medical Robotics and rehabilitation Robotics is growing every year. Rehabilitation Robotics aims to apply robotic technology (sensors, actuators, control) to the rehabilitation and assistance of disabled people. Only some years ago developers were able to implement viable robotic systems to assist a person with a functional limitation. Thus, devices have been developed to assist mobility and the motor functions of the arms and legs, among others.

Tremor is a movement disorder that has a great impact on the quality of life of people who suffer it, mainly to do specific tasks (Rocon et al., 2004). It can affect the head, face, jaw, voice or the upper and lower extremities. In particular, tremor that affects the upper limbs is of major interest, since it can be very disabling to lead an independent life. It is a symptom associated with some abnormal neurological condition or cerebral lesions and degenerative diseases, including Parkinson's disease, essential tremor, orthostatic tremor, cerebellar diseases, ethylic intoxication, among others.

As well as medication, rehabilitation programmes and surgical interventions, the application of biomechanical loading on tremor movement has been shown to be a technique that is able to suppress the effects of tremor on the human body (Rocon et al., 2004). Starting from this principle, the development of upper-limb non-invasive ambulatory robotic exoskeletons is presented as a promising solution for patients who cannot benefit from the use of medication to suppress the tremor. An orthosis is defined as a medical device applied externally to a limb of the human body to establish some kind of functional compensation. In this area robotic exoskeletons have emerged, in the form of orthoses, to provide motor assistance and functional compensation to disabled people.

An exoskeleton is an external structural mechanism whose joints match those of the human body. It adapts to a person so that physical contact between the operator and the exoskeleton enables a direct transfer of mechanical power and information signals. Similarly, it must provide an effective interface between the mechanical structure and the upper limb, bearing in mind the characteristics of the soft tissue of the muscular system, (Ruiz, 2005). Thus, one of the most important specific aspects of rehabilitation robotics is the intrinsic interaction between the human being and the robot. This interaction has two key points: 1) a cognitive interaction with which the human being is able to control the robot while the robot transmits feedback to the human being, 2) a biomechanical

interaction related to the application of controlled forces between the human being and robot.
In the event of reducing tremor, the orthosis must be able to apply viscous or inertial loads and opposing forces to the arm tremor movement, in some joints of the upper limb. As a portable device, exoskeletons must exhibit a number of aesthetic, cosmetic, and functional characteristics (Rocon et al., 2005a). The aesthetic and cosmetic characteristics are directly related to the size, weight and appearance of the robotic device. The functionality of the device is more related to matching the torque, speed and bandwidth required for the system and its robustness during the operation.
In the framework of the DRIFTS project the WOTAS (Wearable Orthosis for Tremor Assessment and Suppression) device was developed, which is a robotic exoskeleton that can apply dynamic internal forces, i.e., without any external reference, on the upper limb and it will be the platform used to evaluate control strategies for tremor suppression by applying biomechanical loads (Manto et al., 2003). In this chapter we will describe the general concept of WOTAS in detail, highlight its special characteristics and the design and selection of system components. Two new control strategies will also be described for tremor suppression. Finally, the results obtained in the exoskeleton clinical trials will be presented.

2. WOTAS

The aim of the WOTAS exoskeleton is to provide a platform to evaluate control strategies for cancelling the tremor with robotic exoskeletons. Furthermore, it constitutes an evaluation and diagnosis tool for patients suffering tremors under the effects of tremor suppression strategies or in non-intervention conditions.

2.1 Mechanical design

The intrinsically dynamic characteristics of tremor mean that the conventional orthotic systems on sale do not suppress tremor because, in these instances, the orthoses tend to lose alignment with the body instead of suppressing the tremor. This loss in alignment can be explained by the fact that when the orthosis tries to apply forces on the arm, the fixation supports tend to rotate over its axis (Rocon et al., 2005a). Accordingly, in the framework of the DRIFTS project the development of a robotic system with specific characteristics for the application of dynamic forces on the arm was posed. The fixation of the orthosis on the upper limb is fundamental because it enables forces to be applied and distributed along the different body limbs involved. Moreover, for the dynamic elements to develop their action, it is necessary to have a base, or rigid structure (the orthosis), which acts as a point for applying those external forces that cause the dynamic effect.
The WOTAS platform was designed for the elbow and wrist joints, so that different control strategies on the flexo-extension movements of the elbow and the wrist and the pronation-supination of the forearm can be applied, (Rocon et al., 2005a). Therefore, the exoskeleton must be adjustable or adaptable to align its joints with the revolute centres of the elbow and wrist joints.
The mechanical design of the joints related to the WOTAS elbow and wrist flexo-extensions are similar to the orthotic solutions found on the market and are based on the biomechanical behaviour of these joints. The elbow joint, like that of the knee, is probably

the joint in the human body which is more like the revolute joint (Kapandji, 1983). This joint has a variable rotation centre but it can be modelled via a simple rotation joint with a fixed rotation centre. The rotation axis of the elbow joint is located on the line between the two epicondyles. The wrist is a highly complex joint because it consists of a very large number of bones. Therefore, the flexion-extension movement of the wrist does not possess a specific rotation axis. However, the same as for the elbow joint, the flexo-extension movement of the wrist can be considered a pure rotational movement with its rotation axis aligned with the capital and lunar bones of the carpus for the modelling (Rocon et al., 2005a). The design of the system for controlling the pronation-supination movement of the forearm is more complicated. The pronation-supination movement of the forearm is a rotational movement of the forearm on its longitudinal axis which engages two joints that are mechanically connected: the upper radioulnar joint (which belongs to the elbow) and the lower radioulnar joint (which belongs to the wrist) (Kapandji, 1983). The WOTAS platform controls the pronation-supination movement with the rotation control of a bar parallel to the forearm. This bar is fixed very close to the olecranon. Thus the bar is fixed to the ulnar position at elbow level. The distal fixation of the bar is done on the radius head.

From the torque estimates and efforts that the exoskeleton structure must support (Rocon et al., 2005b), duralumin was selected as the material to construct the exoskeleton structure. This material was selected in order to build a lightweight structure with sufficient rigidity to support the efforts.

2.2 Application of forces on the arm

To determine the points of the upper limb where the dynamic forces would be applied, i.e, the points where the arm supports would be placed between the actuators and the arm, a number of biomechanical and physiological considerations of the upper limb have to be observed, such as (Rocon et al., 2005a): 1) the forces on the arm tissues must stay in acceptable limits 2) the arm restrictions in order to preserve normal activity, i.e., like applying compensatory forces on the arm without affecting the natural movement patterns of the upper arm, particularly for the elbow and wrist 3) the interaction of the robotic device with the arm, i.e., where the forces will be applied on the upper limb and how the load will be transmitted to the person for optimum comfort.

To respond to these issues a biomechanical study was done of the upper limb. The aim of this study was to determine the limits of comfort regarding pressure, so that there is an upper limit to the total force that can be applied safely to the upper limb, (Markensco & Yannas, 1979). This study analysed two key aspects: the person's perception of the pressure and the maximum pressure tolerance thresholds (Rocon et al., 2005a). The first aspect is important to select the appropriate strategy to apply to the load on the body.

For the development of the mechanical structure, different types of materials for the securing or support elements between the orthotic device and the arm were considered. The mechanical conditions of these elements is critical because they must ergonomically couple the upper limb, and also the rigidity of the material must be greater than the rigidity of the underlying tissues. To securely fix the structure it was decided to use supports made from thermoplastic. With this type of material, supports are obtained that adapt to the morphology of each user's arm, Figure 1. Each support has at least three contact points per segment and thus misalignments are avoided between the orthosis and limb (Rocon et al., 2006).

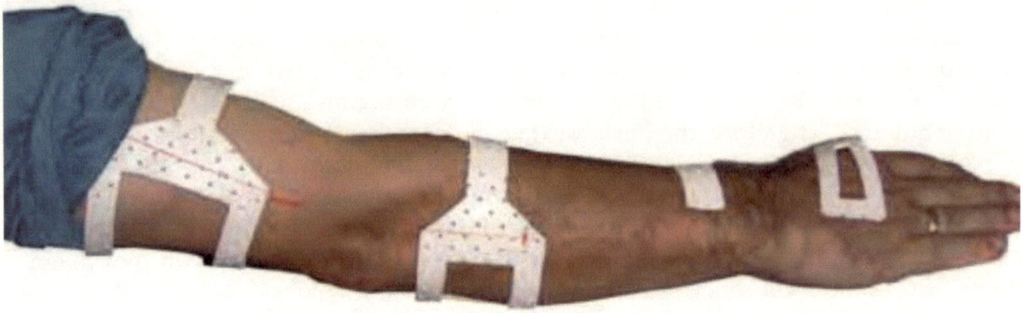

Fig. 1. Illustration of the WOTAS supports on a patient's arm. The supports are manufactured in thermoplastic to best adapt to the morphology of each user's arm.

2.3 Measurement systems

The device is also an evaluation and diagnosis tool for patients who suffer tremors, so it is equipped with kinematic sensors (angular position, speed and acceleration) and kinetics (interaction forces between the orthosis and upper limb). The analysis developed for the selection of sensors and actuators among the several candidate technologies is based on the Dominic method (Rocon et al., 2005a).

2.3.1 Kinematic measurement

Gyroscopes were selected as the technology for the kinematic measurement of the tremor (Rocon et al., 2005a). The main advantages of gyroscopes are that they measure rotational movements (human movements are rotational around the joints), they are not affected by gravity, frequency and amplitude information is precise in a long frequency range, up to DC (zero frequency), the angular position is obtained with an integration, the angular acceleration is obtained with a derivation, they have a high signal/noise relation and do not affect the natural movement of the limb.
An analysis was done of the gyroscopes available commercially and it was decided to use the gyroscope manufactured by Murata GYROSTAR ENC-03J. These gyroscopes are used for stabilising video camera images, so they are expected to be a good alternative for measuring tremor speed. An electronic device was also developed to process the gyroscope signal before it was integrated into the WOTAS system. The basic circuit consists of a bandpass filter with a short frequency between 0.3 Hz and 25 Hz. This is the range of frequencies where nearly all the tremor energy is concentrated, (Rocon et al., 2004).

2.3.2 Kinetic measurement

We selected the strain gauges as the sensor for extracting the kinetic characteristics from the tremor movement. The gauges are responsible for measuring the torque applied by the motors on the WOTAS structure, therefore, they are mounted on the structure so that they only measure the force perpendicular to the motor axis, thus their measurement is not affected by forces caused in undesired directions.
The strain gauges are connected to a Wheatstone Bridge circuit in a combination of four active gauges (full bridge). When a strain is applied to the gauges, there is a change in value of their resistances resulting in an unbalance of the Wheatstone Bridge. This produces an output signal related to the strain value.

2.4 Actuation system

When designing any orthoprosthetic device that works parallel to the human body to suppress the tremor it is of paramount importance to specify the actuators. Vital information for the selection of an actuation technology is the torque and the power required by the application. To obtain these values a study was done with several patients, (Rocon et al., 2005b). Bearing in mind the application requirements, a number of actuators were selected as possible candidate technologies to suppress the tremor, (Rocon et al., 2006). As in the case of the sensors, the Dominic method was used to select the technology to suppress the tremor. From the actuators studied, we selected some for subsequent analysis: Electroactive Polymers (EAPs), Electro- and magneto-rheological fluids (ERF-MRF), DC motors, Shape memory actuators (SMAs), pneumatic muscles and ultrasonic motors. The results of the evaluation process determined that ultrasonic and DC motors are the best solutions for activating the exoskeleton.

A number of experiments were done to evaluate the performance of the ultrasonic motors. The conclusion of our assessment process of the ultrasonic motors is that, although they offer a number of advantages for the rehabilitation robotic field like, for example, their reduced size and silent operation, they are not the right actuators for the exoskeleton proposed in this work due to their poor response to low speeds, which means that they cannot be applied to track slow movements like human movements, (Rocon et al., 2006).

Owing to the problems encountered with ultrasonic motors, a new WOTAS device was implemented using continuous current motors as an actuation element. Continuous current motors are one of the most well-known actuation technologies. We selected the Maxon Motor EC 45 Flat continuous current, which is a very light, small DC motor without brushes that adapts to orthotic applications. In order to match the speed and torque of the DC motor to the application requirements, a gearbox was necessary for the system. This was done via a harmonic drive. In particular, the drive selected for our application was the HDF-014-100-2A. The actuator system configured in this way can apply a maximum torque of 8 N.m. However, the maximum torque was limited electronically to 3 N.m to guarantee user safety. Figure 2 presents the WOTAS version developed from DC motors as actuator elements and coupled to the gearbox (harmonic drive). Similarly all the sensor elements are observed on the mechanical structure and the fixation of the orthosis to the patient's arm. The total weight of the system developed is approximately 850 g, (Rocon et al., 2006).

2.5 Control architecture

The WOTAS control architecture basically consists of 3 components: 1) the orthosis, with its structure, sensors and actuators 2) a control unit, responsible for executing the algorithms in real time to suppress the tremor and the acquisition card for the interface between the sensors, actuators and the controller 3) a remote computer, which in our case executes an application developed to do the interface between all the system and the doctor who is using it.

The WOTAS device operates in three different modes:

1. **Monitoring**. In this operation mode, WOTAS behaves like a system to measure and characterise the tremor qualitatively and quantitatively. Thus it offers no opposition to the patient's voluntary or tremor movement.
2. **Passive intervention**. In this mode, WOTAS behaves like a device that can mechanically damp the tremor movements, simulating the application of viscosity or inertia on the upper limb to dissipate vibrations caused by the tremor and improve the user's voluntary movement.

3. **Active intervention.** In this mode, WOTAS suppresses the tremor dynamically, and estimates the voluntary and tremor movement signals in real time and generates actuation signals proportional to tremor intensity.

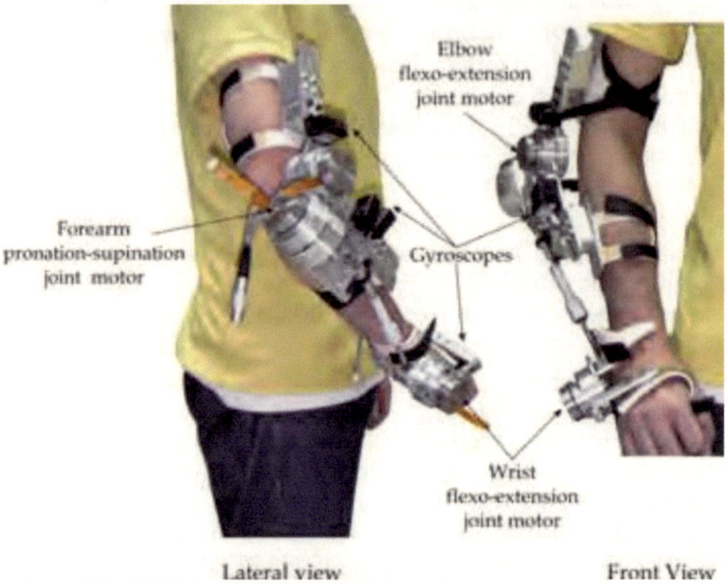

Fig. 2. Final version of WOTAS for the control of three human upper-limb movements: flexion-extension of the elbow, flexion-extension of the wrist and pronation-supination of the forearm.

2.5.1 Computer application

A computer tool was developed to manage the system. The application is installed in an external computer and provides communication with the device, data storage, signal acquisition, information analysis and display, and report generation. As a basic aspect, it evaluates the control algorithms developed in Matlab for tremor suppression to control their execution, monitor algorithm variables and adjust or tune algorithm parameters in real time. Moreover, it implements the specified measurement protocol and the clinical trials defined, and displays quantitative information of the functionality of the algorithms evaluated.

3. Control strategies

The application of biomechanical loading to reduce tremor can be done using portable devices (robotic exoskeletons) and fixed devices (devices mounted on platforms, for example, wheelchairs), (Rocon et al., 2004). The first approach is characterised by applying internal forces on specific joints of the human body, whereas the second is based on applying external forces globally to reduce tremor.

This control strategy can be implemented actively and passively. The passive concept uses a mechanical damper, (Kotovsky and Rosen, 1998), which generates a dissipation force on tremor movement. It is based on increasing the damping of the biomechanical oscillation system where the tremor is generated.

In active systems, (Rosen et al., 1995), actuators generate a movement of equal amplitude but in counter-phase from the estimate in real time of the tremor component of the movement. Thus the system actively cancels and effectively subtracts the tremor from the total movement done by the exoskeleton user. Unlike in the passive approach, where tremor movement energy is dissipated, in active systems, energy is transferred (in counter-phase to tremor movement) to the systems.

After an exhaustive bibliographical review on tremor characteristics and control strategies for the application of forces on the human body, two control strategies were defined to suppress tremor using biomechanical loads, (Rocon et al., 2005a):

1. *Tremor reduction via impedance control.* A strategy is defined to control the impedance of the exoskeleton-upper-limb set. In this instance, the rigidity, damping and inertia parameters of the upper limb are modified to study the effects on tremor in this limb's joints.
2. *Implementation of a notch filter focusing on the frequency of tremor movement.* The use of noise reduction techniques is posed to suppress the pathological tremor actively.

3.1 Tremor reduction via impedance control

The impedance of a system is defined as the relation between the reaction force of the system to the external movement imposed on it and the movement, (Hogan, 1985). Generally, impedance involves three components: rigidity, damping and inertia. In the literature there is evidence that variation in the three components modifies the biomechanical characteristics of the tremor in the upper limb, (Adelstein, 1981).

In this work approach, the musculo-skeletal system (each joint of the upper limb that contributes to the tremor) is modelled as a second-order biomechanical system, (Adelstein, 1981). It is known that the frequency response of a second-order system presents the behaviour of a low-pass filter. The cut-off frequency of this filter is directly related to the biomechanical parameters of the second-order system. The approach proposed consists of selecting the right inertia and damping parameters, so that the cut-off frequency, f_c, of the musculo-skeleton system is immediately above the maximum frequency of voluntary movement, cancelling the tremor component of overall movement.

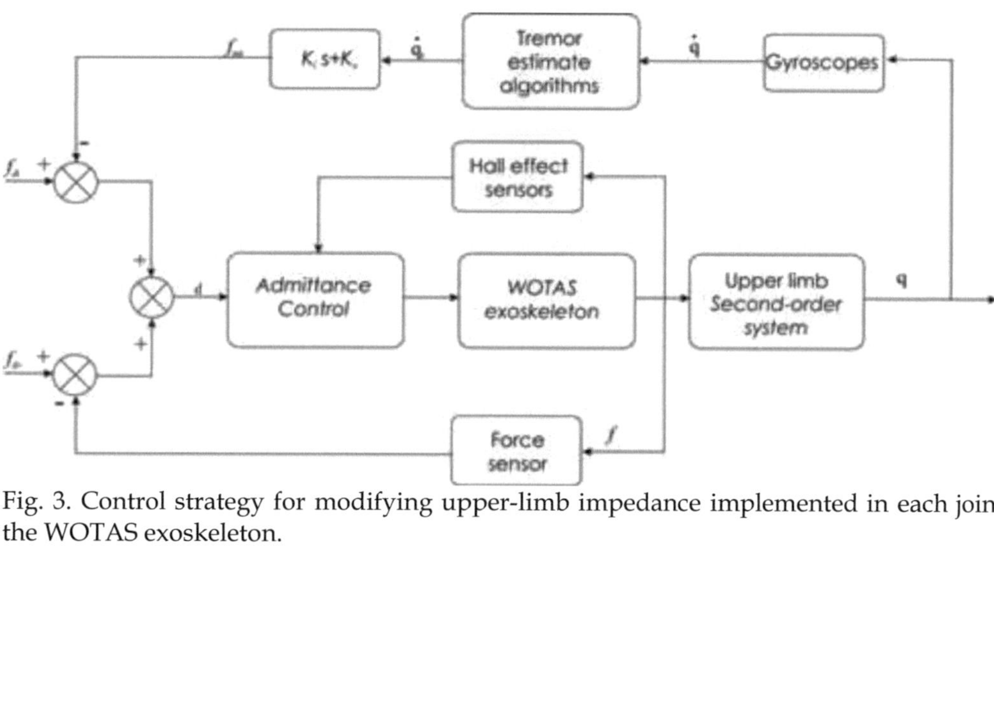

Fig. 3. Control strategy for modifying upper-limb impedance implemented in each joint of the WOTAS exoskeleton.

The control algorithm illustrated in Figure 3 is the one proposed for modifying the biomechanical parameters of the upper limb. As can be observed in the Figure, the force control applied by the exoskeleton on the arm is implemented using external control force loops around an internal speed loop. For each joint, a specific motor controller used in WOTAS undertakes a motor speed internal control loop. Around this internal loop, two external loops are closed: one for feedback and interaction force control between the exoskeleton and the limb (lower loop); the other loop applies forces to alter the biomechanical forces of the upper limb to suppress the tremor (upper loop). The force value, τ_d, which is introduced in the internal force loop is calculated via the sum of actions of the two external loops:

$$\tau_d = f_{dt} - f_{mt} + f_{dv} - \tau = f_{dt} - k_i q_t - k_v \dot{q}_t + f_d v - \tau \qquad (1.1)$$

The upper part of the control loop proposed is the one responsible for modifying the apparent upper limb impedance. The feedback coefficients K_i and K_v define the apparent inertia and damping characteristics of each upper limb joint. The force (f_{mt}) applied on the arm is calculated from the coefficients and the filtered information of the movement of each upper limb joint (so that only the tremor information is re-fed). This force tends to disappear as the tremor is suppressed. Thus, the difference between the calculated force, f_{mt}, and the desired force, f_{dt}, will tend to zero because in our application, the value of f_{dt} was selected as zero.

The lower part of the control loop proposed is responsible for minimising the effects of the exoskeleton on voluntary movements. In this loop, the force sensors measure the interaction between the exoskeleton and the upper limb (τ). In ideal conditions, a patient who does not present tremors must not feel any resistance to the natural movement of his/her arm from the exoskeleton. As a result, the added impedance is adjusted by the lower loop to zero. Accordingly, the consign that defines the force, f_{dv}, applied on the voluntary movement of the user, is adjusted to zero

The control strategy proposed has an adaptive behaviour so that constantly (in real time) it updates the tremor amplitude estimate. Thus the system can respond to the changes produced by the control strategy on the tremor, (Rocon et al., 2003). Moreover, the control strategy proposed is based on an articular control approach because it is simpler and also makes it possible to implement individual control loops in each joint with a high dynamic range, (Tsagarakis & Caldwell, 2003). Furthermore, the fact that each exoskeleton joint tries to suppress the tremor generated in its corresponding anatomical joint is interesting because it guarantees reducing the tremor in each joint. Thus the problem of coupling the tremor between the upper-limb joints is successfully tackled, (Rocon et al., 2005a).

In studies done by the authors, the behaviour and contribution of each joint in the upper-limb tremor were evaluated, (Rocon et al., 2003). This work has shown that in most patients the tremor movement "displaces" along the kinematic chain of the arm when its effects are reduced (by applying biomechanical loads) on one of the arm joints. However, the study of tremor behaviour when its effects are cancelled in different joints of the arm has still not been properly studied, (Rocon et al., 2004). Thus the factors that affect the functioning and stability of the force controller vary more from joint to joint than from Cartesian direction to Cartesian direction. This aspect led to devising active and independent control strategies in each joint. Accordingly, if the cancellation of the tremor in one of the joints increases the tremor in the other joint, the algorithm responsible for controlling the adjacent joint will identify the increased tremor and try to reduce the tremor generated by coupling the upper-limb joints. The aim is thus that the active behaviour of tremor reduction in each joint reaches equilibrium, thereby decreasing the coupling effects of the upper-limb joints.

3.2 Exploitation of the repetitive characteristics of tremor movement

Tremor is usually described in the bibliography as a rhythmic and involuntary contraction characterised by oscillations at a central frequency, (Rocon et al., 2004). Tremor frequency varies according to patient pathology. For patients with essential tremor the frequency range is between 5 and 8 Hz, while for rest tremor the frequency is usually low, between 3 and 6 Hz.

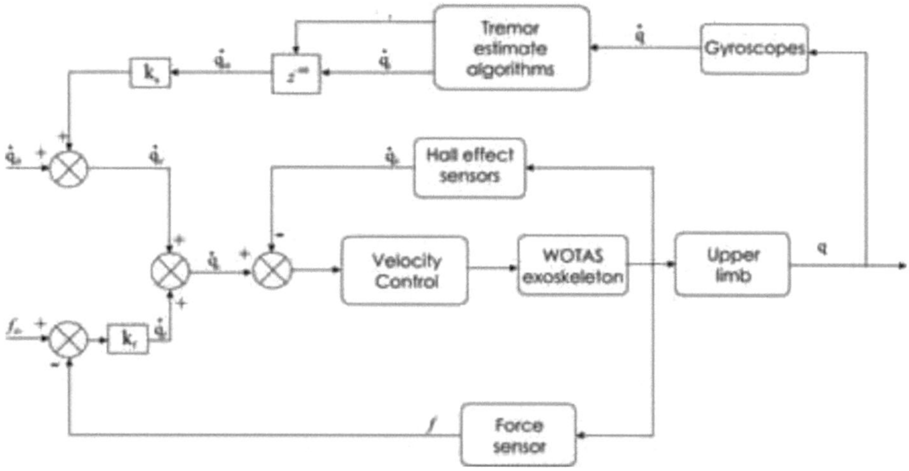

Fig. 4. Repetitive control strategy of speed implemented in the exoskeleton.

Moreover, the frequency varies among patients with a definite pathology, but it tends to be stable in the same patient. This characteristic is explored in this work by implementing a control strategy based on repetitive control (RC), (Inoue, 1998). To implement the active controller from the repetitive control to suppress the tremor, an articular control approach was used, i.e., each joint was controlled independently to minimise tremor-coupling problems in the different upper-limb joints. The control strategy designed and proposed for active control of the pathological tremor is illustrated in Figure 4. In the control strategy proposed the speed of each human upper-limb joint is controlled. The consign speed, q_c which is introduced in the speed control loop is calculated using the following control law:

$$\dot{q_c} = \dot{q_f} + \dot{q_{tr}} = k_f(f_{dv} - f) + (\dot{q_{dt}} + z^{-M_k} \cdot \dot{q_t}) \tag{1.2}$$

As in the passive approach, this strategy also consists of two loops. The upper loop is responsible for the action actively suppressing the tremor, while the lower loop is responsible for reducing the effects of biomechanical loading on natural movement. In the upper loop an estimate is done of the speed of tremor movement, q_t. The amplitude of the speed of tremor movement suffers a time lag of M seconds. The value of this time lag is defined by the frequency of tremor movement, ω_t. Thus, the amplitude of tremor movement, added to a speed consign, q_{dt}, is re-fed to the internal speed controller of the WOTAS exoskeleton. Thus, the WOTAS actuators will describe a speed profile with equal amplitude but in counter-phase to tremor movement, actively cancelling and effectively subtracting the tremor from the user's total movement. Accordingly, in our system the speed consign, q_{dt}, is adjusted to zero. The value of the constant, ka, defines the amplitude of the movement that will be re-fed to the speed controller.

The lower loop is in charge of reducing the application of loads on voluntary movement. Accordingly, an admittance control is implemented, i.e., the sensors measure the force of interaction between the exoskeleton and the upper limb, *f*, which multiplied by the force control loop gain, k_f, defines the speed consign, q_f, which is re-fed to the WOTAS motor internal speed controller. As already mentioned, in ideal conditions, a patient who does not present tremors must not feel any resistance to the natural movement of his/her arm from the robotic device. Accordingly, as in the passive control case proposed above, the consign defining the force applied on the user's voluntary movement, f_{dv}, is adjusted to zero.

As explained in the preceding paragraph, unlike the passive approach, in which tremor movement energy is dissipated, in the active approach energy is transferred (in counter-phase to tremor movement) to the system. The active tremor suppression approach had never been implemented in any system for suppressing tremor. The system proposed is innovative and the evaluation of its effectiveness on suppressing pathological tremor and the effect on users will be presented in the next section of this chapter.

3.3 Tremor estimate

The two control strategies presented in the previous sections require identifying and tracking voluntary movement and tremor movement in real time. The major challenge of this type of treatment, irrespective of the approach used, is the distinction between what is tremor movement and what is voluntary movement before the control strategy applies any type of biomechanical loading on the arm. This process requires estimating both movements in real time.

In the literature, the algorithm most used for estimating tremor movement is the Weighted-frequency Fourier linear combiner (WFLC) developed by Riviere, (Riviere & Thakor, 1998), in his doctoral thesis for filtering the tremor signal caused by physiological tremor in the context of microsurgery. This algorithm models tremor movement as a sinusoidal movement. Its recurrent implementation updates the model parameters at each iteration, which transforms it into a simple algorithm, easy to implement and with low computational cost. These characteristics are very interesting for our application and we have therefore adopted it as our first alternative. The WFLC can be described by equation 1.3, where wk = $[w_{1k} \ldots w_{2Mk}]^T$ is the adaptive vector of the Fourier coefficients, s_k is the input signal, *M* is the number of harmonics of the model signal,μ is an adjustment parameter of the coefficients to be estimated.

$$\varepsilon_k = s_k - \sum_{r=1}^{M} \left[w_{r_k} \sin(r\omega_{0_k} k) + w_{r+M_k} \cos(r\omega_{0_k} k) \right] \tag{1.3}$$

In its recurrent implementation, the WFLC is capable of estimating the amplitude and frequency of the tremor in real time, (Riviere & Thakor, 1998).

$$w_{0_{k+1}} = w_{0_k} + 2\mu_0 \varepsilon_k \sum_{r=1}^{M} r \left(w_{r_k} x_{M+r_k} - w_{M+r_k} x_{r_k} \right) \tag{1.4}$$

Where

$$x_{rk} = \begin{cases} \sin\left(r \sum_{t=1}^{k} w_{0_t}\right), & 1 \le r \le M \\ \cos\left((r-M) \sum_{t=1}^{k} w_{0_t}\right), & M+1 \le r \le 2M \end{cases} \tag{1.5}$$

The WFLC algorithm was evaluated in signals measured in patients suffering tremor, (Rocon et al., 2005c). In the trials done, the algorithm was able to estimate the tremor movement of all the patients with accuracy always lower than 2 degrees. The main disadvantage of the WFLC is the need for a preliminary filtering stage to eliminate the voluntary component of the movement. This filtering stage introduces an undesired time lag for our system when estimating tremor movement.

The ideal solution is to define a method that can estimate human voluntary and tremor movements in real time. The tremor literature (Elble et al., 1990), (Mann et al., 1989), (Riviere & Thakor, 1998), indicates that voluntary movements and tremor movements are considerably different. Voluntary movements are slower while tremor movements are brusquer. This indicates that adaptive algorithms to estimate and track movement would be useful when separating the two movements with an appropriate design. The underlying idea is to design the filters so that they only estimate the less dynamic component of the input signal, which in our case we consider to be voluntary movement, thereby filtering out the tremor movement. Thus, to estimate voluntary movement and tremor movement, the development of a two-stage algorithm is proposed to estimate voluntary movement and tremor movement with a minimum time lag, see Figure 5.

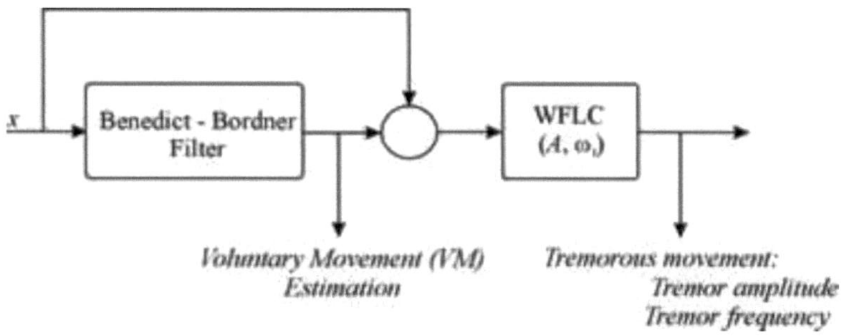

Fig. 5. Two-stage tremor modelling: first, the low frequency content voluntary motion is estimated, secondly, the voluntary motion estimation is subtracted from the original motion, eventually, tremor frequency and amplitude are determined.

First, a set of algorithms was considered to estimate voluntary movement: two point-extrapolator, critically damped g-h estimator, Benedict-Bordner g-h estimator, and Kalman filter. These algorithms implement both estimation and filtering equations. The combination of these actions allows the algorithm to filter out the tremor movement from the overall movement while reducing the phase lag introduced, (Bar-Shalom & Li , 1998). The equation parameters were adjusted to track the movements with lower dynamics (voluntary movement) since tremors present a behaviour characterised by quick movements, (Rocon et al., 2006). The algorithms evaluated were two-degree-of-freedom estimators, i.e., they assume a constant speed movement model. This assumption is reasonable since the sample period is very small compared with the movement speeds (Brookner, 1998), i.e., the sample period adopted was 1 ms and the voluntary movement estimated occurs in a bandwidth lower than 2 Hz. The performance of these algorithms was compared based on their accuracy when voluntary movements of tremor time series from patients were estimated. The result of this analysis indicated that the Benedict-Bordner filter presents the best results with the lowest computational load, (Rocon et al., 2006). This estimation algorithm is a g-h filter with the following tracking update equations:

$$\dot{x}^*_{k,k} = \dot{x}^*_{k,k-1} + h_k \left(\frac{y_k - x^*_{k,k-1}}{T} \right) \tag{1.6}$$

$$x^*_{k,k} = x^*_{k,k-1} + g_k \left(y_k - x^*_{k,k-1} \right) \tag{1.7}$$

and g-h prediction equations, (Brookner, 1998).

$$\dot{x}^*_{k+1,k} = \dot{x}^*_{k,k} \quad (1.8)$$

$$x^*_{k+1,k} = x^*_{k,k} + T\dot{x}^*_{k+1,k} \quad (1.9)$$

The tracking update equations or estimation equations (equations 1.6 and 1.7) provide the joint angular speed and position. The estimated position is based on the use of current measurement as well as past prediction. The estimated state contains all the information that we need from the previous measurements. The predicted position is an estimation of xk+1 based on past states and prediction, equations 1.8 and 1.9, and takes into account current measurement using updated states. The Benedict-Bordner estimator is designed to minimise the transient error. Therefore, it responds faster to changes in movement speed and is slightly under damped, (Bar-Shalom & Li , 1998). The relation between filter parameters is defined by equation 1.10:

$$h = \frac{g^2}{2-g} \quad (1.10)$$

In the second filter stage, the voluntary movement estimated in the first stage is subtracted from the input signal, so it is assumed that the remaining signal is tremor. In this stage the WFLC is used to estimate the amplitude and frequency of tremor movement in real time.
The capacity of the algorithm to estimate the tremor movement parameters was also evaluated in over 40 patients. This study proved that the estimate of tremor movement has a maximum convergence time of 2 seconds and that, after this convergence time, the mean error to estimate tremor movement is always lower than 1 degree. Figure 6 illustrates the functioning of the algorithm with a patient suffering essential tremor when drawing a spiral.

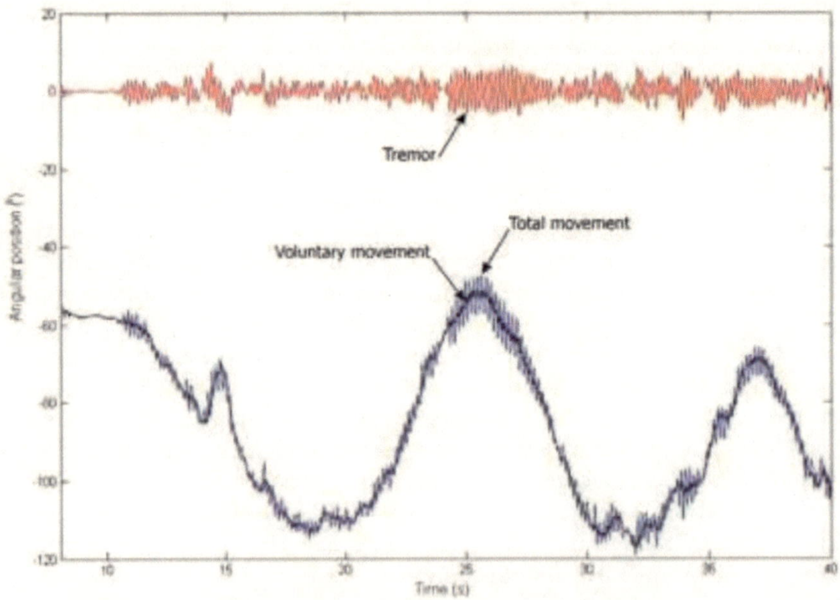

Fig. 6. Illustration of the functioning of the algorithm proposed to estimate voluntary movement and tremor movement with a minimum time lag. The total movement corresponds to the elbow joint of a patient with essential tremor when drawing a spiral. The algorithm consists of two stages, in the first the voluntary movement is estimated using the Bendict-Bordner filter and, in the second stage, the tremor movement is estimated using the WFLC.

4. Measurement protocol

In order to evaluate the capacity of the exoskeleton to suppress the upper-limb pathological tremor, a number of experiments were done. To achieve this aim a protocol was defined for the experiments. These experiments aim 1) to evaluate the hardware platform that was developed 2) to validate the control strategies developed for mechanical pathological tremor suppression 3) to determine the differences between active and passive approaches (control) 4) to determine the best combination of parameters for each approach 5) to evaluate the functionality of the different alternative actuators 6) to estimate the possible impact and acceptance of a future orthotic model to suppress tremor.

The trials were done in two different countries. In the first evaluation stage pre-clinical trials were done at the Department of Neurology at Hôpital Erasme in Brussels, Belgium. The second clinical trial stage was done at the Department of Neurology at the Hospital General in Valencia, Spain. The experiment protocol was approved by the ethical committees at each hospital where the trials were done.

The functioning of the WOTAS exoskeleton was evaluated in 10 patients with tremor-related diseases. The pathology of each patient was first diagnosed by a neurologist at the hospital using the quantification functional scale by Faher et al., (Fahn et al., 1998). There were a total of 7 male patients and 3 female patients. All the patients signed an experiment protocol consent form. They also authorised the data obtained in the experiments to be used for scientific purposes.

During the experiments the only person who knew how the exoskeleton worked was the operator, i.e., the patient, physiotherapist and the doctor did not know whether the orthosis was applying some active or passive strategy to suppress the tremor or whether it was working in free or monitoring mode. This was the approach adopted to reduce the placebo effect obtained in the experiments (Belda et al., 2004).

4.1 Evaluation tasks

In the framework of the project and using a medical base, a set of tasks was selected for patients to do in the evaluation trials. The tasks selected were 1) keeping the arms outstretched 2) taking the finger to the nose 3) keeping the upper limb in a resting position 4) drawing a spiral.

All the tasks done by the patients are clinical and functional trials that neurologists use to diagnose tremor-related diseases. These trials provide relevant amplitude and frequency information that can be used to classify the pathological tremor. Three different measurements for each task and WOTAS functioning mode had to be done to guarantee the repeatability of the data. Similarly, for each of the tasks the time taken to do the task, the time between measurements and a specific file code to be stored on the disk were defined. The total number of repetitions of the tasks was selected so that the total time of the measurement session did not exceed 1 hour to avoid patient fatigue and tiredness during the trials. During the experiments, the different WOTAS functioning modes and tasks were generated randomly. This approach reduced the learning effects and their effect on the analysis of the data obtained, (Rocon et al., 2005a).

4.2 Data analysis

The data used for the analysis come from the gyroscopes placed on each of the joints activated by the WOTAS exoskeleton. The output value of the gyroscopes was sampled at a frequency of 2 KHz. To analyse the values, the data acquired were filtered using a Kernel smoother algorithm and a Gaussian window with 51 width points. The figure of merit selected, R, to evaluate the functioning of the WOTAS exoskeleton is the relation between the spectral power of patient movement with WOTAS operating in monitoring mode, P_{mm}, and the spectral power of patient movement with WOTAS operating in tremor suppression mode P_{ms}, passively and actively, equation 1.10. The bandwidth analysed was between 3 and 8 Hz due to the fact that most pathological tremors occur in this frequency range, (Rocon et al., 2004). Furthermore, voluntary movements related to tasks developed in these experiments occur at frequencies below 2 Hz, (Rocon et al., 2004).

$$R = \frac{P_{ms}}{P_{mm}} \cdot 100 \tag{1.11}$$

Thus, the signal used as a reference is the signal acquired with WOTAS operating in the monitoring mode and the effectiveness of the strategy to suppress the tremor refers to this value. Accordingly, we achieve that both time series (monitoring and suppression) are acquired while the user is wearing the exoskeleton, thereby ensuring that tremor reduction is only due to the action of the tremor suppression strategies and not the mere use of the exoskeleton, (Belda et al., 2004).

5. Experimental results and discussion

Figure 7 illustrates the results obtained from analysing the data generated during the measurement sessions. The abscise axis of the Figure represents the R value in the different experiments with WOTAS operating in the tremor suppression modes actively and passively. The ordinate axis coordinates are related to the patient tremor power obtained when WOTAS operates in the monitoring mode.

In Figure 7 we can check that the robotic exoskeleton has a minimum tremor suppression limit, i.e., if the spectral density of tremor movement is below a lower limit, around 0.15 rad^2/s^3, the WOTAS exoskeleton is ineffective in suppressing the tremor. This spectral energy density corresponds to a tremor with moderate amplitude which is not visually detectable. The existence of a lower WOTAS functioning limit was expected because for tremor amplitudes, the relative movement between the user's skin and the exoskeleton structure acts as a dead zone. Moreover, the system backlash prevents it from acting on tremors with such small amplitudes. The authors believe that this is due to the system backlash and the relative movement between the user's soft tissues and the exoskeleton structure, (Rocon et al., 2005b).

In accordance with the results obtained, it can be said that the mean range of tremor reduction in the active functioning mode is between 3.4% and 95.2%, with a mean reduction value in tremor movement energy of 81.2 %. The results obtained also indicate that when the exoskeleton is functioning in passive mode, the mean range of tremor reduction obtained by the WOTAS exoskeleton is between 12% and 92% and the mean reduction value was 70%. The maximum values of tremor reduction were 92.3% and 97.1% for the passive and active strategies, respectively. When we consider the effect of the exoskeleton on the tremor, irrespective of the strategy applied, we attain a mean reduction of 78.6% in tremor movement energy. Figure 8 illustrates the reduction in tremor energy for a patient with essential tremor. In both instances, actively and passively, the reduction in tremor amplitude is visible. This reduction can also been seen in the frequency domain (graphs on the right of the Figure) which illustrates the power spectral density, calculated by the FFT of the tremor signal, of the same signal. It is important to highlight that the movement frequency has not changed, i.e., the energy associated with tremor movement was significantly reduced but the frequency of the tremor stayed the same. This result is in accordance with the theoretical forecasts, (Adelstein, 1981), since on adding viscosity to the human upper-limb second-order biomechanical model, we alter movement amplitude and do not change its frequency.

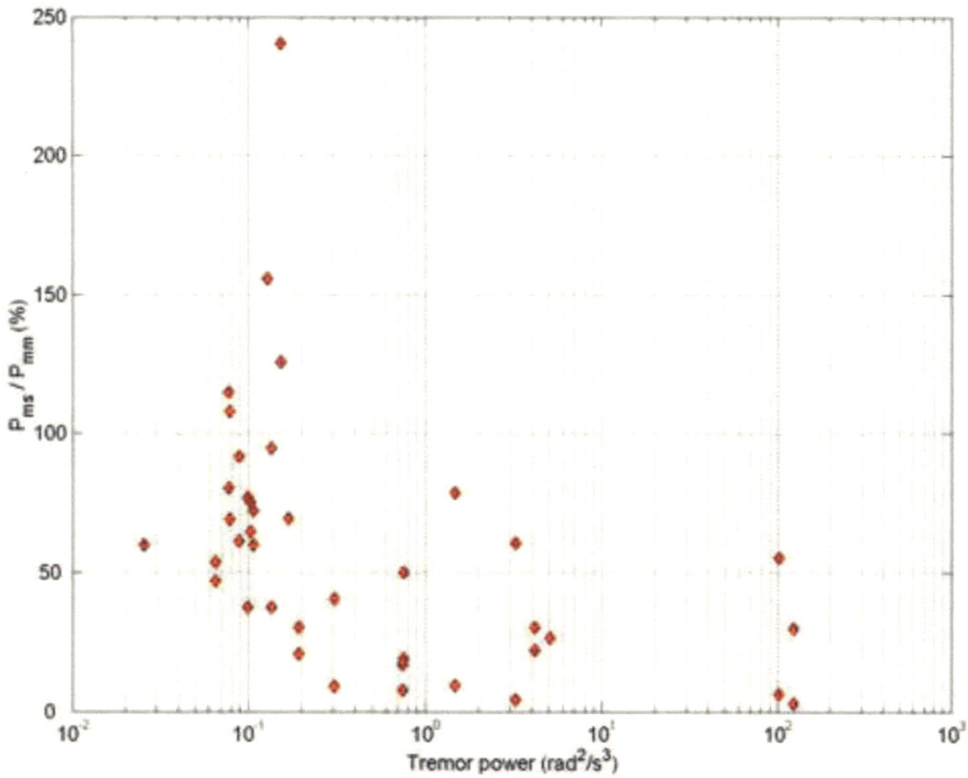

Fig. 7. Relation between the spectral power of patient tremor movement with WOTAS operating in *monitoring* mode, P_{mm}, and the spectral power of patient tremor movement with WOTAS operating in the tremor suppression modes P_{ms}. This relation quantifies the reduction in tremor amplitude with the application of control strategies.

The reduction values attained are very high but the authors believe that not all this reduction is the result of limb tremor reduction. This is due to the fact that the transmission of exoskeleton movement to the limb is not a rigid transmission, i.e., although the tremor in the exoskeleton is reduced 97% (as is shown in the results) the limb tremor is not reduced in this proportion due to the arm movements in relation to the exoskeleton supports. Analysis of the videos recorded during the measurement sessions show that exoskeleton movement was indeed reduced with the application of control strategies, but there was, however, a residual tremor in the limb.

Another interesting point highlighted by three of the ten patients evaluated is that the visual feedback of tremor reduction produces positive effects on the task undertaken. These patients said that it was easier to do the tasks when the exoskeleton was active. In their opinion, the fact that they could see that the tremor was reduced made them tremble less. This indicates that the tremor reduction caused by the robotic exoskeleton stems from two reasons 1) the effect of the control strategies and the application of forces on tremor movement 2) the visual feedback (biofeedback) of tremor reduction due to the action of the control strategies.

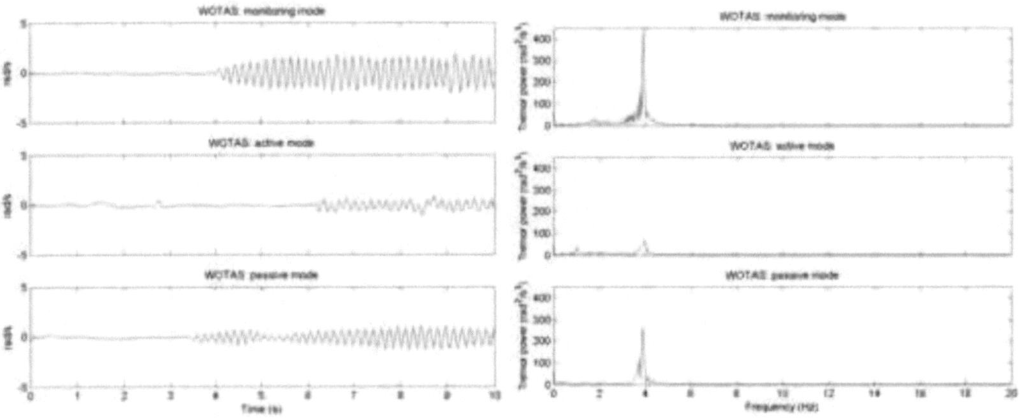

Fig. 8. Time series (left) and power spectral density (right) of the tremor movement of the wrist joint of a patient with essential tremor when taking the finger to the end of the nose using different tremor suppression strategies.

The effect of the visual feedback of tremor reduction on the generation mechanisms was detected in these experiments and will be the subject of future research by the authors. It is important to highlight that this was not detected by the users, which indicates that a study is required to determine the patients who benefit from this feedback.

6. Conclusions

Tremor is the most common movement disorder and is an important source of functional disability, affecting many daily tasks. For cases where treatment is not successful, the path to take is technological aids in the form of mechanisms attached to the arm (robotic exoskeletons).

This article has evaluated the different aspects of the WOTAS robotic exoskeleton. The WOTAS was evaluated with patients in real situations and a number of clinical tasks were defined, which were selected when the evaluation was done with the systems. Ten patients took part in the clinical experimentation stage of the system. The patients wore the device while it operated in three possible operation modes: monitoring, passive suppression and active suppression. Clinical effectiveness (from the variables obtained) and user acceptance were the base for selecting the best combination of algorithm parameters. Flaccidity and white tissue characteristics of the muscular system were the main disadvantages to providing the compensatory force on the arm, at the moment when the algorithms intervened to suppress tremor. However, reductions of approximately 80% in tremor power were obtained in patients suffering severe tremor. From the results and tremor reduction obtained in the system evaluation trials, the importance of these exoskeleton devices was demonstrated.

Thus at the Instituto de Automática Industrial, where this work was done, the aim is to begin developing an exoskeleton device like WOTAS but for a more general application, not only for cancelling tremor but also for generating and applying forces of different kinds on the upper limb to evaluate other types of pathologies and neuro-motor studies.
Robotic devices, like the one presented in this chapter, represent assistance technology to reduce dependency and allow patients to do daily tasks autonomously.

7. References

Adelstein, B.D. (1981). Peripheral mechanical loading and the mechanism of abnormal in tention tremor. PhD thesis. MIT.

Belda-Lois, J.M., Vivas, M.J., Castillo, A., Peydro, F., Garrido, J.D., Sanchez-Lacuesta, J., Barberá, R., Poveda, R. & Prat, J. (2004). Functional assessment of tremor in the upper-limb. In: International Journal of Rehabilitation Research: Proceedings of the 8th Congress of European Federation for Research in Rehabilitation. Ljubljana, Slovenia.

Bar-Shalom, Y. & Li, X.R. (1998) Estimation and Tracking: Principles, Techniques, and Software. Artech House Publishers.

Brookner, E. (1998) Tracking and Kalman Filtering Made Easy. John Wiley & Sons, Inc.

Elble, R., Sinha, R. & Higgins, C. (1990) Quanification of tremor with a digitalizing tablet. Journal of Neuroscience Methods, 33:193–198.

Fahn, S., Tolosa, E. & Marin, C. (1998) Clinical rating scale for tremor. In E. Tolosa J. Jankovic, editor, Parkinson's disease and movement disorders. Urban & Schwarzenberg, Baltimore.

Hogan, N. (1985). Impedance control: An approach to manipulation: Part I - theory. Journal of Dynamics System, Measurement and Control 107, 1-7.

Inoue, T. (1990). Practical repetitive control sys tem design. In: Proceedings of 29th IEEE Conference on Decision and Control. Vol. 3. IEEE. pp. 1673-1678.

Kapandji, I. (1983). The physiology of the joints: Upper limb. Churchill Livingstone, vol. 1.

Kotovsky, J. & Rosen, M.J. (1998). A wearable tremor-suppression orthosis. J. Of Rehabilitation Research and Development.

Mann, K.A., Werner, F.W. & Palmer, A.K. (1989) Frequency spectrum analysis of wrist motion for activities of daily living. Journal of Orthopedic Research, 7(2):304–306.

Manto, M., Topping, M., Soede, M., Sanchez-Lacuesta, J., Harwin, W., Pons, J.L., Williams, J., Skararup., S. & Normie, L. (2003). Dynamically responsive intervention for tremor suppression. IEEE Engineering in Medicine and Biology 22(3), 120-132.

Markensco, X. & Yannas IV (1979). On the stress-strain relation for skin. Journal of Biomechanics 12(2), 127-129.

Pons, J.L., Rocon, E., Ceres, R., Reynaerts, D., Saro, B., Levin, S. & Van Moorleghem, W. (2004). The manus dextrous robotics upper limb prosthesis: mechanical and control aspects. Autonomous Robots 16, 143-163.

Riviere, C.N. & Thakor, N.V. (1998). Modeling and canceling tremor in human-machine interfaces. IEEE Engineering in Medicine and Biology pp. 29-36.

Rocon, E., Bueno, L., Ceres, R., Calderón, L. & Pons, J.L. (2003). Theoretical control discussion on tremor supression via biomechanical loading. In Asistive Technology - Shaping the future, pages 827–831.

Rocon, E., Belda-Lois, J.M., Sanchez-Lacuesta, J.J. & Pons, J.L. (2004). Pathological tremor management: modelling, compensatory tech nology and evaluation. Journal of Technology & Disability 16, 3-18.

Rocon, E., Ruiz, A.F, Pons, J.L., Belda-Lois, J.M. & Sánchez-Lacuesta, J.J. (2005a). Rehabilitation robotics: a wearable exo-skeleton for tremor assessment and suppression. In: International Conference on Robotics and Automation 2005 - ICRA05. pp. 241-246.

Rocon, E., Belda-Lois, J.M., Sánchez-Lacuesta, J.J., Ruiz, A.F. & Pons, J.L. (2005b). Estimation of biomechanical characteristics of tremorous movements based on gyroscopes. In: Asistive Technology - from Virtuality to Reality. AAATE05. Lille , France.

Rosen, M.J., Arnold, A.S., Baiges, I.J., Aisen, M.L. & Eglowstein, S.R. (1995). Design of a controlled-energy-dissipation orthosis (cedo) for functional suppression of intention tremors. J. Of Rehabilitation Research and Development 32(1), 1-16.

Ruiz, A.F. (2005). Robótica aplicada a la rehabilitación y asistencia de discapacitados. Trabajo de Investigación del Curso de Ingeniería de la rehabilitación al servicio de la discapacidad.

Tsagarakis, N.G. & Caldwell, D.G (2003). Development and control of a soft-actuated exoskeleton for use in physiotherapy and training. Autonomous Robots, 15:21–33.

26

Lower-Limb Wearable Exoskeleton

J.L. Pons, J.C. Moreno, F.J. Brunetti, E. Rocon.
Bioengineering Group, Instituto de Automática Industrial - CSIC
Spain

1. Introduction

There are numerous causes that can affect the functioning of the human locomotor system, leading to the appearance of joint disorders in the lower limb and generating atypical gait patterns. The importance of research and development in assistance technologies to compensate pathological gait have been recognised since the beginning of the twentieth century and numerous challenges still lie ahead to make their clinical application a reality. In this section, GAIT, the lower-limb Wearable exoskeleton is presented, conceived as a compensation and evaluation system of pathological gait, for application in real conditions as a combined assistance and assessment methodology of the problems affecting mobility in individuals with neuromotor disorders.

The main technological challenges are discussed with respect to sensing, actuation and control subsystems. Special emphasis is placed on advances in robotic lower-limb orthoses, and biomechanical requirements, structural design considerations and the approaches existing to develop robust real-time controllers for portable solutions with a common aim, human motor control, are analysed.

2. Normal and pathological human gait

Regarding gait disabilities due to neurological, orthopaedic or traumatic conditions, there are different robotic approaches, and a classification of lower-limb robotic exoskeletons is presented in Rehabilitating robots, evaluation and tracking systems, and functional recovery wearable systems.

The cyclical process of events during gait is known as the gait cycle, and it starts and ends the moment when one of the feet come into contact with the ground, and the stance phase begins. While one leg displaces moving the body, the other leg acts as a support; thus, the state of the lower extremity is divided into two phases depending on its situation with regard to the ground: swing phase and stance phase. During gait at normal speeds there is a short period of simultaneous support of both legs. As speed increases a cycle is reached where there are no bipodal supports. Gait can be characterised by a set of parameters: stride length, step length, rhythm and speed. The complexity of the human locomotion process implies studying the cyclical movements that are executed, considering the kinematics and kinetics (forces and moments) and also the work, energy and power engaged in the process. Moreover, to understand all the phenomenon, it is necessary to have knowledge of the principles and neurological movements that control movement, the periphery input or sensory systems that intervene and the mechanisms that command the musculoskeleton system.

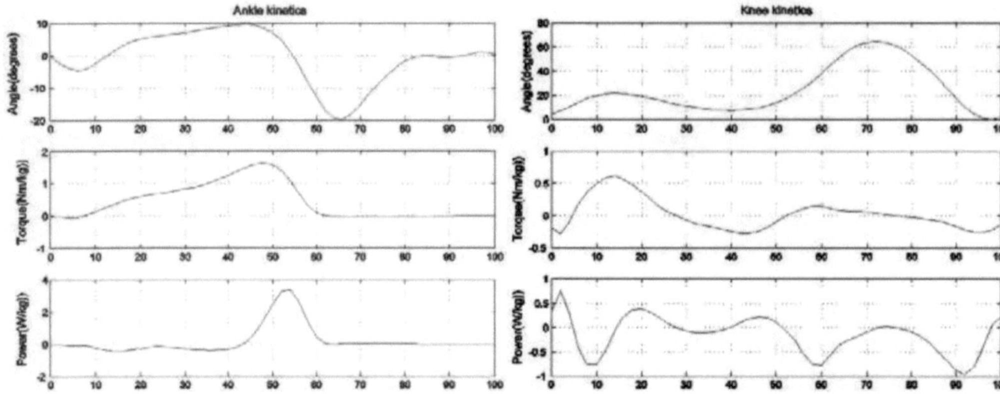

Fig. 1. Normal gait biomechanical data: angles (upper panel), moments (middle panel) and power (lower panel) of the ankle joint (left) and knee joint (right) at natural cadence (105 steps/min).

Typical patterns that characterise the biomechanics of joints obtained from normality average data (Winter, 1991) are shown in Figure 1. The temporary tracking of these variables is used to characterise a gait cycle. During rehabilitation therapies it is frequent to find patients affected at unilateral or bilateral level in the hip, knee and/or ankle joints due to numerous causes. Apart from serious lesions that lead to paralysis of the limbs in charge of locomotion, there are also disorders that restrict mobility, such as restriction of flexion during swing, excessive flexion of the knee and drop foot. These conditions can be treated with orthoses or active exoskeletons. These alterations occur as a result of different aetiologies, including muscular neurological disorders, trauma sequelae, spina bifida and others, and it is cerebrovascular accidents, poliomyelitis and post-poliomyelitis, which have the most impact, apart from other neurological afflictions like multiple sclerosis and cerebral palsy.

2.1. Impact

Individuals with proximal weakness in the lower limb can benefit from compensation using orthoses and functional compensation robotic exoskeletons. It is estimated that in the European Union the percentage of people who suffer diseases associated with reduced muscular capacity is between 0.05% and 1% of the total population. In the United States over 1.5 million people are partially or totally paralysed in their extremities. Many individuals require assistance technologies, and this demand increases with age. There is a notable increase in the frequency of paralysis in the lower limb with age (Irby et. al., 2002). Consequently, mobility in individuals with neuromuscular disorders is one of the aspects most commonly treated by rehabilitation professionals.

Other causes that require technologically advanced systems for the lower limb are neurological disorders, post-traumatic sequelae, spina bifida and others. Joint instability can also be caused by insufficiency of stabilising forces due to ligament or bone disorders. The population of potential users of lower-limb wearable exoskeletons that permit a more natural gait are not restricted to muscular insufficiency cases but include different causes that result in gait disorder.

A lower-limb exoskeleton or robotic orthosis can have several objectives depending on the pathology. Table 1 lists the objectives with the main pathological cases that can potentially benefit from a wearable exoskeleton that applies compensation on the lower limb.

Population	Pathologies		Purpose		
		Knee stability	Support and improvement of gait	Independent locomotion	Support during standing
Neuromuscul ar disorder	Post-polio syndrome, spina bifida	√	√	√	√
Protection/ joint support	Posttraumatic sequelae, osteoarthritis	√	√		
Injury	Spinal cord		√		√

Table 1. Potential objectives for use and/or treatment with lower-limb wearable robotic exoskeletons.

2.2. Functional compensation wearable systems

Neuromuscular disorders and joint disorders that lead to atypical gait patterns are varied and can affect the hip, knee and ankle. In this work we will focus on the compensations applicable to the knee and ankle. We analyse from the functional point of view, the compensation strategies for the lack in strength in the lower-limb proximal muscles. In particular, quadriceps weakness, the possible compensations of knee stability during gait, the mechanical stabilisation means (support systems) and the compensation strategies of ankle instability are analysed.

Lower-limb orthoses, as the most common traditional solution to compensate disorders related to lower-limb muscular weakness affecting the ankle and knees, are the unilateral knee, ankle and foot orthoses. Partial solutions that are commercially available are available which permit knee flexion during the swing phase but completely restrict movement during the stance phase.

The modelling and processing methodologies of the information for controlling pathological gait generally include the application of finite state machines, linear control, neuronal networks, adaptive control and fuzzy control. The measurement methods that can be integrated into an wearable compensation solution can be based on a user's manual control, or rather, on obtaining physical myoelectric, plantar contact, kinematic and/or kinetic signals. Myoelectric proportional control of pneumatic actuators has been proposed by Ferris, for regulation of artificial generation of dorsal flexion and plantar flexion torques, activated proportionally to the amplitude of EMG signals (Ferris et. al, 2006). Variable-impedance control of ankle-foot orthosis to assist drop foot gait, is proposed by Blaya et al., discussing the application of a state machine with selective gait phase-dependent control of the stiffness of a spring, by means of a DC motor, (Blaya & Herr, 2004b). Kazerooni et. al., proposed the application of proportional control of position for the Bleex system, a powered lower extremity exoskeleton for human strength augmentation during locomotion (Kazerooni et. al., 2003). The authors propose the use of proportional control on each joint to cause the exoskeleton joint angles to track the human joint angles.

Computational methods for modelling and processing of sensory information in locomotion control using neuroprothesis are interesting for their application in lower-limb exoskeletons. Orthoses that do not have joint locking capacity at knee level manage to meet the safety requirements, permit mobility and keep the knee rigid during the full gait extension. However, energy requirements increase unnecessarily and the gait patterns that are obtained are not very natural. There are several types of knee joints and systems commercially available that permit flexion of the knee during the swing phase but restrict movement during the stance phase. The evaluation of these orthoses does not exhibit obvious advantages in terms of energy demand for the patient. The loading application at joint level using an exoskeleton robotic system, which compensates gait disorders, is presented as a promising alternative for patients who cannot benefit from the orthoses available. The main technological challenge to make the application of this type of devices reality consists of a design that considers user aspects, such as portability, aesthetics and ease of use on equal terms. It is concluded that the crucial point is the problems related to the applicability to solutions because of integration problems, problems related to robustness, non-linearity and low repeatability of the sensor systems proposed.

3. The GAIT exoskeleton

Interaction with the human neuromotor system to assist locomotion requires adequate design of the components, both the biomechanical and functional aspects. Robotic exoskeletons conceived as an aid to mobility are designed to be used in numerous environments.

The absence of activity in the body segments leads to joint instability and body collapse. To resolve this problem, a robotic exoskeleton should compensate the moment of strength lacking in the joint in order to stabilise and compensate the lack of muscular force. An exoskeleton with an actuation system should appropriately apply the external joint moment on the body segments. The most appropriate force system for knee and ankle joints is analysed below.

3.1. Knee instability compensation

The system should compensate the loss of control of the knee extensors, especially the quadriceps, which put the knee at risk of collapsing under weight. During gait, paralysis of these muscles will tend to have a greater effect just after heel contact. During this period the effect of gravity and the moment of body progression will cause flexion of the knee. Without the quadriceps, the knee would collapse unless stability is maintained with an internal compensation, for example, the use of the hip extensor or trunk flexion during initial stance, or applying an external system.

An exoskeleton should ideally have the following actions:

a) Stance phase: controlling the flexion of the knee and assisting the knee to recover total extension.

b) Swing phase: permitting flexion of the knee during swing and assisting extension at the end in preparation for subsequent foot contact.

This type of stabilisation can be achieved using a three- or four-force system. For the four-point system (Figure 2), the interface forces will be fewer and also the internal moments on the sagital plane.

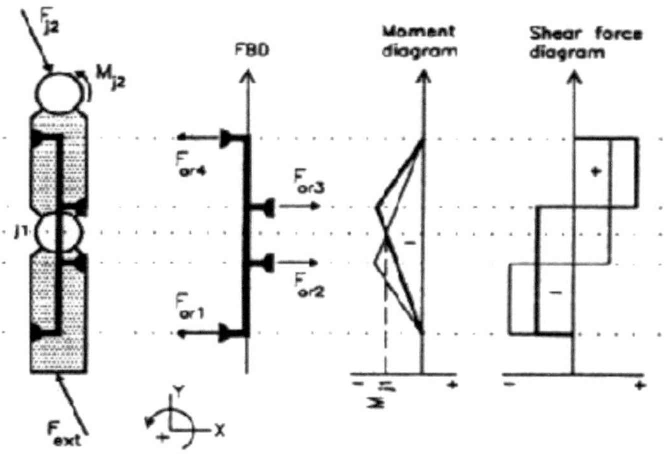

Fig. 2. Exoskeleton four-point support.

3.2. Ankle instability compensation

Ankle compensation requirements are related to the strategies adopted at knee level. In pathological cases with unilateral weakness of the knee extensors, this problem is usually overcome by adopting an internally flexed posture of the trunk to displace the action line of the ground reaction force in front of the knee, thus creating a stabilising moment. The success of this manoeuvre requires sufficient plantar flexion power to prevent dorsal flexion as the patient inclines forward. The exoskeleton should deliver sufficient dorsal flexion power to avoid involuntary plantar flexion. Dorsal flexion can be generated by an external actuation system at ankle level.

3.3. Exoskeleton structure

Depending on the type of interface or adjustment system to the limb, a unilateral or bilateral structure can be used. For example, if the interfaces cannot generate sufficient torque on the transversal plane at the connection points with the lateral bars, a unilateral system is not viable. Conversely, if the interfaces can generate moments on the transversal plane, it is possible to use a unilateral exoskeleton, whose supports are rigid to do the stabilisation on the sagital plane. Alignment in a bilateral solution is a crucial problem because if the two joints are not parallel, friction and undesired effort will be produced at each step. For the design of the mechanical structure a unilateral framework was used, with four loading interfaces on the soft surfaces, as the most appropriate to test the application of compensation strategies. The configuration of the exoskeleton adopted consisted of a included knee and ankle joints, lateral bars joined to the thigh (proximal), the leg (distal) and the foot (support and insole inserted into the shoe), and four securing bands to the limb (see Figure 6).

In the analysis of the mechanical resistance of the exoskeleton for muscular paralysis conditions, we assume that a) internal muscular moments cannot be generated b) internal support forces can be generated and c) most of the forces exercised in the body by an exoskeleton are perpendicular to the local contact surface.

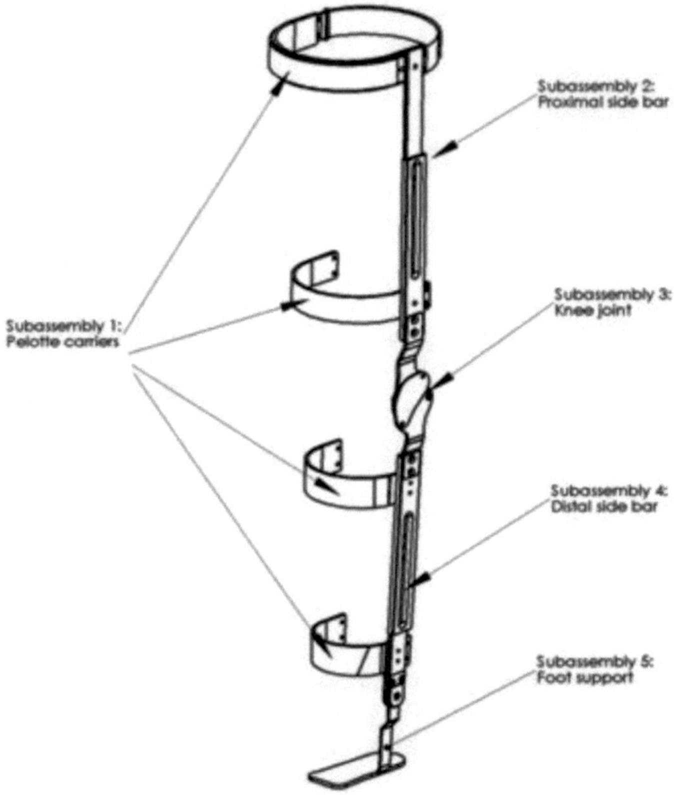

Fig. 6. Exoskeleton structure components.

Exoskeleton-leg system stiffness. When an external load is applied to the exoskeleton-leg system strains are produced. The magnitude and relation between these strains determines the rigidity of the system, which can be defined as the ability to stabilise internal forces with minimum internal strains. If M_{MR} is the external moment on the knee and the variation in the angle of the knee due to strains, the total rigidity of the exoskeleton system can be defined as

$$K_0 = \frac{M_{MR}}{\Delta\phi_{MR}} \tag{1}$$

The most significant strains in the system are:

- Soft tissue strains. In the limb interfaces the soft tissues are subject to loads. The effect of forces on the limb interfaces is soft tissue strain. The tissues react to non-linear loads as a function of time.
- Segment strain due to flexion efforts. The moments per flexion in the segment or proximal bar of an exoskeleton result in bar deflexions, characterised by v_{2b} and v_{3b}, as depicted in Figure 7. The deflections of the interfaces, 2 and 3, depend on the forces, F_1 and F_2, in the interface:

$$v_{2b} = \frac{F_1}{K_{2b1}} - \frac{F_2}{K_{2b2}} - \frac{F_3}{K_{2b3}};\ v_{3b} = \frac{F_1}{K_{3b1}} - \frac{F_2}{K_{3b2}} - \frac{F_1}{K_{3b3}}; \tag{2}$$

where d_n are the distances in agreement with Figure 7, G is the module shear, J is the moment of inertia of the central bar with regard to the y-axis.

- Segment strain due to torsion. The torsion moments in the exoskeleton lead to a specific rotation angle in the proximal bar at the position of the securing bands. Owing to this, there is a slight rotation of the securing bands, which causes a specific change in the position of the point of contact of the interface force. Considering the fixed bar at the ends, the effect of torsion on the strains can be characterised by the deflections, v_2t and $v3t$, at the position and by the forces, F_1 and F_2. It can be expressed generally:

$$v_{2t} = F_1[\frac{R_b^2(d_1-d2)}{GJ_{yc}}] \quad (3)$$

$$v_{3t} = F_1[\frac{R_b^2(d_1+d3)}{GJ_{yc}}] + F_2[\frac{R_b^2(d_2+d3)}{GJ_{yc}}] \quad (4)$$

Theoretically the forces applied on the limb by an exoskeleton can be calculated by modelling the rigidity of all the components as explained in the previous point. For the exoskeleton with four securing bands and forces applied externally, using the moment mean data on the knee given by Winter (Winter, 1991), an approximate estimate can be obtained of the internal forces in a gait cycle, as depicted in Figure 8. This estimate, although it does not include a precise model of soft tissue rigidity, it is useful as a reference to know the state of the interface, design new devices and size transducers to measure strains and forces.

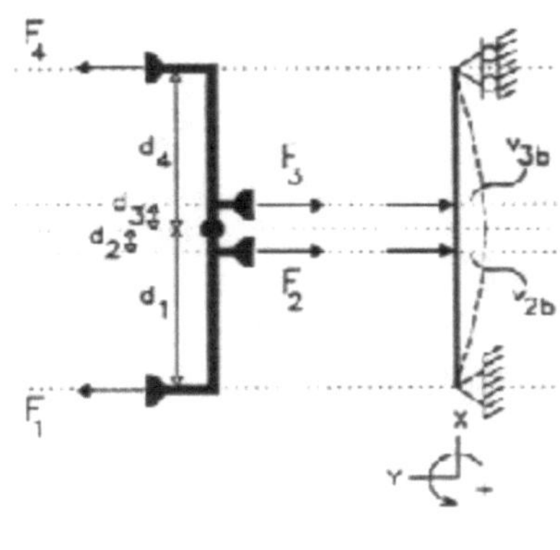

Fig. 7. Deflections in the central bar.

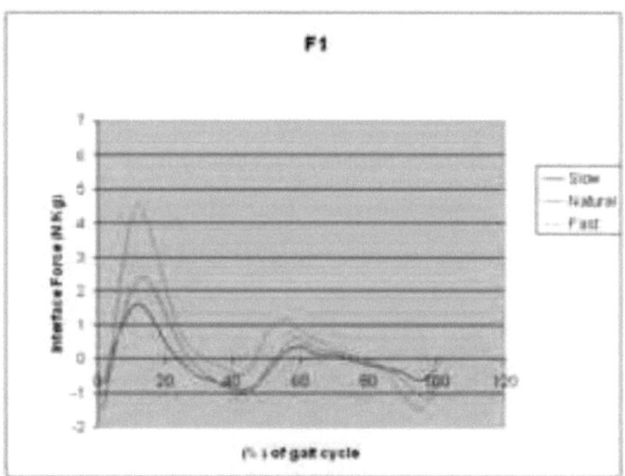

Fig. 8. Model of location of external and middle forces, F_1, during a complete gait cycle.

3.4. Knee joint

The design of the knee joint is a key point in the functioning of the exoskeleton. Several authors (Regalbuto, 1989; Rovick, 1991) consider this joint as the most important component of a pathological functional compensation system. Accordingly, we analyse the anatomy of this joint and its mechanical characteristics in detail. For the design and interaction with the knee it is fundamental to know the knee composition and functioning. The bones of the knee, femur and ankle form a mechanical joint. The lateral menisci help to stabilise the knee. The collateral ligaments are located along the lateral bones and restrict side movement. The anterior crossed ligament connects the tibia to the femur in the centre of the knee. Its function is to restrict rotation and forward movement of the tibia on the transversal plane. The posterior crossed ligament restricts backward movement of the tibia on this plane. These components and the muscles work together to administer the effort that the knee receives during walking, running, jumping and other functional activities.

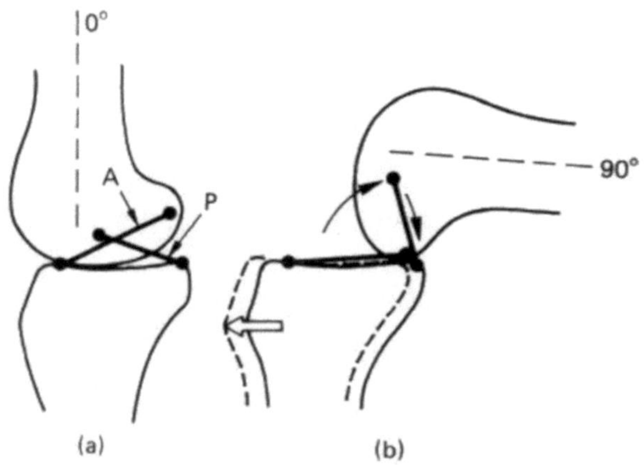

Fig. 9. Crossed ligament role. a) extension b) flexion.

For walking, the knee requires approximately 70 degrees of flexion, a range considerably lower than the total range of movement. It also necessitates the extension or even a slight hyperextension at the moment prior to heel contact. The geometrical place of the instantaneous centre of knee rotation on the sagital plane is not a specific point but a curve, which may be reproduced by a four-bar mechanism that simulates the crossed ligaments and reproduces the combined movement of knee sliding and rolling.

3.4.1. Four-bar mechanism

A four-bar mechanism was chosen for the exoskeleton knee joint, which permits movement in the normal range without restrictions and avoids the generation of migrations or undesired forces. The length and location of the bars was optimised by applying genetic algorithm methodology on the study presented by Baydal, (Baydal et. al., 2006), to track the instantaneous axis of rotation of the knee in the lateral part. The

Kurosawa-Walter model, (Walter et. al., 1985) , defines the instantaneous axis of rotation of the knee, see Figure 10.

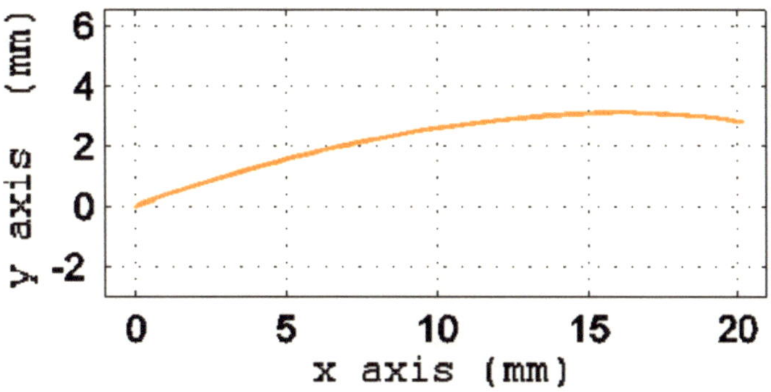

Fig. 10. Displacement of the helicoidal anatomical rotation axis in the lateral part of the knee determined with the Kurosawa-Walter model.

The four-bar mechanism can be fully described by the coordinates of its axes in their natural position to the relative movement of the mechanism. From the solutions obtained in Baydal's work, what best matched natural movement was chosen for the exoskeleton. Figure 11 presents the degree of complete movement of the four-bar mechanism compared with the natural movement of the knee. The knee joint of the exoskeleton based on this mechanism includes two lateral protection plaques to prevent the clipping effect. There are also two mechanical restrictions to maintain the natural range of movement of the knee, i.e., between 0 and +120 degrees (see Figure 12).

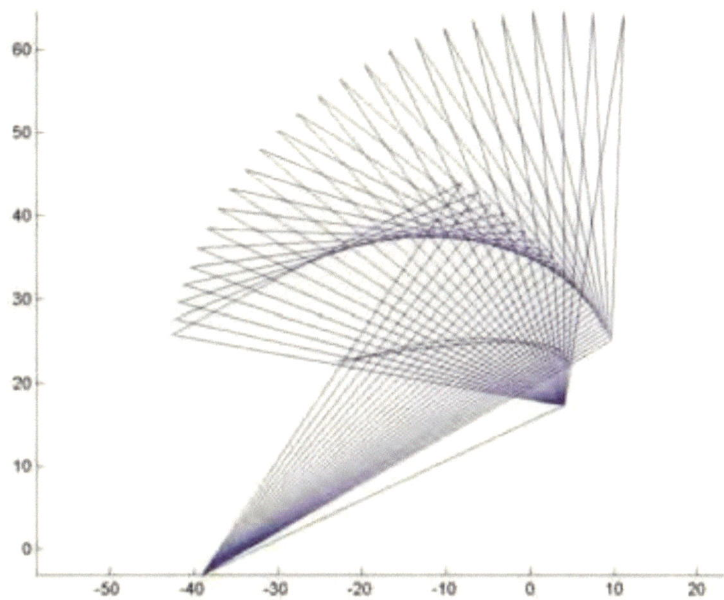

Fig. 11. Comparison of the movement of the natural knee joint (red) and the four-bar mechanism (blue). Displacements on the sagital plane (mm).

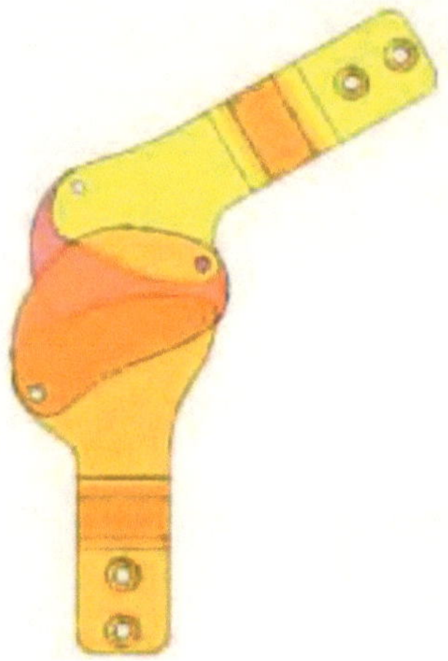

Fig. 12. Knee joint design.

3.5. Ankle joint

The ankle joint plays an important role in the progression and absorption of impact in the gait-stance phase, and helps to clear the ground during stance. In the complete gait cycle, the ankle does two plantar flexion trajectories and two dorsal flexion trajectories alternately. The design considers a monocentric joint adapted to the anatomy. The joint, whose design considers the trajectory of an external actuator element, varies in size depending on the user's anthropometric data. In the GAIT exoskeleton the ankle joint is joined to an insole inside the user's shoe. The shape of the insole follows the curvature of the sole of the foot to achieve effective distribution of the forces and obtain a good support and permit the most natural gait possible. The insole of the exoskeleton was designed with carbon fibre to provide sufficient rigidity to transmit ankle actuator torque and also be an elastic element capable of recovering energy to assist the lifting of the foot from the ground.

3.6. Actuation methodologies

Using an external joint system constant or variable impedance can be obtained. By applying joint locking, i.e., infinite impedance, during gait with quadriceps deficiency, the locomotion capacity can be enabled with joint rigidity. By applying null impedance, with the generation of movement, theoretically it is possible to compensate the absence of torque necessary to generate the joint trajectories. We analyse the functional situation at joint level to the absence of muscular control. The role of the knee extensors, active in the phase prior to stance and the end of the swing phase, is to control the degree of knee flexion which is generated by the ground reaction force. With quadriceps weakness during stance, flexion is uncontrolled and there is the risk of falling. The torque amount necessary will be determined basically by the subject's weight and his/her remaining muscular capacity. Control of joint impedance during the stance phase is a critical aspect of safety which must guarantee stability for stance and flexion flexibility at the right moment in the phase prior to the swing phase. Moreover, assisting leg extension at the end of the swing phase is a requirement for gait with quadriceps deficiency, because it makes subjects adopt undesired compensatory movements to be able to walk. It is possible to provide torque during the final phase to assist extension using an external system or the recovery of energy of the

system during a prior phase. In this respect, the application of control has been researched to restrict the exaggerated extension generated in hybrid gait systems (orthosis + stimulation).
Muscular weakness at quadriceps level typically affects the functioning of the ankle joint. Compensation manoeuvres of patients with deficient control of the knee have consequences on ankle displacements. To compensate gait using an external system at ankle level it will be necessary to provide sufficient plantar flexion to prevent involuntary dorsal flexion and provide dorsal flexion power to prevent uncontrolled plantar flexion.

3.6.1. Technologies

There are different actuation technologies that can be applied to control joint impedance in the knee and ankle joints of an exoskeleton. Regarding the compensation requirements of pathological gait according to a classification of impedance control (braking), infinite impedance (locking) or null impedance (generation of movement), in the state-of-the-art actuation technologies there are clear restricting factors: power, weight, and size requirements.
In particular, DC motors, which are presented as the most favourable actuation technology, present critical restrictions for an ambulatory solution. For example, a flat 50 W motor with nominal power, with a high-energy efficiency series (Maxon) and acceptable dimensions for the application (43 mm diameter, 21 mm thick), can deliver a maximum permanent torque of 8.14 Nm with a continuous current consumption of 2.58 A, a load that no accumulator or battery covers with the portability required. For a subject weighing 80 Kg, from the joint kinetic data of healthy subjects during gait at natural rhythm (Winter, 1991), in the stance phase of the knee joint a moment of approximately 50 Nm is generated, while in the ankle joint during the stance phase the moment increases progressively to exceed 120 Nm in the lifting of the foot. It is possible to conceive a hybrid actuation solution for integration in the exoskeleton. In the GAIT exoskeleton, this approach imitates the basic functionalities of the biological musculoskeleton system: a biomimetic approach.

Biomimetism: Functional analysis of the joints

It is highly unlikely that future actuators (e.g. based on polymers) use the same principles as biological muscle mechanisms. Thus, research currently focuses on designing actuators that imitate muscle functionality based on alternative functioning principles, (Meijer et. al, 2003). Imitation of muscular design can be considered a first step towards a new class of functionally diverse and robust actuators. The following step will require a system integration approach to interpret and imitate the functions of biological musculoskeleton systems during natural movements, (Full & Meijer, 2001). This type of approach will seek to identify the biomechanical principles to be introduced in the artificial model. An approach integrated into actuator design presents great potential for research. As an example, realistic biomechanical models of human limbs for the analysis of locomotion, which focus on interpreting underlying geometries and control problems, offer an interesting base to conceive a system-based approach: extensive groups of complex tendons have been successfully modelled as simple contractile elements in a functional model, (Roberts & Marsh, 2003). Redundancy problems associated with high numbers of muscles are resolved with an appropriate control criterion, (Rehbinder & Martin, 2001).

A biomimetic actuator for the compensation of pathological gait should be versatile and adaptable. The crucial construction needs for this system —and any other type of biomimetic wearable device— are low volume and size, low-energy consumption, low-heat dissipation and a high torque (in natural gait, 3.3 W are required per kilogram of body weight during the initial swing phase); we propose a biomimetic design to achieve these requirements. The weakened musculoskeleton system, in the absence of the quadriceps muscular group, requires assistance for impedance control and power generation (maximum demand during gait, 3.3 w/kg) and other compensations already mentioned (foot dragging, difficulty in lifting toe, etc.) We start from the hypothesis that this type of biomimetic system may increase the functionality level by increasing the integration level of actuation and control systems. In order to model and analyse the dynamic behaviour of the two joints during a gait cycle, we propose their separation into functional ranges where mechanical behaviour or impedance can be identified by each joint. We identify the mechanical functioning by analysing the relations between the rotations and joint moments, extracted from mean data representative of net moments and angles, at natural and low rhythms.

Knee

In the knee (see Figure 13), we can identify three functional ranges. The AB range, while the joint during stance is absorbing the impact and damping the descent of the body, the joint set can be modelled as a linear system since the torque-angle relation represents an elastic behaviour given by

$$T = K_n(\alpha - \alpha_0) \qquad (5)$$

where T is the torque, α the angular position, 0 the initial state, and K_n the elastic constant representing the torque-angle rate that varies depending on the subject's weight and gait speed. The BC range, with flexion and extension trajectories in the swing phase, presents a non-linear relation that can be interpreted as a pseudo-elastic system. This is characterised by an increase in considerable strain with minimum effort applied, once an initial loading effort has been overcome. The CD range, during extension before heel contact, can be characterised mechanically as an elastic system using the K2 elastic constant.

Ankle

In the ankle we identify three ranges (see Figure 14). The first, included between heel contact and a point around maximum flexion, where the joint controls plantar flexion, can be modelled as a linear system because of an elastic relation, which we call K3. During the AB range, dorsal flexion takes place during stance while a T1 absorption zone of energy is observed, and a linear model approximated by a K4 constant elastic can be defined. For the BC range, the plantar flexion trajectory coincides with the maximum energy demand and another approximately linear relation K5 is found, to approach the joint function.

Identification

It can be concluded that joint behaviour can be imitated using elastic devices during certain gait phases. For each functional range, from the data representative of gait normality at natural rhythm, we calculate the coefficients of a first-degree polynomial (A) to linearly adjust p (A(n)) to M(n), using the square-minimum method, where A is the angle of the knee, M the moment of force, n the percentage of the gait cycle.

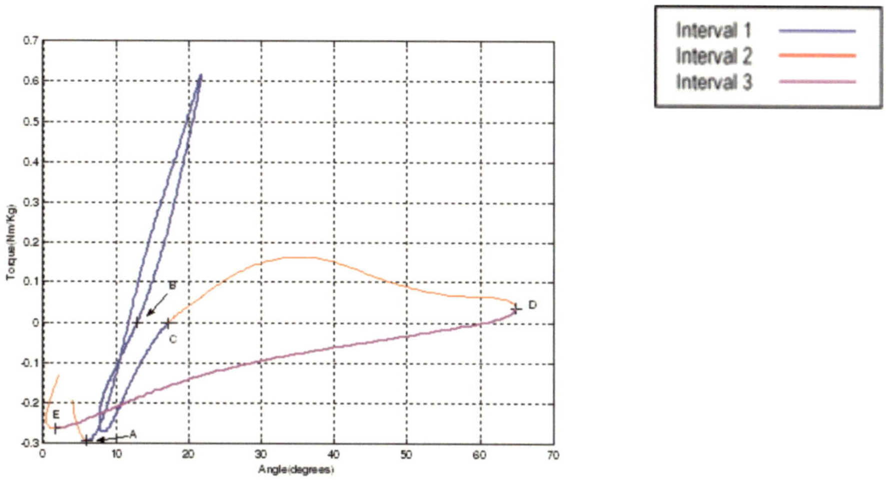

Fig. 13. Torque-angle rate in the knee joint during a complete gait cycle and identification of functional ranges at natural rhythm (Winter's average gait data).

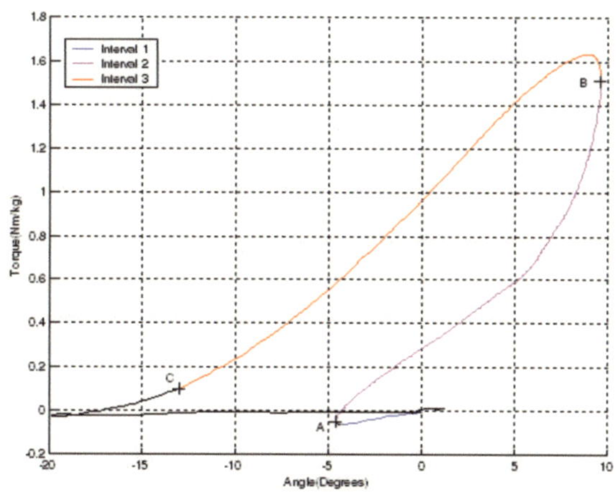

Fig. 14. Torque-angle rate in the ankle joint during a complete gait cycle and identification of functional ranges at natural rhythm (Winter's average gait data).

Range	Coefficients	(N.m/Kg)
A-B	K_1	6.013 x10^{-2}
C-D	K_2	4,26 x 10^{-5}
0-a	K_3	1,4 x 10^{-4}
a-b	K_4	8,9 x 10^{-4}
b-c	K_5	7,4 x 10^{-4}

Table 2. Moment polynomial adjustment coefficients vs. angles calculated for the functional ranges in a gait cycle.

Table 2 presents the values of the coefficients obtained for each linear adjustment, depending on body weight. Proceeding in this way we characterise the functional ranges identified using linear parameters. Based on the biomimetic model of the compensation elements of the actuators, the different operation ranges of the musculoskeleton system are identified functionally and they are modelled using mechanisms. Figure 16 represents the resulting linear adjustments obtained from linear functions with K_1 and K_2 parameters which are calculated theoretically for the knee joint. Figure 15 represents the linear approximations for the moment and angle for the ankle joint. The dotted lines represent the phases when an adjustment to a greater order polynomial would be necessary.

Interaction with the four-bar mechanism: viability analysis

The instantaneous centre of rotation (ICR) in the knee joint must be followed by the rotation centre of the four-bar mechanism joint. The mechanism kinematics is crucial for the functioning but this adaptation leads to more complex kinematics and for this reason we analyse the viability of applying external torques on the four-bar mechanism. In the four-bar mechanism, a rotational actuator should transmit or receive torque on the fixed A- or D-axes (see Figure 18). To evaluate the torque relation to the angle on these application points, we developed a model based on the optimised four-bar joint.

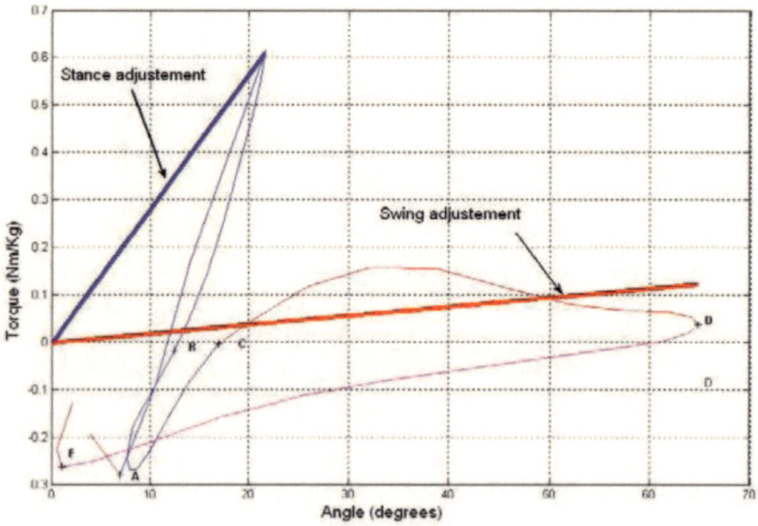

Fig. 15. Linear adjustments (blue solid lines) of the angle and force moment for the knee joint and normality patterns (red).

We generate a free-body diagram of the mechanism depicted in Figure 17. To model the knee joint, we consider the optimised values of limb length and we assume that M torque is applied on the ICR. We formulate a linear system of nine equations with nine variables corresponding to the reaction forces to calculate the torque in A for a gait pattern:

$$A_1 Rb_x - A_2 Rb_y + A_3 Rc_y + A_4 Rc_x + M = 0$$
$$A_6 Rb_y - A_5 Rb_x - Ta = 0$$
$$A_7 Rc_x + A_8 Rc_y = 0$$

$$
\begin{aligned}
Rc_x + Rb_x &= 0 \\
Rb_y + Rc_y &= 0 \\
Ra_x - Rb_x &= 0 \\
Ra_y - Rb_y &= 0 \\
Rd_x - Rc_x &= 0 \\
Rd_y - Rc_y &= 0
\end{aligned} \tag{6}
$$

where A_i are the coefficients that define the moments caused by the reaction forces at the application point. The model output evaluated on D-axis, for a complete cycle, is represented in torque terms and angular displacements in Figure 18. In the period between the load response and the final gait stance phase, the resulting T_d torque on the D-axis, maintains a linear relation with the axis rotation.

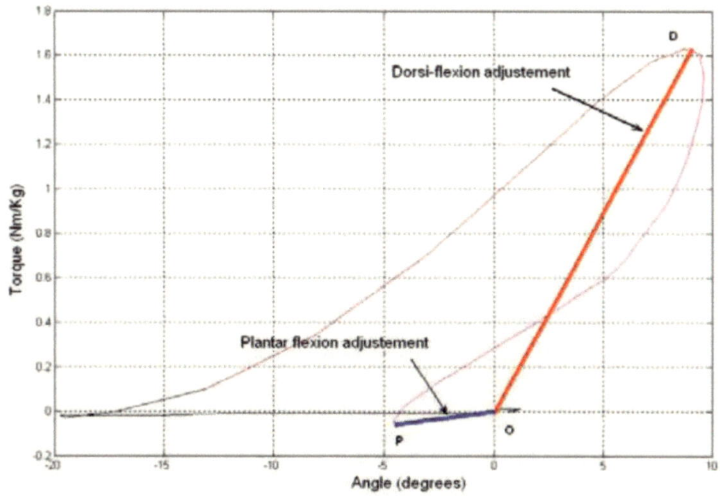

Fig. 16. Linear adjustments (blue solid lines) of the angle and moment of force for the ankle joint and normality patterns (red).

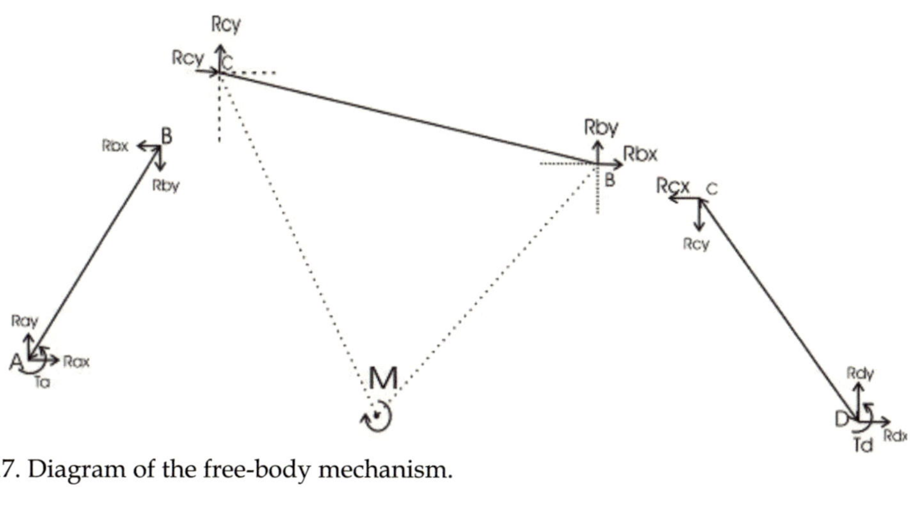

Fig. 17. Diagram of the free-body mechanism.

3.6.2. Biomimetic design of the actuation system

Considering the characterisation and compensations necessary at joint level with the exoskeleton, the design of the actuation system is presented below. The actuation system is conceived as a semi-active solution based on:

- Selective use of mechanical means.
- Transition activated electrically or mechanically between the mechanical means.

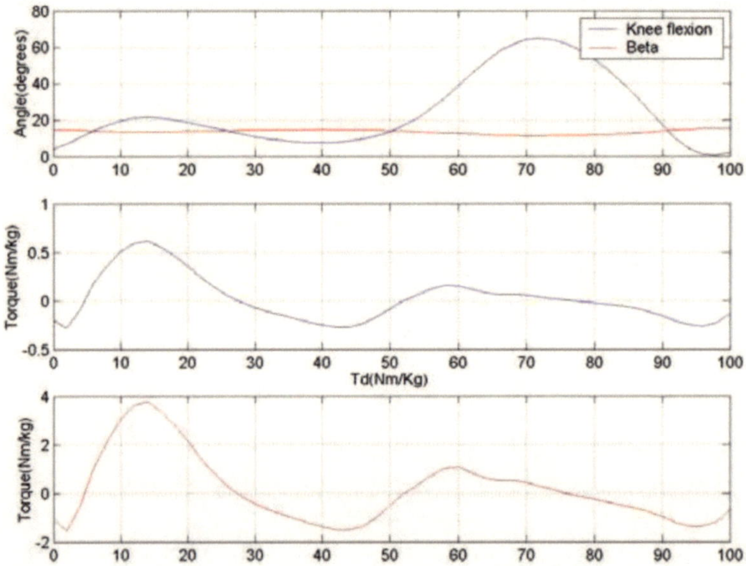

Fig. 18. Comparison of normal pattern of angular torque in the knee (M) and angular torque resulting on the D-axis of angular displacement, in the evolution of the mechanism in a gait cycle.

Knee

Given the linear rotations found that model joint functioning for some phases of the gait cycle, the functioning principle of the knee actuator (see Figure 19) is given by:

- A K2 elastic element that is activated at heel contact, with locking at B1, in the initial stance phase, applying K2 rigidity on the knee with a maximum longitudinal trajectory corresponding to a flexion angle restriction.
- A K1 elastic element (compression spring) is activated at the terminal stance phase, using the unlocking in B1 to release the joint and permit free swing, given that K2 >> K1. The element presents a maximum longitudinal displacement, which corresponds to knee flexion restriction. Total locking at B1 to maintain full leg extension and give security when standing up or going up or down stairs or slopes.

The K2 elastic element, configured using stacked Belleville discs, has a maximum trajectory of 13 mm corresponding to 15 degrees of flexion permitting a safe load response and consequent extension prior to swing. The K1 elastic element presents a maximum displacement of 55 mm, which corresponds to a knee flexion of 95 degrees.

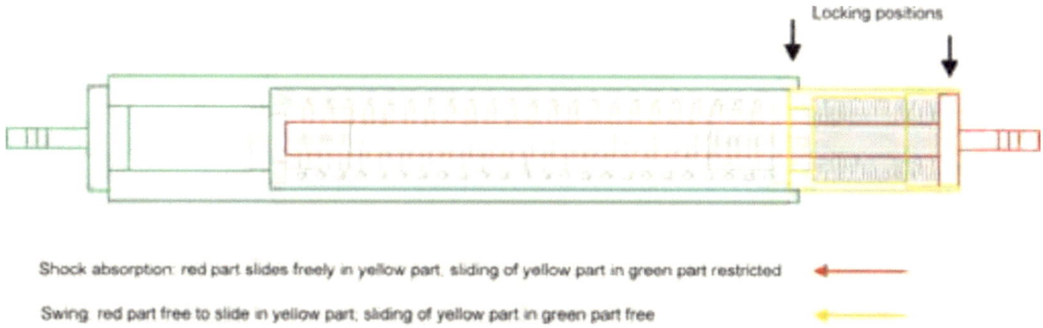

Fig. 19. Functioning of the actuator on the knee joint.

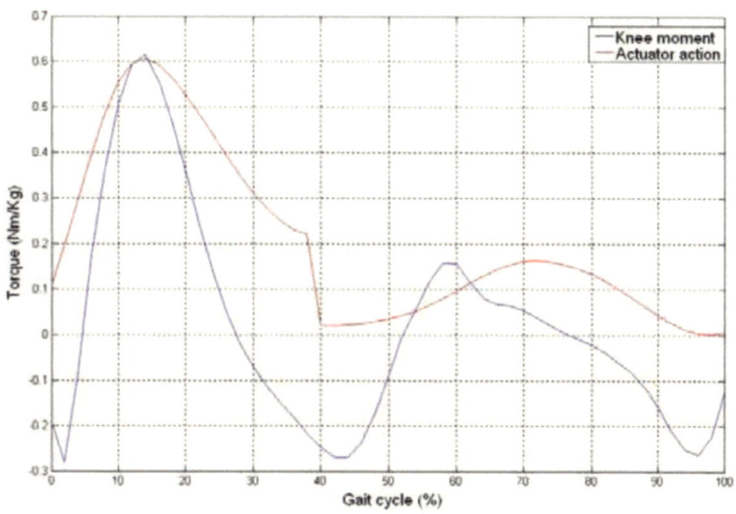

Fig. 20. Actuator-joint model outputs of the knee during the stance and swing phases, in comparison with Winter's mean data (dotted lines).

Locking/unlocking intermittent mechanism

A locking/unlocking mechanism was designed. In extension the linear displacement of the internal cylinder of the actuator is restricted. The unlocking is produced with the rotation of a piece that covers the actuator and this activation is done via a linear solenoid. With the joint model, we theoretically estimate the torques that the system operates during gait with the normality patterns for stance and swing. The K1 and K2 compensations are theoretically depicted for 80 Kg and 100 Kg subjects in Figure 20.

Ankle

The passive system that acts on the ankle contains springs that are sized according to the linear relations given by K3 and K4 which model the joint functioning. The functioning principle of the ankle actuator (see Figure 21) is given by:

- A K3 elastic element that is compressed stores energy and controls dorsal flexion at the stance phase. In compression, K3 has a maximum longitudinal trajectory equivalent to a dorsal flexion restriction of the ankle. The energy stored in dorsal flexion is recovered towards a plantar flexion trajectory prior to swing with the K3 extension.

- A K4 elastic element that adds rigidity to extension to control plantar flexion on stance and avoid the drop of the foot during swing. The element has a maximum longitudinal trajectory equivalent to a plantar flexion restriction of the ankle equivalent to a dorsal flexion restriction of the ankle. The energy stored in dorsal flexion is recovered towards a plantar flexion trajectory prior to swing with the K3 extension.
- A K4 elastic element that adds rigidity to the extension to control plantar flexion on stance and avoid the drop of the foot during the swing. The element has a maximum longitudinal trajectory equivalent to a plantar flexion restriction of the ankle.

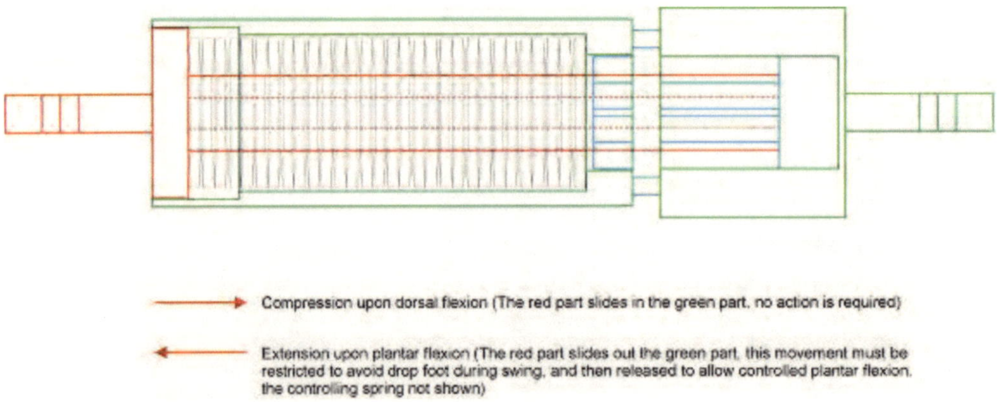

Fig. 21. Functioning of the actuator on the ankle joint.

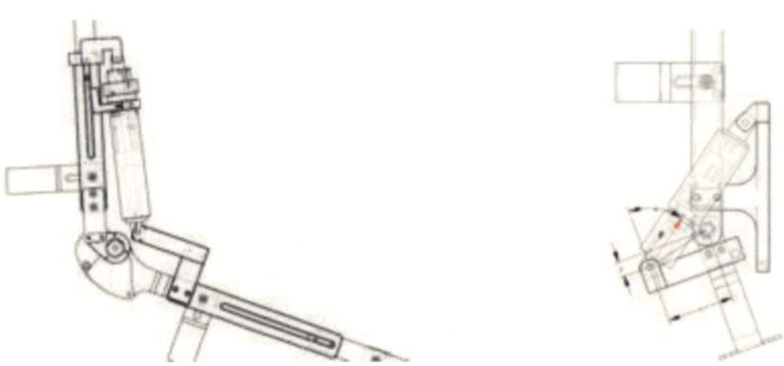

Fig. 22. Knee (left) and ankle (right) actuators attached to the frame.

In particular, for the design of the knee actuator integrated into the ankle joint, the K3 elastic element (stacked Belleville disc) is compressed with a trajectory of 15 mm equivalent to 20 degrees of dorsal flexion of the ankle. The K4 elastic compression element has a maximum displacement in plantar flexion of 6.5 mm, equivalent to 15 degrees. The final design of the biarticular actuation system integrated into the complete structure of the exoskeleton is presented in Figure 22.

3.7. Sensor system

In previous works, the feasibility of inertial sensing for the control of walking was studied, (Baten et. al., 2004), and a particular design was proposed (Moreno et. al., 2006b). The sensors set up for control consist of an initial inertial measurement unit (IMU) on the foot element inside the shoe (below the orthotic ankle joint) and a second unit for the lower bar of the exoskeleton. Each IMU is composed of a) a single miniature MEMs rate gyroscope, sensing Coriolis force during angular rate by measuring capacitance (Analogue Device ADXRS300, volume less 0.15 cc, weight 0.5 gram) with maximum sensitivity +/- 300/s; and b) a complete dual-axis (surface micromachined) 200mV/g accelerometer (ADXL202 5x4.5x1.78 mm). Units are housed in boxes attached to foot and shank orthotic bars, (as depicted in Figure 23), sensing rotational motion, tilt, tangential and radial segment accelerations in orthogonal directions (X and Y), while the majority of orthotic rotations at the level of joints and bars take place on the locomotion progression plane (sagittal), due to mechanical constraints imposed by the structure. Movements of interest occur at normal (2.6 km/h) and low (2 km/h) gait speeds, and therefore, signals outside the band frequency related to gait kinematics (0.3–20 Hz) are rejected from the sensor outputs with -3 dB low-pass filters, while lowering noise floor by bandwidth restricting. A precision angular position sensor, with an effective electric range of 340 degrees is fixed at one rotation axis of the four-bar mechanism of the knee joint, for continuous tracking of the knee joint angle on the sagittal plane. A resistive pressure sensor (5 mm in diameter active area, 0.30 mm thickness) is used to monitor the knee locking mechanism status.

Each IMU is housed in boxes with straight angles and standards, useful for the assembly and development of calibration protocols. Moreover, the robustness of electric connections is another important factor due to the fact that each device will be subject to a high number of flexions, movements, impacts and efforts. The unit on the ankle bar measures rotational movements, inclination and tangential and radial accelerations of the limb in orthogonal direction on the sagittal plane. The same rotations and movements are measured in the leg by the second unit, mounted on the lateral side of the bar. A IMU is on the foot bar that is introduced into the subject's shoe (under the ankle joint); a second IMU is on the foot bar (on the ankle joint). Figure 23 depicts the locations. The IMU signals are digitalised using a 10-bit analogical-digital converter, sampled at 100 Hz, with a reference voltage of 3.3 V and a resolution of 2.92 mV/bit. Robust fixation and solid movement are assumed. The output of an accelerometer with its measurement axis aligned on the i-axis can be represented by

$$A_i = a_i(t) - g + n \tag{7}$$

a_i being the sensor linear acceleration, g, the gravity, and n, white noise. Additionally, from the combination of signals of the accelerometers mounted tangentially, a measurement of the angular acceleration of the limb can be obtained. Using the Coriolis force, F_c, the gyroscope directly measures the angular speed *s(t)*, which can be represented by the relation

$$F_c(t) = 2mv(t)s(t) \tag{8}$$

where *m* is the sensor mass and *s(t)* its speed. Thus, the sensor output corresponds to its rotation rate. In a later step and during cyclical gait, the orientation angle of the sensor can be calculated from the signal integration, in periods between consecutive steps, reinitiating the process to eliminate the cumulative error. Integration unbalance can be calculated during the quasi-static conditions detected (e.g. the foot segment during the stance phase, speed equal to zero). The relative angular speed of ankle joint rotation can be calculated from the subtraction between the foot and leg speeds.

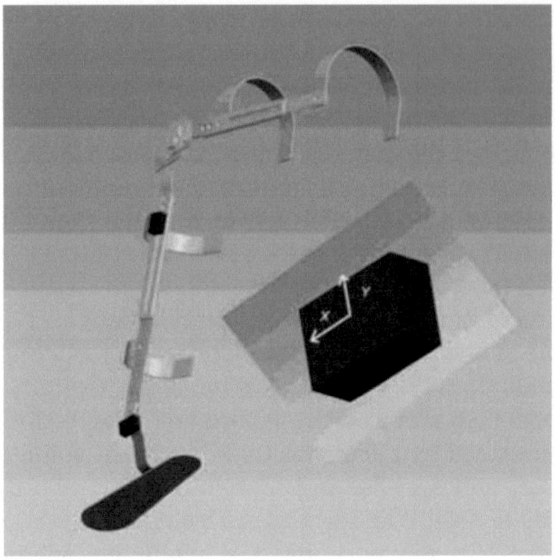

Fig. 23. Configuration of the IMUs in the structure.

3.8. Gait controller

The strategies that can be applied to functionally compensate pathological gait can be classified according to their implementation a) position control b) impedance control and c) intermittent joint control. We propose selective control of joint rigidity by modifying the joint rigidity of the exoskeleton with exchanged external means. The control strategies implemented in ambulatory means have to be highly robust and should guarantee safe interaction between the human being and the machine. This section discusses the implementation of a strategy based on intermittent joint control.

3.8.1. Functional compensation using intermittent control

All the aspects related to the design and application of intermittent control for functional compensation of gait with the exoskeleton developed are analysed. We consider the lower-limb system consisting of the thigh, leg and foot segments. Weakened quadriceps will provide minimum or null torque amount in the knee. The system is designed to apply torque on the sagittal plane and is restricted by the construction of exoskeleton joints. In the exoskeleton the ankle actuator is designed to passively compensate, i.e., without any need for a control action, and the elastic components (K3 and K4) of the device are customised to match the user's weight. The spring with K3 is compressed to store energy during the stance phase and control dorsal flexion during the swing phase, and the spring with K4 applies rigidity to control the drop of the foot during the swing phase.

The functional objectives of a gait cycle in the exoskeleton-limb system using the actuator control of the knee consist of approximating the characteristic conditions of natural human gait (Figure 24). The compensations using the ankle actuator affect foot movement with consequences on the configuration of all the kinematic chain of the limb and its state in relation to the ground. At knee level, the actuator reacts and generates the transition between the K1 and K2 compensations and passes from knee with restricted flexion to free flexion where the elastic element is loaded that recovers energy to assist the extension. The appropriate transition moment between the actuator components occurs in the phase prior to swing and coincides with a specific dorsal flexion of the ankle and a period when the direction of rotation of the leg changes to the knee forward movement direction.

3.8.2. Discrete controller

The intermittent mechanism on the knee has two possible states, R0 and R1, during the cyclical gait. The correct intermittent transition of the system between these states permits the locomotion and application of joint compensation. The R0 to R1 transition is achieved via linear solenoid action. The R1 to R0 transition is done automatically using mechanical means, when the complete extension of the knee is recovered.

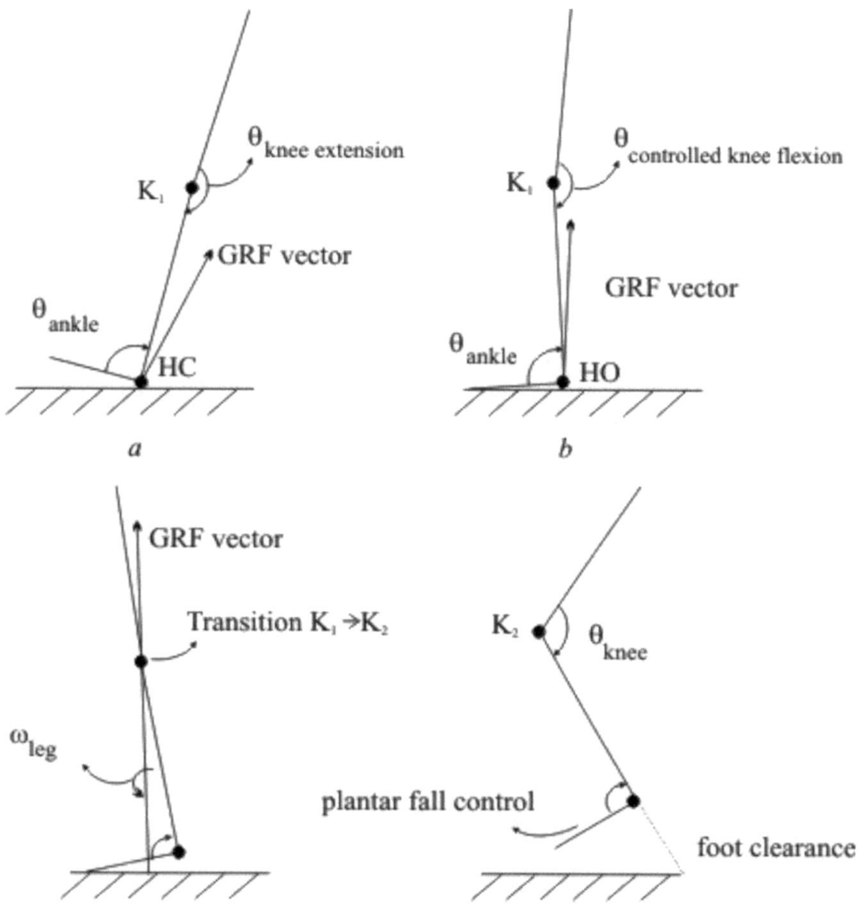

Fig. 24. Partial objectives of knee control in a gait cycle: (a) heel contact (HC) with controlled plantar drop after knee extension stabilised using K1 at the end of the swing phase (b) heel lift (HL) in the stance phase after controlled knee flexion trajectory in the range of 15° (c) in the phase prior to swing, the direction of leg rotation is inverted. Using the K1 to K2 transition the joint is released (d) leg rotation in response to knee flexion. Control of the plantar drop avoids dragging the toe and K2 is enabled to assist the extension in the air and the end of a cycle.

The aim of the discrete controller is to detect the transition moment (TI) using real time evaluation, at a sampling frequency of 100 Hz, of the information obtained from the inertial measurement units (IMUs) of the exoskeleton. The inertial system embarked directly measures on the sagittal plane, the angular speed of the leg, ω_{pierna}, the angular speed of the foot, ω_{pie}, and the linear acceleration of the foot limb, ay_{pie}, on the y-axis, where y is parallel to the upper-lower axis of the exoskeleton foot bar. The condition for detecting TI is defined in the cyclical gait discrete controller based on the speed of the segments using the following equation:

$$(\underset{.}{U}\omega_{pie} < \omega_{pie} < \dot{U}\omega_{pie}) \wedge (\underset{.}{U}\omega_{pierna} < \omega_{pierna} < \dot{U}\omega_{pierna}) \wedge (ay_{pie} < \underset{.}{U}ay_{pie}) \quad (9)$$

with the $\underset{.}{U}\omega_{pierna}$ and $\dot{U}\omega_{pierna}$ thresholds. The algorithm verifies the rotation of the foot segment by dorsal flexion of the ankle in the margins given by $\underset{.}{U}\omega_{pie}$ and $\dot{U}\omega_{pie}$, and in turn verifies the trajectory of the lifting of the foot from the ground using the $\underset{.}{U}ay_{pie}$ threshold. Additionally, the algorithm evaluates the state of the system and degree of flexion of the knee in the swing phase to ensure that no undesired activations of the solenoid occur at the final swing phase.

3.8.3. Activation

The TI detector output in each cycle is a square pulse with a variable width, and a time-rise edge T after TI. This pulse produces activation and displacement of the linear actuator that causes the transition to R1 in the intermittent mechanism.

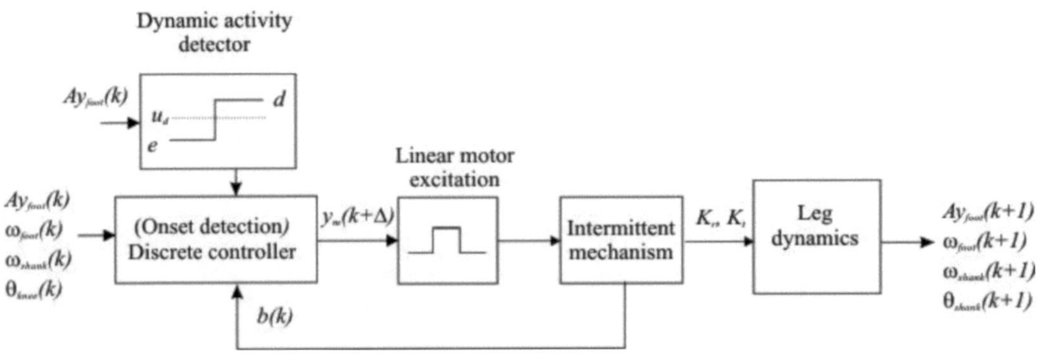

Fig. 25. GAIT exoskeleton control system.

Ideally, the width of the pulse should be sufficient to ensure that the knee is free the time necessary to initiate the flexion and maximum of half of the magnitude of the swing period. We define as an activation criterion in the gait cycle n, the function:

$$P_{act}(n) = P_{act}(ini) + P_a(n) - \frac{[R(n-1)P_a(n-1)+P_a(n-2)]}{2} \quad (10)$$

which evaluates the activation state of the previous cycle, the stance phase of the current cycle and the two stance phases immediately before, in order to adjust the $P_{act}(n)$ activation period of the actuator to match the gait rhythm trend. A $P_{act}(ini)$ is defined a priori, which should correspond to the mean activation period adjusted to a mean rhythm expected.

3.8.4. Preliminary results

A version of the GAIT exoskeleton operated mechanically has been developed. This mechanical solution is cable-driven exoskeleton (CDE) that switches the state of the knee joint, based on the degree of ankle dorsal flexion. The first results with the (CDE) produces response errors on 2.4% of occasions in technical validation trials of 100 steps. Comparatively, according to the trial data with a normal subject, the controller significantly reduces the rate of errors and obtains 99% success in the functioning of all the trials at low and medium rhythm.

4. Experimental trials

A left-leg unilateral exoskeleton was customised to two patients with post-polio syndrome. The construction of the joints restricted movement at the sagital plane. Special attention was paid to achieving the right mechanical adjustment and adaptation of the exoskeleton to guarantee comfort and the appropriate transmission of forces, with the continual assistance of an expert in orthopaedics. The securing pieces were strained and material was added to adjust to the anatomical form until no marks were left on the skin after using the system for twenty-minute periods. The height of the ankle and toe were adjusted using additional material on the shoe insole, when it was necessary. Each protoype was made with the actuators consisting of the springs built to offer the compensations calculated according to the moment polynomial adjustment coefficients against angle, depending on the subject's weight (according to the results in Table 2).

For the intermittent mechanism of the knee actuator a traction solenoid was anchored (12 Vdc, 10 W, Belling Lee) which transmits the force necessary (up to 700 g, 3 mm trajectory) for the switching between springs and joint unlocking during the stance phase. The solenoid was fed electrically from a lead-sealed battery (Serie Dryfit 1.2Ah, 12V, Sonnenschein) and controlled digitally using a switching circuit in pulsated mode to reduce power consumption. The circuit implements the discharge via a capacitor to offer rapid unlocking. The exoskeletons were made with the set of sensors consisting of the inertial measurement units, the angular position sensor and the resistive pressure sensor (active area of 5 mm and 0.30 mm of thickness) on the unlocking mechanism to detect the state of the knee joint (R0: locking in extension [K1]; R1: free swing [K2]).

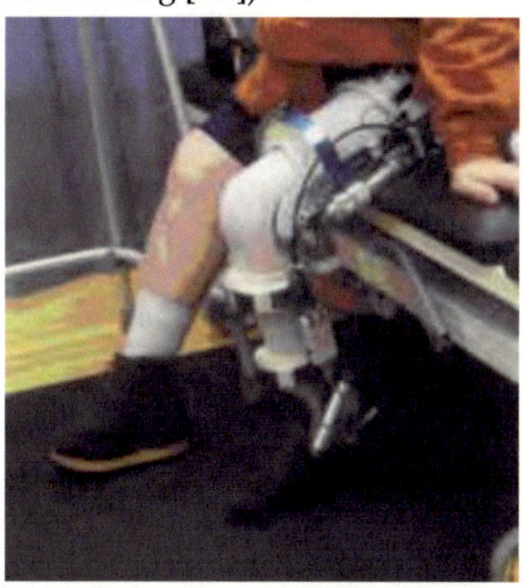

Fig. 26. Image of the wearable exoskeleton on a patient after fitting to the anatomy.

The monitoring and control unit included two buttons for direct control by the subjects, offering the possibility of disabling the control strategy and thus totally unlocking the knee at any moment. The exoskeleton with the actuators, batteries, set of sensors and the monitoring and control unit weighed a total of 2.71 Kg.
The ambulatory unit (Atmega128, Atmel Inc.; sampling frequency 100 Hz) was used as a real-time control interface with implementation of the control algorithm that generates the real-time control signals (pulses of 12V of amplitude) of activation and activation time of the linear solenoid to compensate gait.

4.1. Protocol

In the first approach of the exoskeleton on the patients the passive prototype version was used which controls the exchange mechanism on the knee actuator using the cable connected to the ankle joint, dorsal flexion control (CDE). With this system functioning the practical session was completed which consisted first of bipedal trials and after walking on flat ground with the patients' normal aids. One controller was tuned following a sequential procedure from an initial adjustment. The electronically-controlled exoskeleton (ACE) could be disabled remotely from one-base unit at any moment to prevent joint unlocking. Adaptation was expected from the subject after a specific number of trials. In the event that the patient adapted and achieved complete gait cycles, and at the same time increased his/her perception of trust in the body weight support on the exoskeleton (stance phase) and after prior consent, 5 free-gait trials were done with the ACE without external supports.

4.2. Results

4.2.1. Effects on kinematics

Patient S2 usually uses a knee and ankle orthosis to be able to walk. The orthosis has the knee joint locked while the ankle joint restricts plantar flexion and dorsal flexion mobility. The gait pattern with her orthosis is with the knee locked during the stance and swing phases. Immediately after the stance response, there is a dorsal flexion movement greater than normal in the ankle. During the swing phase the foot is protected from the plantar drop with the restriction imposed by the exoskeleton. To put the foot forward, the patient compensates with his body on the transversal and frontal plane.
Using the exoskeleton with CDE, subject S2 required a training time of 30 minutes to walk with the crutches instead of standing on the parallel bars used in the first tuning trials of the cable-driven mechanism. After 30 minutes, the patient was able to walk with free swing of the knee (maximum flexion mean of 50°) with the two crutches, and although the speed adopted was low, the knee clearly reaches extension at the end of the swing phase (see Figure 27). After a short time, the patient learnt to manage joint locking at the beginning of stance, used only one crutch and felt sure without any risk of falling.
On examining the ankle angle, dorsal flexion, excessive with the subject's habitual orthosis, progresses appropriately during the stance phase from the action of the ankle actuator. Regarding plantar drop, it is restricted by a maximum of 5° (mean of 4.5°). It was found that assistance to knee extension during the swing phase with the actuator functions considerably well, as can be observed in the mean knee flexions (Table 3).

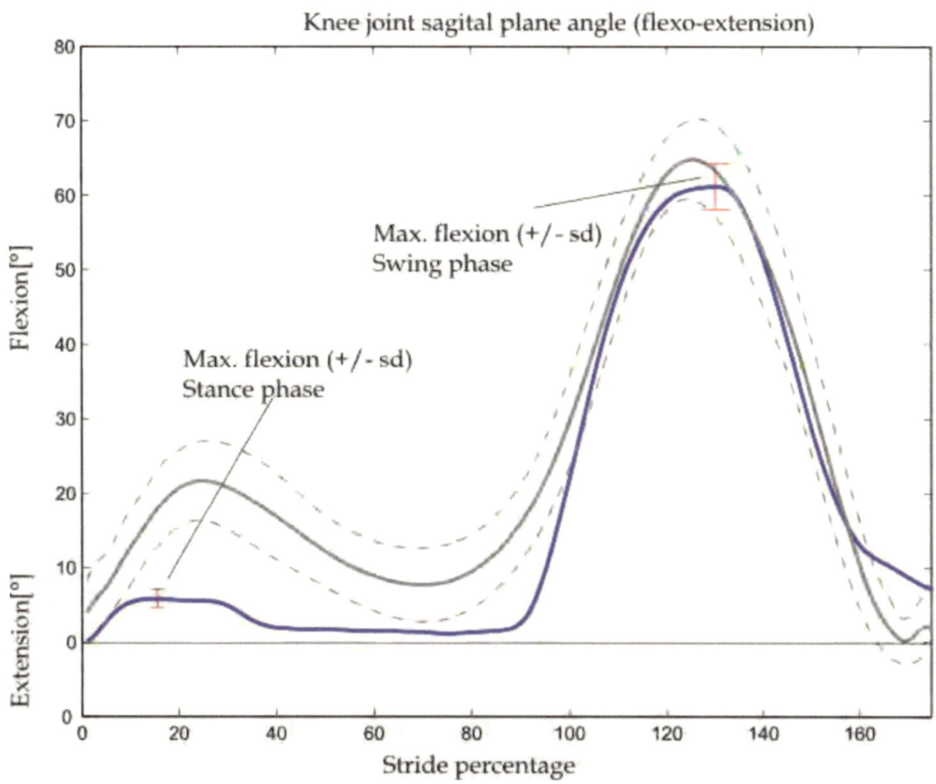

Fig. 27. Effects (average values) on joint kinematics.

The maximum mean values of knee flexion and ankle flexion for the swing and stance phases are represented in Table 3, and correspond to trials under final training conditions. The number of trials with CDE was reduced to measurements of 5 gait cycles, because of the fatigue problems mentioned earlier.

	CDE (5 cycles)	ACE (25 cycles)
Peak knee flexion in stance [°]	5.5 ± 2	5.5 ± 1
Peak knee flexion in swing [°]	61 ± 5	61 ± 3
Peak dorsiflexion in stance [°]	6 ± 3	5 ± 2
Peak dorsiflexion in stance [°]	22 ± 5	20 ± 3

Table 3. Mean values of maximum joint flexions for the stance and swing phases under final training conditions.

4.2.2. Kinetics

From the mean values of the ground reaction forces a reduction in mediolateral forces can be observed in patient S1 when automatic gait control is used. In Figure 28 this reduction in mediolateral forces can be observed in the initial stance phase, which avoids lateral movement, typical in the gait of patients with post-polio syndrome.

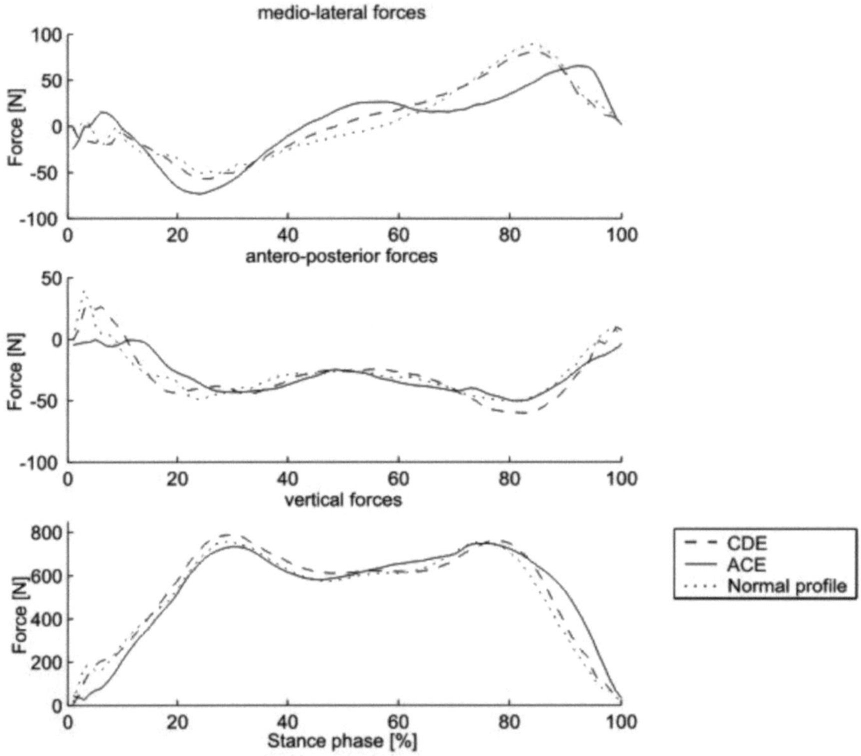

Fig. 28. Mean values of the ground reaction forces of evaluation data set of patient S1, under CDE and under ACE, and normality pattern with exoskeleton calculated for the subject's weight.

The pattern obtained of vertical ground reaction forces with the exoskeleton with CDE approximates the normality pattern calculated for the subject with a correlation factor of 0.94. An increase was observed in the level of lift force with ACE in comparison to CDE.

5. Conclusions and discussion

The differences found in the patients' kinematic gait patterns during the application of functional compensation on the lower limb showed significant differences regarding the subjects' usual gait. In both patients rapid adaptations were observed and new motor commands were learnt necessary for managing the exoskeleton with the constraints imposed on the limb. The benefits of the correct release of the knee in both instances is clear evidence of approximating their gait patterns to the normality pattern depicted in Figure 27, with the compensations of the biomimetic actuation system by applying intermittent impedance (K1 and K2).

The GAIT exoskeleton made it possible for patient S1 to walk for the first time without compensation with the hip movement, necessary with the knee-locking orthosis. Assistance to the extension of the knee actuator using energy recovery is obvious and is effectively reached before contact with the ground, as can be observed in the mean values of Figure 27, when a low and constant gait speed is maintained. It is uncertain what percentage of

assistance to the knee extension is due to the actuator action and what percentage is determined by movement inertia. It can thus be hypothesised that the recovery spring for extension acts against movement at the beginning of extension.
The results with patient S2 give an indication of the functioning of the ankle actuator for the partial recovery of energy —stored during stance by the spring with K3— in combination with the carbon fibre insole recovery of energy in the shoe if the resulting lift forces are observed with regard to the subject's insufficient muscular capacity.
The system was designed taking the weight to the most proximal part. Although the subjects' first impression was that the system was a slightly heavy, with time this impression changed and the level of acceptance gradually improved. The cyclical control gait system applied is based on the speed of rotation of the limbs. It is important to highlight how at the end of trial, patient S2 preferred to use the ACE and rejected the CDE, which operates under the same principle of commercial orthotic systems. The importance of flexibility in the initial adjustment of the algorithm to be customised to the subject's gait is clear. In the trials, it was observed that patient S2 had reduced mobility in the ankle, so the controller conditions were modified and the $U\omega_{pierna}$ and $U\omega_{pierna}$, thresholds reduced to detect the transition moment. It was observed that, although the algorithm monitored the state of the knee joint in order to avoid undesired activations of the solenoid, this condition was not sufficient, and it was necessary to change the adjustment of the P_{act} activation period consign.
The results found in this study show that the patterns with ambulatory assistance using the robotic exoskeleton are significantly better than those offered by traditional orthoses or basic aids. Each pathological case has its own intrinsic characteristics, and the mechanical adaptation and control system therefore necessitate customisation of the robotic solution. The evidence obtained with both subjects with post-polio show the viability of the gait compensation concept using wearable robotic exoskeletons on the improved quality of daily life in subjects with lower-limb joint disorders.

6. References

Baten, C., de Vries, W., Moreno, J. & Freriks, B (2004). Use of inertial sensing in an intelligent orthosis. - A feasibility study, *Esmac Conference*, Warswaw, 2004.

Blaya, J. & Herr, H. (2004b). Adaptive Control of a Variable-Impedance Ankle-Foot Orthosis to Assist Drop Foot Gait. *IEEE Trans Neural Syst Rehabil Eng,* Vol. 12, No. 1, (march, 2004), 24-31.

Irby, S., Kaufmaun, K., Wirta, R. & Sutherland, R.. (1999). Optimization and application of a wrap spring clutch to a dynamic knee-ankle-foot orthosis. *IEEE Transactions on Rehabilitation Engineering*, Vol. 7, No. 2, 130-4.

Ferris, D.; Gordon, K., Sawicki, G. & Peethambaran, A. (2006). An improved powered ankle foot orthosis using proportional myoelectric control. Gait and Posture 23(4), 425-428.

Ferris, D.; Gordon, K., Sawicki, G. & Peethambaran, A. (2006). An improved powered ankle foot orthosis using proportional myoelectric control. Gait and Posture 23(4), 425-428.

Kazerooni, H., Steger, R., & Huang, L. (2003). Hybrid control of the Berkeley lower extremity exoskeleton. *The International Journal of Robotics Research,* 25(4-6), 561-573.

Moreno, J.C., Rocon E., Ruiz, A., Brunetti, F., & Pons, J.L. (2006b). Design and implementation of an inertial measurement unit for control of artificial limbs: application on leg orthoses. *Sensors and Actuators B,* 118(1-2), 333-337.

Moreno, J.C., Brunetti, F., Cullell, A., Forner-Cordero, A. & Pons, J.L. (2006c). Simulation Of Knee Function During Gait With An Orthosis By Means Of Two Springs Of Different Stifnesses. *Gait and Posture,* 21(Sup1), S140.

Rehbinder H. and Martin C. (2001). A control theoretic model of the fore arm. Journal of Biomechanics 34(6), 741-748.

Rocon, E., Belda-Lois, J.M., Sánchez-Lacuesta, J.J., Ruiz, A.F. & Pons, J.L. (2005b). Estimation of biomechanical characteristics of tremorous movements based on gyroscopes. In: Asistive Technology - from Virtuality to Reality. AAATE05. Lille , France.

Winter, D.A. (1991). *The biomechanics and motor control of human movement,* University of Waterloo, 2nd edition.

27

Exoskeleton-Based Exercisers for the Disabilities of the Upper Arm and Hand

[1]Ioannis Sarakoglou, [1]Sophia Kousidou, [2]Nikolaos G. Tsagarakis and [2]Darwin G. Caldwell

University of Salford[1], Manchester, UK

Italian Institute of Technology[2], Genoa, Italy

1. Introduction

The impact of disability on society is great not only on direct treatment costs. Invaluable loss of human creative activity and mental wellbeing as well as productivity losses reflect the indirect impact on the disabled individual as well as on society as a whole.

Stroke is the leading cause of disability in the industrialised countries. Every year, over 130,000 people in the U.K. suffer strokes, with 13,000 under retirement age. Ischemia or haemorrhage in the brain may be the cause of cerebral vascular accidents which result in strokes (Parker et al., 1986). Fortunately over 65% of patients survive but the majority does have residual disabilities with up to 1/3 having severe disabilities particularly in the upper limb and hand. Hemiplegia, the most common impairment resulting from stroke, leaves the survivor with a stronger unimpaired arm and a weaker impaired one (hemiparesis). Traumatic injuries as well as conditions like muscular dystrophy, arthritis and regional pain syndromes, also add to the major causes of disability and functional dependence. Deficits in motor control and coordination synergy patterns, spasticity and pain are some of the most common symptoms of these conditions (Parker et al., 1986).

In the case of stroke victims, it is widely accepted that spontaneous recovery accounts for the motor and functional restoration taking place within the first months after the stroke incident. Recent evidence has shown that further improvement can be achieved if neural organisation is modified. Partially damaged neural pathways can be reinstituted and neurons not normally involved in an activity can be engaged. Neuroplasticity is use-dependent; therefore it has been shown that intensive and repetitive physiotherapy may be necessary to modify neural organization (Carr & Shepherd, 1987) and recover functional motor skills. In the case of other disability victims, repetitive physiotherapy is also the key for regaining motor control, as it contributes in regaining muscle strength as well as in restoring the joints' range of motion.

Despite the benefits of intensive physiotherapy, upper limb and hand disability are seldom considered life-threatening; therefore they rate relatively low on the priority list for urgent medical assistance. In addition to that, manipulative physiotherapy procedures are labour-intensive with hundreds of arm flexing movements per day forming part of a rehabilitation regime that is no untypical. Manipulation requires high levels of one to one attention from highly skilled medical personnel, but there is an international shortage of physiotherapists. Finally, patients must receive individualised treatment. The need for longer treatment periods, more intensive regimes and the shortage of trained stuff means that robotic and

power assistive techniques are increasingly viewed as a potential replacement for the physical labour leaving the therapists with greater time to develop the treatment plan.
Computer generated three-dimensional environments (VEs) can provide visual, auditory and physical (haptic) interactions in a way that engages a patient's attention while at the same time keeping him/her motivated. Motivation is a key factor in successful rehabilitation. If an impaired person lacks motivation, he/she may use the unimpaired arm/hand in performing activities of the daily living (ADLs) and therefore hamper the functional restoration of the impaired arm/hand (Nakayama et al., 1994). The role of VEs in rehabilitation can be considered as dual: they provide the therapists with a set-up for repetitive functional ADL training while at the same time giving quality feedback to the patients helping them control their physiological responses in an engaging and entertaining way.
There has been a lot of work on power-assisted device therapy and as a result, there is an increasingly wide and diverse range of systems. These systems range from simple powered 2-link orthoses to industrial robots and from simple data gloves in VEs to complicated hand exoskeletons. They use a variety of actuation methods and control strategies and they are targeted at different disabilities.
The next two sections explore the art in rehabilitation exoskeletons for the upper arm and hand. Sections 4 and 5 present work that is undergoing at the University of Salford. More specifically, Section 4 presents a rehabilitation system using Salford Rehabilitation Exoskeleton as a medium for delivering therapy whereas Section 5 presents a Hand Rehabilitation Exoskeleton. Section 6 concludes with a brief discussion including the authors' view regarding future directions in the area of Rehabilitation Robotics.

2. Upper Arm Rehabilitation Exoskeletons

The major findings in robot-mediated rehabilitation come from two systems that have undergone extensive clinical trials: the MIT-MANUS robot (Hogan et al., 1992; Volpe et al., 2000) and the Palo Alto/VA Stanford Mirror Image Motion Enabler (MIME) (Burgar et al., 2000). Due to the fact that both systems are using robots rather than exoskeletons to deliver therapy to stroke patients, they will not be the subject of detailed presentation here. The main findings of these clinical trials however, indicated a significant improvement in patients' motor abilities while there was no significant improvement in their functional skills.
The orthoses/exoskeleton systems presented below are targeted mostly at patients with muscular weakness or multiple sclerosis. Some of them have been clinically tested but none of them has undergone extensive clinical trials.

2.1 ARMin

ARMin (Mihelj et al., 2006) is a 6 DOF exoskeleton developed at the Swiss Federal Institute of Technology in Zurich. It is specifically designed for neurological rehabilitation; as a device-therapy medium as well as a tool to test existing rehabilitation strategies and find the best rehabilitation practice. ARMin is a semi-exoskeleton solution in the sense that its structure is fixed on the wall via an aluminium frame and the patient's wheelchair can be placed beneath figure. 2.1. Its kinematic structure is depicted in figure 2.2. The exoskeleton has 3 DOF at the shoulder permitting horizontal, vertical and internal/external shoulder rotation, 1 DOF for elbow flexion extension, 1 DOF for forearm pronation/supination and finally, 1 DOF for wrist flexion/extension.

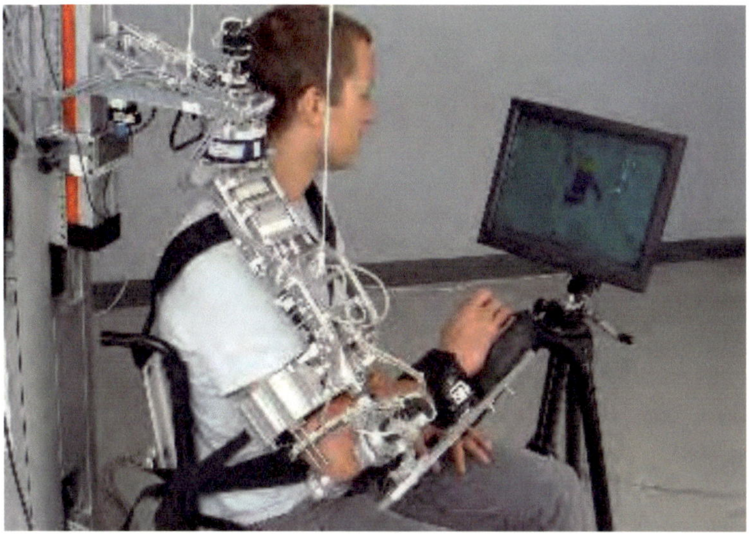

Fig. 2.1. ARMin. The image depicts the semi-exoskeleton structure. (Mihelj et al., 2006).

Impedance control is used to ensure compliant behaviour and many safety features have been incorporated in order not pose danger to the patient in case of malfunction. Its modes of operation are currently three. In the *movement therapy mode*, the therapist guides the patient's arm to form trajectories which can be repeated by the exoskeleton with different velocities. This mode is targeted at preserving joint range of motion and preventing joint degeneration. The *game therapy mode* strives to motivate the patient with simple games such as catching a virtual ball. If the patient is able to play the game, ARMin just compensates its weight. If the patient cannot play the game then it guides the patient's arm with an adjustable force towards the ball position. Finally, in the *ADL training mode*, the patient can train in ADL tasks like eating or grasping. In this mode the patient generates the trajectory in the sense that based on the patient's position and speed, ARMin predicts the required forces and torques.

In a pilot study with ten healthy subjects and five patients, comfort, functionality and acceptance was tested out. During the movement therapy, trajectory recording and repetition at different velocities was well performed and the robot support for the game therapy mode was adequate. The subjects assigned a grading of 8.5 to the therapy modes and an increase in their performance was noted progressively.

2.2 Wearable Orthosis for Tremor Assessment and Suppression (WOTAS)

WOTAS (Ruiz et al., 2006) is an upper limb exoskeleton specifically designed to measure and compensate for movement disorders such as tremor. It is actuated by electric motors at the wrist and elbow and its sensory system comprises of chip gyroscopes (which measure tremor force constantly) and kinetic sensors. The total weight of the system is roughly 850 gr. Impedance control strategy is used and real-time filtering algorithms distinguish between intended motion and tremor.

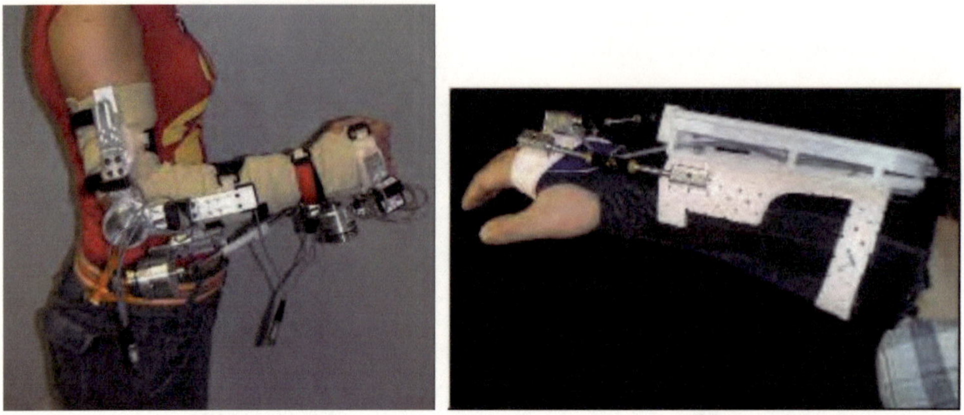

(a) (b)

Fig. 2.2. WOTAS. Image (a) shows a subject wearing the exoskeleton (Ruiz et al., 2006) while image (b) shows the forearm module.

Tremor is suppressed with the means of an actuator based on magneto-rheological fluids (whose viscosity can change by applying a magnetic field and therefore act as an effective damper).

Initial studies were performed with subjects wearing the exoskeleton while executing various tasks of the daily living. It was reported that WOTAS did not affect the subjects' range of motion. At the second stage of the study, the system added viscosity and inertia in order to suppress tremor (passive control strategy) and was able to estimate and measure tremor parameters. It was estimated that the system could suppress 30% of the production of tremor power. The reduction of the tremor power was sustained in the order of 80% in patients with severe tremor.

2.3 Motorized Upper Limb Orthotic System (MULOS)

MULOS (Motorized Upper Limb Orthotic System) (Johnson et al. 2001) was developed under a project funded by the Technology Initiative for Disabled and Elderly (TIDE) program of the Commission of European Communities and it was intended as stroke rehabilitation as well as an assistive. MULOS is a 5 DOF powered orthosis for the upper limb which allows the movement of the shoulder (3 DOF), the elbow and the forearm. It was designed to provide single joint exercise and operates in 3 modes:

a) Assistive, to compensate for loss of muscular action caused, for instance, by muscular dystrophy of high-level spinal cord injury.
b) Continuous Passive Motion, to provide physical therapy to selected joints of the arm.
c) Exercise, to provide graded resistance in order to allow exercise therapy to people with muscle weakness.

The shoulder structure is a 3 DOF mechanism having intersecting axes to allow it to behave as a spherical joint with a centre approximate coincident with that of the user's shoulder. The structure has sufficient compliance to allow a full range of motion at the shoulder. The joints are powered by cable drives in such a way as to keep the electric motors as close to the first joint as possible and thus, keep required torques to a minimum.

The elbow joint has one degree of freedom providing flexion/extension and a separate power unit positioned at the wrist provides elbow pronation/supination. The system can achieve a maximum output torque of 7 Nm and maximum speed of 9.5 rpm. An integral slip clutch between the motor and the elbow drive ensures safety of operation. A potentiometer for position control is located in line with the lower arm section of the orthosis.

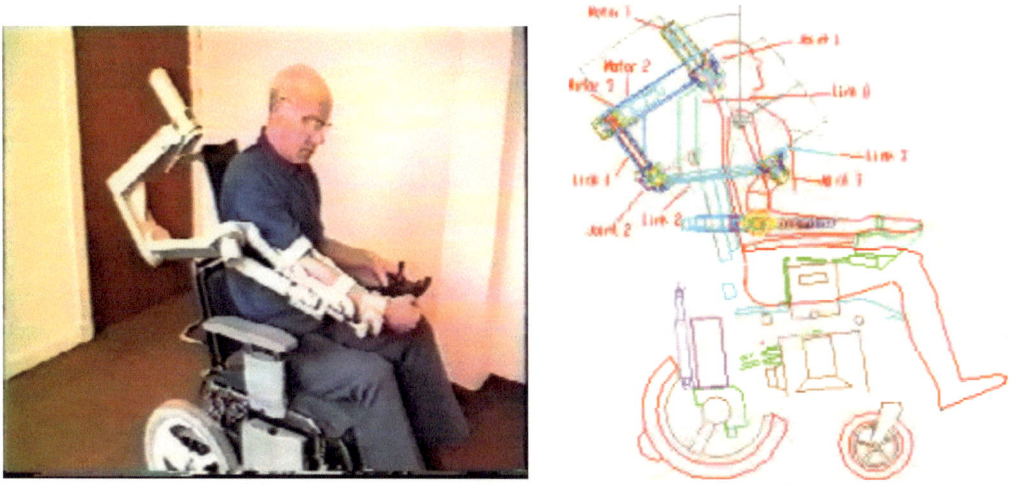

(a) (b)

Fig. 2.3. Motorised Upper Limb Orthotic System (MULOS). (a) shows a patient wearing the exoskeleton (b) a rough sketch of the position of motors, joints and links (Johnson et al., 2001).

Control hardware is mounted at the back of the wheelchair and the available control strategies are:

a) Point-to-point, using a 4 DOF joystick with the unimpaired limb to control the movement of the impaired limb
b) Joint-by-joint control
c) Walk-through programming in which trajectories can be pre-programmed moving the orthosis through a particular trajectory on a passive mode.

Although the device seemed to have good potentials, its development stopped in 1997.

2.4 FUNCTIONAL UPPER ARM ORTHOSIS

Functional Upper Limb Orthosis (Rahman et al., 2000) was a joint project between Alfred I. DuPont Hospital for Children and the School of Biomedical Engineering, Science and Health Systems at Drexel University. It was targeted at people with limited strength in their arms as a result of muscular dystrophy, spinal muscular atrophy and partial spinal cord injury.

The goal of the particular orthosis was to provide a sense of "floatation" that would allow a person with neuromuscular weakness to move his/hers arms. This was accomplished by gravity-balancing the entire arm - hand, forearm and upper arm - for all positions in 3D space. It had four DOF - two at the shoulder and two at the elbow. Three prototypes have been developed and evaluated

The orthosis had been tested on 10 patients. It was mounted on an adjustable stand and was placed so that the subject's shoulder joint was just above the anatomical shoulder. The patients were asked to put their right arm in the orthosis trough and a Velcro strap then secured the arm. The orthosis bungee cords were then stretched or relaxed based on their observed "floatation". After being able to move their arm at their own will, they were asked to perform activities of daily living. The responses from the patients varied during this first series of trials but the functionality of the device as far as the size adjustability is concerned was expressed repeatedly by all patients.

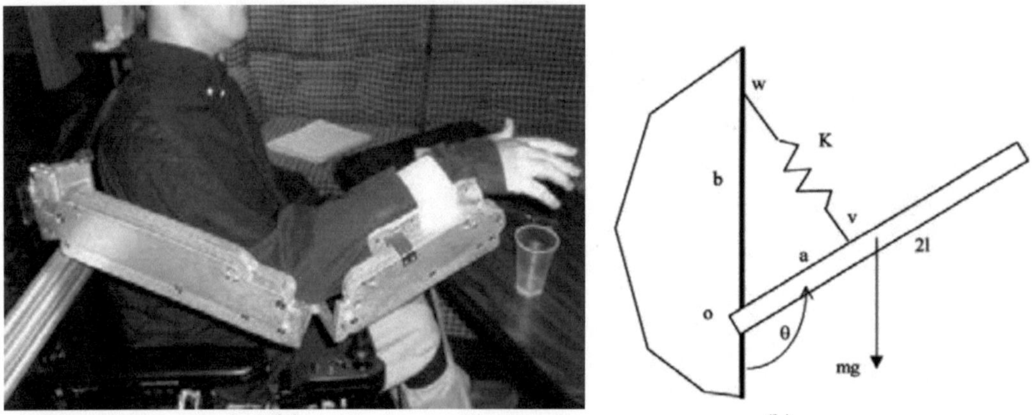

(a) (b)

Fig.2.4. Functional Upper Arm Orthosis. (a) shows a patient wearing the exoskeleton (b) depics the gravity compensation model (Rahman et al., 2000).

Due to the inexact gravity compensation (in vertical movement), the device is rarely prescribed. The majority of the BFO users settle only for planar motion and rely on compensatory body movements to achieve vertical motions.

2.5 ROBOTIC ASSISTANT OF UPPER LIMB EXERCISE

Alastair Cozens, while he was with the Rheumatology and Rehabilitation Research Unit at the University of Leeds, performed a study in which a robot assisted an active single limb exercise (Cozens, 1999). Robot assistance was demonstrated using torque applied to an individual joint, with electromyographic (EMG) data to confirm active exercise and monitor the pattern of activity within the antagonistic muscle pair.

During the experiments, the patient sat with the shoulder flexed forward to 90 degrees. The forearm was fastened to a lever, which could rotate in the horizontal plane about an axis aligned with the elbow. The upper arm was immobilized so that the lever could only be moved by elbow flexion/extension. Around the lever circumference target lamps were placed at locations corresponding to 10 degrees and 80 degrees elbow flexion denoting the targets towards which the lever should be aimed during extension and flexion. The angular movement of the lever was monitored by an electrogoniometer and an accelerometer whereas EMG activity in biceps and triceps was monitored via surface electrodes. The lever was set into motion by means of a servomotor, which assisted flexion/extension of the elbow. The motor had a maximum preset torque of 2 Nm for safety reasons.

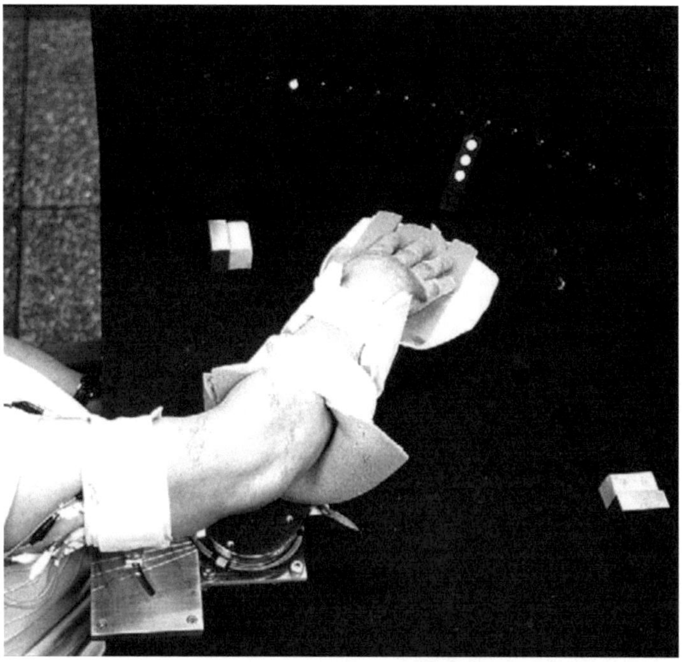

Fig. 2.5. Robotic Assistance of Upper Limb Exercise. The image depicts the orthoses, the contact points with the arm and the target towards which the lever should be aimed during extension and flexion of the elbow (Cozens, 1999).

Experiments using this arrangement were performed on ten stroke and multiple sclerosis patients of ages between 47 and 69. Each of these patients exhibited a weakness of the upper limb such as they could move the lever a little but were unable to complete an unassisted ten-cycle exercise with full movement between target lamps on every cycle. Some patients exhibited spasticity. During a ten cycle experiment, it was observed that the patients completed two cycles with extreme effort and biceps spasticity offered resistance to the elbow movement. When the motor assisted the elbow extension, the patients were able to achieve a full extension/flexion range in all ten cycles.

2.6 BALANCED FOREARM ORTHOSIS

Balanced Forearm Orthosis (Alexander et al., 1992) is a body-powered device that was developed in 1965. It was designed for people with muscular weakness and provided with the ability to move their arms in a horizontal plane.

Movement was accomplished via two linkages having joints along the vertical axes. One end of the orthosis was mounted on a wheelchair and the other end was connected to a trough into which a person placed his/her forearm. In the cases where the shoulder was depressed, the hand elevated via a fulcrum at mid-forearm. The orthosis allowed a person to move horizontally, for example over a lap tray, and to use compensatory movements to attain limited movement in the vertical direction.

An enhanced version of the Balanced Forearm Orthosis allowed vertical movement by providing a horizontal joint at the base. The weight of the arm was compensated by means of rubber bands. In 1975, Burke Rehabilitation Centre modified the orthosis by adding actuators (dc motors). Control was maintained through use of a joystick, control pad, or various micro-switch assemblies and it provided 5 DOF to the system.

2.7 HYBRID ARM ORTHOSIS

Hybrid Arm Orthosis (HAO) was developed by Benjuya and Kenney in 1990 (Benjuya & Kenney, 1990). It was targeted for patients who are wheelchair bound due to post-polyomyelitis, high-level spinal cord injury or stroke. The purpose of the HAO was to restore hand/arm functions.

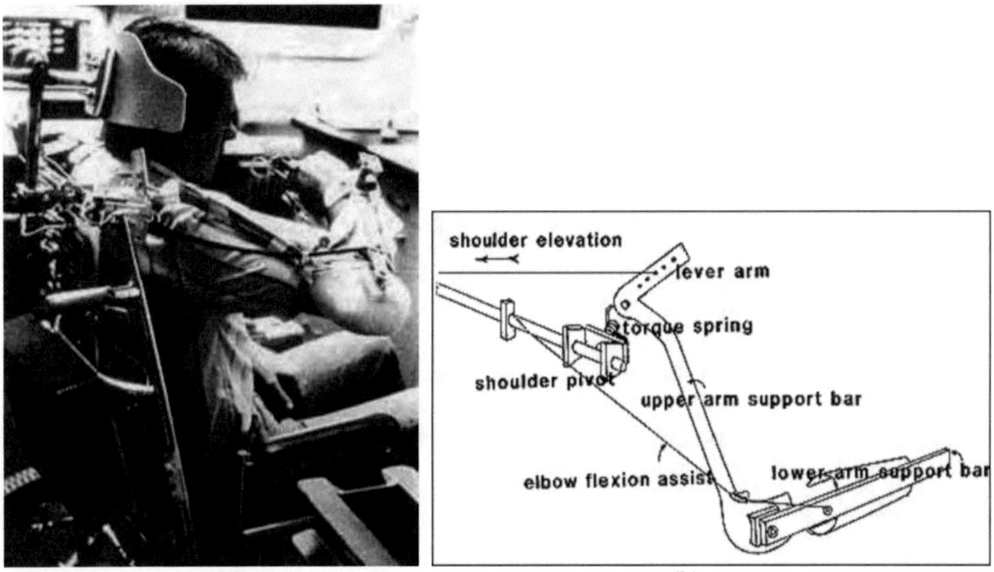

(a) (b)

Fig. 2.6. Hybrid Arm Orthosis. (a) shows a patient wearing the exoskeleton (b) depicts the orthosis structure (Benjuya & Kenney, 1990).

HAO achieved two major functions by using two different power sources. The shoulder and elbow joints were interconnected and simultaneously abduct and flex, respectively, by contra lateral shoulder elevation. The wrist supination and three-point jaw chuck pinch was generated by two separate switchable DC motors in sequence. In order to activate the motors, the patient slightly pressed air-switches that were located on the headrest of the wheelchair.

Clinical evaluation was limited to quadriplegics of C3-4 level. The patients tested daily-living activities, such as self-feeding, with relative ease after minimal training (1-2 hours). In developing the HAO the feasibility and ease of modifying parts of the system for individuals with different needs was tested with success.

3. Hand Exoskeletons

Successful impairment diagnosis and continuous monitoring of progress are two important parameters of effective hand rehabilitation. Manual measurement of hand parameters is a timely and subjective task prone to errors. Sensing gloves could be a potential tool for increasing the efficiency and reliability of performing a rehabilitation task. Sensing gloves

seem to be very effective in diagnosing hand disability because they provide excellent measurement of hand parameters and they don't require the presence of a medical specialist. Initial evaluation of a patient's impairment can be performed, which can be, accurately, repeatedly and objectively compared to follow up measurements.
Even though sensing gloves have been applied to hand diagnosis and rehabilitation they are unable, on their own, to apply resistive or assistive forces on the patient's hand. Forced mobilisation of joints is usually a necessary part of the treatment process. Researchers are addressing this with the application of robotic exoskeletons previously applied in Virtual Reality and Master-Slave telerobotics. Hand exoskeletons in particular have been in the centre of research due to their ability to apply forces to individual fingers and in some cases to multiple finger joints. Their multiple degrees of freedom offer increased quality and dexterity in finger joint mobilisation resulting to better therapy.
A review of the most relevant hand rehabilitation systems that have contributed by demonstrating a blend of technological advances and clinical outcomes is presented.

3.1 VPL DATAGLOVE AND THE MOVEMENT ANALYSIS SYSTEM

The first sensing glove to be applied to hand diagnosis was the DataGlove, developed by VPL. This was a thin lycra glove employing optic fibres as sensor elements for the measurement of finger positions figure 3.1. In its standard version it utilised two optic fibres per finger for the measurement of flexion and extension of the metacarpal and proximal interphalangeal joints. The principle of operation was measurement of light intensity attenuation as light travels through the optic fibre. The optic fibre's cladding was treated at the position of the measured finger joint so that its refractive index in combination with that of the core material allowed attenuation of light when the structure was bent. Therefore flexion of a joint can be measured by means of light intensity attenuation in the respective optic fibre.

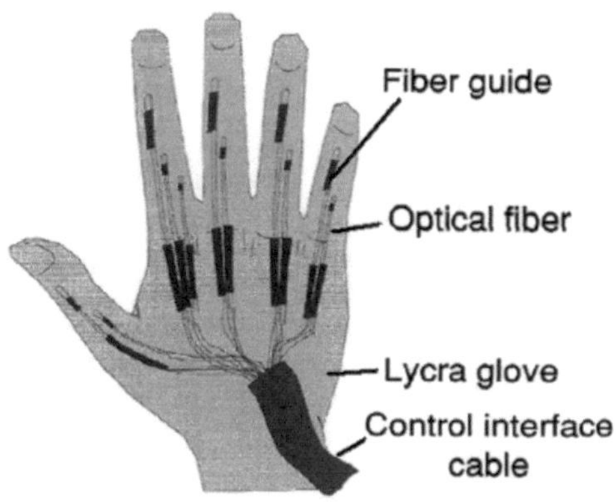

Fig. 3.1 The first version of the VPL DataGlove. Adapted from Burdea & Coiffet, 1994.

Greenleaf Medical Systems was first to incorporate a sensing glove into a commercial hand diagnostic system (Greenleaf, 1992). This system called Movement Analysis System adapted the DataGlove's fibre optic technology and linked it with new software to create a tool for quantitative assessment of upper-extremity function.

3.2 CYBERGLOVE AND THE RUTGERS MASTER EXOSKELETON

The Human-Machine Interface Laboratory at Rutgers has been a pioneer in the development of force feedback interfaces and was one of the first to develop a light weight portable hand exoskeleton (Burdea et al., 1992 b). This exoskeleton called Rutgers Master I (RMI) was the first to demonstrate high portability combined with relatively high force output. In 1992 Burdea and his colleagues first proposed the idea of a system for both diagnostic and rehabilitation of the hand (Burdea et al., 1992 a). The Rutgers Master II New Design (RMII-ND) is the latest version based on the RMII exoskeleton device that applies forces to the user's fingertips figure 3.2. It uses non-contact position sensors to measure the fingertip position in relation to the palm. Lightweight custom pneumatic actuators are attached to the tips of the thumb, index, middle, and ring fingers with force output up to 16N (Bouzit et al., 2002).

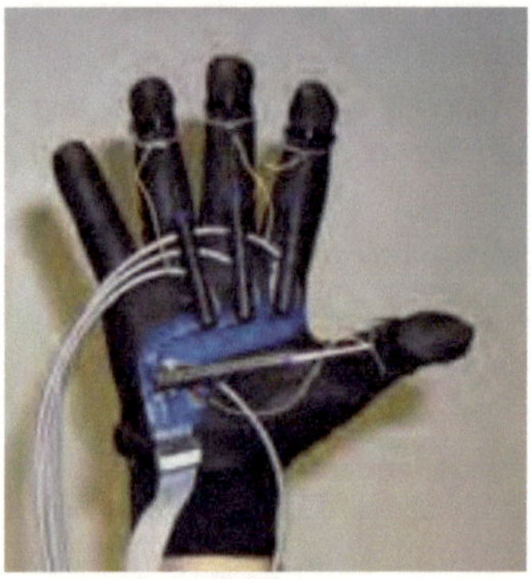
(a)

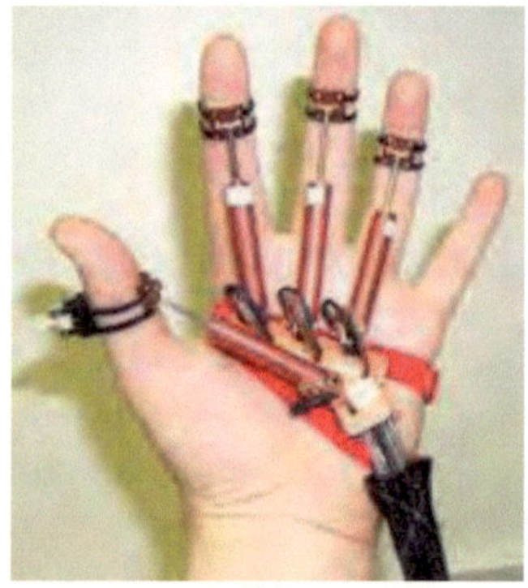
(b)

Fig. 3.2. (a) The Rutgers Master II force feedback glove, (b) The Rutgers Master II-New Design glove. Copyright Rutgers University.

In 2001 Jack et al proposed a hand rehabilitation system for stroke survivors (Jack et al., 2001; Boian et al., 2002; Adamovich et al., 2005). The aim of the proposed system was to offer dedicated exercises for finger range of motion, speed, fractionation and strength. The proposed system employs two devices to perform the aforementioned exercises. A Rutgers Master II-ND force feedback glove is used for exercises concerning finger strength, while a CyberGlove is used for the finger range, speed and fractionation exercises.

The Cyberglove is a sensing glove produced by the immersion corporation and is currently accepted to be the industry standard in hand tracking figure 3.3. The CyberGlove uses custom resistive bend sensors to measure the deflection of each finger. The 18-sensor model features two bend sensors on each finger, four abduction sensors, plus sensors measuring thumb crossover, palm arch, wrist flexion and wrist abduction.

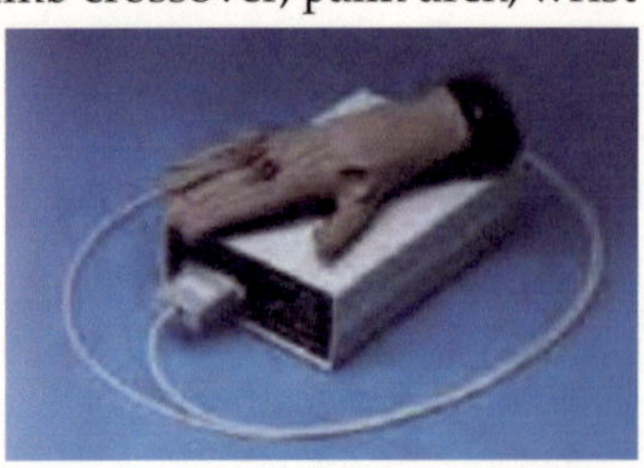
(a)

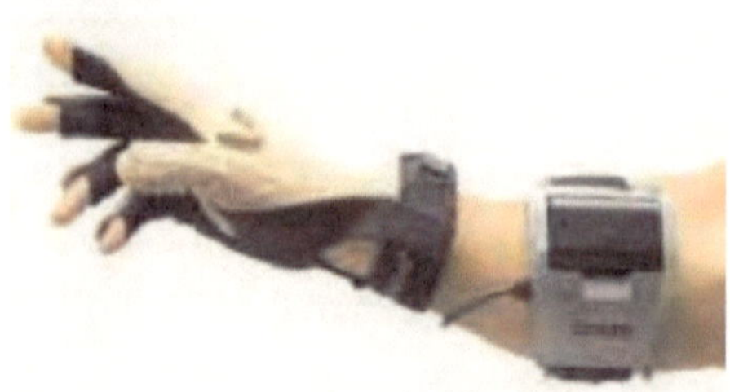
(b)

Fig. 3.3. The Cyberglove sensing Glove (a) Desktop version (b) Bluetooth wireless version. Picture Immersion Corporation.

Treatment with this system is facilitated in a VR environment with game like tasks. Also web interconnectivity with patient progress databases, treatment parameter updates, video conferencing for telerehabilitation and online synchronous monitoring of multiple patients are some of the developed features. Automatic report generation of patient progress with detailed graphs has been also a part of this research.

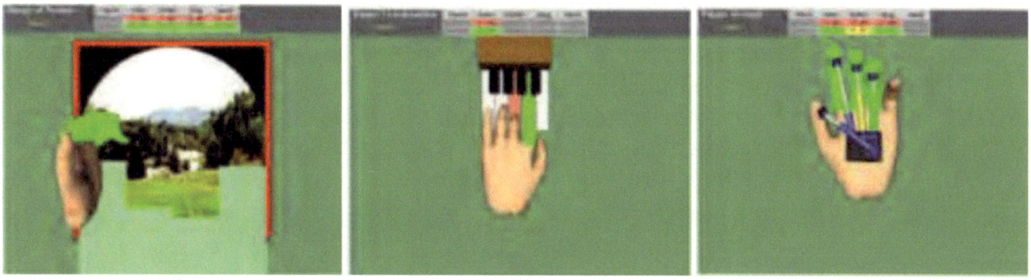

(a) (b) (c)

Fig. 3.4: Screen snapshots for the four VR exercises for post-stroke rehabilitation. (a)Range of Motion (b)Finger fractionation (c)Finger strength. Adapted from (Boian et al., 2002).

The four exercises were designed with World toolkit software development package. For the range-of-motion exercise, the patients have to flex their fingers to reveal pleasing images figure 3.4(a). In the speed exercise, the patients try to "chase away " a butterfly in the virtual scene by quickly flexing their fingers or thumb. In the fractionation exercise, the patients play a virtual piano keyboard pressing one key at a time figure 3.4(b). For the strengthening exercise, which is performed with the RMII-ND the patient has to push down a piston with the thumb, index, middle, and ring fingers against a constant force figure 3.4(c). During exercise the patients receive auditory, visual, and numerical feedback about their target goal and their current performance. The target goals of the VR exercises are calculated automatically by the system, based on the patient's previous results (Adamovich et al., 2005).

To determine whether the skills gained in the VR environment transferred to real-world movements, two generalization tests were utilized, a clinical evaluation using the Jebsen Test of Hand Function and kinematic analysis of prehension movements. On average, the task was performed 22% faster after the intervention, illustrating transfer of their improvement in VR to a functional task (Adamovich et al 2005).

3.3 P5 GAME GLOVE

Rehabilitation and diagnostic systems based on high fidelity VR equipment like the DataGlove and Cyber glove are expensive and their cost may not be justified for general health care practice. In an effort to minimise this cost and to make VR therapy attractive for a more generalised use, (Morrow et al., 2006) proposed a system built around commercial video gaming equipment.

After successfully testing VR rehabilitation using high-end equipment in a clinical environment (Adamovich et al., 2005), the Rutgers group proceeded into applying the same therapeutic principles and exercises via alternative, more economical hardware. The CyberGlove was replaced by a P5 game glove while the PC formally responsible for graphics processing was substituted by an Xbox game console. The P5 game glove is a 5DOF finger tracking glove which also incorporates 6DOF hand tracking. It employs one

bend sensor on the dorsal side of each finger for flexion tracking with a resolution of 3°. With this configuration tracking of individual joint flexion is not performed rather a single value representing the total flexion is obtained. Hand tracking is performed by means of an optical infrared tracker. In this application tracking was limited to finger flexion while hand position and orientation in space was not implemented.
The aim of this project was to replicate the same finger velocity and range of motion exercises previously applied through a superior and more expensive system (Adamovich et al., 2005). Java 3D simulations were chosen to emulate the exercises initially developed with WorldToolKit graphics development platform alleviating the high cost of the latter. Also extensive interventions on both Xbox's hardware and software have been performed in order to allow interconnection of hardware and compatibility with the Java 3D VR application. Figure 3.5 presents the system components.

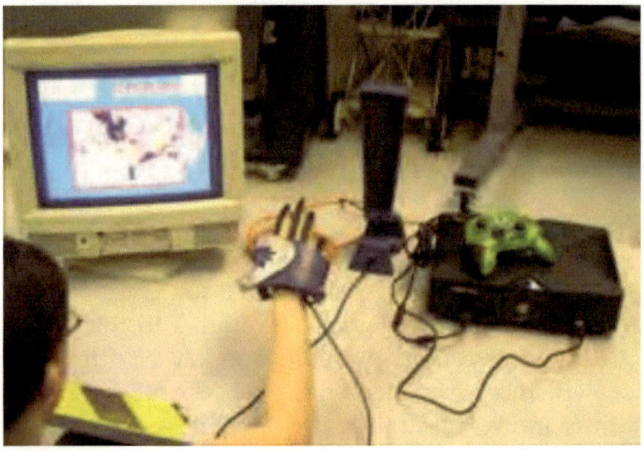

Fig. 3.5. Overall view of the experimental low-cost finger training system. Adapted from (Morrow et al., 2006).

According to the researchers this approach had been proven to be highly cost effective since it produced a system costing only $549, 32 times cheaper than its precursor. Nevertheless, overall business running costs for the adaptation of a bulk of such systems have not been calculated and thus a final price figure remains to be seen. As expected the claimed cost savings come at a trade-off in functionality and accuracy since CyberGlove is definitely offering superior performance to the gaming P5 Glove. If further clinical testing proves that such a system is beneficial to post-stroke hand rehabilitation, it will provide an answer to the cost related scepticism towards VR and tele-rehabilitation systems.

3.4 HAND WRIST ASSISTING ROBOTIC DEVICE (HWARD)

Recent encouraging findings of research on motor retraining following a cerebrovascular accident have motivated researchers at the University of California to develop a hand assisting robotic device for stroke rehabilitation (Cramer et al., 2007). The system called HWARD (Hand Wrist Assisting Robotic Device) is a 3 DoF device that exercises flexion and extension of the hand as well as some wrist movement. The aim was to retrain hand grasping and releasing movements while simultaneously using real objects during therapy. This is achieved by providing an unobstructed palm area where various objects can be offered for interaction during exercise. In this manner assisted grasping and releasing of objects can be combined with tactile stimuli, which is useful for associating and retraining tactile sensation in grasping.

HWARD is a pneumatic actuated desk mounted exoskeleton that supports the patients arm and is attached on the thumb and fingers as shown in figure 3.6. The device can flex or extend all 4 fingers together about the metacarpophalangeal (MCP) joint, the thumb at the MCP joint, and the wrist. Joint angle sensors in the structure are used to measure the movement of the exoskeleton's joints, and hence, movement of the subject's limbs when attached to the device.

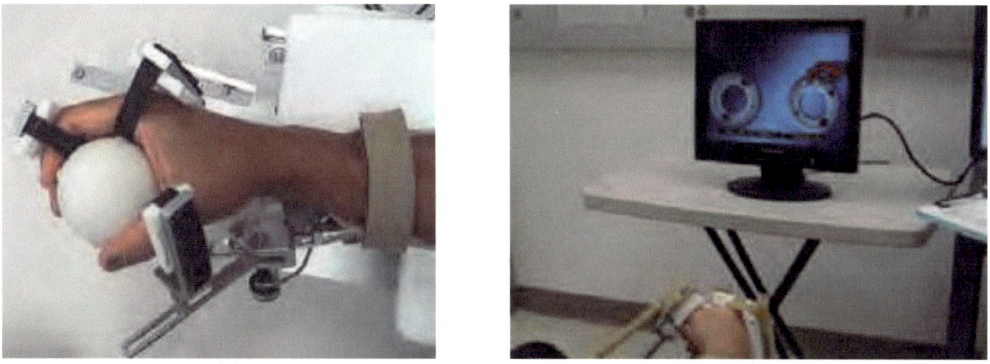

(a) (b)

Fig. 3.6. HOWARD hand exoskeleton. (a)The exoskeleton allows practice of grasping with real objects; (b) practice of grasping in a VR environment. Adapted form (Cramer et al 2007).

A therapy program based on this device was developed and emphasised right hand movement speed, force, precision, timing, and repetition, and included virtual reality/games.

In a pilot study to assess the efficacy of the system, a selection of thirteen patients of an average age of 63 received 15 two-hour therapy sessions spread over three weeks. During treatment all subjects worked with HWARD. The sessions were a mixture of grasp/release protocols of real/virtual objects. Seven of the subjects received full support from the system throughout each session. For the remaining six patients full assistance in the grasping and releasing exercises was offered only in the second part of each session.

To objectively measure the effect of therapy all patients were assessed prior and post treatment using three tests. These tests were Action Research Arm Test, Box-and-Blocks Test and the standard occupational therapy assessment tool called the Fugl-Meyer score. At the end of treatment the results showed an average improvement of 10 and 20 percent in the first two tests respectively, which assess occupational functionality and dexterity, while they were all rated as less disabled according to the Fugl-Meyer score. An increase of 17 percent in the range of motion was also observed. Comparing the average gains of the two groups of patients, in the three assessment tests, researchers observed a twofold increase, in all test, in the group that had received full assistance throughout each session. These changes in functionality within each subject before and after the three week treatment were assessed as highly significant. An interesting finding of this study supported by functional MRI tests was that functional gains obtained for practised motions did not extend to unpractised motions. This close association of gain and practiced task indicates the need for both intensive and diverse VR therapy in order for a generalised functional improvement.

3.5 THE HAND MENTOR

The hand mentor is the first commercial hand rehabilitation *Active Repetitive Motion™* therapy system produced by Columbia Scientific LLC. The hand Mentor is a single degree of freedom device that provides a controlled resistive force to the hand and wrist figure3.7. The applied force can oppose flexion or assist extension of the hand. It incorporates sensors that monitor the position of wrist and fingers during flexion-extension motions as well as force sensors to measure the force applied on the hand by the system actuator.

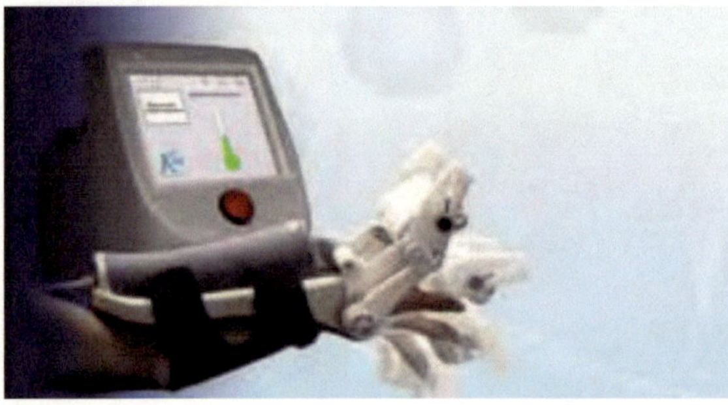

Fig. 3.7. Hand Mentor, the first commercial Active Repetitive Motion™ hand therapy device. Adapted from Columbia Scientific LLC.

The actuator is a compliant air muscle actuator with a combination of high power and high compliance (Caldwell et al., 1994). The device incorporates surface electromyography (EMG) recording electrodes in contact with the patient's muscles and an EMG level display. In an exercise with the Hand Mentor the patient initially works towards a target without any assistance from the device while observing the EMG indication display. Observation of the EMG level display provides a reliable feedback of muscle firing that can gradually train the patient to intuitively achieve muscle coordination. When the patient reaches the limit of his motion range the device actively assists the motion. Stretching beyond this limit helps to reduce spasticity and muscle tone.

In order to investigate the potential of the hand mentor as a clinical tool for hand rehabilitation post stroke, a clinical study was carried out (Kinetic Muscles Inc. 2005). The study protocol consisted of eight patients attending sessions five days a week for three weeks for 3 hours a day. The device was used for 1.5 hours each day and 1.5 hours were spent on repetitive task practice with a clinician. The assessed hypotheses were weather Mentor could work in a clinical study, the effectiveness of Active Repetitive Motion Therapy in restoration of hand function, and the cost effectiveness of such a system.

The Mentor was well accepted by patients. The therapy was assessed to work in a clinical setting. ARM therapy was effective in restoring function in the selected sample of stroke patients. By using therapist time more efficiently, the therapy seemed to be cost-effective compared to conventional CI therapy. This device's portability and reasonable cost could allow for a lending regime for home therapy where the patient can exercise intensively in his own time at the convenience of his home. This would reduce travel cost and expensive clinic time.

4. Salford Rehabilitation Exoskeleton

Tsagarakis *et al* at the University of Salford (Tsagarakis et al, 2003) have designed and built a multi-jointed gravity compensated upper arm assistive exoskeleton. The use of novel pneumatic actuation techniques (Caldwell et al., 1994) provides a design with accurate position and forced controlled paths, compliance and a high level of inherent safety that is capable of controlled path and force trajectories in a complex 3D workspace. SRE's mechanical design, figure 4.1, has 7 degrees of freedom (DOF). Three of these DOF are located at the shoulder permitting flexion/extension, abduction/adduction and lateral/medial rotation. Two are located at the elbow permitting flexion/extension and pronation/supination of the forearm. The remainders are located at the wrist permitting flexion/extension and abduction/adduction. More details about the mechanical structure can be found here (Tsagarakis & Caldwell, 2003).

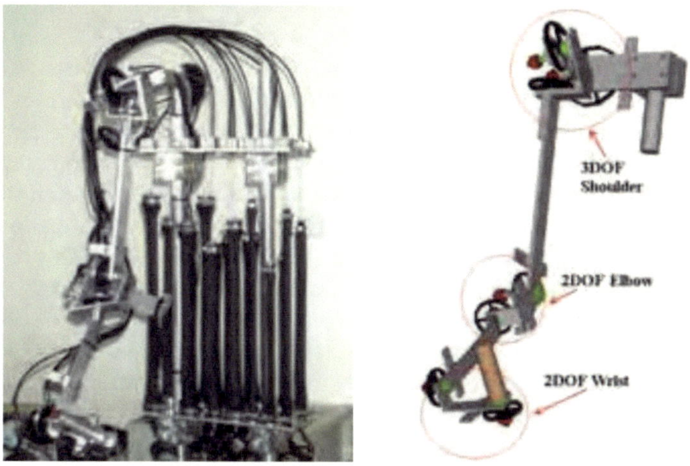

(a) (b)

Fig. 4.1. Salford Rehabilitation Exoskeleton. (a) The arm exoskeleton; (b) 3Dimensional model of the exoskeleton structure (Tsagarakis et al., 2003).

The exoskeleton framework is light due to its fabrication in aluminium with stressed components in steel (approx. weight 2kg) although the use of gravity compensation means that a user does not need to support any load if this is required. It is attached to the user at the elbow via a Velcro strip which makes it comfortable to wear, easily fitted and more acceptable to the patients. The workspace of the system permits motion over 75% of the volume of normal operation (Tsagarakis & Caldwell, 2003) permitting excellent duplication of the motions needed in completion of real world tasks. Dedicated software permits the control of the exoskeleton in three different modes: joint position control, joint torque control and impedance control respectively (Tsagarakis & Caldwell, 2003).

Rehab Lab is a computer generated therapy environment (Kousidou et al., 2006) that supports task-based therapy and through which, therapists can synthesise therapeutic protocols. In order to synthesise a protocol, a therapist combines a number of tasks with information about the number of repetitions, the interval after each repetition and the resting period between the different tasks. The tasks can vary from simple (i.e. shoulder flexion/extension) to more complicated (e.g. reaching tasks). Rehab Lab enables SRE to operate in three modes. These modes vary from full assistance from the exoskeleton to no assistance (recording and monitoring only), according to the recovery stage the patient is in. The modes are: Full Assistive mode (FA), Partial Assistive mode (PA), Non Assistive mode (NA).

During the first stages of recovery and while the patient cannot move his/her limbs without assistance, the *full assistive mode* can be used in order for the protocols to be executed with full assistance from the exoskeleton. All protocol tasks are executed at a constant speed (which can be adjusted for different tasks). This mode extends the concept of isokinetic machines already used in rehabilitation and has been evaluated in (Kousidou et al., 2003). While isokinetic machines offer only single joint exercises, Rehab Lab can exercise multiple joints simultaneously. Start and stop angles as well as speed, are the necessary parameters for trajectory generation of single joint exercises. For multi-joint exercises, trajectories are produced by recording a motion using the exoskeleton and then playing it back. *Partial assistive mode* is implemented with the help of a force/torque (F/T) sensor attached to the wrist of the exoskeleton. The sensor detects intention of movement (through a sensitivity scaling of the sensor's values) and Rehab Lab moves SRE accordingly. In *non assistive mode,* the exoskeleton is configured to simulate the forces generated by an exercise. This mode of therapy can be used when the patient has regained enough strength to complete a protocol on his/her own. In this mode, an impedance controller accepts as input the torques produced by the user and the control mode changes from position to impedance control.

Rehab Lab also contains a Virtual Environment (VE) figure 4.2. The VE provides the setup for the tasks to be performed but can also be manifested as a means of biofeedback. Currently, only one set-up exists which contains a table and a number of objects placed on its surface. After the therapist selects the suitable protocol for the patient, he/she can preview it in the VE. A female avatar is demonstrating the protocol so that the patient has a better idea of the sub-tasks to be performed. Once instructed in the protocol, the exoskeleton is fitted to the patient and the patient is asked to complete the tasks.

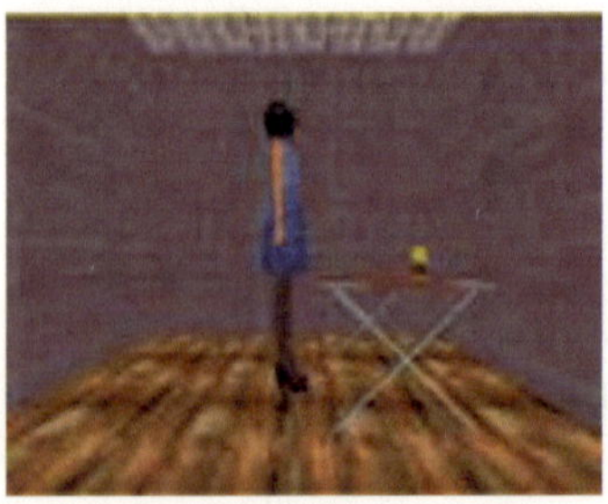

Fig. 4.2. The VE in Rehab Lab. The figure depicts a female avatar getting ready to perform a reaching task.

During the protocol, the patient can see a reflection of his/her movements in the virtual environment. That is, a virtual character is sitting in exactly the same position as the patient and his arm is moving exactly the same way as the patient's. The virtual character's arm position is updated by the exoskeleton's position sensors. This awareness helps them establish the boundaries of their limb with respect to the environment and the objects they have to manipulate and therefore learn how to control their responses.

In a pilot study involving healthy subjects, reaching tasks were performed (with no, partial and full assistance form the exoskeleton) in order to test the system's ability to replicate complex input trajectories. The results were encouraging as position sensing showed that output trajectories for reaching tasks were well correlated with inputs to the exoskeleton. EMG evaluation demonstrated the successful switching between the various modes of exercise. Results for a typical reaching task are shown in figure 4.3 and figure 4.4.

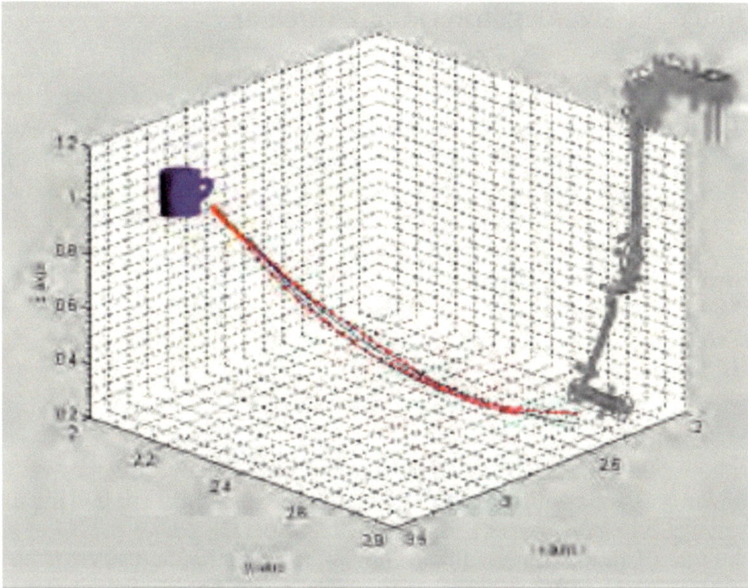

Fig. 4.3. Typical reaching task. The thin blue line denotes the input trajectory and the red thick line the actual exoskeleton trajectory as the task was performed. As seen, the red line follows the blue line with a high degree of correlation. (Kousidou et al., 2006)

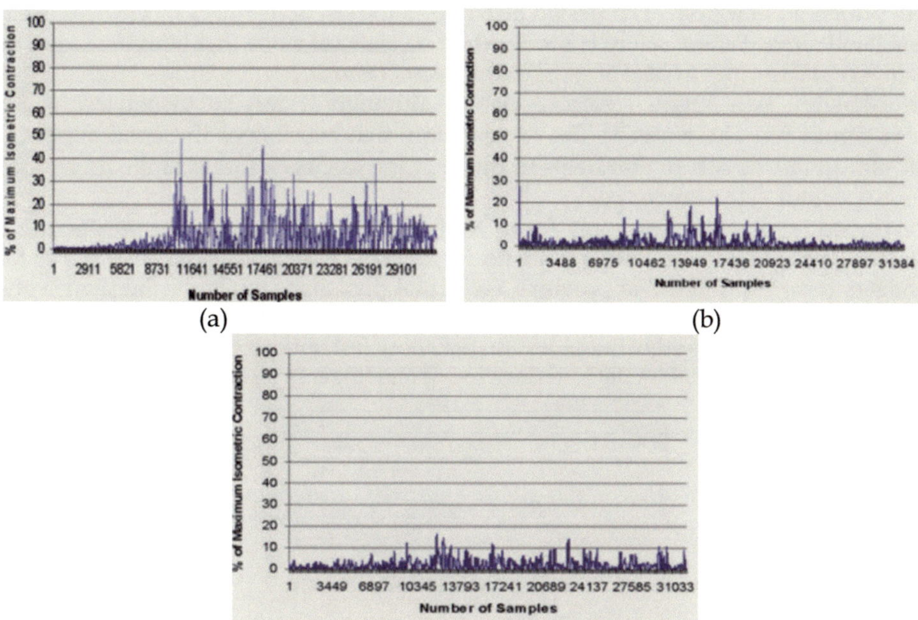

(a) (b)

(c)

Fig. 4.4. Typical reaching task. (a) is a typical muscle activity snapshot during non-assistive mode; (b) during a partial assistive mode and (c) during full assistive mode. (Kousidou et al., 2006)

5. Salford University Exoskeleton Hand Exerciser

A common problem of the presented hand exoskeletons is their inadequacy to combine different modalities such as hand parameter diagnosis and exercise assortment with qualities such as finger dexterity and satisfactory finger range of motion. Sarakoglou et al (Sarakoglou et al., 2004) have proposed an exoskeleton exerciser that combines dexterity with a good range of motion. The system enables the execution of finger therapy regimes and can also be used as a motion analysis and lost finger mobility diagnosis tool. The overall aim of this system is to provide physiotherapy regimes in an interactive virtual environment using a hand exoskeleton based exerciser.

As far as the therapeutic functionality of this system is concerned it provides facilities for hand motion tracking, recording and analysis as well as ability of execution of both occupational and physical therapy exercises.

5.1 Mechanical Design

The mechanical structure of the hand exerciser provides 7 active degrees of freedom. The Exoskeleton resides on the dorsal side of the hand and the forces are applied from that direction. The forces are generated by dc motors mounted in a low profile power pack and are transmitted to the fingers by low friction tendons. Finger force reflection that is generated by DC motors is accurately controlled by means of strain gauge based sensors. Measurement of the finger flexion is achieved by a combination of flexible resistive sensors integrated in a soft lycra glove and custom made linear electromagnetic sensors embedded in the exoskeleton's metallic structure. The incorporated glove unlike other systems is part of the exoskeleton structure and thus it is faster to put on and take off. The design also allows for fast adjustment of the exoskeleton for different hand sizes. Patient safety is provided by mechanical stops that limit the finger motion to within acceptable range in case of exoskeleton loss of control.

This exoskeleton is a single wearable device although it can be visualised as 3 main modules, figure 5.1. These are: 1) The exoskeleton, that consists of the hand support plate and the aluminium structure that helps to transmit the feedback forces to the finger joints, 2) the glove unit and 3) the Power pack.

The developed exoskeleton can apply forces to the index, middle and ring fingers and to the thumb. The applied forces can either resist flexion or assist extension of the fingers. For the first three fingers force is provided to proximal and distal phalanges while for the thumb only the distal phalanx is currently active. The exoskeleton is designed to fit a range of hand sizes and for this purpose it incorporates adjustment levers that allow fast and easy adjustment of the metallic structure for the three fingers. A 3D Cad drawing of one finger is presented in Figure 5.2.

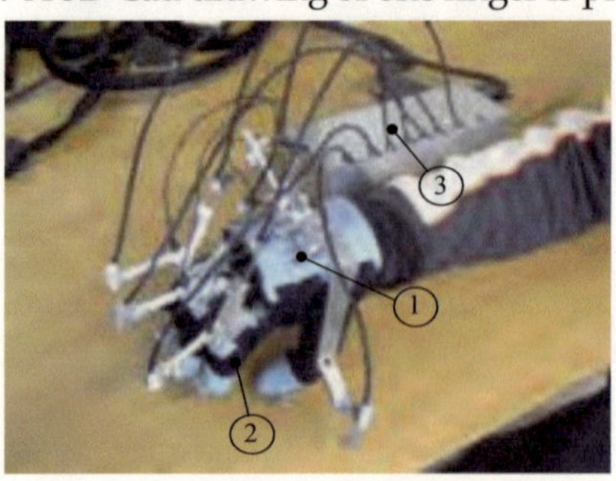

Fig. 5.1. The hand exoskeleton indicating the three basic modules. Adapted from (Sarakoglou et al., 2004).

To address the requirement for accurate finger tracking the hand exoskeleton employs a combination of input sensors. As mentioned previously it incorporates a lycra glove, which facilitates the housing of seven resistive flex sensors that measure finger flexion. Four flex sensors measure the flexion angle of the middle joints of the three fingers. The angles of the distal inter-phalangeal joints θ_3 (equation (1)) of the fingers are calculated from the middle joint angle θ_2 which is directly measured by a flex sensor (Gomez et al., 1995). Another three sensors monitor the flexion, rotation, abduction and adduction of the thumb.

$$\theta_3 = 0.46 \cdot \theta_2 + 0.083 \cdot \theta_2^{\ 2} \qquad (1)$$

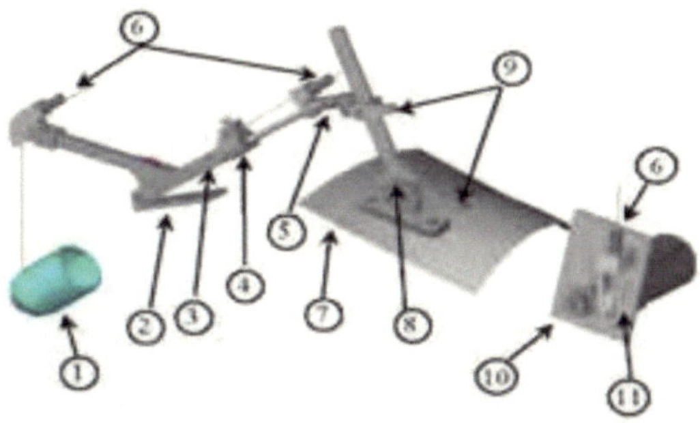

Fig. 5.2. Main components of the exoskeleton: 1-Finger Cup, 2-metalic plate attached with Velcro to the proximal phalanx,3-Structure for support and finger flexion measurement, 4-Steel rod & linear bearing, 5-Universal Joint, 6-Pull cables for force transmission, 7-Cushioned thermoplastic plate for exoskeleton support on the hand, 8-Adjustable Support, 9-Adjustment levers, 10-Motor module, 11-Strain gauge for measurement of force applied to the fingers. Adapted from (Sarakoglou et al., 2004).

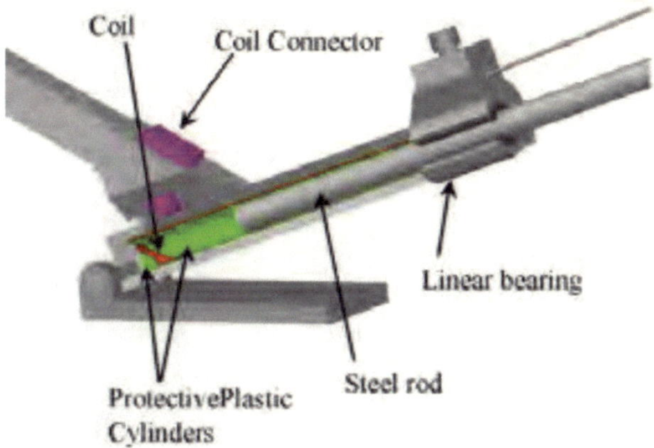

Fig. 5.3. Linear electromagnetic sensor integrated in the metallic structure. Adapted from (Sarakoglou et al., 2004)

Because of the obstruction posed by the mechanical structure placed on the back of the hand and on the proximal phalanges, the flexion of the proximal joint is not performed with flex sensors. Instead a custom made linear electromagnetic sensor is employed that is embedded in the metallic structure, figure 5.3.

5.2 System Integration and Therapeutic Environment

To enable the execution of hand therapy exercises the system was integrated within a Hand Therapy System. This therapy system, which is shown in figure 5.4 formed the test-bed where a clinician can customise and perform both finger motion evaluation tests and hand therapy regimes. The later resemble real tasks as much as possible particularly in terms of mechanical movements.

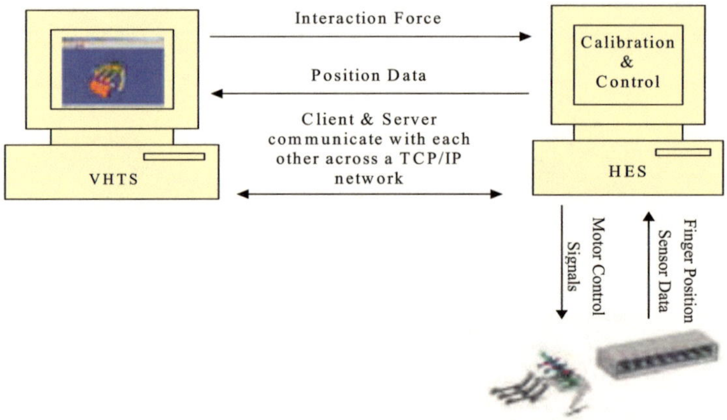

Fig. 5.4: Hand Therapy System Configuration. Adapted from (Sarakoglou et al., 2004).

The Hand therapy system consists of the Virtual Hand Therapy Station (VHTS) and the Hand exerciser Server (HES). The VHTS consists of a dedicated graphics machine that is responsible for the execution of the software relating to the exercise customisation and visualization. The HES is realized using a dedicated PC, which executes the software modules associated with the Hand Exerciser device calibration and control. Communication between the (VHTS) and (HES) is performed using a dedicate TCP/IP link. The aim of the Virtual Hand Therapy system is to perform hand rehabilitation using simple tasks. Since the exact type of deficiency can vary tremendously from patient to patient, even with the same diagnosis, the system was designed to be flexible so that the training can be adjusted to the needs of different patients. The virtual exercises resemble the real tasks as much as possible with the care that very complex, realistic or fanciful graphics and fast-paced game formats may be overwhelming for patients. In contrast, a very simple display, with few movements may help a patient to focus on the task at hand and enhance learning.

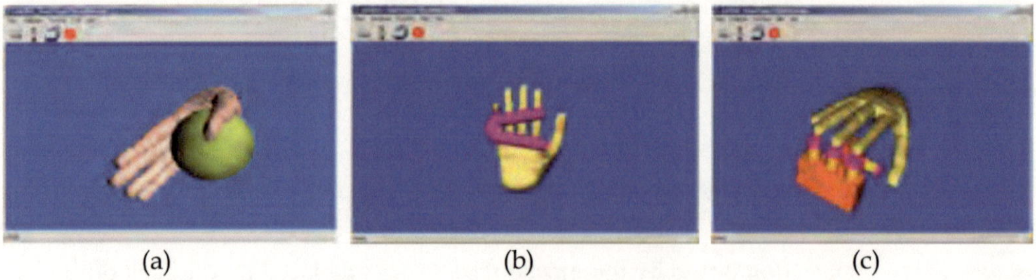

Fig. 5.5. Implemented VR Exercises: (a) Simulation of elastic ball exerciser, (b) Simulation of hand grip exerciser, (c) Simulation of trumpet keys exerciser (fractionation exercise). Adapted from (Sarakoglou et al., 2004).

In this respect existing therapy regimes constitute the basic principles in designing the VR physical exercises. Based on these existing physiotherapy methods recommended by physicians, three initial exercise regimes were developed. Figure 5.5(a) and figure 5.5(b) present VR Exercises simulating the action of existing manual exercisers. The aim of these exercises is to strengthen grip and increase hand motion. In the third exercise figure 5.5(c) the patient is required to push down the virtual model of a trumpet key. In order to do so, the patient must resist the opposing force of the virtual spring in the piston and flex his fingers. The stiffness of the VR objects is increased as the patient's therapy progresses.
A number of experimental trials were carried out to evaluate the performance of the system. Although the tests were performed by healthy subjects, they indicated that the system is reliable enough to undergo further clinical trial.

6. Discussion and conclusions

In this chapter we have stated the need for power-assisted and robotic tools as means of providing intensive, cost-effective and objectively measured physiotherapy. We presented the state-of-the-art as well as early exoskeleton systems targeted at upper arm and hand disabilities. We also presented work that is undergoing at the University of Salford, UK, an upper arm and a hand exoskeleton that can be used as potential tools for delivering device-mediated rehabilitation. Clearly, device-mediated rehabilitation is an active area of research whose findings have great impact on our society's well-being.
One could argue that the systems reviewed in the previous sections define or have already defined, in one way or another, future trends in rehabilitation robotics. Based on the advantages and drawbacks of the systems presented, we can draw some rough design and functionality requirements of an effective rehabilitation system.
The number of degrees of freedom is important for a rehabilitation facility as it allows for a broad range of tasks to be performed. Exoskeletons are expected to play a big role in the future of physical and occupational therapy as they offer a more natural way of interaction with real or virtual environments. The latter happens due to the fact that they utilise most of the human physical workspace. The weight and the volume of the system are also important. Adequate force/torque output, adequate range of motion and accurate position tracking are also required for such systems. Safety mechanisms at mechanical, electrical and software level need to be incorporated in order for a system to become commercial.
Virtual environments are also increasingly considered as a key component in rehabilitation: they can provide visual and auditory interactions and when used in conjunction with haptic feedback, they can engage a patients' attention while at the same time keeping them motivated. VEs also provide therapists with a set-up for repetitive functional ADL training or any other form of intensive training while at the same time giving quality feedback to patients helping them control their physiological responses in an engaging and entertaining way. EMG measurements can monitor levels of muscle activity and therefore can be included in a rehabilitation system as an indicator of recovery levels.
What is clearly missing from the prior art though, is a standard method of delivering therapy consisting of a unified way of synthesising therapeutic protocols and which could potentially be used as a common platform by researchers and therapists. A common platform such as this could promote a better insight into the nature of disability treatment as it would create the opportunity for keeping a certain number of variables constant (such as exercise type and parameters) while exploring others.

Device-mediated rehabilitation is an active area of research whose findings have great impact on our society's well-being. There are many problems that need to be solved but the cause of producing effective rehabilitation systems is very important and therefore worth persisting upon.

7. References

Adamovich S., Merians, A., Boian, R., Tremaine, M., Burdea, G., Recce, M., & Poizner, H. (2005). A Virtual Reality Based Exercise System for Hand Rehabilitation Post-Stroke. Presence, Special Issue on Virtual Rehabilitation, Vol.14, No.2, April 2005 pp.161-174, ISSN:1054-7460

Alexander, M.A.; Nelson, M.R. & Shah, A. (1992). Orthotics, Adapted Seating and Assistive Devices, Pediatric Rehabilitation 2nd Edition, pp. 186-187, Baltimore MD, 1992, Williams and Wilkins (eds)

Benjuya, N. & Kenney, S.B. (1990). Hybric Arm Orthosis, Journal of Prosthetics and Orthotics, Vol. 2, No. 2 (2nd Quarter, 1990), pp. 155-163, ISSN 1040-8800

Boian, R., Sharma, A., Han, C., Merians, A. S., Burdea, G., Adamovich, S., Recce, M., Tremaine, M., & Poizner, H. (2002). Virtual Reality-Based Post Stroke Rehabilitation, Proceedings of Medicine Meets Virtual Reality 2002, pp. 64-70, IOS Press, January 2002, Newport Beach CA.

Bouzit, M., Popescu, G., Burdea, G, & Boian, R. (2002). The Rutgers Master II-ND Force Feedback Glove, Proceedings of VR 2002 Haptics Symposium, pp. 145-152, Orlando FL, March 2002, IEEE, Orlando FL

Burdea, G & Coiffet, P. (1994). Virtual Reality Technology, 1st Ed, John Wiley & Sons, Inc., ISBN 2-8666601-386-7, New York:

Burdea, G., Roskos, E., Silver, D., Stone, R., & Dipaolo, D. (1992 a). Diagnostic / Rehabilitation System using Force Measuring and Force Feedback Dexterous Masters, Proccedings of Medicine Meets Virtual Reality 5 Conference, pp.18-10, June 1992, San Diego, CA

Burdea, G., Zhuang, J., Roskos, E., Silver, D., & Langrana, N. (1992 b). A portable dextrous master with force feedback. Presence: Teleoperators and Virtual Environments Vol. 1, No. 1, (Jan. 1992),pp 18-28, ISSN1054-7460

Burgar, C.G.; Lum, P.S.; Shor, P.C. & Van der Loos, M. (2000). Development of robots for rehabilitation therapy: the Palo Alto VA/Stanford experience, Journal of Rehabilitation Research and Development, Vol. 37, No. 6. (November/December 2000), pp. 663-73, ISSN 0748-7711

Caldwell, D.G.; Medrano-Cerda, G.A. & Goodwin, M.J. (1994). Characteristics and adaptive control of pneumatic muscle actuators for a robotic elbow, Proceedings of IEEE International Conference on Robotics and Automation, pp. 3558-3563, US, May 1994, San Diego, IEEE, California

Carr J.H. & Shepherd, R.B. (1987). A motor Relearning Programme for Stroke, Butterworth Heinemann, ISBN 0871893126, Oxford

Cozens, J.A. (1999). Robotic assistance of an active upper limb exercise in neurologically impaired patients, IEEE Transactions on Rehabilitation Engineering, Vol. 7, No.2 (June 1999), pp. 254 – 256, ISSN 1063-6528

Cramer, S.C., Takahashi, C.D., Der-Yeghiaian, L., See, j., Motiwala, R.R. & Le, V. (2007). Robot-Based Hand Motor Therapy after Stroke, Presented in the International Stroke Conference, Feb. 2007, San Francisco, CA

Gomez, D., G. Burdea & N. Langrana. (1994). The Second Generation Rutgers Master - RM II, Proceedings of Automation'94 Conference, Vol. 5 pp.7-10, Taipei, July 1994. Taiwan

Greenleaf, W. J. (1993). DataGlove, DataSuit and Virtual Reality Advanced Technology for People with Disabilities, Proceedings of Virtual Reality and Persons with Disabilities. California State University, 1993, Northridge, CA

Hogan, N.; Krebs, H. I.; Charnnarong, J.; Srikrishna, P. & Sharon, P. (1992). MIT-MANUS: A workstation for manual therapy and training, Proceedings of IEEE Workshop on Robot and Human Communication, pp. 161-165, 0-7803-0753-4, Japan, September 1992, IEEE, Tokyo

Jack, D., Boian, R., Merians, A. S., Tremaine, M., Burdea, G. C., Adamovich, S. V., Recce, M. & Poizner, H. (2001). Virtual Reality-Enhanced Stroke Rehabilitation. IEEE Transactions on Neural Systems and Rehabilitation Engineering, Vol.9, No.3, September 2001, pp 308-318, ISSN:1534-4320

Johnson, G.R.; Carus, D.A.; Parrini, G.; Scattareggia Marchese, S. & Valeggi, R. (2001). The design of a five-degree-of-freedom powered orthosis for the upper limb, Proceedings of the Institution of Mechanical Engineers Part H-Journal of Engineering in Medicine, Vol. 215, No. 3 (2001), pp. 276 – 284, ISSN 0954-4119

Kinetic muscles Inc. (2005). Active Repetitive Motion™ (ARM) Therapy for Increasing the Function and Independence of Stroke Patients,Report Submitted for NIH Grant Approval 2005

Kousidou, S.; Tsagarakis, N.G. & Caldwell, D.G. (2003). Evaluation of a "soft" exoskeleton for rehabilitation and physiotherapy of the upper limb Proceedings of IEEE International Conference on Advanced Robotics, pp. 1080-1085 Portugal, June 2003, IEEE, Coimbra

Kousidou, S.; Tsagarakis, N.G. & Caldwell, D.G. (2006). Assistive Exoskeleton for Task-Based Physiotherapy in 3-Dimensional Space, IEEE International Conference on Biorobotics and Biomechatronics, pp. 266- 271, Italy, February 2006, IEEE, Pisa

Mihelj, M.; Nef, T. & Riener, R. (2006). ARMin – Toward a Six DoF Upper Limb Rehabilitation Robot, IEEE International Conference on Biorobotics and Biomechatronics, pp. 1154- 1159, Italy, February 2006, IEEE, Pisa

Morrow, K., Docan, C., Burdea, G. & Merians, A. (2006). Low-cost Virtual Rehabilitation of the Hand for Patients Post-Stroke, Proceedings International Workshop on Virtual Rehabilitation, pp 6-10, ISBN: 1-4244-0280-8, August 2006, New York, NY

Nakayama, H.; Jorgensen, H.S; Raaschou, H.O. & Olsen, T.S. (1994). Recovery of upper extremity function in stroke patients: the Copenhagen Stroke Study, Archives of Physical Medicine and Rehabilitation, Vol. 75, No.4 (April 1994), pp. 394-8, ISSN 0003-9993

Parker, V.M.; Wade, D.T. & Langton, H.R. (1986). Loss of arm function after stroke: measurement, frequency, and recovery, International Rehabilitation Medicine, Vol. 8, No.2 (1986), pp. 69-73, ISSN 0379-0797

Rahman, T.; Sample, W.; Seliktar, R.; Alexander, M. & Scavina, M. (2000). A Body-Powered Functional Upper Limb Orthosis, Journal of Rehabilitation Research and Development, Vol. 7, No. 6. (November/December 2000), pp. 675-680, ISSN 0748-7711

Ruiz A.F.; Forner-Codrero, A.; Rocon, E. & Pons, J.L. (2006). Exoskeleton for Rehabilitation and Motor Control, IEEE International Conference on Biorobotics and Biomechatronics, pp. 601- 606, Italy, February 2006, IEEE, Pisa

Sarakoglou, I., Tsagarakis, N.G. & Caldwell, D.G. (2004). Occupational And Physical Therapy Using A Hand Exoskeleton Based Exerciser, Proceedings of Intelligent Robots and Systems, (IROS 2004), Vol: 3, pp 2973- 2978, ISBN: 0-7803-8463-6, Sept.-Oct. 2004 IEEE/RSJ, Sendai, Japan

Tsagarakis, N.G. & Caldwell, D.G. (2003). Development and control of a physiotherapy and training exercise facility for the upper limb using soft actuators, Proceedings of IEEE International Conference on Advanced Robotics, pp. 1092-1097, Portugal, June 2003, IEEE, Coimbra

Volpe, B.T.; Krebs, H.I.; Hogan, N., Edelstein, L.; Diels, C. & Aisen, M. (2000) A novel approach to stroke rehabilitation: robot-aided sensorimotor stimulation, Neurology, Vol. 54, No. 10 (May 2000), pp. 1938-44, ISSN 0028-3878

28

Stair Gait Classification from Kinematic Sensors

Wolfgang Svensson & Ulf Holmberg
Halmstad University
Sweden

1 Introduction

Gait measurement is of interest for both orthopedists and biomechanical engineers. It is useful for analysis of gait disorders and in design of orthotic and prosthetic devices. In recent years portable sensors have been studied as a complement to vision based (Morris & Paradiso, 2002). They have been used to measure both the kinematics of gait such as accelerations and angles as well as kinetics such as torques and forces. The main contribution of using portable sensors is the possibility of long time measurement of daily life situations. But the technique has also been included in active control of foot for rehabilitation. The research has mainly been focusing on the area of drop foot control see e.g. (Pappas et al., 2001: Veltink et al., 2003). The objective is to provoke foot lifting just in time for swing phase. The time to control is estimated often from gyros and force sensitive resistors. An alternative approach is to actively control foot ankle orthosis (Blaya & Herr, 2004). Recently also an active controlled foot ankle in a foot prosthesis has been studied (Svensson & Holmberg, 2006) for adapting to hill variations. But the existing systems are still limited in their capability of adapting to stair climbing. Just as orthoses, many prosthetic feet have fixed ankle position and attempting to move the body's center of mass forward may cause a sense of instability. With pressure sensors, characteristics of stair climbing and descending can be detected as the "foot down" often differs to horizontal walking. In a typical case of a sound person with two biological feet going up a stair, peak plantar pressures increase in the rear foot sensors. While at down stair there is a significant increased rate of pressure change in the frontal part. But both speed of gait and size of staircases can influence the accuracy of classification. Gyros or accelerometers have typically been attached to the waist, hip or shank. The sensors detect compensations made for different walking situations. But internal noise and temperature sensitivity of kinematical sensors tend to drift the angle estimation.

In this chapter an algorithm is presented to suit estimation of one foot angle in the sagital plane, independent on gait conditions. Only one gyro is used during swing and two accelerometers are needed for calibration during stance. Also, the sensor placement at the front of the foot avoids the need for heel strike for stance transition. Stair walking can therefore be studied. From the estimated swing trajectory three different gait conditions: up stair, horizontal and down stair are classified.

2 Stair walking

2.1 Ascending

Movements during gait in stairs have been studied earlier (see e.g. (Andriacchi et al., 1980: McFayden et al. 1988) at hip, knee and ankle during stair walking. Normal stair ascending can be divided into three phases: weight acceptance, pull-up and forward continuation. During weight acceptance and pull-up the knee dominates with support of the hip and ankle. While, during forward continuation the ankle generates a large amount of energy. The ankle angle differs from horizontal walk mostly at the late swing phase and at the early stance. At the lift up to next staircase the edge is avoided by a small dorsiflexion and moving the knee backwards.

2.2 Descending

Also in down stair the ankle angle differs from horizontal in the swing phase when moving the limbs down (Andriacchi et al., 1980: McFayden et al. 1988). In the early stance the toes are put down before the heel. At this stage most of the energy is transferred in the knee and ankle. The hip is only dominant at the end of the downward movement of the leg into next staircase. At push-off not so large force is needed since the leg almost only has to fulfill the swing. In horizontal walk decreases the dorsiflexion when the ankle passes the lowest position during forward swing in preparation for heel down, while in stair descending this is not so crucial. Less muscle activity for vertical movements is also needed when descending.

2.3 Fixed ankle angle

Walking with fixed ankle angle, e.g. ankle foot orthoses, AFO or prostheses compensations are made with hip and knee. Studies of AFO stair walking has been done on children with neuromuscular disorders (Nahorniak et al., 1999: Thomas et al., 2002). Although there was some discrepancy found depending on test group caused by different movement strategies, differences to able-bodied could be found. An AFO prevents normal plantar flexion during weight acceptance. As solid AFO blocks dorsiflexion during forward continuation this is compensated with reduced knee flexion. Compensations at the pelvis, hip and knee mainly occurred at the late stance when lowering opposite foot to next stair. Then also the ankle flexor moment was reduced resulting in a less effective push into the next step.

There are not so many studies published about stair ambulation using prosthetic feet. But it has been observed that transtibial amputees using the *Seattle lightfoot* prosthesis have a slower velocity and asymmetrical gait pattern compared to non-amputees (Power & Boyd, 1997). This asymmetry between limbs was shown to be more significant in stair ambulation than level walking. Kinetic analysis determined significant limitations in the prosthetic ankle motion which necessitated compensatory functions at hip and knee (Schmaltz et al., 2007: Yack et al., 1999).

It has previously been reported that the dynamic-elastic-response (DER) design store energy, which is released during forward progression making it easier to run or jump and it appears not to be any significant difference between different designs during normal gait. In a study of the five most commonly used prostheses for below-knee amputation it was shown that prosthetic stair walking differs from biological (Torburn et al., 1994). But, their results showed that the dynamic response did not improve stair walking. They conclude that the reason could be that the individuals do not roll the forefoot over in the same manner as in e.g. jogging. This can be seen in the decrease in step length which restricts body weight from loading the energy storing forefoot. The shorter step length requires an increased dorsiflexion when ascending, mostly in the early stance. The limitation in the prostheses also causes a limited plantarflexion at the end of the stance phase. This is compensated by the amputees with larger anterior pelvic tilt (hip movement). Going down the DER prostheses where dorsiflexed while a biological foot is plantarflexed during heel down. But during the forward movement the flexion increased faster with a biological foot giving a larger dorsiflexion than the prosthetic. This is compensated by the amputees by less knee flexation and larger flexation in the hip.

3 Classification of stair walking

Pressure sensors have been used to characterize stair climbing and descending (Wervey et al., 1997). In comparison to level walking the stair climbing peak plantar pressures showed significant increase at the lateral foot sensors and significant decrease at all other locations. While at down stair there was a significant increased rate of pressure change in the frontal part. This work was done to understand how different particular walking activities influence the force distribution and may be useful in preventing injury to the foot.

A related area is classification of stair and level walking for monitoring daily activities especially by disabled people. Coley et al. attached a gyroscope to the shank and with wavelet transformation they were able to detect both toe-off and heel-strike (Coley et al., 2005). Furthermore, in stair descent as well as level walking there is a forward rotation of the shank about the ankle during stance while for ascent a backward rotation also is seen during foot-flat. The sign of the gyroscopic data was used to separate stair ascending from other walking conditions. The system was used on elderly hospitalized as well as healthy people in non-lab bounded surroundings. The results show that the two types of walking could be correctly classified in more than 97 percent of the cases.

With one accelerometer on each hip and ankle Kern and Schiele correctly estimated 84 percent ascending and 80 percent descending on one person. The estimator was a Bayes classifier using the mean and variance from a data window (Kern & Schiele, 2003).

Sekine et al. used a tri-axial accelerometer attached to the waist. With the wavelet transformation they were able to classify level, up and down stair walking (Sekine et al., 1998). The three types of walking patterns were categorized by comparing powers of wavelet coefficients in the vertical direction in the anterior-posterior direction. This was shown to be effective for young people (99 percent correct classification) but not for elderly people since gait changes with age. This is especially significant in lower heel down acceleration and also the shuffle which elderly do while walking. Therefore they included variance estimation and a larger difference between walking cases could be seen (Sekine et al., 2002). This was especially important looking at older people, as well as with Parkinson decease.

We propose the use of kinematical sensors attached to the shoe sole or orthosis sole. The features of using kinematical sensors are

- Foot-to-ground angle can be estimated both during stance and swing.
- The sensors do not wear out since the physical contact is limited.
- Less sensitive than pressure sensors to quality of stance phase e.g. surface roughness, balance of wearer or sensitivity in foot/skin.

By combining the signals from gyro and acceleration sensors the foot motion can be estimated and be used for classification of gait characteristics.

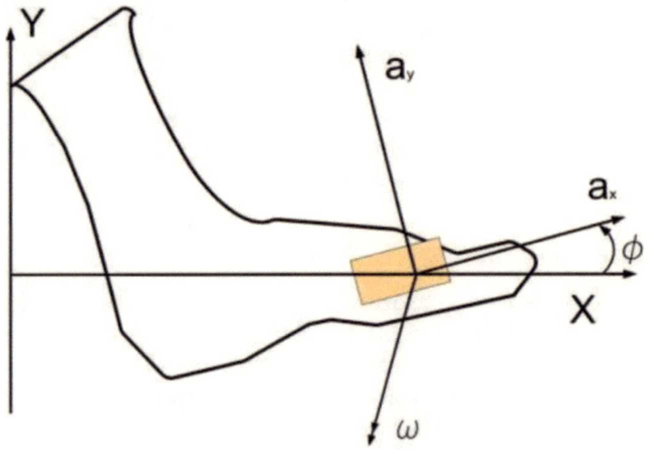

Fig. 1. Sensor setup: a gyroscope measuring ω and a two dimensional accelerometer a_x , a_y. The foot moves in the global coordinate system of X, Y.

4 Methods

The foot movement was estimated by mounting a sensor system close to the toe as shown in Fig.1. The sensor system consists of one gyroscope measuring the angular velocity, ω and accelerometers measuring a_x and a_y.

The sensors measure in a moving frame and the signals can be rotated to the fixed frame as

$$\begin{aligned} a_X &= a_x \cos\phi - a_y \sin\phi \\ a_Y &= a_x \sin\phi + a_y \cos\phi - g \end{aligned} \quad (1)$$

4.1Stance estimation

In the stationary case when the foot is at inclination ϕ the accelerometers measures are a_x = g sin ϕ and a_y = g cos ϕ respectively and where g is the gravitational constant. The resulting angle is then

$$\phi = \arctan \frac{a_x}{a_y} \quad (2)$$

Thus the foot-to-ground angle is defined positive for foot dorsi flexion. Since the foot is stationary during stance the angle ϕ can be estimated using the accelerometers using eq(2). The placement guarantees that the sensors are stationary during stance for all possible gait situations, even in stairs.

During swing, however, the accelerometers do not only measure the gravitational acceleration but also the acceleration of the foot. Therefore eq.(2) cannot be used for estimation of ϕ during swing. Instead, integration of the gyro signal$\omega = d\phi/dt$ can be used as an estimate.

A complete foot movement estimator should include a switching procedure between stance and swing phases.

A low pass filtered gyro signal is used to switch between the two phases:

$$\Omega_k = \frac{1}{7}\sum_{n=-3}^{3} |\omega_{k+n}| \tag{3}$$

The instance estimation motivates a symmetric low pass filter and ω is zero during stance. The detector uses $|\omega|$ since during change of rotational directional or linear movement during stair walking ω would be zero without being at stance. The transitions between the gait phases are detected by the following conditions:

- Stance: ground estimation phase. The whole foot or only the frontal part is stationary. Stance starts at sample k_{FD} when W consecutive samples of Ω are limited as

$$\begin{aligned} \Omega_k &\le \gamma_s, k = k_i, \ldots, k_{i-1+W} \\ k_{FD} &= \min_i k_i \end{aligned} \tag{4}$$

  The threshold $\gamma_{S,}$ is chosen to be larger than the noise level at stance.
- Transitions to Swing starts with heel lift which occurs at sample k_{HL} when the condition (4) no longer is fulfilled.

Thus, the mean angle during stance is

$$\bar{\phi} = \frac{1}{M}\sum_{k=Tstart-M}^{Tstart-1} \arctan\frac{a_{x,k}}{a_{y,k}} \tag{5}$$

Where M=kHL-kFD and T_{start} is the start of the swing phase.

4.2 Swing estimation

At sample k and discrete time h swing integration of the gyro signal is

$$\hat{\phi}_{k+1} = \hat{\phi}_k + \omega_k h, \qquad k = T_{start}, \ldots, T_{end} \tag{6}$$

where $\hat{\phi}_{Tstart} = \bar{\phi}_{Before}$ angle at stance before swing starts from eq(5). But, to reduce the inherent bias effect, (Sabatini et al. 2005) proposed two adjustments: *i*) assuming that a step angle is almost same at the start and end the difference can be assumed to be cause by an equal noise effect. *ii*) The angle is to be adjusted during each stance using the accelerometers. A modified estimation, includes ground inclination variations between stance instances

$$\phi_k = \hat{\phi}_k \frac{T-k}{T} + \bar{\phi}_{After}\frac{k}{T}, \qquad k = T_{start}, \ldots, T_{end} \tag{7}$$

and where $\bar{\phi}_{After}$ is angle at the stance phase directly after swing and $T=T_{end}-T_{start}+1$ is the swing time.

From eq.(1) a_X , a_Y can be estimated and since the velocity is zero at stance, can by integration, v_X and v_Y be estimated as

$$\begin{aligned} \hat{v}_{X,k+1} &= \hat{v}_{X,k} + a_{X,k}h \\ \hat{v}_{Y,k+1} &= \hat{v}_{Y,k} + a_{Y,k}h \end{aligned} \tag{8}$$

which also is compensated for bias effect as

$$v_{X,k} = \frac{T-k}{T}\hat{v}_{X,k} \tag{9}$$

$$v_{Y,k} = \frac{T-k}{T}\hat{v}_{Y,k}$$

Finally is the swing position relative the stance in the X and Y direction found with an integration of the velocity

$$y_{k+1} = y_k + v_{Y,k}h \tag{10}$$

$$x_{k+1} = x_k + v_{X,k}h$$

4.4 Classification of a step

Non gait swings are discriminated by requiring the forward movement to be large than the foot length. To further reduce the influence of estimation error the resulting inclinations was used for classification. Thus, the resulting classification variable, when x_T>0.2m is

$$\mathrm{Q_T} = \frac{\mathrm{y_T}}{\mathrm{x_T}} \tag{11}$$

Classification of stair up stair up, horizontal and stair down is then made by thresholding

Up: $\gamma_U < Q_T$
Horizontal: $\gamma_D < Q_T < \gamma_U$
Down: $Q_T < \gamma_D$

4.5 Classification during swing

It would be interesting to investigate if it is possible to classify a step while it is taken. If so, it would open the possibility for online adjustment of controllable orthoses and prostheses. At the end of forward swing the largest part of vertical motion also is completed. Using the forward acceleration sensor this *swing end* can be detected. First, a time instant just before the forward acceleration is passing a lower threshold γ_L

$$\mathrm{k_L} = \min_k \arg\{a_x(k) < -\gamma_L\} \tag{12}$$

Then the time τ in swing, corresponds to the first proceeding acceleration maximum is calculated as

$$\tau = \min_k \arg\{a_x(k) > a_x(k \pm 1)\} \tag{13}$$

The foot angle can then be estimated by eq.(5-7) by replacing T with τ and assigning $\overline{\phi}_{After} = \overline{\phi}_{Before}$. In the same way the velocities $v_{X,\tau}$ and $v_{Y,\tau}$ and the positions $x_{\square}$ and $y_{\square}$ are estimated from eq.(8-9) and eq.(10) respectively. Thus, the resulting classification variable, when $x_{\square}$>0.2m is

$$Q_\tau = \frac{y_\tau}{x_\tau} \tag{14}$$

Classification of is also here made by thresholding.

4.6 Measurement system

The sensor system consists of one gyroscope *Murata ENC-03J* measuring the angular velocity, ω and a two dimensional accelerometer *ADXL 311* measuring a_x and a_y. Signals are sampled at 50 Hz with 10 bit AD converters with a low cost, off the shelf, 40 MHz PIC18F microprocessor. The signals are smoothed by a first order analog low-pass filter with cut-off frequency of 50 Hz. Furthermore, to analyze the system performance on-line, a *Bluetooth* unit enables logging of data to a PC.

4.7 Experiments

The evaluation was performed by letting four healthy men walk in a corridor and up and down stairs in the lab building at self selected speeds. In average each person walked 40 steps in the lab corridor. When walking in the stairs only one foot was put on each staircase. Each staircase was 17cm high and 31cm deep. The stair consisted of 10 staircases where only one foot was placed per staircase. Halting was not considered in this study. Each person walked six stairs up and six down. In between the stairs was a small platform resulting in one or two horizontal steps. Measurements were done with and without wearing a foot-ankle orthosis. Walking down stairs with an orthosis this foot was partly put in front of the staircase thereby avoiding the limitation which the ankle stiffness causes.

5 Results

The test showed several occurrences where the using |ω| avoids erroneous stance starts where the gyro signal is zero during several samples. At high speed walking though, it was hard to detect stance phases. Decreasing the window size *W*makes it easier to detect stance but resulting in poor ground angle estimations.

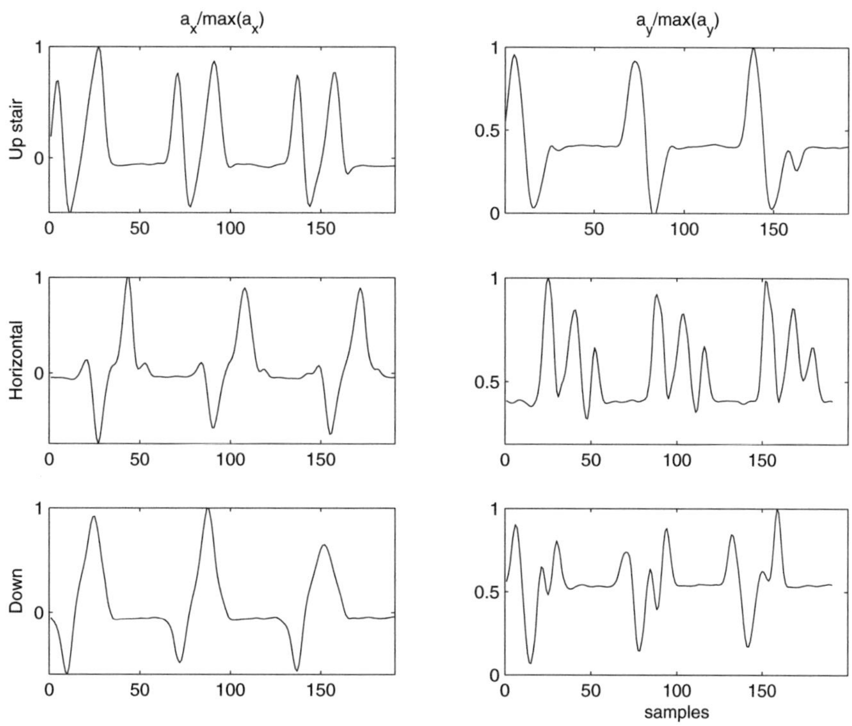

Fig. 2. Sensor signals a_x *and* a_y at different gait conditions.

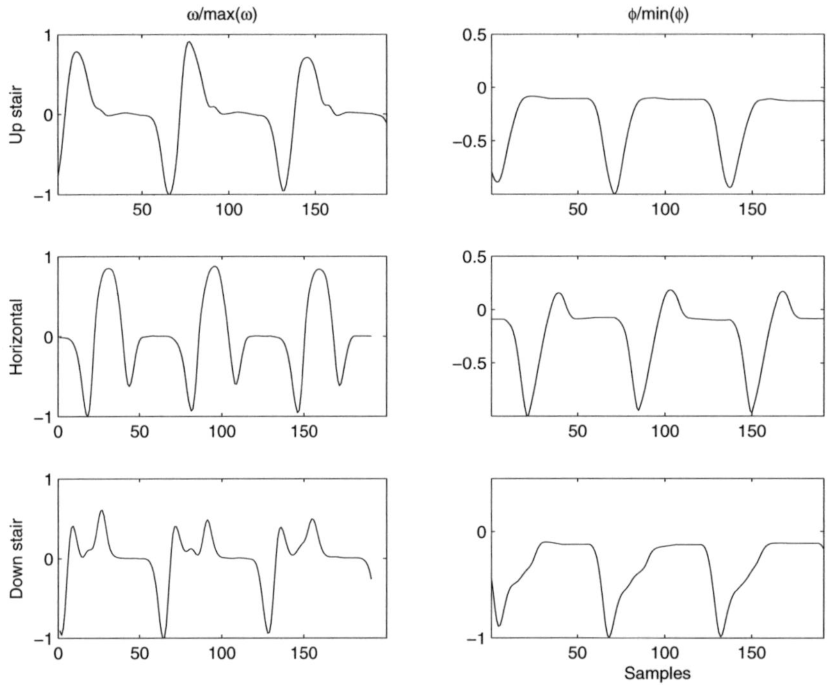

Fig. 3. Gyro signals and estimated foot-to-ground angle at different gait conditions.

From the angle estimation, as shown in Fig. 3 (Horizontal) it can be observed that the angle reaches its minimum when the heel lift phase is completed. This is followed by a calf pendulum movement forward in the swing phase which ends when the angle is maximal. The heel touches ground and the foot blade is brought down. The foot lift is similar for stair walking. During ascending is no maximum observed since the foot mostly is brought down with the toes first. Often only the frontal part is in contact with the staircase.

At descending the foot is not largely flexed since the foot forward motion brings clears the toe from ground. Here it can also be seen that the foot is adjusted so that the toe is brought down first. The time for first foot contact to ground is approximately the same for ascending and descending. The lack of heel down is seen as reduced variations at foot down.

Walking with orthoses no larger differences appear in the sensor data for the horizontal case. At ascending is the heel or at least the whole foot down. The reason why there are no more differences support the previous studies that knee and hip compensate for ankle stiffness. But at descending the foot is clearly brought down with the heel first. At stance end the foot rolls over the staircase edge and the frontal part moves down at foot lift. Only a small lift is needed to clear from the stair and start the downward motion. This rolling is partly caused by the ankle stiffness and makes the stance phase period a bit shorter.

The estimation of a_Y shows in Fig 4. a large increase when ascending to lift the foot up to next staircase. In the same way is a large descending causing a large decrease. During horizontal walk the foot accelerates upward during lift and then down during the initial forward swing. At the last part of the swing it again accelerates upwards preparing for heel down. Comparing the horizontal accelerations a_X reveal no large differences between different gait conditions and are therefore omitted.

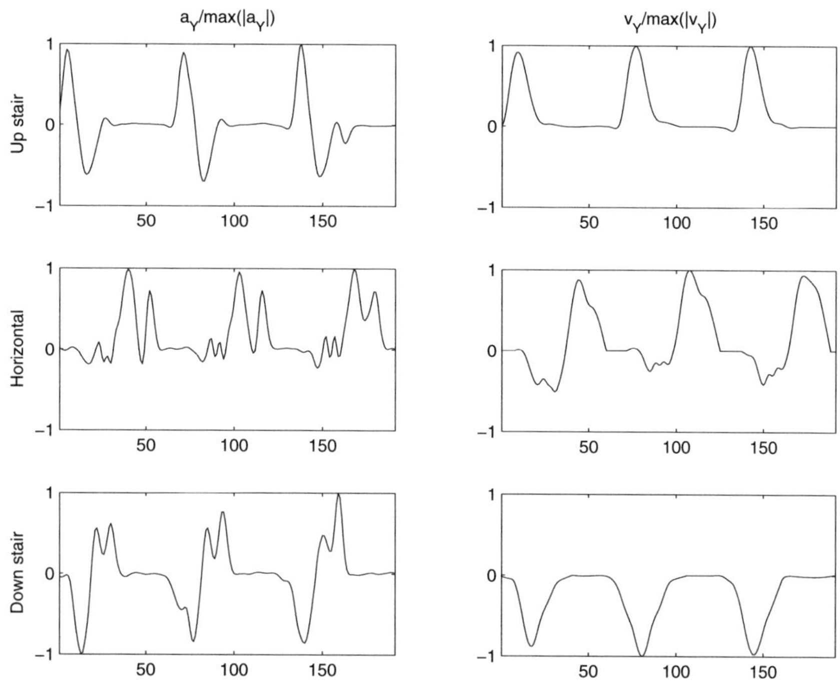

Fig. 4. Estimated vertical acceleration a_Y and velocity, v_Y at different gait conditions.

For the same reason v_X is not shown. But in the vertical velocity, as shown in Fig. 4, are the differences in gait conditions even more apparent. The positioning of the sensor causes a velocity variation which at a first glance may as if the foot was moving downwards. But this is only the sensor (due to a rounded front foot) and since the final position is of interest this is assumed to not cause any misclassifications.

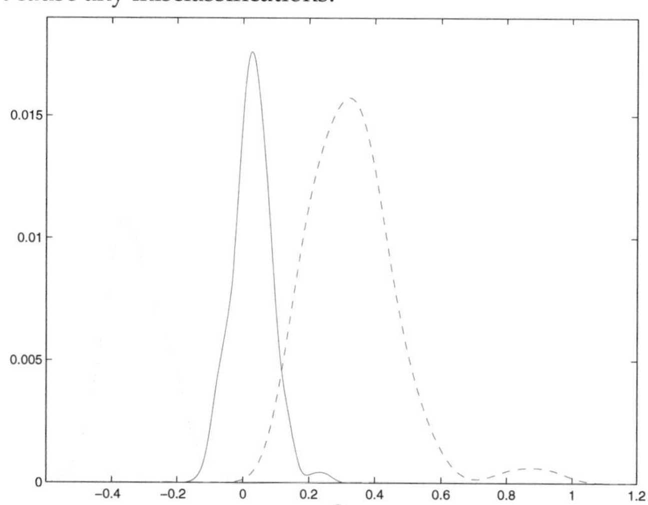

Fig. 5. Histogram of the classification quotient QT plotted using the complete step walking up-stair (red --), horizontal (blue solid) and down stair (green dotted).

In Fig. 5 is the histogram of the classification quotient Q_T plotted. The averages differ distinctly. The deviation at horizontal walk is not large. It was noted that some of the deviations were caused by rotations and sliding of the feet when walking in curves, especially at the platforms in the stairs. Possible boundaries for a Bayesian classifier and their probabilities are

Ascending : $P(Q_T > 0.12 \mid \text{Ascending}) = 96\%$
Horizontal: $P(-0.12 < Q_T < 0.12 \mid \text{Horizontal}) = 92\%$
Descending: $P(Q_T < -0.12 \mid \text{Descending}) = 93\%$

$P(Q>\gamma \mid C)$ denotes the probability of $Q>\gamma$ given class C.

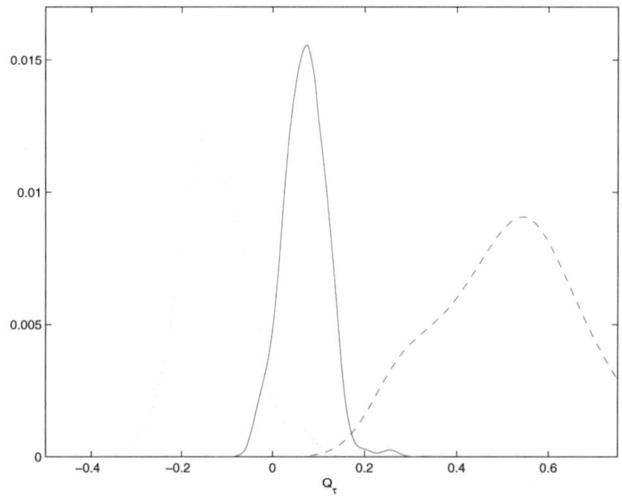

Fig.6. Histogram of the classification quotient Qt when estimating during swing step walking up-stair (red --), horizontal (blue solid) and down stair (green dotted).

Also when an estimation of motion during swing is used the different gait conditions can be separated.

Possible classification boundaries and probabilities are

Ascending: $P(Q_\tau > 0.17 \mid \text{Ascending}) = 99\%$
Horizontal: $P(-0.02 < Q_\tau < 0.17 \mid \text{Horizontal}) = 94\%$
Descending: $P(Q_\tau < -0.02 \mid \text{Descending}) = 91\%$

The estimation instance τ of using an early detection is 45 % descending, 43% horizontal and 65% at ascending of the total swing time *T*. Available control time is approximately 30% of *T* if the adjustment is to be done before the foot hits ground.

Tests were also done without using bias compensation (7) and (9). These results showed, at descending the deviation from average is too large to be used for classification. This motivates the use of a bias compensating weight. It is interesting to notice that the classification improves for ascending and horizontal gait when classifying during swing is used rather than waiting for the complete step. The bias compensator in these cases seems appropriate.

6 Discussion

This chapter describes a compact portable measuring system which both can be used for analysing able-bodied as well as foot orthosis control. Mounting the sensors on the frontal part of the foot enables detection of stance phase from the gyro signal in stair walking. By sensor fusion a model-free gait classifier be can used. Also an on-line motion estimator makes classifying during swing possible.

7 Future research

Test on able bodied people have shown promising results. Sekine et al. recognized that people with malfunctioning lower extremities are harder to classify. Further studies on patients should be done to show if orthotic walk is distinct. Moreover, a complete system has to include classification of gait or no gait conditions. Finally has the usability for control to be developed.

8 Reference

Andriacchi, T.P.; Andersson, G.B.; Fermier, R.W.; Stern, D. & and Galante J.O. (1980). A study of lower-limb mechanics during stair-climbing. *The Journal of Bone and Joint Surgery*, 62-A(5), pp. 749-757.

Blaya, J. & Herr, H. (2004). Adaptive control of a variable-impedance ankle-foot orthosis to assist drop-foot gait. *IEEE Transactions on neural systems and rehabilitation engineering*, 12(12), pp. 24-31.

Coley, Brian; Najafi, Bijan; Paraschiv-Ionescu, Anisoara & Kamiar, Aminian (2005). Stair climbing detection during daily physical activity using a miniature gyroscope. *Gait and Posture*, 22(4), pp. 287-294.

Kern, Nicky & Schiele, Bernt (2003). Multi-sensor activity context detection for wearable computing. *In proceedings of European Symposium on Ambient Intelligence*, Eindhoven, The Netherlands, November 2003.

McFayden, B.J. & Winter D.A.(1988). An integrated biomechnical analysis of normal stair ascent and descent. *Journal of Biomechanics*, 21(9), pp 733-744.

Morris, S.J. & Paradiso, J.A. (2002) Shoe-integrated sensor system for wireless gait analysis and real-time feedback. *Proceedings of the second Joint EMBS/BMES Conference*, pp. 2468--2469.

Nahorniak, Maureen T.; GortonIII, George E.; Ganotti, Mary E. & Masso, Peter D. (1999). Kinematic compensations as children reciprocally ascend and descend stairs with unilateral and bilateral solid afos. *Gait and Posture*, (9), pp. 199--206.

Pappas, P.; M.,P.;, Keller, T.; Dietz, V. & M.M. (2001). A reliable gait phase detection system. *IEEE Transactions on Neural Systems and Rehabiltitation Engineering*. 9(2), pp. 113-125.

Powers, C. & Boyd, L. (1997). Stair ambulation in persons with trantibial amputation: An analysis of the seattle lightfoot. *Journal of Rehabilitation Research and Development*, 34(1), pp9--18.

Sabatini, A.; Martelloni, C.; Scapatello, S. & Cavallo Filippo. Assessment of walking features from foot inertial sensing.*IEEE Transactions on biomedical engineering*, 52 (3):1--9, 2005.

Schmaltz, Thomas; Blumentritt, Siegmar & Marx, Björn (2007). Biomechanical Analysis of stair ambulation in lower limb amputees. Gait & Posture, (25), pp. 267-278.

Sekine, Masaki; Tamura, Toshiyo; Ogawa, Mitsuhiro; Togawa, Tatsuo & Yasuhiro, Fukui (1998). Classification of acceleration waveform in a continuous walking record.

Proceedings of the 20th Annual international Conf. of the IEEE Engineering in Medicine and Biology Society, 20(3), pp. 1523-1526.

Sekine, Masaki; Tamura, Toshiyo; Akay, Metin; Fujimoto, Toshiro; Togawa, Tatsuo & Yasuhiro, Fukui (2002). Discrimination of walking patterns using wavelet-based analysis. *IEEE Transactions on neural systems and rehabilitation engineering*, 10(3), pp. 188-196.

Svensson, Wolfgang & Holmberg, Ulf, (2006). An autonomous control system for a prosthetic foot ankle. *The 4th IFAC-Symposium on Mechatronic Systems*. Heidelberg, Germany, pp. 856-861, 2006.

Thomas, Susan S.; Buckon, Cathleen E.; Jakobson-Huston, Sabrina; Sussman, Michael D. & Aiona, Michale D. (2002). Stair locomotion in children with spastic hemiplegia: the impact of three different ankle foot orthosis (afos) configurations. *Gait and Posture*, (16), pp. 180--187.

Torburn, L.; Schweiger, G.; Perry, J. & Powers, C. (1994). Below-knee amputee gait in stair ambulation. *Clinical Orthopeadics and Related Research* (303), pp. 185-192.

Veltink, P.; Slycke, P.; Hemsens, J.; Buschman, R.; Bulstra, G. & Hermens, H. (2003). Three dimensional inertial sensing of foot movement for automatic tuning of a two-channel implantable drop foot simulator. *Medical Engineering and Physics*, Vol. 25, pp. 21-28.

Wervey, Roy A.; Harris, Gerald F. & Wertch, Jaqueline, J.(1997). Plantar pressure characteristics during stair climbing and descent. *Proceedings 19th International conference IEE/EMBS*, pages 1746--1748.

Yack, J.; Nielsen, D. & Shurr, D. (1999). Kinetic patterns during stair ascent in patients with transtibial amputations using three different prostheses. *Journal of Prosthetics and Orthotics*, 11(3), pp. 57-62.

The ALLADIN Diagnostic Device: An Innovative Platform for Assessing Post-Stroke Functional Recovery

Stefano Mazzoleni[1], Jo Van Vaerenbergh[2], Andras Toth[3], Marko Munih[4], Eugenio Guglielmelli[5], Paolo Dario[1]
[1] ARTS Lab, Scuola Superiore Sant'Anna, Pisa, Italy
[2] Arteveldehogeschool, Gent, Belgium
[3] Department of Manufacturing Engineering, Budapest University of Technology and Economics, Budapest, Hungary
[4] Laboratory of Robotics and Biomedical Engineering, Faculty of Electrical Engineering, University of Ljubljana, Ljubljana, Slovenia
[5] Laboratory of Biomedical Robotics & EMC, Campus Bio-Medico University, Rome, Italy

1. Introduction

Each year 920,000 new stroke cases are reported in Europe, and of that number more than 100,000 benefit from comprehensive inpatient rehabilitation. Transcranial magnetic stimulation, computed tomography, positron emission tomography (PET), functional magnetic resonance imaging (fMRI), electroencephalography (EEG), electromyography (EMG) and evoked potentials all have shown that cortical reorganisation after stroke exists, however it remains poorly understood which complex regulating system hides behind functional restoration.

Many years ago, robots and mechatronics technology were successfully introduced (Aisen, 1997; Reinkensmeyer, 2000) to support and quantify functional recovery (Krebs, 1998). However, the ability of classifying stroke patients according to a specific recovery profile is scarcely out of the egg.

As the emphasis in stroke rehabilitation is on the improvement of functional performance, an ideal measuring tool should use Activities of Daily Living (ADL) tasks as principle for its quantitative measurements. ADL tasks such as "Drinking a glass of water", "Picking up a spoon", "Turning a key", "Lifting a bag", "Reaching for a bottle" and "Bringing a bottle to the opposite side" are well described and emphasized in textbooks for physical and occupational therapists (Bobath, 1978; Brunnstrom, 1970; Carr, 1998; Perfetti, 1997).

An improved execution of these tasks is depending on changing neural control parameters and in line with important functional milestones that stroke patients acquire during recovery. The basic assumption inspiring this research work is that the initiation of goal intended movements has some of the functional properties as performing the task (Clark, 2004; Dechent, 2004; Ehrsson, 2003; Jackson, 2003; Johnson-Frey, 2004; Kilner, 2004; Lehericy, 2004; Wolpert, 2001). The focused interest in the very first goal directed muscle contractions after stroke motivated an isometric approach for post-stroke functional assessment. Till now this knowledge has never been implemented in a measuring instrument; this is the ultimate goal of the effort being carried out by a multidisciplinary team of European researchers whose achievements so far are partly reported in this chapter.

2. Background

Nevertheless the existence of a vast number of studies dealing with brain reorganization and recovery, it was never investigated whether information derived from the very first, nearly invisible goal intended movements could conceal information about future functional performance and brain reorganization. Considering these very weak contractions as loose building blocks of a movement initiation pattern on their way for a meaningful blend, an acceptable idea might be that during recovery these blocks move from a disorganized to an organized status. An attractive hypothesis is that this so called organized status is reached far before recovery becomes obvious and contains information on the remaining internal sensory motor representation of a particular task (Buchanan, 1996; Dewald, 1995; Koo, 2003).
This is acceptable because it takes only the early start of the global movement into consideration and might be conceptualized as the fingerprint for a movement execution. However an organized status does not necessary stand for good recovery, it only tell something about how stable a reached condition is, it can be either good or bad, unless we know what an organized status means for able bodied people (Sejnowski, 1998; Wolpert, 2001). The good news is that with this approach a condition shortly after a stroke can be compared with a condition also present in normal controls.
To test the hypothesis that precocity of sensory motor reorganisation in functional movement initiation after stroke is demonstrable far before a complete movement becomes possible, a special device was developed for the analysis of movement onset of the six earlier described routine ADL tasks.

3. The ALLADIN system

A diagnostic platform using an isometric approach for recording forces and torques from the whole body during the movement imagination and initiation of ADL tasks was designed and developed. This methodology has never been implemented so far: it represents an original contribution in the domain of functional assessment in neurorehabilitation.
The following paragraphs presents the clinical requirements, the functional specifications, the design methodology of the Alladin Diagnostic Device (ADD) and the Alladin software: the system reveals great potentials as a platform for clinical practice and as a tool for research in Neuroscience.

3.1 Clinical requirements

An interactive design process involved rehabilitation specialists and engineers toward the definition of specifications for an innovative diagnostic device. According to the state-of-the-art in the domain of Neuroscience and to the above mentioned specifications, the novel platform had to meet the following basic requirements:

- able to record forces/torques (F/T) data from the thumb, index finger and middle finger, from the arm, the trunk, the seat, from the whole foot and, separately, from the big-toe from a patient seated on a standard wheelchair. The measurement input ranges have been derived partly on the basis of existing references about typical data on human subjects (Mathiowetz, 1985; Deutsch, 2004; Bozec, 1997; Walsh, 1996) and partly on the basis of preliminary measurements;

- easy and quick to adjust for different anthropometrical characteristics of the population;
- to be used on both the right and the left body side;
- requiring a minimum of physical effort and time to the operator;
- able to record measurements in different postures;
- to be a modular system.

3.2 Functional specifications

The ADD is capable of measuring isometric F/T trajectories during the imagination and initiation of the selected ADL tasks. Stroke patients have been invited to perform six different ADL tasks according to a protocol which will be described in paragraph 3.4. The isometric F/T patterns have been simultaneously measured by 6-axis F/T sensors at different body segments during the imagination and initiation of each ADL task. The main objective of the isometric F/T measurements is to obtain quantitative evidence for recovery from stroke during rehabilitation.

Every isometric measurement is used to determine the actual status of the patient. Therefore, it was necessary to measure a large number of patients with the same device and in the same anatomical starting position. This assured a high reproducibility during the entire period of data acquisition in clinical trials. The data acquisition system has recorded isometric F/T data from:

- the trunk (at the patient's back),
- the lower trunk (at the patient's fundament),
- the impaired lower arm,
- the impaired foot and toe,
- the impaired middle finger, index finger and thumb.

ADL tasks to be performed during isometric F/T measurements are listed in the following sequence, together with the corresponding object:

1. *Drinking a glass (no reaching)*: the arm is placed close to the body, close to the midline, the position of the foot is standard, the fingers of the hand are prepared for a cylindrical grasp. *Object*: glass placed close to the hand.
2. *Turning a key*: the starting position is the same as for grasping the glass. *Object*: a key in a lock located in front of the hand. The key should be oriented horizontally in the lock.
3. *Taking a spoon*: the starting position is the same as for grasping the glass. The reaching movement towards the spoon is measured. The position of the foot is standard. *Object*: a spoon is placed a bit higher than the glass and on the side of the back of the hand.
4. *Lifting a bag*: the starting position of the arm is at the side of the body, the elbow is in a natural position (slightly flexed), the position of the hand and the foot are standard, the fingers of the hand are prepared for a cylindrical grasp. *Object*: a bag placed on the ground.
5. *Reaching for a bottle*: the starting position is an almost extended arm over the midline. The starting position of the hand is the same as for drinking the glass. The position of the foot is slid backward, and the back should be leaned forward. *Object*: a bottle placed in front of the hand.
6. *Bringing the bottle to the other side*: the starting positions of the arm, hand, and the foot are the same as for reaching for a bottle. *Object*: a bottle placed in front of the affected shoulder at arm reach distance.

ADL tasks are performed during isometric F/T measurements in three different positions: position 1 covers ADL task #1, ADL task #2 and ADL task #3, position 2 is related to ADL task #4, and position 3 covers ADL task #5 and ADL task #6. The anatomical angles in position 1, position 2 and position 3 are listed in Table 1, Table 2 and Table 3 respectively, except those that are in neutral position. The above functional specifications have been included into the design methodology presented in the following section.

Articular movement	Anatomical angles (degree)
Shoulder abduction	15
Shoulder flexion	50
Shoulder internal rotation	45
Elbow flexion	35
Thumb abduction	50
Finger metacarpophalangeal flexion	15
Finger proximal interphalangeal flexion	20
Finger distal interphalangeal flexion	20
Hip flexion	90
Knee flexion	90

Table 1. The anatomical angles in position 1.

Articular movement	Anatomical angles (degree)
Shoulder abduction	5
Shoulder extension	7
Elbow flexion	12
Thumb abduction	50
Finger metacarpophalangeal flexion	15
Finger proximal interphalangeal flexion	20
Finger distal interphalangeal flexion	20
Hip flexion	90
Knee flexion	90

Table 2. The anatomical angles in position 2.

Articular movement	Anatomical angles (degree)
Shoulder flexion	100
Shoulder internal rotation	45
Elbow flexion	20
Thumb abduction	50
Finger metacarpophalangeal flexion	15
Finger proximal interphalangeal flexion	20
Finger distal interphalangeal flexion	20
Lumbar-thoracic flexion	30
Lumbar-thoracic rotation	20
Lumbar-thoracic lateral flexion	18
Hip flexion	90
Knee flexion	110
Ankle dorsiflexion	8
Toe metatarsophalangeal flexion	7

Table 3. The anatomical angles in forward reaching tasks (position 3).

3.3 Design methodology

A human-centered mechatronic design approach has been followed by starting from anthropometrical considerations and iteratively refining the design choices in a tight debate with end-users (i.e., therapists, patients). Simulations, mock-ups and early prototypes have been extensively used to obtain a direct feedback from end-users and to enable experimental preliminary tests in the real application domain.

The proposed method for isometric F/T measurements requires fixed, very stiff, anatomically standard and, at the same time, repeatable individual setting of the device for each patient in order to ensure reproducibility, reliability and good precision in the isometric measurements.

Design requirements of the platform arose from three different areas. Firstly, standardisation of the measurement, secondly safety standards, as well as medical certification requirements.

Finally, space limitations in hospitals regarding the room where the device was used and the location where the wheelchairs was stored when they are not in use, have been taken into account. Standardisation of the posture and measurement procedure assures reliability and validity to the recorded F/T measurements.

As a reference position, the user is seated on a wheelchair at height of 580 mm from the floor of the platform. The back of the user is 330 mm back from the rear side of the device. In this configuration, isometric contractions in two reference postures of the lower extremities can be performed by using the proposed platform (Figure 1). In the former, the user is seating in a neutral posture. This position is typical for the initiation of most common tasks, such as lifting or grasping an object: it is the starting position for ADL task #1, ADL task #2, ADL task #3 and ADL task #4. The latter takes into account a different posture, as the user moves the trunk forward and the feet backward. Starting from this position, other tasks, such as a forward reaching tasks, can be performed: it is the starting position for ADL task #5 and ADL task #6.

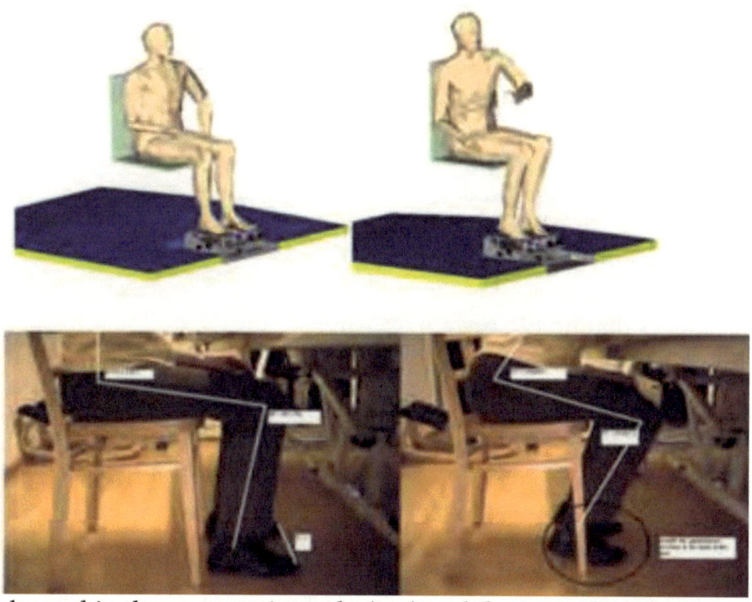

Fig. 1. CAD models used in the ergonomic study (top) and the two selected postures for the lower extremities and the feet (bottom).

The anthropometric data of the European population was studied for such design (Peebles, 1998). The ergonomic study was performed through CAD simulations (Pro/Engineer): a 3D mannequin model, created by using the Mannequin Pro tool, has been inserted into the CAD environment with the aim of (i) simulating the different postures according to the gender and percentile and (ii) fitting the design of the platform to the anatomical positions accordingly.
The results of this study enlightened the possibility of implementing a limited number of discrete settings on the platform, henceforth named S (Small), M (Medium) and L (Large), corresponding to the percentile values of the 25%-ile female (S size), the mean of the 50%-ile male and 50%-ile female (M size), and the 75%-ile male (L size).
Therefore, the device can be set without error to the above mentioned percentiles of the population, which represents a vast majority of the population. The adjustability of the device to the three discrete patient sizes was implemented.
The adjustability of the device to the three discrete patient sizes was implemented as follows. To minimize the error in the anatomical angles to be set at each of the six ADL tasks, as well as to keep the handling complexity of the diagnostic device on a tolerable level for the operating physiotherapist, the patients recruited for the isometric F/T measurements have been classified into three groups according to their height. During the measurements the appropriate size accessories and device settings must be used. The size groups are denoted by the S, M, L labels and colour codes have been used in order to make the operations easier (Table 4).

Label	Colour code	Height (h)
S	Yellow	h <1625 mm
M	Green	1625 mm < h < 1751 mm
L	Blue	h >1751 mm

Table 4. Definition of the three groups of patients sizes.

As a consequence of the mentioned approach, the set of the anatomical angles described in subsection 3.2 is fixed for any patient size. The calculated deviation from the ideal anatomical angles remains in the range ±0.5°.
The anthropometrical and ergonomic design approach, by identifying only a very limited number of adjustments required to the therapist, clearly simplified the design and the development of the overall system, presented in the following section, and represents a benefit for the therapists.

3.4 The ALLADIN diagnostic device (ADD)

The main objective of the mechatronic platform here presented is to perform valid and reliable isometric F/T measurements at stroke patients during the execution of the 6 ADL tasks. The ADD has to provide repeatable and accurate results: given this important requirement, the patients were precisely positioned to the same set of ADL positions for each measurement during the clinical trials, started in February 2005 and ended in September 2006.
The standardisation achieved both in terms of the mechanics of the device, the F/T sensor unit, the measurement control software and the unambiguous guidelines on the operation of the device have resulted in high reproducibility and comparability of the force torque measurements.

Since April 2004 a complete product design and development cycle which included the computer aided design, the development of three early prototypes and the feedback from the testing were implemented. Refinement and detailing of the conceptual design was a natural result of this cyclic process. The eight 6-axis F/T sensors are respectively installed behind the trunk, below the posterior, at the affected lower arm, at the affected thumb, index and middle finger, at the affected foot and toe (Figure 2).

They output detailed data on the ADL tasks to be performed. Table 5 shows the basic characteristics of the 6-axis F/T sensors (50M31A-I25, 67M25A-I40, 90M40A-I50, 90M40A-I50, 90M40S-I50, 90M40A-I50, 50M31A-I25; JR3 Inc., Woodland, USA). The orthogonal reference frame for the force and torque vectors is located inside the sensor. The platform has three positional settings for the patient according to the tasks to be performed. The first operational position is associated to the ADL task #1, ADL task #2 and ADL task #3, a second position is selected for the ADL task #4 task and a third for the ADL task #5 and ADL task #6. All operating instructions are presented on a screen in front of the patient. A first instruction is the video presentation of the task to be initiated by the patient; the second instruction is an invitation to "memorize the task" and then to "execute it". The measured behaviour is the combined output of 48 channels representing the x, y, z F/T data for all eight F/T sensors.

The diagnostic device includes the following main units (Figure 2):

1. Accessory storage board
2. Transit lying wheelchair
3. Monitor for the patient
4. Podium
5. Trunk Device
6. Foot Device
7. Arm Device
8. Finger Device
9. Seat Device

The Arm Device, the Finger Device and the Foot Device are shown in Figure 3. A customized software has been developed in order to allow the recording of different types of data: F/T data, clinical scales and natural language descriptions made by the physiotherapists (See subsection 3.5). Several young volunteers participated in a preliminary testing that aimed at verifying the output of the proposed isometric procedure. Altogether 250 subjects (150 hemiplegic patients and 120 normal control) were recruited during the clinical trials at the three hospitals. The centres participating in the multi-centre clinical trials were:

- Algemeen Ziekenhuis Maria Middelares Sint-Jozef Hospital (AZMMSJ), Gent, Belgium,
- Adelaide & Meath Hospital (AMNCH), Tallaght, Dublin, Ireland,
- Szent János Hospital, Budapest, Hungary.

All the three clinical trial centres obtained the approval of the relevant ethics committees. An informed consent was obtained from the subjects participating the clinical trials.

Subjects were measured and assessed twice a week during the first two months period and once a week during four consecutive months. They were seated in a special designed wheelchair and driven into an anthropometrical adaptive measuring instrument characterized by the above mentioned three discrete positions (Small, Medium and Large).

Appropriate size accessories and device settings were also used to ensure that the error in the anatomical angles is minimal, as well as to keep the handling complexity of the diagnostic device on a tolerable level for the operating physiotherapist (See the accessory storage board in Figure 2).

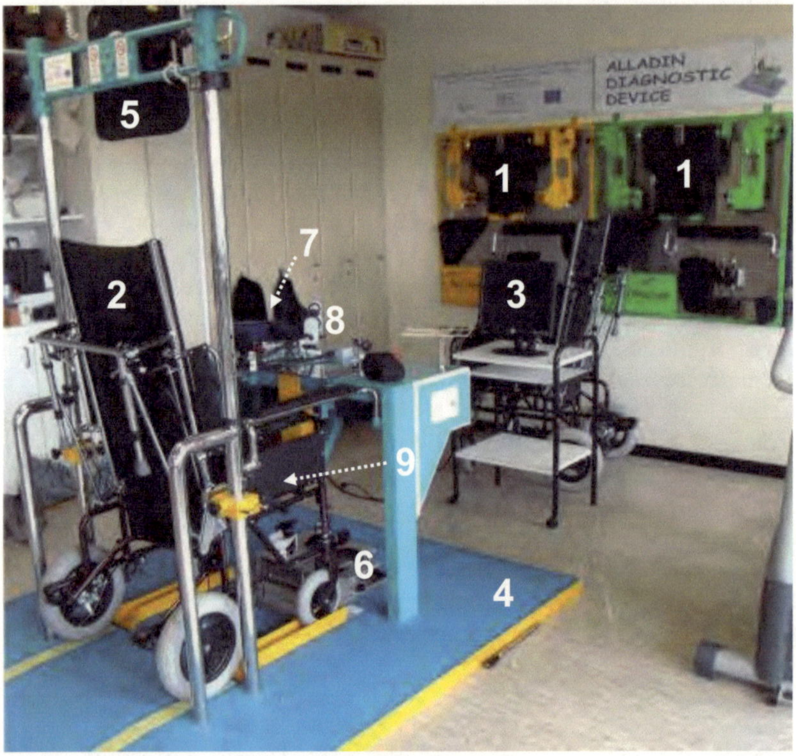

Fig. 2. The components of the Alladin diagnostic device.

Description	Quantity	Lateral forces (Fx, Fy)	Axial force (Fz)	Torques (Tx,Ty, Tz)	Dimensions
Type-H(and)	3	150 N	300 N	8 Nm	Ø 50 x 31 mm
Type-A(rm)	1	150 N	200 N	10 Nm	Ø 67 x 35 mm
Type-B(ack)	1	250 N	250 N	20 Nm	Ø 90 x 40 mm
Type-P(osterior)	1	550 N	1100 N	50 Nm	Ø 114 x 40 mm
Type-F(oot)	1	400 N	800 N	25 Nm	Ø 90 x 40 mm
Type-T(oe)	1	150 N	300 N	8 Nm	Ø 50 x 31 mm

Table 5. Basic characteristics of the 6-axis F/T sensors.

The postures chosen for the measurements represents a trade-off between a good approximation of the natural posture and the anthropometric characteristics of the subject. This choice assures sufficient conditions of repeatability to the measurements.

The clinical assessment was performed through the Fugl-Meyer Scale (Lindmark adaptation), the Motor Assessment Scale and the Stroke Impact Scale. The physiotherapists used a Portable Digital Assistant (PDA) in order to record the score for each assessment scale and patients' functional recovery.

The aim of the study is to identify if there are significant links between the recovery that occurs post stroke as measured by the diagnostic device and this recovery as measured by clinical scales and natural language descriptions. As described in section 3.2, six different ADL tasks with a varying complexity were used for F/T measurements.

The data acquisition followed a detailed protocol (Van Vaerenbergh et al., 2004). For each task, the patient watches a video showing the movement (recording #1). Secondly he is asked to mentally imagine and reproducing it with open eyes (recording #2). Finally, for three times he actually tries to perform it, exerting the forces at a comfortable level (recording #3, recording #4 and recording #5).

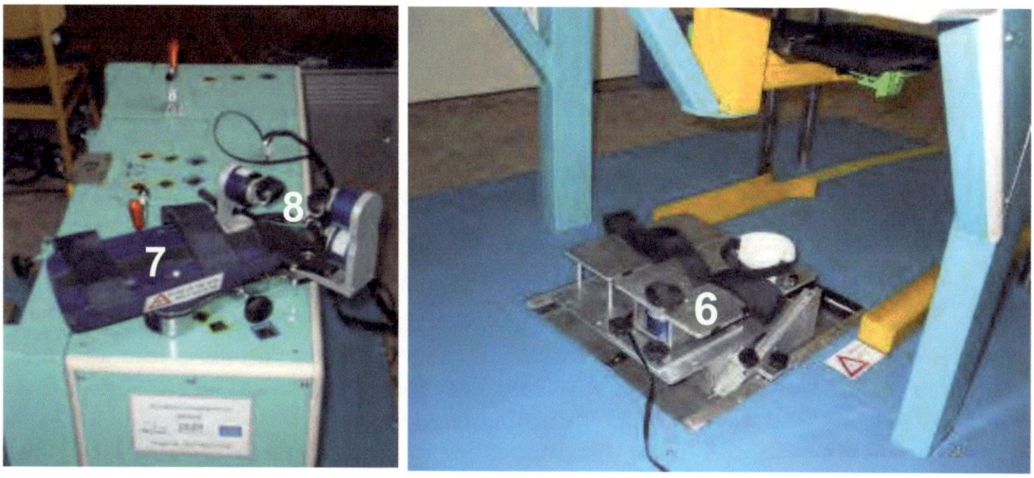

Fig. 3. Devices for measurements on the upper limbs and lower limbs. Left: the Arm Device (7) and the Finger Device (8). Right: the Foot Device (6).

3.5 The ALLADIN software

This section presents in detail the functional and technical specifications and the design approach of the software of the diagnostic device and describes the implementation of the different software modules as well as for their integration.

A general architecture of the diagnostic device software has been defined according to the functional specifications of the diagnostic device defined reported in previous section, and also taking into account the additional information provided through a close collaboration with end users (i.e., clinicians and physiotherapists) on this specific topic (Figure 4).

Specifications of the Database Module were given using the UML (Cantor, 1998) notation and diagrams in order to provide a definition of the functionality of this module which can be easily interpreted both by the software developers and by the clinicians. UML notation was also used to define the interface between the Cover Application (CA) module and the Database (DB) module. All other modules, i.e. Data acquisition (DAQ), Data viewer, Automatic Speech Recognition (ASR), were described by using simpler notations, such as flowcharts or direct presentation of the low level functions definition.

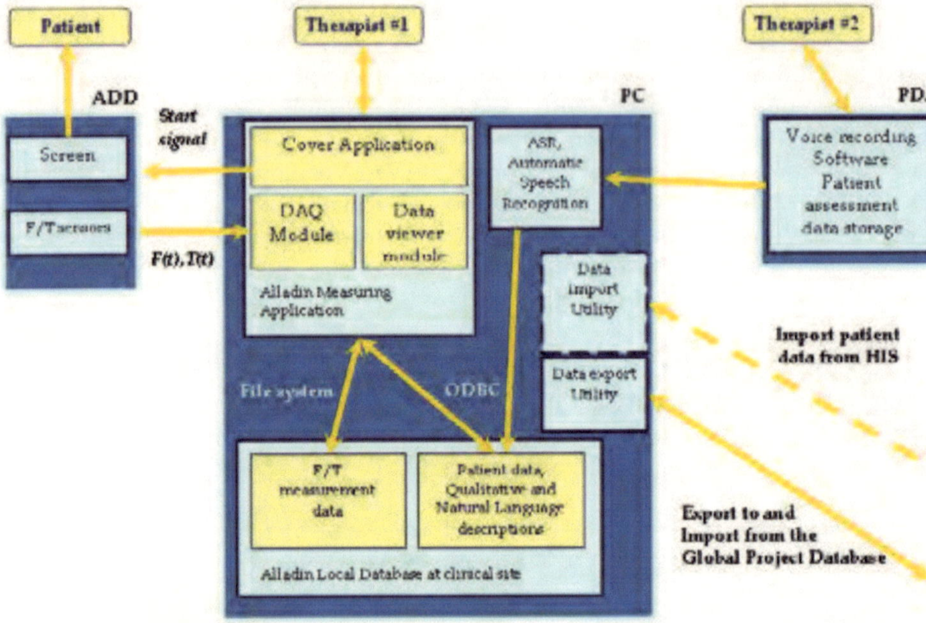

Fig. 4. The ALLADIN Software Architecture.

The software has been based on the general user requirements and specifications which have been defined in a preliminary phase. The software allows to manage all the functionalities provided by the ADD, including the recording and exchange of different kind of data between the CA module and the other modules and between the CA module and the DB. The main data to be collected and managed are:

- Patient data and case history
- Standard Outcome Measure (SOM)
- Natural language descriptions of the patient's status
- Voice records of the descriptions
- F/T measurement records of the ADL tasks

All data, after having been collected, are uploaded to the Local Database (Figure 4).

The main software requirements and specifications formed the framework for the Cover Application software design and development.

The CA was implemented using the Microsoft Visual Basic (VB) Environment Release 6.0, which allows the creation of friendly graphical user interfaces and simplifies the integration of modules developed with heterogeneous techniques. In particular it provides a means to connect the CA module with the ALLADIN database and with the other ADD modules, as for instance, the dynamic link libraries (DLLs) which implements the DAQ module and the Data Viewer Module. The DB was implemented in Microsoft Access 2000 and the other software modules were developed according to the CA module specifications in terms of I/O interfaces and functionality. The CA module allows the user to create, retrieve and modify records by queries on the patient information and clinical assessment in the DB.

The CA module was developed in order to allow the user to record the different information related to each patient and the data which come out from the measurements.

The main menu (Figure 5), offers different functionalities, such opening a patient record, starting a new session of measurements, creating a new patient record, editing and creating an user's profile, synchronizing with the global DB, system settings adjustment and remote assistance.
Four different types of users were identified (ADD physiotherapist, Natural language physiotherapist, Principal Investigator and System administrator); for each user profile an access rights policy was defined.

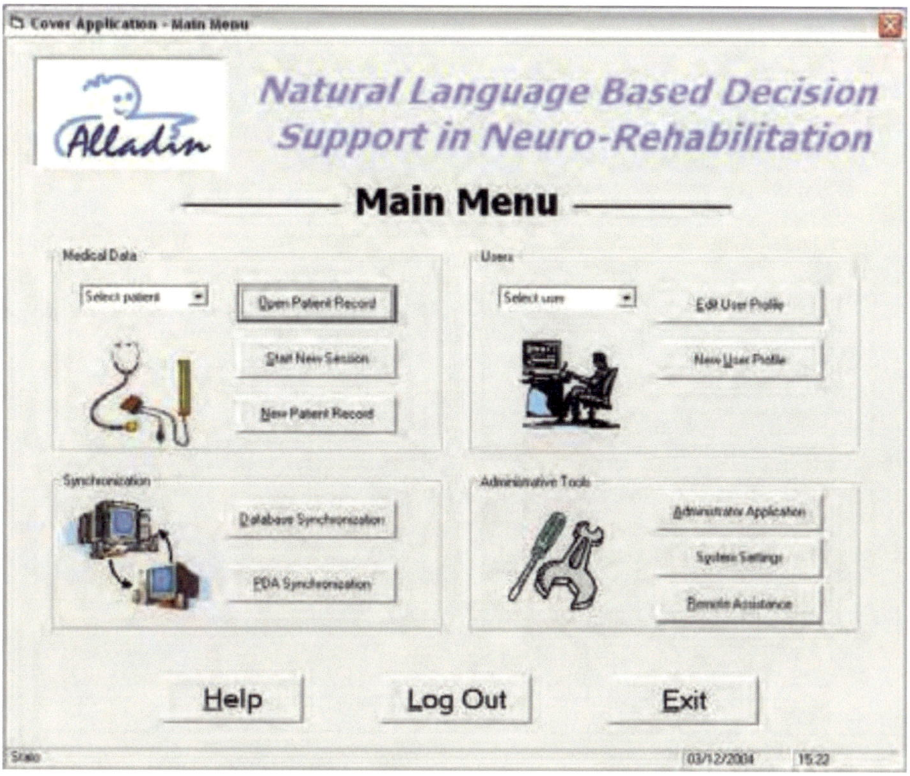

Fig. 5. The Cover Application main window.

4. Results and discussion

Some preliminary results from a normal control subject and a pathological subject are here presented. The choice of the task and the sensors is based on the preliminary results of data mining algorithms applied to the pre-processed data (Van Djick et al. 2006). Let's consider the task *"Drinking"* in a normal control (AHS-028, male, 45 years old, right dominant hand, measurement of the left side) and in a pathological subject (AHS-064, male, 43 years old, right dominant hand, right side of hemiparesis, date of stroke 15/12/2005, measurement on the right side), 25 days and 131 days following the stroke onset. The number of samples from force measurements shown in Figure 6-8 is 5400: as already stated, the sample frequency for data acquisition is 100 Hz, therefore the task lasts 5.4 seconds. Figure 6 show the force measurements from the thumb in the normal control (top plot), in the hemiplegic patient, 25 days following the stroke onset (middle plot) and 131 days following the stroke onset.

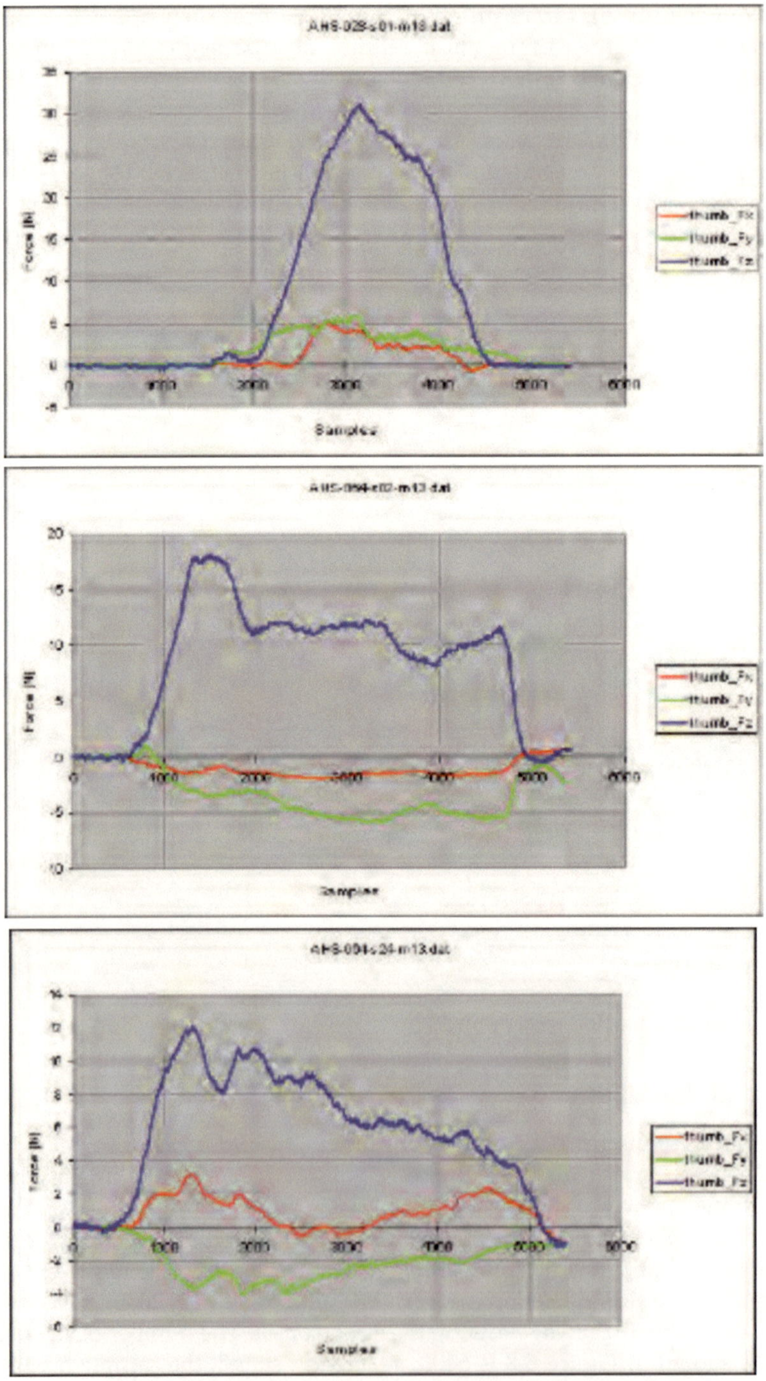

Fig. 6. Force measurements from the thumb in a normal control subject (top), in a hemiplegic patient, 25 days following the stroke event (middle) and 131 days following the stroke event (bottom) for the task *"Drinking"*.

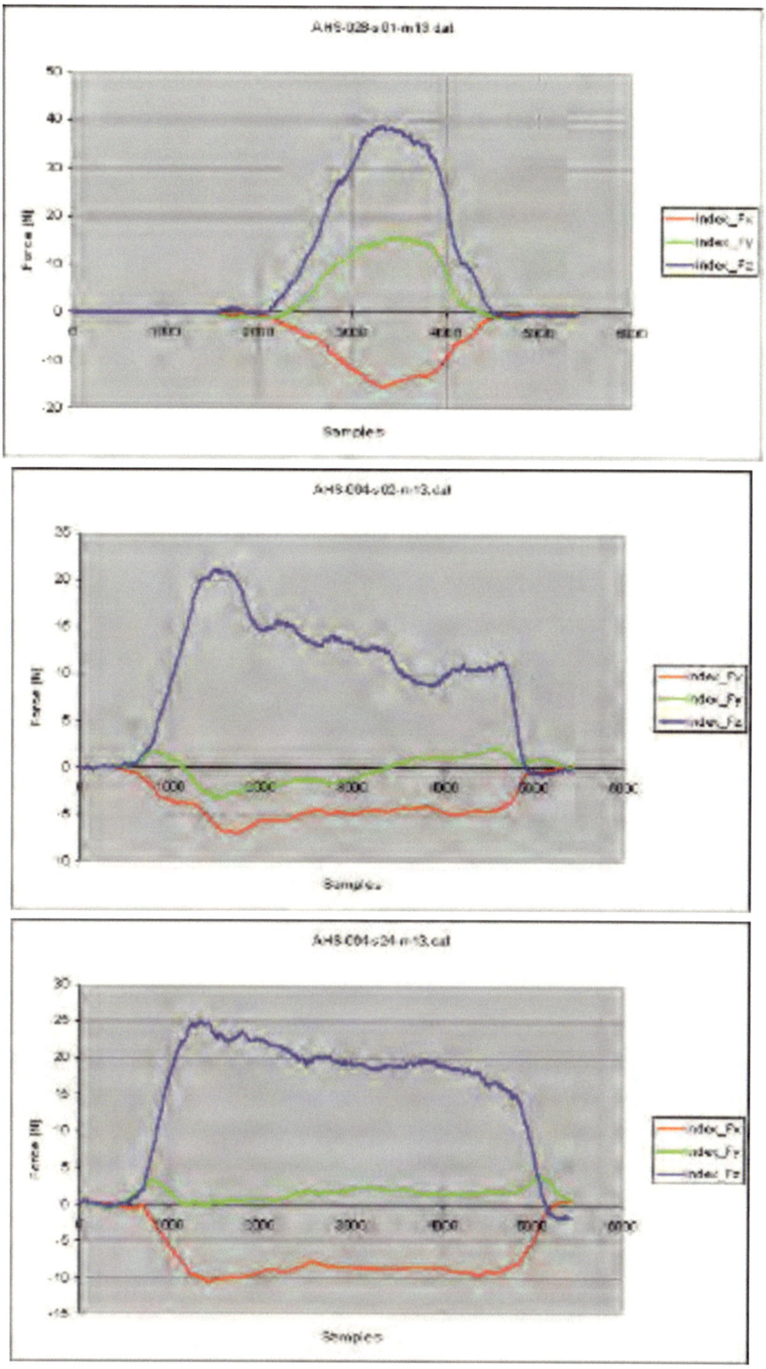

Fig. 7. Force measurements from the index finger in a normal control subject (top), in a hemiplegic patient, 25 days following the stroke event (middle) and 131 days following the stroke event (bottom) for the task *"Drinking"*.

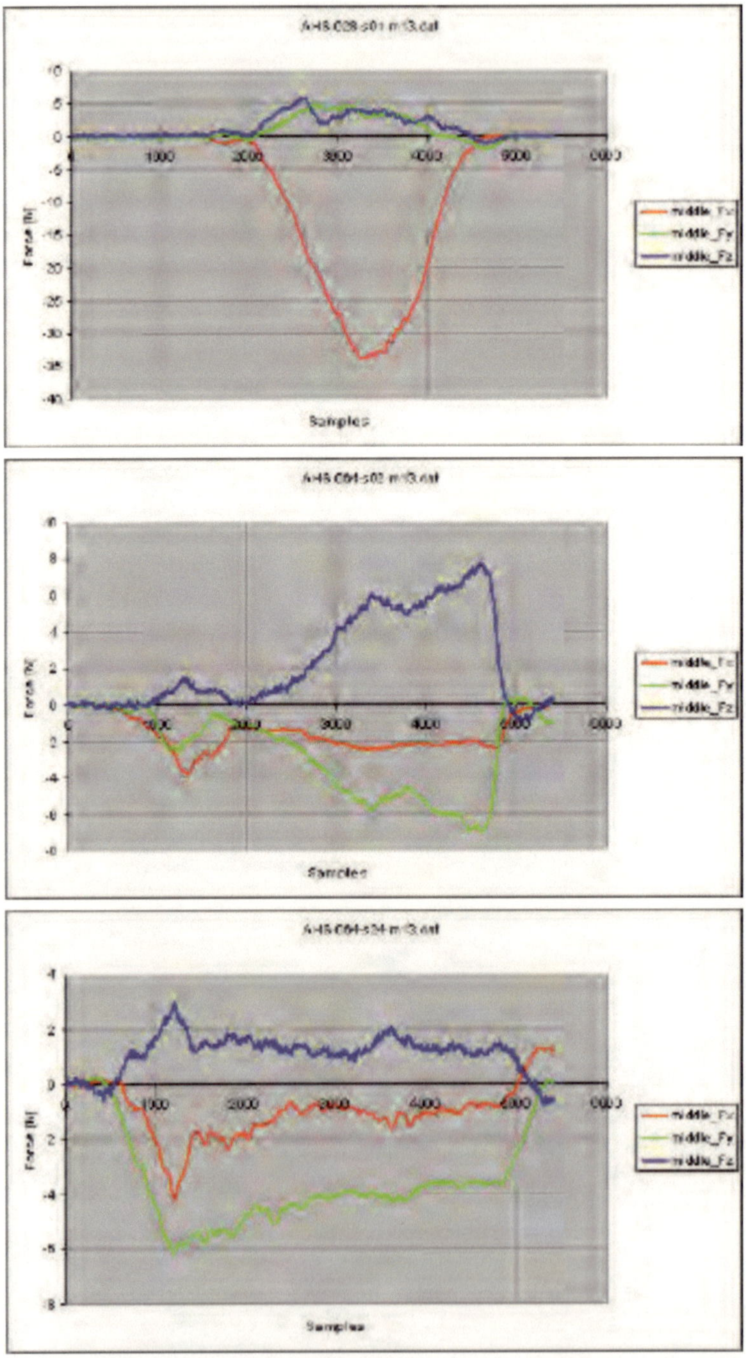

Fig. 8. Force measurements from the middle finger in a normal control subject (top), in a hemiplegic patient, 25 days following the stroke event (middle) and 131 days following the stroke event (bottom) for the task *"Drinking"*.

In the normal control, positive values in the F_x-direction can be observed. In normal circumstances, for a grasping movement, the thumb will be brought to the point where the index and the middle finger touch each other. In the diagnostic device, the thumb is fixated on the same height as the index finger. This causes a downwards movement of the thumb when the subject grasps the glass to drink. The positive values in F_y-direction means that the subject moves the thumb forwards when he positions the fingers around the glass to drink. The positive values for F_z-direction points out that the subject grasps the glass to drink.

The force measurement from the thumb recorded 25 days following the stroke onset show negative values on the x-axis: the force is directed in the opposite direction than the motor performance in the normal control subject, pointing out that the subject moves the thumb upwards to bring the glass to the mouth, instead of moving downwards. The negative values observed along the F_y-direction mean that the subject pushes the thumb forwards to bring the glass to the mouth. The positive values along the z-axis allow to conclude that the subject tries and grasps the glass to drink. The force is exerted in advance than the normal control subject and it lasts till to the end of the attempt.

The force measurement from the thumb recorded 131 days following the stroke onset show the positive values on the x-axis, same direction as the motor performance in the normal control subject, meaning that the subject moves the thumb downwards to bring the glass to the mouth, even if the force reaches the zero at about the half of the measurement, before still rising to positive values. The negative values observed along the y-axis point out that the subject pushes the thumb forwards to bring the glass to the mouth. The positive values along the z-axis mean that the subject tries and grasps the glass to drink. The force is exerted in advance than the normal control subject and it lasts till to the end of the attempt.

Figure 7 show the force measurements from the index finger in the normal control (top plot), in the hemiplegic patient, 25 days following the stroke onset (middle plot) and 131 days following the stroke onset.

In the normal control subject, the negative values along with the x-direction point out that the subject moves the index upwards to bring the glass to the mouth, while the positive values along with the y-axis points out that the subject moves the index backwards to bring the glass to the mouth. The positive values along with the z-axis means that the subject grasps the glass to drink.

The force measurement from the thumb recorded 25 days following the stroke onset show negative values along with the x-direction: the subject moves the index in the same direction as the normal control subject (upwards) to bring the glass to the mouth, even if with lower values and for a larger range of time. The positive, negative and positive values along with the y-axis points out that the subject first moves the index forwards, backwards and then forwards to bring the glass to the mouth. The positive values along with the z-axis means that the subject grasps the glass to drink, even if the exerted force doesn't shows a bell shaped form, as in the normal control subject. It shows a peak and then a falling to a lower value.

The force measurement from the thumb recorded 131 days following the stroke onset show negative values along with the x-direction: the subject moves the index in the same direction as the normal control subject (upwards) to bring the glass to the mouth, approaching the force values of the normal control subject even if for a larger range of time. The rather positive values along with the y-axis points out that the subject first moves the index forwards to bring the glass to the mouth, with a less fragmented trend, compared to the measurement recorded 25 days following the stroke onset. The positive values along with the z-axis means that the subject grasps the glass to drink, with a quite bell shaped form, as in the normal control subject.

Figure 8 show the force measurements from the middle finger in the normal control (top plot), in the hemiplegic patient, 25 days following the stroke onset (middle plot) and 131 days following the stroke onset. In the normal control, the negative values on the x-axis means that the subject moves the middle finger upwards to bring the glass to the mouth. The positive values observed along the F_y-direction point out that the subject pulls the middle finger backwards to bring the glass to the mouth. The positive values along the F_z-direction means that the subject grasps the glass to drink.

The negative values on the x-axis recorded from the hemiplegic patient, 25 days following the stroke onset means that the subject moves the middle finger upwards to bring the glass to the mouth, showing lower amplitude values than the normal control. The negative values observed along the F_y-direction and the positive values along the F_z-direction mean that the subject pulls the middle finger backwards to bring the glass to the mouth and grasps the glass to drink respectively, but showing a fragmented trend. The negative values on the x-axis from the middle finger force measurements recorded 131 days following the stroke onset means that the subject moves the middle finger upwards to bring the glass to the mouth, showing lower amplitude values and a more fragmented trend than the normal control.

The negative values observed along the F_y-direction and the positive values along the F_z-direction point out that the subject pulls the middle finger backwards to bring the glass to the mouth and grasps the glass to drink respectively, with a more regular trend if compared to the force measurements recorded 25 days following the stroke onset.

5. Future directions and conclusions

A large set of features characterizing the clinical recovery have been extracted from the data according to the preliminary results from data mining techniques (Van Djick et al., 2006b) in order to track the recovery process through milestones and to foresee the rehabilitation outcome through predictive markers.

The positive results obtained so far through the extensive use of the proposed diagnostic device during the clinical trials for functional assessment of post-stroke patients allow to foresee new possible scenarios for the neurorehabilitation domain. The use of the diagnostic device together with systems for brain imaging (PET, fMRI, MEG) and techniques for monitoring brain activity (EEG) will allow to monitor the degree of learning and the changes in motor performances induced by the rehabilitative treatments through traditional and robotic therapies. Alternative applications for the proposed platform are:

- isometric motor exercise. Many clinical protocols for motor therapy of different type of patients prescribe the execution of isometric exercises. The proposed system could allow to accurately tune, monitor, measure and record the forces/torques exerted by the patient during such exercises. To this aim, a self-calibration routine will be added to the system, such that forces/torques due to the body's weight will be automatically set to zero at the start of the motor therapy;

- human-machine interface. The proposed system can be associated to a virtual reality environment for motor rehabilitation, as recently implemented with similar devices for isometric measurements in the upper limb (Kurillo et al., 2005) or it can be used as novel human-machine interface for many different applications where the use of the hand and the foot is required, e.g. pedal and handle interfaces for game, surgical robots, vehicles for enabling independent living to citizens with residual abilities.

Further possible developments comprise also:

- a migration to a mechatronic platform embedding actuators to produce perturbations and assisted constrained motion of the affected limbs;
- the application of the proposed platform for research in neuroscience, e.g. by comparing isometric performance of healthy controls and different patients, and for studying anticipative and high-level planning capabilities based on the study of whole-body dynamics in isometric conditions at the inception of voluntary movements.

The proposed platform is the first device which acquires a great deal of different data (F/T data, clinical scales, natural language descriptions made by the physiotherapists) till now. It is a versatile research tool, which records heterogeneous fields in a complete and detailed way. It has been used in clinical trials in order to verify the clinical hypotheses.

The proposed platform, which has been validated in three different clinical centres in Europe, proved to be effective as a tool for experimental use in novel functional assessment procedures of post-stroke patients, according to the original specifications provided by the medical doctors and therapists. The platform has also a range of other potential applications, from motor therapy to human-machine interface.

The reduction of its level of complexity and the development of an optimized version for clinical uses are the next steps, after the completion of the analysis of data collected during the clinical trials. The use of actuators in the platform can be also considered as a further development of the platform as tool both for functional assessment and rehabilitative treatment.

6. Acknowledgment

This work was partly supported by the European Commission - 6th Framework Programme under the grant N. 507424 (ALLADIN - Natural Language Based Decision Support in Neuro-rehabilitation).

The ALLADIN project is co-ordinated by Jo Van Vaerenbergh, Arteveldehogeschool (Gent, Belgium). The other partners of the ALLADIN project are: Language and Computing NV (Belgium), Budapest University of Technology and Economics (Hungary), School of Electrical Engineering of the University of Ljubljana (Slovenia), Zenon SA Robotics and Informatics (Greece), Multitel ASBL (Belgium), Trinity College Dublin (Ireland), National

Institute for Medical Rehabilitation (Hungary), Scuola Superiore Sant'Anna (Italy) and Campus Bio-Medico University (Italy).
The authors greatly acknowledge the inputs received from all the people participating in the ALLADIN project in many project meetings and internal working groups activities.

7. References

Aisen, M. L.; Krebs, H. I.; Hogan, N.; McDowell, F. & Volpe, B. T. (1997). The effect of robot assisted therapy and rehabilitative training on motor recovery following stroke. *Arch Neurol,* Vol. 54, No. 4, April 2000, pp. 443-446.

Bobath, B. (1978). *Adult hemiplegia: evaluation and treatment,* William Heinemann Medical Books, London.

Bozec, S. L.; Goutal, L. & Bouisset, S. (1997), Dynamic postural adjustments associated with the development of isometric forces in sitting subjects, *C R Acad Sci III,* Vol. 320, No. 9, pp. 715-720.

Brunstrom, S. (1970). *Movement therapy in hemiplegia: a neurophysiological approach,* Harper and Row, New York.

Buchanan, T. S. & Shreeve, D. A. (1996). An evaluation of optimization techniques for the prediction of muscle activation patterns during isometric tasks. *J. Biomech. Eng,* Vol. 118, No. 4, November 1996, pp. 565-574.

Cantor, M. R. (1998), *Object-Oriented Project Management with UML,* John Wiley & Sons, New York.

Carr, J. & Shepard, R. (1998). *Neurological rehabilitation,* Butterworth-Heineman, Oxford.

Clark, S.; Tremblay, F. & Ste-Marie, D. (2004). Differential modulation of corticospinal excitability during observation, mental imagery and imitation of hand actions. *Neuropsychologia,* Vol. 42, No. 1, pp. 105-112.

Dechent, P.; Merboldt K. D. & Frahm J. (2004). Is the human primary motor cortex involved in motor imagery? *Brain Res Cogn Brain Res,* Vol. 19, No. 2, April 2004, pp. 138-144.

Deutsch, J. E.; Merians, A. S.; Adamovich, S.; Poizner, H. & Burdea, G. C. (2004), Development and application of virtual reality technology to improve hand use and gait of individuals post-stroke, *Restor Neurol Neurosci,* Vol. 22, No. 3-5, pp. 371-386.

Dewald, J. P.; Pope, P. S.; Given, J. D.; Buchanan, T. S. & Rymer, W. Z. (1995). Abnormal muscle coactivation patterns during isometric torque generation at the elbow and shoulder in hemiparetic subjects. *Brain,* Vol. 118, Pt 2, , April 1995, pp. 495-510.

Ehrsson, H. H.; Geyer, S. & Naito, E. (2003). Imagery of voluntary movement of fingers, toes, and tongue activates corresponding body-part-specific motor representations. *J Neurophysiol,* Vol. 90, No. 5, November 2003, pp. 3304-3316.

Jackson, P. L.; Lafleur, M. F.; Malouin, F.; Richards, C. L. & Doyon J. (2003). Functional cerebral reorganization following motor sequence learning through mental practice with motor imagery. *Neuroimage,* Vol. 20, No. 2, October 2003, pp. 1171-1180.

Johnson-Frey, S. H. (2004). Stimulation through simulation? Motor imagery and functional reorganization in hemiplegic stroke patients. *Brain Cogn,* Vol. 55, No. 2, July 2004, pp. 328-331.

Kilner J. M.; Paulignan, Y. & Boussaoud, D. (2004). Functional connectivity during real vs imagined visuomotor tasks: an EEG study. *Neuroreport,* Vol. 15, No. 4, March 2004, pp. 637-642.

Koo, T. K.; Mak, A. F.; Hung, L. & Dewald, J. P. (2003). Joint position dependence of weakness during maximum isometric voluntary contractions in subjects with hemiparesis. *Arch Phys Med Rehabil,* Vol. 84, No. 9, September 2003, pp. 1380-1386.

Krebs H. I.; Hogan N.; Aisen M. L. & Volpe B. T. (1998). Robot-aided neurorehabilitation. *IEEE Trans Rehabil Eng,* Vol. 6, No. 1, March 1998, pp. 75-87.

Kurillo, G.; Mihelj, M.; Munih, M. & Bajd, T. (2005). Grasping and manipulation in virtual environment using 3by6 finger device, *Proceedings of the 9th IEEE International Conference on Rehabilitation Robotics,* pp. 131-134, Chicago, IL, USA, 2005.

Lehericy, S.; Gerardin, E.; Poline, J. B.; Meunier, S.; Van de Moortele, P. F.; Le Bihan, D. & Vidailhet, M. (2004). Motor execution and imagination networks in post-stroke dystonia. *Neuroreport,* Vol. 15, No. 12, August 2004, pp. 1887-1890.

Perfetti C. (1997). *Der hemiplegische Patient. Kognitiv-therapeutische Ubungen.* Richard Pflaum Verlag GmbH & Co, München.

Peebles, L. & Norris, B. J. (1998) *Adultdata. The handbook of adult anthropometrical and strength measurements - Data for design safety,* Department of Trade and Industry, London, UK.

Reinkensmeyer, D. J.; Hogan, N.; Krebs, H. I.; Lehman, S. L. & Lum, P. S. (2000). *Rehabilitators, robots, and guides: new tools for neurological rehabilitation, biomechanics and neural control of posture and movement,* J. Winters and P. Crago, Springer-Verlag, pp. 516-533.

Sejnowski, T. J. (1998). Making smooth moves. *Nature,* Vol. 394, No. 6695, August 1998, pp. 725-26.

Van Dijck, G.; Van Hulle, M. M. & Van Vaerenbergh, J. (2006). Statistically Rigorous Human Movement Onset Detection with the Maximal Information Redundancy Criterion, *Proceedings of 28th IEEE EMBS Annual International Conference,* pp. 2474-2477, New York City, USA, August 2006.

Van Dijck, G.; Van Hulle, M. M. & Van Vaerenbergh, J. (2006). Hybrid feature subset selection for the quantitative assessment of skills of stroke patients in activity of daily living tasks, *Proceedings of 28th IEEE EMBS Annual International Conference,* pp. 5699-5703, New York City, USA, August 2006.

Van Vaerenbergh, J. et al. (2004), Deliverable D1.1: Methodology for multi centre trial, ALLADIN Project, IST-2002-507424.

Walsh, S.; Saltzman, C.; Talbot, K.; Aper, R. & Brown, T. (1996), In vivo validation of in vitro testing of hallucal flexor mechanics, *Clin Biomech,* Vol. 11, No. 6, pp. 328-332.

Woldag, H. & Hummelsheim, H. (2002). Evidence-based physiotherapeutic concepts for improving arm and hand function in stroke patients: a review. *J.Neurol,* Vol. 249, No. 5, May 2002, pp. 518-528.

Wolpert, D. M.; Ghahramani, Z. & Flanagan, J. R. (2001). Perspectives and problems in motor learning. *Trends Cognitive Sciences*, Vol. 5, No. 11, November 2001, pp. 487-494.

30

Synthesis of Prosthesis Architectures and Design of Prosthetic Devices for Upper Limb Amputees

Marco Troncossi & Vincenzo Parenti-Castelli
DIEM – Dept. of Mechanical Engineering of the University of Bologna
Italy

1. Introduction

This chapter presents a procedure for the Determination of the Optimal Prosthesis Architecture for upper limb amputees (DOPA). The presented approach can consistently manage both the clinical aspects and the technical issues involved in the design of electromechanically actuated prostheses. The procedure is composed on one hand of algorithms useful for analyzing the patients' requirements and on the other hand of algorithms that perform kinematic and kinetostatic simulations of several architectures of artificial arms attempting to fulfil important activities of daily living. The systematic evaluation of the prosthesis models' performance can methodically guide designers in the synthesis of the optimal prosthesis that best suits the patients' requirements.

1.1 Prosthetic rehabilitation of upper limb amputees

The loss or the congenital deficiency of an upper limb part represents a serious physical and psychological trauma, apart from having an evident and considerable restriction on personal autonomy in everyday living. Rehabilitating an amputee with a proper device allows the patient to recover (part of) the lost autonomy and the sense of psychophysical integrity, and thus to enable his/her reintegration in domestic, working and social environments.

The prosthetic intervention is a complex process which involves technical aspects and clinical issues strictly dependent on the amputee to be treated; prosthetic rehabilitation is therefore carried out by a multidisciplinary team including physicians, technicians, therapists and psychologists which operates with the aim of providing the amputee with the device and the services that best match his/her different requirements. The first step the rehabilitation team must face is to investigate the individual needs of every amputee. The choice of the best prosthesis for a given patient depends on several aspects, all of which must be taken into account (Atkins & Meyer, 1989):

- amputation level
- mono- or bi-laterality of the amputation
- patient's age
- patient's gender
- stump conditions (shape, muscle strength, skin conditions, pain…)
- range of motion of the residual limb

- presence of other diseases
- personal motivations for rehabilitating and expectations regarding the prosthesis
- psychological status
- home environment and family support
- subject's particular characteristics
- ...

Even if it is glaringly obvious that the evaluation of these aspects is strictly patient-dependent, it is generally possible to state that for mono-lateral amputees the sound limb becomes dominant and the prosthesis works mainly as an auxiliary device for bimanual activities. On the contrary, for bilateral amputees the prostheses are strictly necessary to perform those activities of daily living that allow the patient not to be completely dependent on others' help thanks to the acquisition of a certain level of functional autonomy. Obviously, the higher the level of amputation the greater the importance of the prosthetic devices. The right selection of the proper prosthesis for a given patient relies on the assessment of the patient's characteristics and must be made by experienced personnel.
In order to satisfy the patient's needs the features that a prosthesis must have are:

1. the highest possible dexterity
2. good performance (in terms of velocity and forces/torques)
3. appropriate robustness
4. efficient control
5. a humanlike appearance
6. a light weight
7. proper size and proportions
8. good comfort for the wearer
9. easy control for the amputee
10. extremely reliable components of the artificial system
11. a low noise level
12. sufficient autonomy of the energy source to allow the prosthesis to work all day

It is possible to summarize the features required of a prosthesis as good *functionality* of the artificial arm on one hand (features 1–4) and good *wearability* for the patient on the other (features 5–9). The last specifications, 10 to 12, concern technological issues and the level of their observance depends basically on the component design, the materials used and the state of the art of both the electronic and the mechanical fields. It is worth noting that functionality and wearability are basically contrasting features; for instance, a device which has to provide high forces and speed must supply an appropriate power, implying a size of actuators far from lightweight. When selecting the appropriate prosthesis for a given amputee, the importance to be allocated to every single factor strictly depends on the evaluation of the patient's characteristics and requirements.

1.2 Upper limb prostheses

There are various kinds of prosthesis to be evaluated and chosen from. The "externally powered prosthesis", i.e. a robotic arm where the artificial limb segments are driven by electromechanical joints, is the most advanced. The joint motors are directly activated by the amputee by means of input commands that are collected by specific sensors located in the socket of the prosthesis, the socket being the interface by means of which the prosthesis is suspended on the patient's stump. The command signals are processed by a programmable electronic circuit which carries out the control strategy to operate the device. Rechargeable batteries power all these components. Some passive friction joints are sometimes included in the system and are useful to give the prosthetic limb an optimal pre-determined configuration when performing certain tasks. The passive joints are operated by applying external forces by means of the sound limb or resting the artificial segments on fixed points, before or after the action of the active joints.

Currently, the most common electromechanical prosthetic components available on the market are many kinds of terminal devices (each with one degree of freedom - DoF - for grasping), the elbow joint, the wrist prono-supination unit (which allows the terminal device to rotate around the longitudinal forearm axis), and the wrist flexion unit. Many other active articulations have been studied and proposed as prototypes but they have not yet been distributed commercially. Among the recent interesting research results, the authors would like to mention: the multi-fingered prosthetic hands (Kyberd et al., 2001; Pons et al., 2004; Yang et al., 2004), which provide the terminal device with more than one DoF, thus making different grip patterns available (one of these seems ready to be commercialized[1]); a powered humeral rotator (Weir & Grahn, 2005) which allows the forearm segment to rotate around the longitudinal humeral axis (this is a novelty, because most above-elbow prostheses are equipped with passive humeral rotators); a shoulder joint with one DoF for upper arm elevation (Gow et al., 2001); a shoulder joint with two DoFs which is based on a differential mechanism and provides upper arm elevation and abduction (Cattaneo et al., 2001).

There are several ways of controlling electrically-powered prostheses, the most popular being myoelectric control: electromyographic signals (EMG, i.e. electrical signals associated with the muscle contractions), measured on the skin by myoelectric electrodes located in the socket, are properly amplified and filtered, and then processed by the controller that switches the motors on or off in the active joints to produce movements and functions. Although theoretically possible, the *simultaneous and independent* contraction of distinct bundles of muscles, that would generate EMG signals able to operate different functions at the same time is very difficult and stressing for the patient. The myoelectric control scheme is therefore generally based on the sequential activation of the prosthetic articulations one at a time, resulting in a not very natural control. In this context, some recent results seem to be promising to overcome this limitation (Kuiken et al., 2004).

The good qualities of this prosthesis are sufficient functionality, good performance and a pleasant appearance. The critical aspects are the weight and the volume of the physical structure, and the intricate control, due to the sequential activation of both the active and passive joints. Finally, it is proven that electrically-powered prostheses provide a high level of technology but at a high cost.

1.3 New prosthesis design and overview of the presented method

In order to provide high level disarticulated patients with a comfortable, humanlike and user-friendly prosthesis, not all the physiological joint movements can be replicated, thus limiting the functionality of the artificial arm. When compared to the human arm, the

[1] http://www.touchbionics.com/page.php?pageid=12&section=3.

dexterity of current commercial prostheses is very poor and amputees generally have to resort to compensatory movements of the residual limb, or even of other parts of the body as well as to auxiliary aids to execute many motor tasks. For patients with very high level amputations (bilateral above all), who have an extremely restricted residual movement ability, current prostheses could be inadequate to guarantee the functionality needed to reach a satisfactory level of autonomy. In order to solve this deficiency and to improve the quality of life of this amputee population, the development of new electrically powered prostheses with greater mobility, advanced control and good "wearability" is thus required.

It is authors' firm belief that the same observations that guide the rehabilitation team in the selection of the proper device for a given patient must also be considered by engineers and technicians when designing new prosthetic devices. Computer-based simulations represent a useful tool, in this perspective, for the development of new mechanical systems. In particular, the work presented in (Romilly et al., 1994) shows how the kinematic simulations of artificial arm models attempting to execute given trajectories can guide the development of powered orthoses with less than six DoF.

This chapter presents a methodology for the synthesis of new prosthetic architectures for patients with high level amputation, based on a procedure for the determination of the best compromise between the contrasting features required of a prosthesis, taking into account the different needs of diverse patient profiles. "Architecture" is intended here as the geometry and the topology of a robotic arm model, i.e. the number and type (active/passive) of its joints and their arrangement.

With the proposed procedure, the characteristics, the needs and the goals of a generic patient are formalised and organised in such a way as to be systematically analysed by means of specifically developed algorithms. Based on the collected data, further algorithms then perform the kinematic and kinetostatic simulations of several robotic arm architectures with one up to six active joints differently arranged (and considering the possible presence of passive joints as well) when carrying out some activities of daily living considered important for a given amputee. The models with less than six DoF correspond to simpler robot architectures and are thus appreciated from the wearability viewpoint; on the other hand, their performance is poorer than those of the six DoF models, because they normally carry out the manipulation tasks with an error which increases as the number of active joints decreases. The structure simplification of these robots and the corresponding worsening of their global functionality are evaluated with respect to the quality of life assigned to the patient profile. For this purpose, some indices have been specifically developed to properly weigh up both the clinical aspects (depending on the patient) and the technical factors (depending on the robotic models).

The approach is subject-oriented, foreseeing a single patient as input and providing his/her optimal prosthesis as output. However, the final application of the methodology can supply more general design guidelines, suitable to determine a limited number of prosthesis architectures able to match the requirements of many different amputees.

Finally, the results of the kinematic and kinetostatic simulations can provide the mechanical design specifications (e.g. the joint range of motion, the power of the actuators) of the new devices that will prove fundamental in overcoming the limitations of the existing prostheses.

2. The DOPA procedure

The procedure receives a given patient's information as input and provides his/her corresponding optimal prosthesis model as output (Fig. 1). It is based on a database and a number of algorithms which make it possible to choose the optimal robot arm architecture able to fit patient's *specific* needs and limitations. On one hand the database (database *DB-T*) collects upper limb activities of daily living and the corresponding trajectories which model them - hereinafter "Reference Trajectories", normally requiring six DoF for positioning and orienting tasks - and on the other hand (database *DB-R*) several kinematic models of upper limb prostheses with one up to six active revolute joints differently arranged and possible revolute or spherical passive joints (Fig. 3). The procedure can be considered as a process of three sequential steps, running automatically once that the appropriate amputee data have been entered.

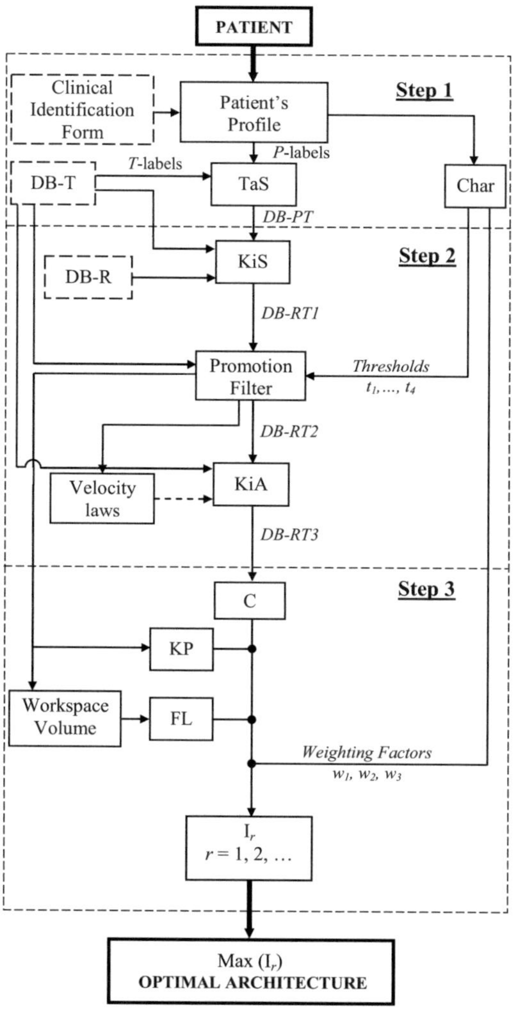

Abbreviation	Meaning
T-labels	Markers of motor tasks
P-labels	Markers of the patient profile
DB-T	Upper Limb Activities Database
TaS	Task Selection Algorithm
DB-PT	Upper Limb Activities selected for the patient
Char	Characterization Algorithm
DB-R	Robotic Models Database
KiS	Kinematic Simulation Algorithm
DB-RT1	Robotic models kinematic performance
Promotion Filter	Model kinematic performance evaluation
DB-RT2	Promoted models kinematic performance
KiA	Kinetostatic Analysis
DB-RT3	Promoted models dynamic performance
C	Complexity Index
KP	Kinematic performance Index
FL	Flexibility Index
I	Overall Index

Fig. 1. The DOPA procedure schematic layout.

Step 1 - The compilation of the patient's *Clinical Identification Form* is the starting point of the procedure. It collects all the information necessary to classify the amputee's needs; different aspects are investigated in order to identify a patient's profile useful to portray a personalized level of life quality to be achieved after the prosthetic rehabilitation plan. An algorithm (*TaS*) based on the processing of this profile determines which upper limb activities are most significant for the given patient from the viewpoint of reaching a satisfactory functional autonomy in everyday living. The prosthesis will be designed aiming at performing these selected functional tasks. A further algorithm (*Char*) determines the values of the parameters involved in the selection of the optimal architecture by balancing the relative importance of the different factors which contribute to define the amputee's quality of life (e.g. expected level of functional autonomy, simplicity of the structure, easiness of control, etc.).
Step 2 - Kinematic simulations (*KiS*), performed for all the models in *DB-R*, generate the trajectories performed by the robot when attempting to fulfil the tasks assigned by *TaS*. The models with less than six DoF (hereinafter "Deficient Robots"), corresponding to simpler, less massive robot architectures (thus appreciated from the wearability viewpoint), execute the Reference Trajectories with a certain error which increases as the number of active joints decreases.
If the error overcomes the acceptable value fixed for every given task, then the robot model is considered not adequate to perform that activity. Only the robotic models which fulfil a given number of tasks, dependent on the functionality required by the subject (*Thresholds* $t_1,\ldots, t_4$), will move on to the next phases, whereas the others will be discarded. The structural simplification of the Deficient Robots and the corresponding worsening of their global functionality have to be evaluated with respect to the quality of life assigned (by means of the *Char* algorithm) to the given patient. A further kinetostatic analysis (*KiA*), performed for the "promoted" robots, provides the values of torque and power that all the actuated joints must generate to perform the successfully-executed tasks, defining the size of the actuators in a first approximation.
Step 3 - The artificial arm models are assessed in the last step of the procedure: their performance and the complexity of their architecture are evaluated by means of three purpose-built indices, all ranging from 0 to 1, named as *KP*, *FL* and *C* which, properly combined in an overall index *I*, univocally determine the optimal prosthesis architecture, i.e. the robotic arm with the simplest and lightest structure possible which can best satisfy the patient's personal requirements:

$$I = w_1 \cdot KP + w_2 \cdot FL - w_3 \cdot C \qquad (1)$$

where $w_1, w_2, w_3 \in [0,1]$ are weighting factors which depend on the patient's profile.
The model with the maximum value for *I* designates the optimal architecture of the prosthesis associated with the given patient.
The main elements and algorithms of the DOPA procedure will be explained, in such a way to make their comprehension easy for the reader. In particular they will be outlined as if the procedure must guide the design of an ad-hoc prosthesis for a single patient; the intended implementation is actually different (see Section 3).

CLINICAL IDENTIFICATION FORM			
Label	*Definition*	*Value*	*Definition*
P1	Gender	P1.1	Female
		P1.2	Male
P2	Age	P2.1	0 - 15 years old
		P2.2	16 - 35
		P2.3	36 - 65
		P2.4	> 65
P3	Body-build	P3.1	Small
		P3.2	Medium
		P3.3	Large
P4	Non-dominant limb level of amputation *	P4.1	Distal upper arm amputation
		P4.2	Medial upper arm amputation
		P4.3	Proximal upper arm amputation
		P4.4	Shoulder disarticulation
		P4.5	Forequarter amputation
P5	Dominant limb level of amputation *	P5.1	Healthy (single extremity amputation)
		P5.2	Distal upper arm amputation
		...	...
		P5.6	Forequarter amputation
P6	Patient preferences about the prosthesis	P6.1	High predilection for comfort and appearance
		P6.2	Moderate predilection for comfort and appearance
		P6.3	No preference
		P6.4	Moderate predilection for device functionality
		P6.5	High predilection for device functionality
P7	Living situation	P7.1	He/she lives with someone else who can aid him/her
		P7.2	He/she lives alone, but someone is often present
		P7.3	He/she lives alone, someone is occasionally present
		P7.4	He/she lives alone in complete autonomy
P8	Work	P8.1	None
		P8.2	Houseman/housewife
		P8.3	Administrative employment
		P8.4	Technical employment
P9	Other activities (*All the activities not related to work*)	P9.1	None
		P9.2	Cooking (and kitchen-related activities)
		P9.3	Housework
		P9.4	Doing the shopping
		P9.5	Driving the car
		P9.6	Using home appliances (stereo, computer...)
		P9.7	Home maintenance and workshop activities

* "Non-dominant" (ND) is the injured upper limb of a monolateral amputee or the limb with the severest injury for a bilateral amputee; "dominant" (D) is the other limb. ND and D prostheses are the corresponding artificial arms that will replace the missing limb(s). An ND prosthesis should perform functions of support (simpler) to the D limb (natural or artificial).

Table I. A schematic layout of the *Clinical Identification Form* with the *P-labels* meaning.

2.1 Clinical Identification Form: determination of the patient's main characteristics

Let us suppose we are going to rehabilitate an amputee with a custom-made prosthesis developed according to his/her personal requirements. The design process is thus subject-oriented and, for the sake of its significance and effectiveness, it should be objectively repeatable with a standard protocol for other amputees too; this means that proper information concerning the patient's expectations and impediments have to be systematically collected in a way suitable to automatic processing. This is possible by properly codifying the responses to the queries reported in the patient's *Clinical Identification Form* (Table I) by means of specific markers (called hereinafter *P-labels*). The form is actually a questionnaire and has to portray a well-defined patient profile upon which the architecture synthesis of his/her prosthesis will be based. Different aspects are investigated and, for all the fields, the patient is asked to tick off his/her choice among a number of pre-defined answers, in order not to fall into ambiguities.

The labels *P1–P3* refer to the patient's gender, age and body-build and are useful to determine potential upper limits on the prosthesis size; the kind of amputation (*P4, P5*) defines the subject's disease and thus his/her restrictions. The patient is also asked to point out his/her preference between functionality and wearability of the prosthesis (or a compromise), giving a direct indication useful to evaluate the robotic models (*P6*). In addition, with the purpose of defining the level of functional autonomy requested by the amputee, the field *P7* focuses on his/her living situation, since the same concept of functional autonomy depends on this aspect too: e.g. the personal needs of an amputee living alone are somewhat different from those of an amputee living with a person who can constantly give him/her aid. Finally, information related to work and other activities (*P8, P9*) draft the patient's expectations, making it possible to subsequently select activities more appropriate than others for the given subject. Labels *P9*, that can have more than one answer, guide the "patient-tasks" association performed by the *TaS* algorithm.

The fields in the form have been chosen trying to make them identify the main factors which condition the rehabilitation team's decisions when selecting an *existing* prosthesis for a given amputee, i.e. to translate the decision process into a technical systematic language. Based on the *Clinical Identification Form*, the procedure, which is intended to guide the design of *new* prostheses, can be repeated for many patient profiles according to the same protocol.

Once the *Clinical Identification Form* has been compiled, it is possible to represent the given patient's profile by means of an unequivocal alphanumeric code, suitable for processing by proper algorithms. A possible form of the codified patient's profile can be a "Structure" (i.e. arrays with "data containers" –called fields– which can house any kind of data), whose fields contain the patient's answers to the *Clinical Identification Form* (i.e. the values of the *P-labels*). An example makes it easier to understand: let us suppose we are going to rehabilitate a monolateral shoulder disarticulated amputee, a male, 57 years old, medium body size, who expresses a moderate preference for prosthesis functionality with respect to its wearability, even if he prefers not to return to work after his injury. Let us assume that he lives alone, very close to some relatives, and that he would like his prosthesis to allow him to cook and to do the housework without others' help. His profile is therefore represented by the univocal structure shown in Table II.

Structures have been chosen to represent the patients' profile because it is possible to add, remove and/or modify fields (that can contain information of various kinds) without entailing radical modifications of the algorithms that manage them.

Structure	*Fields*	*Value*
Patient =	Gender:	*P1.2*
	Age:	*P2.3*
	Body-build:	*P3.2*
	Non-dominant limb amputation:	*P4.4*
	Dominant limb amputation:	*P5.1*
	Preference about prosthesis:	*P6.4*
	Living situation:	*P7.2*
	Profession:	*P8.1*
	Non-work-related activities:	*P9.2, P9.3*

Table II. Structures can represent the patients' profile.

2.2 DB-T database and TaS algorithm

Several activities were picked out from different literature sources (Anglyn & Wyss, 2000) and then completed and processed in order to characterize all the main upper limb functions by means of basic movements (motor tasks) as simple and general as possible. The activities were stored in the database *DB-T* along with associated markers (*T-labels*) which outline their main distinguishing characteristics (Table IIII).

In particular, the label *T1* provides the motor task identification code which is univocally linked to the task name, e.g. T1.1 = "Drinking from a glass". *T2* represents the activity macro-area, that is the general functional sector that the activity belongs to.

Since not all the activities have the same priority from the functional autonomy point of view, a prosthesis can be allowed to fail the performance of a certain number of tasks of minor importance and still be considered acceptable for a given subject. Based on their priority, the tasks have been ranked in five different groups corresponding to the *T3* values:

- T3.0: basic and minimal activities of primary importance that any prosthesis is compelled to perform satisfactorily. The ability to perform these tasks allows the patient to autonomously eat and go to the bathroom. The activities of this group are intended as performed by the subject also with the aid of supportive devices or special arrangements, and with large compensatory movements (the Reference Trajectories that model them, see below, respect these control strategies);
- T3.1: high relevance activities dealing with feeding and hygiene (limited to face and private parts). Use of supportive devices, special arrangements, and large compensatory movements is considered;
- T3.2: activities which allow the subject to autonomously take care of total body hygiene and dressing, and activities which make it possible to do without those special arrangements and devices potentially necessary to perform the motor tasks of the previous groups (e.g. the ability to "Cut food with a knife" makes it possible to do without special cutlery);
- T3.3: activities which allow the patient to carry out the most important operations concerning his/her work and non-work-related activities (for which special arrangements and devices are considered) and to live a normal social life (e.g. "Using the telephone"); activities relative to dressing which make it possible to do without special expedients (e.g. "Fastening buttons" allows the amputee not to wear shirts with special Velcro fasteners);
- T3.4: activities which make it possible to do without all the special expedients potentially required for the motor-tasks mentioned in the previous two groups.

The label *T4* establishes how many extremities are intrinsically involved in the activity. The label *T5* indicates the duty cycle of the motor task: the value for this label has been set considering reasonable temporal intervals for performing activities that an amputee can consider acceptable. Finally, the label *T6* indicates the possible payload acting on the end effector to carry out the task, mainly[2] intended as the weight of an object held in the hand. Four weight levels have been set: none, light, medium, and heavy (0 N, 1 N, 5 N, 10 N).
DB-T also collects the end effector Reference Trajectories that model the performance of a motor task, normally requiring six DoF for positioning and orienting tasks. Every trajectory is provided by means of a certain number of nodes through which the terminal device must go with a given orientation; these nodes are fixed according to different criteria, mainly due to obstacle avoidance and humanlike movement replication. Different reasons (Section 2.5) have been suggested to represent the pose (position and attitude) of the terminal device by means of the spatial position of three points properly selected fixed to the end effector (Fig. 4a). Therefore, for every node of the trajectory, the terminal device pose is represented by nine coordinates, that provide the spatial positions of these points with respect to the fixed coordinate system; the nine coordinates are constrained by three equations expressing the constant relative distances (l_{12}, l_{23}, l_{13}) between the three points, and thus only six of them are independent:

T-label	Definition	Value	Definition
T1	Motor task name	T1.*i*; *i* = 1,2,…	
T2	Macro-area	T2.1	Feeding
		T2.2	Hygiene care
		T2.3	Dressing
		T2.4	Kitchen-related task
		T2.5	Housework
		T2.6	Doing the shopping
		T2.7	Driving the car
		T2.8	Using computers
		T2.9	Office/school tasks
		T2.10	Workshop task
T3	Priority	T3.0	First-priority task
		T3.1	High-priority task
		T3.2	Medium-priority task
		T3.3	Moderate-priority task
		T3.4	Auxiliary task
T4	Limb(s) involved	T4.1	Single extremity task
		T4.2	Bilateral task
T5	Duty Cycle [s]	Δt	Time to execute the task
T6	Payload [N]	T6.1	0 N
		T6.2	1 N
		T6.3	5 N
		T6.4	10 N

Table III. *T-labels* and their meaning.

[2] Some tasks require a different model of the payload: e.g. "Opening a drawer" foresees the exertion of a horizontal force. These special cases are treated separately.

Structure	*Fields*	*Examples*	
Task(i) =	Name (*T1*):	T1.1 (Drinking from a glass)	T1.47 (Fastening a zipper)
	Macro-area (*T2*):	T2.1	T2.3
	Priority (*T3*):	T3.1	T3.3
	Limbs involved (*T4*):	T4.1	T4.2
	Duty Cycle (*T5*), [s]:	6 (seconds)	5
	Payload (*T6*), [N]:	1 (Newton)	0
	Reference Trajectory:	$\mathbf{H}_{T1.1}^{ref}$	$\mathbf{H}_{T1.47}^{ref}$
	Position Tolerance in the destination node (*Tl1*):	*II*	*II*
	Position Tolerance in intermediate nodes (*Tl2*):	*III*	*II*
	Orientation Tolerance in the destination node (*Tl3*):	*I*	*II*
	Orientation Tolerance in intermediate nodes (*Tl4*):	*I*	*II*

Table IV. Examples of structures that compose the *DB-T* database.

$$(\mathbf{P}_i - \mathbf{P}_j)^T \cdot (\mathbf{P}_i - \mathbf{P}_j) = l_{ij}^2; \qquad i,j = 1,2,3; i \neq j \qquad (2)$$

For a sound human limb, performing these Reference Trajectories is not the only way to perform the tasks satisfactorily: for each motor task, a tolerance on the actual path of the end effector with respect to the Reference Trajectory was thus introduced in *DB-T* (see also Section 2.6). The tolerance values were established taking into account the intrinsic accuracy required by each task; four levels of tolerance were defined:

I. low tolerance (high accuracy is required)
II. medium tolerance
III. high tolerance (low accuracy is accepted)
IV. infinite tolerance (nought accuracy is accepted).

In conclusion, all the labels, the Reference Trajectory and the tolerable errors of a motor task are gathered in a structure (Table IV).

The information stored in *DB-T* is needed by several algorithms of the procedure. In particular, the Task Selection algorithm (*TaS*) associates a set of upper limb activities with the considered patient: the purpose is to customize the synthesis of the prosthesis architecture according to the functional needs of the amputee, orienting the design process to the opportunity to use the resulting prosthesis to perform a finite number of motor tasks considered as more important than others for the given patient. The tasks that are not regarded as significant will be ignored hereinafter in the application of the other algorithms for the examined patient.

The *TaS* compares the *P7–P10* labels characterizing the patient's functional needs with the *T2* label which identifies the task functional macro-area. Moreover, the comparison between the *P5* value and *T4* (Table V) makes it possible to determine whether the prosthesis to be designed for the given patient should follow the Reference Trajectories of the Non-Dominant (ND) and/or the Dominant (D) limbs (see note in Table I). For instance, for a

monolateral amputee (*P5* = P5.1) the prosthesis (ND) to be designed is not required to perform the task "Drinking from a glass" (for which *T4* = T4.1), because it is presumed that he/she can perform the activity with the sound limb.
On the other hand, in order to "cut food with a knife and fork " (*T4* = T4.2) the two prostheses for a bilateral patient (*P5* ≠ P5.1) should allow him/her to hold the food with a fork with the ND artificial arm and to cut it with the D arm.

	T4.1	T4.2
P5 = P5.1	-	ND
P5 ≠ P5.1	ND	ND and D

Table V: Determination of the Reference Trajectories to be associated with a given patient according to the comparison between *P5*- and *T4-labels*.

The output of *TaS* is the selection of N_{PT} motor tasks collected in *DB-T* that the prosthesis should be able to perform in order to satisfy the patient's functional needs. This selection will be referred to as *DB-PT* hereinafter. Fig. 2 outlines a schematic representation of the operation performed by the *TaS* algorithm. Let us define n_{ti} as the number of tasks with label *T3* = T3.*i* (*i* = 0, 1, …, 4), now gathered in corresponding groups G_{ti}, associated with the given patient; it holds that:

$$\sum_{i=0}^{4} n_{ti} = N_{PT} \tag{3}$$

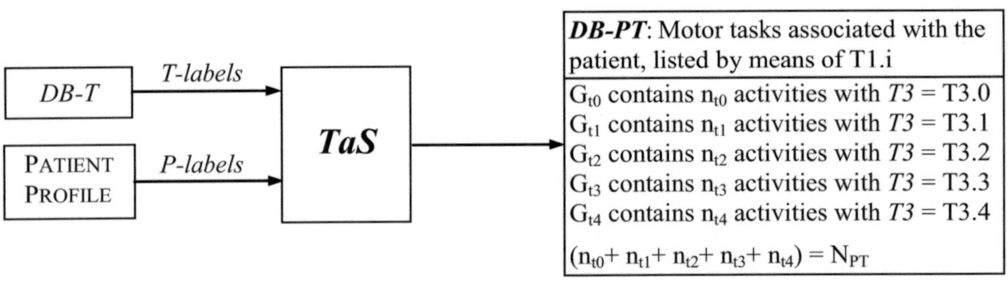

Fig. 2. Input and output of the Task Selection Algorithm.

2.3 Char algorithm: determination of "functionality vs. wearability parameters"

This algorithm processes the patient's profile and provides the value of some parameters involved in other algorithms of the procedure, thus determining another factor of personalization of the prosthesis synthesis process that characterizes the present method. In particular, two sets of parameters are determined: the *Thresholds*, involved in the *Promotion Filter* algorithm, and the *Weighting Factors*, used in the final evaluation of the prosthesis architectures.
Not all the activities selected for a given patient have the same importance from the functional viewpoint; for this reason the task label *T3* allows the motor tasks to be ranked in five groups according to their intrinsic priority; during the kinematic simulations, a prosthesis is allowed to fail the correct performance of a certain number of tasks (apart from those with *T3* = T3.0) and yet it can still be considered as acceptable. The limit on task failures is provided by the threshold $t_1,\ldots, t_4$ which are the ratios with respect to $n_{t1},\ldots, n_{t4}$ of

the tasks that a prosthesis must perform correctly[3]. For instance, if *Char* provides $t_1 = 0.85$, $t_2 = 0.7$, $t_3 = 0.6$ and $t_4 = 0.45$ for a given patient, a prosthesis model is still considered acceptable even if it fails to perform up to:

- $(0.15 \cdot n_{t1})$ tasks of group G_{t1} (those with labels T3.1)
- $(0.30 \cdot n_{t2})$ tasks of group G_{t2} (those with labels T3.2)
- $(0.40 \cdot n_{t3})$ tasks of group G_{t3} (those with labels T3.3)
- $(0.55 \cdot n_{t4})$ tasks of group G_{t4} (those with labels T3.4)

whereas no tasks with label T3.0 can be failed. The higher the priority of the task group (i.e. the lower the order of the *T3* label value), the greater the corresponding threshold with respect to the others. *Char* assigns the value to the thresholds $t_1,\ldots, t_4$ with a monotonic decreasing function by means of a proper process of the *P-labels*.
Similarly, *Char* determines the value of the factors w_1, w_2, w_3 that weight the relative importance of the investigated aspects in the final evaluation of the prosthesis architectures (kinematic performance, flexibility and complexity of the prosthetic devices; see Section 2.8). *Char* chooses the values in such a way that $w_1 + w_2 + w_3 = 1$.
The labels upon which *Char* assigns the parameter values are those representing the functional requirements of a given patient (P_7, P_8) and possible intrinsic upper limits for the complexity of the device (P_2, P_3), and, above all, the direct preference about functionality vs. wearability expressed by the amputee (P_6).

2.4 DB-R: robotic model database

This database collects the prosthesis architectures that will be simulated. The robotic models are serial kinematic chains with four links and a number of revolute joints differently arranged to form the three limb articulations (Fig. 3). In particular the links are the terminal device, the artificial forearm, the artificial upper arm, and the trunk which is considered as fixed to the global reference frame S_0. The Y and Z axes of S_0 belong to the patient's body sagittal plane, Y being vertical (pointing upward) and Z horizontal (pointing backward); the X axis is determined to form a right-handed triad. The origin of the frame is set at ground level at the intersection between the sagittal and the frontal plane. Each link is associated with an embedded reference frame whose origin is at the centre of its proximal joint (apart from the trunk frame that coincides with S_0) and whose axes are parallel to the S_0 axes when the upper limb is in its rest position (fully extended with the hand span turned inside): S_H, S_F, S_U are the frames fixed to the hand, forearm and upper arm respectively. The artificial segment dimensions, as well as those of the other body segments and other vector entities, were defined according to average anthropometrical proportions (Pheasant, 1996) and scaled to a unitary patient's height (i.e. considering $H = 1\ m$ in Fig. 3). The prosthetic models have from one up to six active joints (all actuated revolute joints) and up to two possible passive friction articulations at the middle of the forearm and upper arm segments respectively. Fictitious links with zero length are considered in the geometry of the articulations in order to connect the revolute joints (Figs. 3 and 4b).

[3] Threshold t_0 has not been introduced here, because $t_0 = 1$ for every amputee.

The passive joints, if they are present in a given model, replicate the spherical and/or revolute friction joints currently mounted in some prostheses for high level amputees, and they will not be part of the design, being already available[4]. Their possible presence was considered due to their essential contribution in performing some important activities, giving the artificial upper limb proper configurations before or after the activation of the powered joints. The passive spherical joints (Fig. 4b) were modelled as three consecutive revolute joints having concurrent and orthogonal axes (Fig. 4c). With this choice it is possible to represent the configurations of the passive joints by means of a (6×1) vector $\boldsymbol{\psi}$ which collects the elementary rotations:

$$\boldsymbol{\psi} = [\psi_{U1}, \psi_{U2}, \psi_{U3}, \psi_{F1}, \psi_{F2}, \psi_{F3}]^T \quad (4)$$

where $\psi_{U(F)1} = \psi_{U(F)2} = 0$ if the upper arm (forearm) passive joint is revolute (Fig. 4d) and $\psi_{U(F)1} = \psi_{U(F)2} = \psi_{U(F)3} = 0$ if there is no passive joint at the upper arm (forearm). It is therefore possible to associate every robotic model in a generic configuration with a vector that gives information about the configuration of the passive joints.
Prosthetic active shoulders and wrists with up to three DoF are considered: the corresponding model of the spherical joints by means of three consecutive revolute joints is not unique. In fact, different arrangements of the three revolute joints form distinct actuated articulation models, different both from the kinematic and kinetostatic viewpoint.
All the possible combinations of the active and passive joints generate the prosthetic architectures of *DB-R*. A model containing d actuated joints (d = 1,..., 6) will be referred to as a d-DoF model; "Deficient Robots" will be generically called all the models with less than six DoF. The active joint motion variables of a model r are gathered in the vector $\boldsymbol{\theta}_r$. All the robot models were systematically named in such a way to univocally define their architecture, and are then stored in *DB-R* with their associated (4×4) homogeneous matrices **A** which express the orientation and the position of the reference system S_H embedded in the end effector with respect to the global frame S_0 - that is fixed to the thorax (Paul, 1981). Matricx $\mathbf{A}_r$, calculated by means of the Denavit-Hartenberg parameters (Denavit & Hartenberg, 1955), depends on the geometry of the artificial arm models (link lengths and arrangement of the joint axes, depending also on the configuration of the passive joints $\boldsymbol{\psi}_r$) and their motion variables $\boldsymbol{\theta}_r$.
The hand pose is represented by means of Natural Coordinates (De Jalon et al., 1986), i.e. the spatial position of three points, $\mathbf{P}_1$, $\mathbf{P}_2$, $\mathbf{P}_3$, attached to the rigid body (Fig. 4a). In particular, $\mathbf{P}_1$ corresponds to the grasping point of the hand and was chosen as the point expressing the position of the terminal device; $\mathbf{P}_2$ is in the centre of the connection between the terminal device and the forearm; $\mathbf{P}_3$ was selected to form a rectangular triangle in a proper plane. The relative position of $\mathbf{P}_2$ and $\mathbf{P}_3$ with respect to $\mathbf{P}_1$ in the global frame univocally determines the orientation of the end effector. The coordinates in S_0 of the three points attached to the end effector of the generic robot model r can be determined with the following relation:

$$^{S_0}\boldsymbol{p}_i = \mathbf{A}_r(\boldsymbol{\psi}_r, \boldsymbol{\theta}_r) \cdot {}^{S_H}\boldsymbol{p}_i, \quad i = 1, 2, 3 \quad (5)$$

[4] The ball-and-socket joints can describe a cone with semi-angle of about 35° and weight 275 g. The revolute passive joints move in the range [0°-360°] and weigh a few dozen grams.

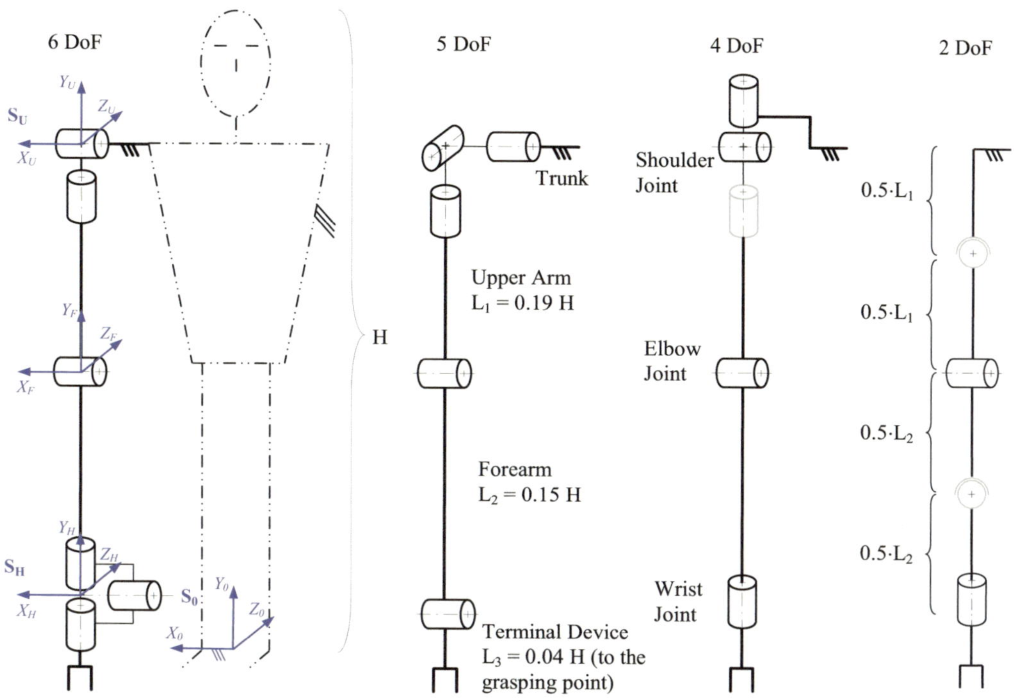

Fig. 3. Examples of prosthetic architectures; passive friction joints are drafted grey.

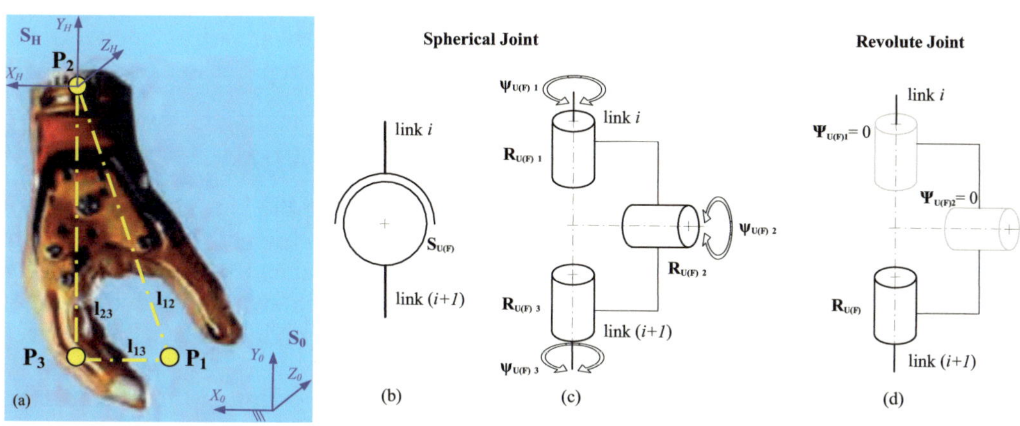

Fig. 4. (a) Three points are selected to represent the terminal device. (b) Passive spherical joint introduced at the middle of the Upper arm (S_U) and or the Forearm (S_F). (c) Alternative model of a spherical joint. (d) A passive revolute joint can be considered as a particular case of the spherical model of (c), with coplanar axes.

where ${}^{S_0}\boldsymbol{p}_i$ and ${}^{S_H}\boldsymbol{p}_i$ are (4×1) vectors that collect the homogeneous coordinates of $\mathbf{P}_i$ expressed respectively in S_0 and S_H (in S_H they are known and constant). The vectors $\boldsymbol{p}_i$ can be gathered in a (4×3) matrix **H** for a more compact hand pose representation:

$$^{S_0}\mathbf{H}={}^{S_0}\begin{pmatrix} p_{1x} & p_{2x} & p_{3x} \\ p_{1y} & p_{2y} & p_{3y} \\ p_{1z} & p_{2z} & p_{3z} \\ 1 & 1 & 1 \end{pmatrix} = \mathbf{A}_r(\boldsymbol{\psi}_r,\boldsymbol{\theta}_r)\cdot {}^{S_H}\begin{pmatrix} p_{1x} & p_{2x} & p_{3x} \\ p_{1y} & p_{2y} & p_{3y} \\ p_{1z} & p_{2z} & p_{3z} \\ 1 & 1 & 1 \end{pmatrix} = \mathbf{A}_r(\boldsymbol{\psi}_r,\boldsymbol{\theta}_r)\cdot {}^{S_H}\mathbf{H} \tag{6}$$

The Reference Trajectory of a generic task T1.i, that collects the desired hand pose at a discrete set of nodes, can thus be represented by a multidimensional (4×3×N_n) matrix ${}^{S_0}\mathbf{H}^{ref}_{T1.i}$ (where N_n is the number of the trajectory significant nodes). The generic term n_j gathers the desired homogeneous coordinates of the hand points $\mathbf{P}_1$, $\mathbf{P}_2$, $\mathbf{P}_3$ when correctly passing through the node n_j of the trajectory T1.i [5].

$$^{S_0}\mathbf{H}^{ref}_{T1.i}(n_j)={}^{S_0}\begin{pmatrix} p^{ref}_{1x} & p^{ref}_{2x} & p^{ref}_{3x} \\ p^{ref}_{1y} & p^{ref}_{2y} & p^{ref}_{3y} \\ p^{ref}_{1z} & p^{ref}_{2z} & p^{ref}_{3z} \\ 1 & 1 & 1 \end{pmatrix}_{T1.i,n_j}, \quad n_j = 1, \ldots, N_n$$

2.5 KiS: Kinematic Simulation algorithm

The *KiS* algorithm calculates the actual trajectory ${}^{S_0}\mathbf{H}^{act}_{T1.i}$ performed by the robotic models of *DB-R* when attempting to follow the Reference Trajectory ${}^{S_0}\mathbf{H}^{ref}_{T1.i}$, for each motor task T1.i (i = 1,…, N_{PT}) selected for the amputee and stored in *DB-PT*. The core of the *KiS* algorithm is formed by the inverse kinematic analysis which calculates the active joint variables $\boldsymbol{\theta}_r$ for the generic model r and for a desired pose of the terminal device in the trajectory node n_j of the task T1.i. In a few words, the algorithm solves the inverse position problem associated with the following system:

$$^{S_0}\mathbf{H}^{act}_{T1.i}(n_j) = \mathbf{A}_r(\boldsymbol{\psi}_r,\boldsymbol{\theta}_r)\cdot{}^{S_H}\mathbf{H} = {}^{S_0}\mathbf{H}^{ref}_{T1.i}(n_j) \tag{7}$$

solved for $\boldsymbol{\theta}_r$ ($\boldsymbol{\theta}_r = \boldsymbol{\theta}_{r,T1.i,nj}$ is the solution). The vector $\boldsymbol{\psi}_r$ collects the kinematic variables of the possible passive joints and must be considered as a parametric entity to be set before carrying out the inverse kinematic analysis. The value of the scalars that it contains can be changed and the analysis can be solved again, thus providing a different solution in terms of $\boldsymbol{\theta}_r$. The simulation of a task T1.i requires to solve Eq. 7 for every node of the trajectory; each trajectory must be simulated by all the prosthetic models.

A generic task normally requires six DoF for positioning and orienting the end effector; therefore the 6-DoF models correctly perform the tasks. In particular, the equation

$$^{S_0}\mathbf{H}^{act}_{T1.i} = {}^{S_0}\mathbf{H}^{ref}_{T1.i} \tag{8}$$

[5] Hereinafter the superscript S_0 will be omitted, unless necessary.

holds for all the T1.i associated with the patient.
In a general case the Deficient Robots are not able to perfectly follow the Reference Trajectory of a given task, due to the lack of the necessary DoF. In fact, the system of equations that represents the position kinematics of the manipulators (Eq. 7) generally has no solution for the models with less than six DoF. The difference between the actual end effector pose and the reference one must be minimized at every node n_j of the trajectory in such a way that the error committed on the actual pose of the terminal device can be considered acceptable for a satisfactory performance of the motor task, even if not perfect (see par. 2.6). The "Error Matrix" $\mathbf{E}_{T1.i}$ is defined as:

$$\mathbf{E}_{T1.i}(n_j) := \mathbf{A}_r(\boldsymbol{\psi}_r, \boldsymbol{\theta}_r) \cdot {}^{S_H}\mathbf{H} - {}^{S_0}\mathbf{H}^{ref}_{T1.i}(n_j) \tag{9}$$

The inverse kinematic analysis that provides an optimal solution for the indeterminate system of equations is based upon the Non-linear Least Squares Method, and solved by means of the Levenberg-Marquardt numerical algorithm (Dennis & Schnabel, 1996). In the analysis, the manipulator links are forbidden to interfere with external obstacles, in particular with the subject's body. Here, the trunk and the upper limb segments, that are modelled on the basis of average anthropometrical proportions, are schematically represented by clusters of spheres in order to be able to implement a known technique for the collision detection [6] required to tackle and solve the problem.
The scalar function f to be minimized in order to find an optimal solution is:

$$f = \sum_{k=1}^{3} [\alpha_k \cdot (\boldsymbol{p}_k^{act}(\boldsymbol{\theta}_r) - \boldsymbol{p}_k^{ref}(n_j))^{\mathrm{T}} \cdot (\boldsymbol{p}_k^{act}(\boldsymbol{\theta}_r) - \boldsymbol{p}_k^{ref}(n_j))] + \Gamma \tag{10}$$

The parameters a_1, a_2, a_3, ranging from 0 to 1, are weights that make it possible to balance the minimization according to proper criteria. For instance, for tasks that do not require a specific orientation of the hand when passing through the nodes, $\alpha_2 = \alpha_3 = 0$. Γ is a scalar which depends on the collision response and gives f a large positive contribution when two body segments interfere. Therefore, the solution $\boldsymbol{\theta}_r = \boldsymbol{\theta}_{r,T1.i,nj}$ corresponds to the configuration of the manipulator that minimizes the squared distance of the actual position achieved by the three points of the hand with respect to the desired values, and that make the manipulator avoid obstacle interferences.
It is possible to change the value of the parameters $\boldsymbol{\psi}_r$ of the kinematic variables of the passive joints – within their range of motion, to repeat the inverse analysis and to find a new solution for $\boldsymbol{\theta}_r$. This iteration makes it possible to optimise the solution also in terms of the passive joints configuration: the optimal value for $\boldsymbol{\psi}_r$ is the one that provides the minimum value of the error at the destination point of the trajectory.
The choice to represent the position and the orientation of the end effector by means of the spatial position of three embedded points was made taking into account the cost function f of Eq. 10. Indeed, if the pose representation of S_H had been based on the spatial position of its origin and three angles (e.g. Euler angles), the function to be minimized in order to find an approximated solution for the Deficient Robots kinematics (and an exact solution for the 6-DoF models) would have included non-homogenous terms. The elements of the Jacobian matrix would have proved sensitive to scale-factors and adding distance and angles is not actually very sensible (Duffy, 1990). Moreover, the three angles representing the orientation depend on the succession of the elementary rotations that they correspond to, and this would

[6] The technique is based on Computer Graphics algorithms well known in the literature (Jimnez, 2001).

create problems in the definition of the orientation errors. Other techniques used in robotics to represent the orientation of a reference frame suffer from similar problems. The technique used in this study was inspired by the Natural Coordinates method (De Jalon et al., 1986).
The output of the *KiS* algorithm is a transient database *DB-RT1* that collects the kinematic performance of the robot models simulating the trajectories associated with the N_{PT} motor tasks selected for the patient. *DB-RT1* is structured in such a way to save all the actual trajectories performed by all the robotic models, expressed both in the "Cartesian space" and in the "Joint space".

2.6 Promotion Filter algorithm: evaluation of the kinematic performance of the robots

This algorithm establishes whether a prosthesis architecture satisfies the minimum level of functionality required by the amputee; among all the simulated robots, the models that do not prove adequate will be discarded at this stage, whereas only those remaining will be "promoted" to the subsequent steps of the procedure.
For each node n_j of the generic trajectory T1.i a "Tolerance Matrix" $\mathbf{T}_{T1.i}(n_j)$ is assigned on the basis of the tolerance levels *Tl1*, ..., *Tl4* associated with the task T1.i (Section 2.2):

$$\mathbf{T}_{T1.i}(n_j) = [t_{lm}(n_j)]_{\mathrm{T1.i}}\,; \qquad t_{lm}(n_j) := ((p_{lm}^{act}(n_j) - p_{lm}^{ref}(n_j))^2)_{\max} \tag{11}$$

where l, m = 1, 2, 3 (m corresponds to x, y, z). The element l, m of $\mathbf{T}_{T1.i}(n_j)$ represents the maximum squared difference between the actual and the reference values of the coordinate m of the hand point $\mathbf{P}_l$ considered still acceptable for a correct positioning and orienting of the terminal device at the node n_j of the task T1.i.
Let us consider the following step as performed for each single prosthetic architecture r (the subscript will be omitted); the algorithm compares the actual Cartesian trajectories with the Reference Trajectories of all the motor tasks associated with the patient, i.e. for each node n_j of the generic T1.i trajectory the actual Error Matrix $\mathbf{E}_{T1.i}(n_j)$ is calculated:

$$\mathbf{E}_{\mathrm{T1.i}}(n_j) = [e_{lm}(n_j)]_{\mathrm{T1.i}} = [(p_{lm}^{act}(n_j) - p_{lm}^{ref}(n_j))]_{\mathrm{T1.i}}\,, \qquad l, m = 1, 2, 3 \tag{12}$$

The matrix $\mathbf{T}_{T1.i}(n_j)$ collects the upper limits that the squared value of $\mathbf{E}_{T1.i}(n_j)$ elements can assume in order to consider the actual pose of the terminal device still acceptable with respect to the reference one. For every node n_j composing the trajectory T1.i the *Promotion Filter* algorithm checks whether the robotic model r is able to position and to orient its end effector with a sufficient accuracy, that is it must hold:

$$e_{lm}^2(n_j) \le t_{lm}(n_j)\,, \qquad \forall l, m = 1, 2, 3 \tag{13}$$

If the tolerance on the error is maintained for every node n_j of the Cartesian path, then the robotic model r is considered suitable to perform the task T1.i satisfactorily. This operation is repeated for all the tasks stored in *DB-PT* and for all the simulated models.
A "flag" $\boldsymbol{\delta}_{r,T1.i}$ describing the capability of the robot r to perform the task T1.i is set and saved: $\boldsymbol{\delta}_{r,T1.i}$ = 1 if the robot performance is satisfactory, $\boldsymbol{\delta}_{r,T1.i}$ = 0 in the opposite case. The tasks associated with the patient can be gathered in five groups G_{ti}, i = 0, 1,..., 4 (Fig. 2), so that it is possible to calculate how many tasks with label $T3$ = T3.i (i = 0, 1,..., 4) are correctly performed.
Let us define k = 1,..., n_{ti} as a pointer of a generic task of the group G_{ti}; the quantity:

$$\Delta_{ri} = \sum_{k=1}^{n_{ti}} \delta_{r,k}\,, \qquad \mathrm{i} = 0, 1, 2, 3, 4 \tag{14}$$

represents the number of G_{ti} tasks that are correctly performed.

The architecture r can be promoted from the functional viewpoint if:

$$\Delta_{ri} \geq t_i \cdot n_{ti}, \quad \forall i = 0,1,2,3,4; \; t_0 = 1 \tag{15}$$

Finally, it is possible to build up another temporary database *DB-RT2* that collects information stored in *DB-RT1* relative to the promoted models only and that also reports the values of $\boldsymbol{\delta}_{r,T1.i}$ and $\Delta_{r0}, \ldots, \Delta_{r4}$ for each model r.

2.7 Kinetostatic analyses (KiA algorithm) and Workspace calculation

For a given promoted robot, velocity laws corresponding to each successfully performed task are calculated: this is possible by interpolating the values of the active joint variables at the path nodes and taking into account the duty cycle that has been presumed for each task. It is then possible to perform kinetostatic analyses of the robot, considering the mass of the robot links and joints (hypothetical values) and the force acting on the terminal device potentially required by the tasks. The analyses are carried out by means of the Newton-Euler recursive algorithm for all the promoted robots and their corresponding correctly performed tasks The dynamic performances of the prosthetic architectures, in terms of torques and powers of their active joints when accomplishing the tasks, are summarized in a new database, *DB-RT3*, structured like *DB-RT1* and *DB-RT2*. Based on these outcomes, it is possible to evaluate a rule of thumb approximation of the size of the gearmotors that drive the articulations: for this purpose, for each robot model r and for each of its active joints l, the maximum power required of the actuator, $W_r(l)$, is calculated and stored in *DB-RT3*.
The reachable workspace volume (WS_r) of each promoted robot r is also calculated. The numerical algorithm used for this purpose, based on a very common technique known in the literature (Huang et al., 1996), considers the geometry of the manipulator, the arrangement of the joints and their range of motion as well as the presence of the subject's body, considered for the interference avoidance in the calculation. The joint ranges of motion of a promoted prosthetic architecture are calculated taking into account only the correctly performed tasks, whereas the joint excursions corresponding to a failed task are ignored.

2.8 Definition of the indices for the global evaluation of the arm architectures

This is the last step of the procedure, where the artificial arm models are evaluated: their functionality and the complexity of their architecture are assessed by means of proper indices which are not intended for applications outside this context. Their purpose is to provide a comparison between manipulators that operate under the same boundary conditions (determined by the patient, the input of the whole procedure) in order to identify the model that provides the optimal compromise between functionality on one hand and wearability, whose concept is defined specifically in this study, on the other.
The three indices presented here range from 0 to 1, in order to normalize the minimum and the maximum "values" (even if theoretical) of the features that they must portray.

KP: Kinematic Performance Indicator

The promoted robotic models guarantee at least the lowest level of functionality, fixed by means of $t_0, \ldots, t_4$ thresholds and checked at the *Promotion Filter* (Eq. 15). It is now necessary to determine how well a robot satisfies the given functional specifications, in order to distinguish which prosthetic architectures are better than others. For this purpose a *Kinematic Performance Indicator* KP_r is defined for each model r. By referring to the definition of n_{ti} (Section 2.2) and Δ_{ri} (Eq. 14), the quantity

$$\sum_{i=1}^{4} \frac{\Delta_{ri}}{n_{ti}} \tag{16}$$

globally measures how well the model overcomes the minimal level of functionality (associated with the distinct G_{ti} groups) evaluated by the *Promotion Filter* algorithm. The thresholds $t_1, \ldots, t_4$ were set with the aim of differentiating tasks having different levels of importance. It is reasonable to extend this concept here, by weighting the terms of the previous sum with the same parameters $t_1, \ldots, t_4$, in order to assign a higher relevance to the accomplishment of important tasks in this evaluation too. KP_r is thus defined as:

$$KP_r = \frac{\sum_{i=1}^{4} \frac{\Delta_{ri}}{n_{ti}} \cdot t_i}{\sum_{i=1}^{4} t_i} \tag{17}$$

Since all the promoted robots can successfully perform the tasks with label $T3$ = T3.0, the term $(\Delta_{r0} \cdot t_0 / n_{t0}) = 1$ was not introduced, being meaningless in this evaluation step.

FL: Functional Flexibility Index

In order to provide an index related to the flexibility of the manipulator model with respect to the accomplishment of whatever activities, the reachable workspace volume was considered as a measure of the capability to perform a generic task. The *Functional Flexibility Index* FL_r is defined for each model r as:

$$FL_r = \frac{WS_r}{\max_r (WS_r)} \tag{18}$$

The denominator, corresponding to the promoted robot with the widest workspace, was introduced in order to set the maximum value of FL_r at 1.

C: Complexity Index

Functionality is not the only specification required of a good prosthetic device: the system complexity, the weight and the cost also play an important role in a prosthesis design. For this purpose, the number of the actuated joints and the size of the gearmotors driving them is assumed in a first approximation as a global estimation of these aspects. For each promoted d_r-DoF model r, the maximum values of power that its active joints must be able to provide in order to perform all the satisfactorily completed tasks were calculated (and collected in *DB-RT3*, Section 2.7). In this study, the power required of an actuator $W_r(l)$ is defined as a rule of thumb measure of the complexity of the joint l that it drives. Let us define the scalar

$$TW_r = \frac{\sum_{l=1}^{d_r} W_r(l)}{\eta^{d_r}} \tag{19}$$

which represents the sum of the maximum powers of the active joints; $\eta \in [0,1]$ is a sort of "efficiency" that can be introduced to penalize to a greater extent models with many actuated joints (see Eqs. 20 and 21). It is possible to define the *Complexity Index* C_r as:

$$C_r = \frac{TW_r}{\max_r (TW_r)} \tag{20}$$

The index can vary from 0 to 1: the minimum value is only theoretical, because it is not likely that a prosthesis with only passive joints will pass the *Promotion Filter*. The maximum value is associated with the most complex architecture.

I: Overall Index
All the above defined indices can be combined to provide an overall index I_r whose value indicates the response of the promoted robot model r to the personal specifications of the patient, both in terms of functionality and wearability:

$$I_r = w_1 \cdot KP_r + w_2 \cdot FL_r - w_3 \cdot C_r \tag{21}$$

where $w_1, w_2, w_3 \in [0,1]$ are the weighting factors that depend on the patient's profile and are determined in the *Char* algorithm by means of the *P*-labels. I_r can assume negative values for those models that prove extremely complex with respect to their functional performance and/or with respect to the patient's requirements. The model with the maximum value for I_r designates the optimal architecture of the prosthesis associated with the given patient, i.e. the artificial arm which provides the best trade-off between the contrasting features required:

$$\max_r (I_r) \rightarrow \text{OPTIMAL PROSTHETIC MODEL} \tag{22}$$

3. Effective application of the DOPA procedure

The procedure has been presented as if it must be applied to a single amputee's profile, in order to personalize the synthesis of his/her optimal prosthesis architecture. As an immediate application, the results of this approach can guide practitioners in choosing the appropriate solution for a given high-level patient, on the basis of a systematic process. It may be the case that the architecture selected for him/her does not correspond to any device available on the market. The design of new components to be introduced in commercial prosthetic systems is thus required. The outlined method is useful for this aim too, defining which new active articulations must be designed (Fig. 5). In particular, the arrangement of the joints in the arm models determines the kind of motion which the new articulations must accomplish.
Morevoer, the results of the kinematic simulations (saved in *DB-RT1*) define the required range of motion of the joints. Finally, the KiA algorithm could be performed on a more detailed model of the chosen prosthetic architecture by referring to the actual patient's anthropometric data in order to determine the performance that the electromechanical actuators of the joints must provide (in terms of torques and powers), so as to correctly carry out the target functional tasks. The fundamental mechanical specifications are thus determined and the subsequent design activity can be started.
However, it is not feasible to design an ad-hoc prosthesis for each patient, as it would be too expensive a process. The DOPA procedure is thus intended to be applied to a huge number of patient profiles (theoretically, considering all the possible combinations of the *P-labels*) in order to define a limited selection of optimal or "sub-optimal" prosthesis architectures suitable to match different amputee requirements. "Sub-optimal" is intended as a degree of quality of the architectures associated with a single patient comparable with the optimal model (although

lower) characterized by a high value of the overall index *I* even if not the highest. Prosthesis models that prove sub-optimal for many amputees are more attractive from a global perspective than architectures being optimal for only a few patients. From a feasibility viewpoint, the choice of a good versatile architecture is actually more sensible than aiming to provide each subject with the best prosthetic device designed according to every single patient's personal needs.

The generation of a "patient population" by means of the permutation of all the possible values of the *P-labels* can be performed automatically (due to the "predefined-answer" nature of the *Clinical Identification Form*). In this perspective, it should not be surprising that an alternative arrangement of the algorithms and elements of the procedure was conceived in a slightly different way from what is presented above, being more appropriate for an automatic and iterative implementation (Troncossi, 2006).

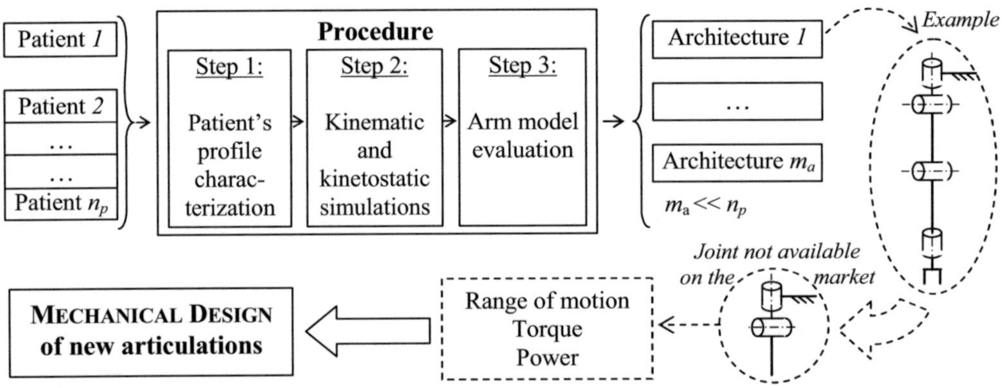

Fig. 5. Scheme of the intended application of the procedure.

4. Discussion and conclusion

The DOPA procedure presented in this chapter was developed in order to formalize principles for decision making in the choice and/or the design of upper limb prostheses for amputees with a high level disarticulation. The method makes it possible to tackle the problem of prosthetic rehabilitation from a general perspective, consistently taking into consideration both the clinical aspects and the technical issues involved in the design of upper limb prostheses. The DOPA algorithms make it possible to guide the synthesis of the artificial arm model that achieves the optimal compromise between a given patient's contrasting requirements in terms of functionality and wearability of the device. This is possible by means of a systematic investigation of the amputee's personal characteristics which generates a specific profile and by proper analyses and evaluations of many prosthetic solutions. The procedure is intended to be applied to a huge number of amputee profiles for a feasible application of its results. The generation of a "patient population" through the permutation of all the possible values of the *P-labels* can be performed automatically (due to the "predefined-answer" nature of the *Clinical Identification Form*) and the presence of real amputees is not strictly necessary to make the procedure run. Hence, the method can be systematically applied without the need to have real patients available; the method was actually devised for this purpose too.

The critical aspect of the approach is that the evaluation of the prosthetic models is deeply affected by parameters ($t_1, \ldots, t_4, w_1, w_2, w_3$) whose value strictly depends on the authors' choices when compiling the *Char* algorithm and that are discriminating for the significance of the final outcomes. A validation process to calibrate these parameters and to prove the real effectiveness of the method is thus required. This is actually the forthcoming step of the project, which entails clinical testing application of the tool and a comparison with the clinical experience for proper updating.

Moreover, it is the authors' opinion that a very good feature of the DOPA procedure is that it can be modified, simplified or expanded (for a more sophisticated use) with little effort, due to the "open" nature of both the algorithms and the internal database.

The effective use of the procedure is intended to provide a database which collects patients' profiles, their associated optimal prostheses and the performance of these with respect to certain functional tasks. This database will be useful to guide the design of new electromechanical articulations, by defining which joints are more important than others to satisfy the given requirements of many amputees (e.g. a humeral rotator rather than a flexion wrist, or vice versa, or both) and by providing technical specifications of the mechanisms to be designed (e.g. range of motion and power of the actuators).

A simplified version of the DOPA procedure was applied with the aim of providing the design guidelines of a novel actuated prosthetic shoulder. Details on this design process can be found in (Troncossi, 2006).

5. Acknowledgements

The authors wish to thank INAIL Prosthetic Centre for financial support and for use of the facilities, and Dr. M. Chiossi and Dr. C. Borghi for the valuable assistance.

6. References

Anglyn, C. & Wyss U.P. (2000). Review of arm motion analyses. *Proc Inst Mech Eng [H]*, Vol. 214, No. 5, pp. 541–555, ISSN: 0954-4119

Atkins, D. J. & Meier, R.H. III (1989). *Comprehensive Management of the upper-limb amputee*, Springer-Verlag, ISBN: 0-3879-6779-6, New York

Cattaneo, B.; Casolo, F.; Camposaragna, M. & Lorenzi V. (2001). An innovative shoulder complex with two active axes for artificial upper limbs, *Proc. of the 28th Congress of the International Society of Biomechanics*, p. 221, Zurich (Switzerland), July 2001

Denavit, J. & Hartenberg, R. S. (1955). A kinematic notation for lower-pair mechanisms based upon matrices. *J. Appl. Mechanics*, Vol. 77, pp. 215-221, ISSN: 0021-8936

Dennis, J.E. & Schnabel, R.B. (1996). *Numerical Methods for Unconstrained Optimization and Nonlinear Equations*, SIAM, ISBN: 0898713641, Philadelphia (USA)

Duffy, J. (1990). The fallacy of modern hybrid control theory that is based on orthogonal complements of twist and wrench spaces. *Journal of Robotic Systems*, Vol. 7, No. 2, pp. 139–144, ISSN: 0741-2223

Gow, D.J.; Douglas, W.; Geggie, C.; Monteith, E. & Stewart D. (2001). The development of the Edinburgh modular arm system. *Proc Inst Mech Eng [H]*, Vol. 215, No. 3, pp. 291–298, ISSN: 0954-4119

Huang, E.J. ; Luh, C.M. ; Adkins F.A. & Wang, J.Y (1996). Numerical algorithms for mapping boundaries of manipulator workspaces. *Trans. of the ASME – Journal of Mechanical Design*, Vol. 118, No. 2, June 1996, pp. 228–234, ISSN: 1050-0472

Jimnez, P.; Thomas, F. & Torras, C. (2001). 3D Collision detection: a survey. *Computer & Graphics*. Vol. 25, No. 2, April 2001, pp. 269–285, ISSN: 0097-8493

Kuiken, T. A.; Dumanian G.A.; Lipschutz, R.D. , Miller, L.A. & Stubblefield, K.A. (2004), The use of targeted muscle reinnervation for improved myoelectric prosthesis control in a bilateral shoulder disarticulation amputee. *Prosthetics and Orthotics International*, Vol. 28, No. 3, pp. 245–253, ISSN: 0309-3646

Kyberd, P. J.; Light, C.; Chappell, P. H.; Nightingale, J. M.; Whatley, D. & Evans, M. (2001). The design of anthropomorphic prosthetic hands: A study of the Southampton Hand. *Robotica*, Vol. 19, No. 6, pp. 593–600, ISSN: 0263-5747

Paul, R.B. (1981). *Robot Manipulators: Mathematics, Programming, and Control (Artificial Intelligence)*, MIT Press, ISBN: 026216082X, Cambridge (Massachusetts, USA)

Pheasant, S. (1996). *Bodyspace – anthropometry, ergonomics and the design of work*, Taylor and Francis LTD, ISBN: 0748403264, London (Great Britain);

Pons, J.L.; Rocon, E.; Ceres, R.; Reynaerts, D.; Saro, B.; Levin, S. & Van Moorleghem, W. (2004). The MANUS-HAND Dextrous Robotics Upper Limb Prosthesis: Mechanical and Manipulation Aspects. *Autonomous Robots*, Vol. 16, No. 2, March 2004, pp. 143–163, ISSN: 1573-7527

Romilly, D. P.; Anglin, C.; Gosine, R. G.; Hershler, C. & Raschke, S. U. (1994). A functional task analysis and motion simulation for the development of a powered upper-limb orthosis. *IEEE Transactions on Rehabilitation Engineering*, Vol. 2, No. 3, September 1994, pp. 119-129, ISSN: 1063-6528

Troncossi, M. (2006). A Procedure for the Synthesis of Upper Limb Prostheses. A case study: Prototype Manufacturing of a Novel Two–DoF Myoelectric Shoulder, PhD Thesis, University of Bologna, Italy

Weir, R. F. ff. & Grahn, E. G. (2005). Powered Humeral Rotator for Persons with Shoulder Disarticulation Amputations, *Proceedings of MEC'05*, ISBN: 1-55131-100-3, New Brunswick (Canada), August 2005, (CD-ROM)

Yang, J.; Pitarch, E. P.; Abdel-Malek, K.; Patrick, A. & Lindkvist, L. (2004). A multi-fingered hand prosthesis. *Mechanism and Machine Theory*, Vol. 39, No. 6, June 2004, pp. 555–581, ISSN: 0094-114X